Veterinary Virology: A Clinical Approach

Veterinary Virology: A Clinical Approach

Editor: Zoe Lucas

STATES
ACADEMIC PRESS
www.statesacademicpress.com

States Academic Press,
109 South 5th Street,
Brooklyn, NY 11249, USA

Visit us on the World Wide Web at:
www.statesacademicpress.com

ISBN: 978-1-63989-559-5 (Hardback)

Cataloging-in-Publication Data

Veterinary virology : a clinical approach / edited by Zoe Lucas.
p. cm.
Includes bibliographical references and index.
ISBN 978-1-63989-559-5
1. Veterinary virology. 2. Veterinary medicine. I. Lucas, Zoe.
SF780.4 .V48 2022
636.089 601 94--dc23

Table of Contents

Preface

The main aim of this book is to educate learners and enhance their research focus by presenting diverse topics covering this vast field. This is an advanced book which compiles significant studies by distinguished experts in the area of analysis. This book addresses successive solutions to the challenges arising in the area of application, along with it; the book provides scope for future developments.

Veterinary virology is a sub-discipline of veterinary medicine. It deals with the study of disease causing viruses and disorders in animals and non-human species. Viruses cannot reproduce independently, they can only reproduce inside the living cells of an organism. Most viruses contain single molecule of nucleic acid, surrounded by a protein coat known as capsid. Foot-and-mouth disease virus (FMDV), Bluetongue virus, influenza virus, African swine flu viruses are some of the causative agents of disease in animal species like pigs, cats, dogs and cattle. Viruses can also change the behavior of animal species to their own advantage. This book unravels the recent studies in the field of veterinary virology. It also provides interesting topics for research which interested readers can take up. This book, with its detailed analyses and data, will prove immensely beneficial to professionals and students involved in this area at various levels.

It was a great honour to edit this book, though there were challenges, as it involved a lot of communication and networking between me and the editorial team. However, the end result was this all-inclusive book covering diverse themes in the field.

Finally, it is important to acknowledge the efforts of the contributors for their excellent chapters, through which a wide variety of issues have been addressed. I would also like to thank my colleagues for their valuable feedback during the making of this book.

Editor

1

Unrecognized circulation of SAT 1 foot-and-mouth disease virus in cattle herds around Queen Elizabeth National Park in Uganda

Moses Tefula Dhikusooka[1], Chrisostom Ayebazibwe[1], Alice Namatovu[1,2], Graham J. Belsham[3], Hans Redlef Siegismund[4], Sabenzia Nabalayo Wekesa[5,6], Sheila Nina Balinda[6], Vincent B. Muwanika[6] and Kirsten Tjørnehøj[3*]

Abstract

Background: Foot-and-mouth disease (FMD) is endemic in Uganda in spite of the control measures used. Various aspects of the maintenance and circulation of FMD viruses (FMDV) in Uganda are not well understood; these include the role of the African buffalo (*Syncerus caffer*) as a reservoir for FMDV. To better understand the epidemiology of FMD at the livestock-wildlife-interface, samples were collected from young, unvaccinated cattle from 24 pastoral herds that closely interact with wildlife around Queen Elizabeth National Park in Uganda, and analysed for evidence of FMDV infection.

Results: In total, 37 (15 %) of 247 serum samples had detectable antibodies against FMDV non-structural proteins (NSPs) using a pan-serotypic assay. Within these 37 sera, antibody titres ≥ 80 against the structural proteins of serotypes O, SAT 1, SAT 2 and SAT 3 were detected by ELISA in 5, 7, 4 and 3 samples, respectively, while neutralizing antibodies were only detected against serotype O in 3 samples. Two FMDV isolates, with identical VP1 coding sequences, were obtained from probang samples from clinically healthy calves from the same herd and are serotype SAT 1 (topotype IV (EA-I)). Based on the VP1 coding sequences, these viruses are distinct from previous cattle and buffalo SAT 1 FMDV isolates obtained from the same area (19–30 % nucleotide difference) and from the vaccine strain (TAN/155/71) used within Uganda (26 % nucleotide difference). Eight herds had only one or a few animals with antibodies against FMDV NSPs while six herds had more substantial evidence of prior infection with FMDV. There was no evidence for exposure to FMDV in the other ten herds.

Conclusions: The two identical SAT 1 FMDV VP1 sequences are distinct from former buffalo and cattle isolates from the same area, thus, transmission between buffalo and cattle was not demonstrated. These new SAT 1 FMDV isolates differed significantly from the vaccine strain used to control Ugandan FMD outbreaks, indicating a need for vaccine matching studies. Only six herds had clear serological evidence for exposure to O and SAT 1 FMDV. Scattered presence of antibodies against FMDV in other herds may be due to the occasional introduction of animals to the area or maternal antibodies from past infection and/or vaccination.
The evidence for asymptomatic FMDV infection has implications for disease control strategies in the area since this obstructs early disease detection that is based on clinical signs in FMDV infected animals.

Keywords: Livestock-wildlife interface, Foot-and-mouth disease virus, SAT 1, Young cattle, Uganda

* Correspondence: kitj@vet.dtu.dk
[3]National Veterinary Institute, Technical University of Denmark, Lindholm, Kalvehave DK 4771, Denmark
Full list of author information is available at the end of the article

Background

Foot-and-mouth disease (FMD) is a highly contagious viral disease affecting a wide range of domestic and wild cloven-hoofed animals [1, 2]. It is known to cause substantial economic losses, directly from the effect of the virus on animal health and indirectly through control efforts including quarantines and trade restrictions [2].

The disease is caused by infection with a single stranded, positive sense, RNA virus (FMDV) belonging to the genus *Aphthovirus* within the family *Picornaviridae.* This virus occurs in seven distinct serotypes namely: O, A, C, Asia 1, SAT 1, SAT 2 and SAT 3, each having multiple strains [3, 4]. All serotypes, except Asia 1, have been reported in eastern Africa, however, serotype C was last detected in Kenya in 2004 and may be extinct [5, 6]. Serotypes O and A are considered endemic in most parts of Africa, while the three SAT serotypes have usually been restricted to sub-Saharan Africa [7], where they are commonly diagnosed [7–9]. However, incursions of SAT 1 into the Middle East (1961–1965 & 1970), and SAT 2 into Saudi Arabia (2000), Libya (2003) and more recently into Egypt and Libya (2012) have been reported [7, 10].

The maintenance of the three FMDV SAT serotypes in cattle in southern and eastern Africa has been associated with contact with wildlife, especially African buffalo (*Syncerus caffer*) [11]. FMDV has been demonstrated to persist in individual buffalo for up to 4–5 years and in isolated buffalo herds for up to 24 years [11]. In southern Africa, it has, in some cases, been concluded that buffalo have been the source of FMDV infections in cattle and impala (*Aepyceros melampus*) [8, 12, 13]. As a result, FMD control policies in southern Africa are centred on isolating the buffalo, in the National Parks and game reserves, away from the surrounding livestock populations, and vaccinating cattle kept in buffer zones around these areas against the FMDV serotypes that are carried by the nearby buffalo [14].

In eastern Africa, FMD was first reported in cattle in 1932 [15] and since then, the marketability of livestock and animal products within, and outside, the region has been negatively affected [16]. The maintenance of FMDV in the region has been attributed to various factors including: the presence of numerous wildlife reservoirs [7, 17–19], communal and pastoral grazing systems that enable contact between livestock and wildlife [20], poor diagnostic capacity in the region [9], emergence of new strains [21–23], transboundary animal movements and traditional cultural practices such as the exchange of live animals for dowry and gifts [24, 25]. East African countries have tried to control the disease mainly by quarantine and post outbreak vaccination. However, these measures have been difficult to enforce and sub-optimal use of vaccines [26] has resulted in large parts of the FMDV susceptible animal populations remaining at risk [9, 27]. Recently, the countries in this region have established a network to combine their control efforts to move towards freedom from FMD by 2020 following the progressive control pathway (PCP) for FMD as described [28]. The PCP defines six steps in the process of achieving freedom from FMD including effective monitoring of circulating serotypes, vaccination and improved biosecurity measures [28]; this strategy has been adopted by all countries in the region, including Uganda [29].

In Uganda, SAT 1 FMDV was first reported in 1959, and since then, FMD outbreaks caused by serotypes O, A, SAT 1 and SAT 2 [7, 9, 24, 27, 30–33] have been regularly reported in livestock. In addition, for the first time, serotype SAT 3 FMDV has been recently isolated from a clinically healthy long horned Ankole calf shortly after its introduction into the area close to the Queen Elizabeth National Park (QENP) [34]. Ugandan buffalo are only infrequently sampled for FMDV, and thus the virus has only been isolated from them during two studies in QENP; these yielded serotypes SAT 1 and SAT 3 in 1997 [35] and SAT 1 and SAT 2 in 2007 [36]. Moreover, in a post-outbreak study conducted on adult cattle and goats in the same area, concurrently with the 2007 buffalo sampling, only serotype O FMDV was isolated. Furthermore, 11 herds of cattle had animals with higher antibody titres against serotype O than against the SAT serotypes, while only one had convincing serological evidence of infection with SAT FMDV [22, 31]. Thus, although wildlife within the Ugandan National Parks are often blamed for being the source of FMD outbreaks in their surroundings [37], this could not be proven for the major 2006 FMD outbreak in the QENP area [31, 36]. Moreover, although it is clear that FMDV can pass from buffalo to cattle [13], recent attempts in Uganda and Kenya to establish the role of the African buffalo in the epidemiology of FMD in domestic species in eastern Africa have so far not settled this [36, 38].

The objective of this study was to assess the presence of FMDV in young, unvaccinated cattle grazing in close proximity to African buffalo in the QENP (Fig. 1) and to establish whether these buffalo play a major role in the maintenance of FMD in livestock around the National Park.

Methods

This study was designed in compliance with REFLECT guidelines and was approved by the Ugandan Ministry of Agriculture, Animal Industries and Fisheries (MAAIF) (Reference LHE 199/01, Uganda) and Makerere University (MU) "School Higher Degrees and Research Committee". The sampling was carried out by MAAIFs National Animal Disease Diagnostics and Epidemiology Centre (NADDEC) in collaboration with Kasese District Veterinary Office in accordance to the guidelines from MAAIF. The

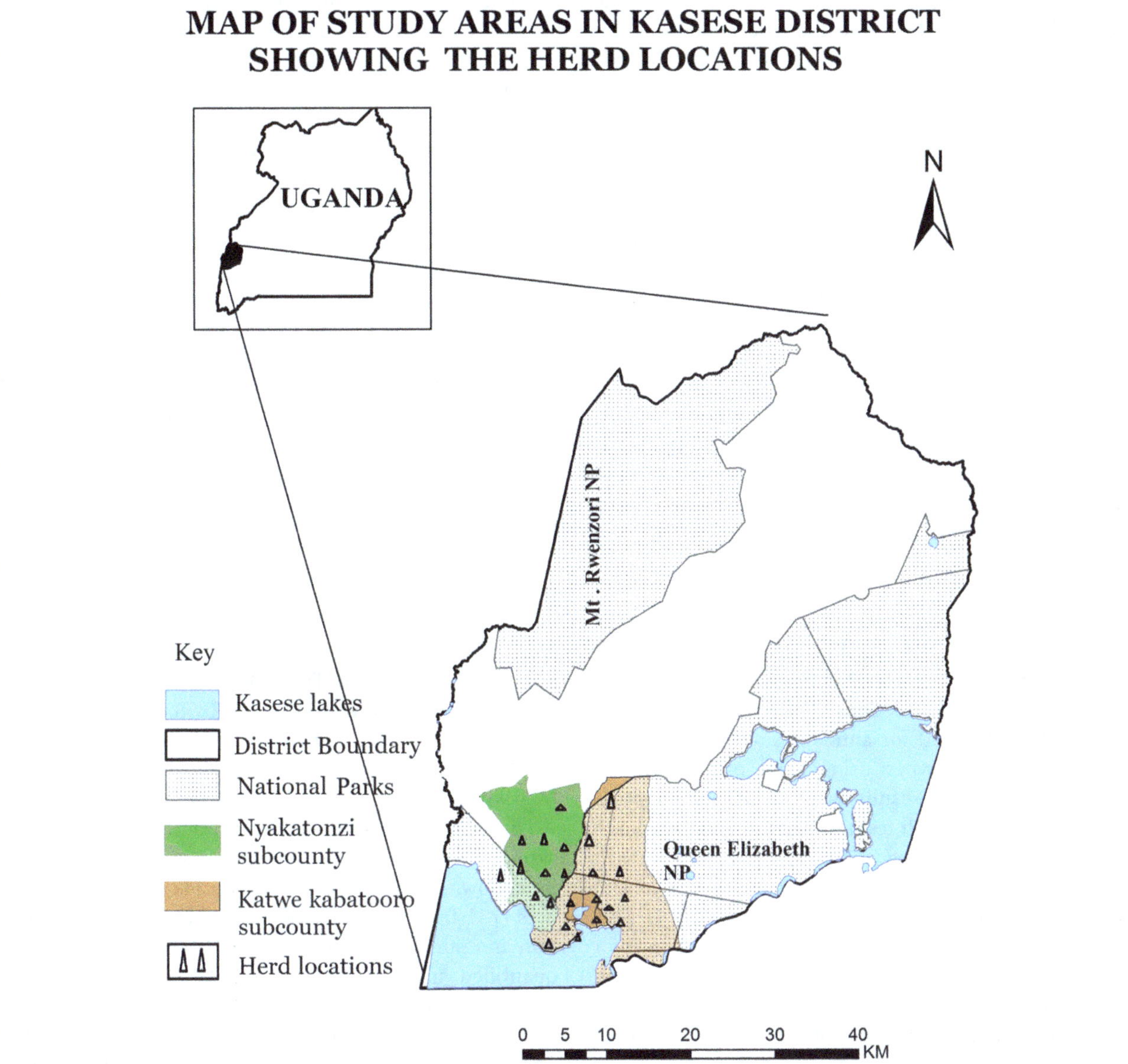

Fig. 1 Map of the study area: Queen Elizabeth National Park (QENP) and its surroundings. Generated using QGIS, version 2.6.1

study included meetings for the herd owners where the purpose of the project was described and informed consent to the sampling, and to participation in the questionnaire survey, was obtained from the individual herd owners.

Sampling approach

A cross-sectional study was conducted in Katwe Kabatooro and Nyakatonzi subcounties of Kasese district in Uganda (Fig. 1) during August-September 2011 to assess the presence of FMDV and antibodies against this virus. The sampled herds were usually grazed communally close to (and inside) the QENP, where the animals, according to the herd owners, regularly moved/grazed/drank within 2–10 m of wildlife. FMD was last reported from this area in 2006–2007, and no vaccinations against FMDV had been carried out in this area since 2007.

The two sampled subcounties had an estimated cattle population of 30,000 head of cattle distributed in approximately 50 herds (personal communication, DVO Dr. V. Kalule, based on [39]). Moreover, it was estimated that approximately 1/6 of these, i.e. 5,000, were unvaccinated 6-24-month-old cattle. A sample size of 296 was calculated using Win Episcope 2.0 software [40] at a 5 % precision level and 95 % confidence level and assuming antibody prevalence of approximately 12 % [41].

At the sampling, both unstabilised blood and oropharyngeal fluid (OP) samples were collected from each of 247 heads of 6-24-month-old cattle. The cattle belonged to 24 settled pastoralists, who in total owned 1171 cattle within this age-cohort, and in each herd, sampled animals were randomly selected. Due to the field conditions, the calculated number of samples was not entirely met; however, the number of cattle in the sampled age-group in the 24 sampled herds was also lower than estimated (2400), so this was evaluated as adequate.

The OP samples were immediately divided into two aliquots: one placed in phosphate buffered saline (PBS) and another in RLT buffer (Qiagen, Hilden, Germany) and kept in liquid nitrogen until stored at −80 °C in the laboratory, while serum was extracted in the field and kept on ice until stored at −20 °C in the laboratory.

Information on: vaccination history, laboratory confirmed FMD outbreaks, unreported observation of clinical symptoms of FMD, farming characteristics, history of contact between cattle and wildlife, age group mostly affected in the event of FMD outbreaks and FMD control methods was collected from the herd owners using a semi-structured questionnaire (Additional file 1).

Serology

Sera were screened for the presence of antibodies against FMDV NSPs using PrioCHECK® FMDV NS ELISA test kits (Prionics, Lelystad, The Netherlands) according to the manufacturer's instructions. Positive samples were tested (at 1:10 dilution) for antibodies against the seven different FMDV serotypes using solid phase blocking ELISAs (SPBEs) [42]. Results were read as the optical density (OD) of wells with test samples and expressed as a percentage of the mean optical density (ODP) of four wells with a known negative control serum. Sera were considered positive, if the ODP was < 50 % for serotypes O, SAT 1, SAT 2 and SAT 3, < 45 % for serotype A, and < 35 % for serotypes C and Asia 1. Due to expected cross-reactions, all sera giving positive reactions in the initial screening were titrated in two-fold dilution series from 1/10 to 1/1280 and titres expressed as the reciprocal of the highest positive dilution [42]. Nineteen samples with titres ≥ 80 in the SPBEs were tested in the relevant virus neutralization tests (VNTs) as described in the OIE Manual [43], while twelve sera with SPBE titres ≤ 40 were not tested further. FMDV strains used for VNT comprised O Manisa, A Iraq 24/64, C Noville, Asia 1 Shamir, SAT 1 BOT/68, SAT 2 ZIM 5/81 and SAT 3 ZIM 4/81; VNT titres ≥ 45 were considered positive, titres of 15–44 inconclusive and titres ≤ 14 negative.

Detection of FMDV RNA and isolation of FMDV from OPs

Thirty two OP samples collected from the animals with antibodies against FMDV NSP were initially screened for FMDV RNA using the 5'-untranslated region (UTR) targeted quantitative reverse transcription PCR (RT-qPCRs) [43, 44] and 22 of these with threshold cycle values (C_T values) ≤ 39 were inoculated onto primary bovine thyroid cells (BTY) and propagated through two cell culture passages [32, 36, 43]. Cultures with cytopathic effect (CPE) were harvested and stored at −80 °C. The 3D coding region targeted RT-qPCR assay was then performed on RNA extracted from the cell harvests as described previously [45] and samples with $C_T < 32$ were interpreted as FMDV RNA positive while C_T values ≥ 32 were considered negative [45, 46]. The presence of FMDV in CPE-positive harvests was analysed using an in-house antigen ELISA, which also determined the serotype of positive isolates as previously described [32, 36, 43].

Sequencing of VP1 coding region from FMDV isolates

RNA was extracted from FMDV antigen positive cell culture harvests as described above, and cDNA synthesized using Ready-To-Go You-Prime First-strand Beads (GE Healthcare Life Sciences, Uppsala, Sweden) with random hexamer primers ($pd(N)_6$) [27]. The cDNA was diluted to 150 µl from which an aliquot was used for VP1 coding region amplification as follows: 5 µl 10X PCR buffer, 4 µl 25 mM $MgCl_2$, 25.1 µl dH_2O, 0.5 µl Amplitaq Gold® DNA Polymerase (Applied Biosystems Foster City, USA), 0.4 µl 10 mM dNTPs, 5.0 µl of each of forward (13 KPN-100 [5′GGGTGGBBGTSTWMCAGRTSACMGACAC 3′]) and reverse (FMD KS2B58 [5′-ACAGCGGC CATGCACGACAG 3′] primers, where B = (C or G or T); S = (C or T); W = (A or T); M = (A or C) and R = (A or G) [47], with 5 µl of cDNA [36, 48].

The PCR was run in a thermocycler (Gene Amp-PCR system 3700 version 3.0 Applied Biosystems) using the touchdown technique as described [48]. The PCR products (731 bp) were purified using QIAquick® gel extraction and purification kit (Qiagen, Hilden, Germany), and quantified using a Nanodrop®1000 spectrophotometer (Fisher Scientific, Waltham, MA, USA). Sequencing of the PCR products was performed using a BigDye® Terminator v 3.1 Cycle Sequencing kit (Applied Biosystems, Foster City, CA, USA), using the same primers as used in the PCRs, according to the manufacturer's instructions, and ran on an automated DNA sequencer (ABI PRISM® 3730 DNA Analyser (Applied Biosystems, Foster City, CA, USA).

Sequence assembly and analysis

Nucleotide sequences were assembled and edited using SeqMan Pro™ software (DNAStar Lasergene 10.0, Madison, WI, USA). The resulting consensus sequences were compared to others using the Basic Local Alignment Search Tool (BLAST) in MEGA 5 (www.megasoftware.net [49]). They were then aligned with 19 other published nucleotide sequences obtained from GenBank (Table 1) in MUSCLE incorporated in MEGA software version 6.06, and trimmed to correspond to the 657 nt encompassing the complete VP1 coding region. Phylogenetic trees were

Table 1 SAT 1 VP1 coding sequences included in this study

Species	Isolate Identity	GeneBank accession no.	Year of sampling	Country	Topotype
Cattle	UGA/116/13**	KP025678	2013	Uganda	IV (EA-1)
Cattle	UGA/161/13**	KP025679	2013	Uganda	IV (EA-1)
Buffalo	UGA/10/70	KF219681	1970	Uganda	IV (EA-1)
Buffalo	UGA/21/70	KF219682	1970	Uganda	IV (EA-1)
Buffalo	UGA/1/97	AY442012	1997	Uganda	VIII (EA-3)
Unknown	UGA/7/99	AY442011	1999	Uganda	IV (EA-1)
Buffalo	UGA/1/07	HM067706	2007	Uganda	IV (EA-1)
Cattle	UGA/13/74	AY442010	1974	Uganda	VII (EA-2)
Cattle	ETH/19/07	FJ98156	2007	Ethiopia	IX
Cattle	ETH/21/07	FJ798157	2007	Ethiopia	IX
Cattle	KEN/11/91	AY441994	1991	Kenya	I (NWZ)
Cattle	KEN/9/91	AY441995	1998	Kenya	I (NWZ)
Cattle	KEN/28/06	HQ267529	2006	Kenya	III (WZ)
Cattle	KEN/66/80	HQ267520	1980	Kenya	I (NWZ)
Cattle	TAN/2/77	AY442008	1977	Tanzania	I (NWZ)
Cattle	TAN/155/71 (Vaccine)	HQ267519	1971	Tanzania	I (NWZ)
Cattle	TAN/19/96	AY442005	1996	Tanzania	I (NWZ)
Cattle	TAN/60/99	AY442002	1999	Tanzania	III (WZ)
Cattle	NIG/2/79	AF431728	1979	Nigeria	VI
Cattle	KNP/196/91	DQ009716	1991	South Africa	II (SEZ)

**: sequences obtained as part of this study

estimated using the Neighbor Joining (NJ) method [50], with 1000 bootstrap replicate samplings and used to determine the topotype clusters for the aligned sequences. The amino acid sequences were deduced from the nucleotide sequences using the standard genetic code and the extent of amino acid relatedness in the VP1 coding regions determined using the same program in MEGA 6 [51].

Results

Clinical signs of FMD were not observed in any of the sampled animals or herds.

Serology

In total, 37 of 247 sera collected from 24 herds in Nyakatonzi and Katwe Kabatooro subcounties tested positive for antibodies against the NSPs of FMDV (Table 2) giving an overall antibody prevalence of 15 % with herd antibody prevalences ranging from 0 to 60 % (median 11 %; Inter Quartile Range (IQR) 0–26 %). In the 14 positive herds, the antibody prevalences in the NSP antibody test ranged from 6 to 60 % (median 23 %; IQR 16–30 %).

Screening of the 37 anti-NSP antibody positive samples in SPBEs resulted in 17, 4, 2, 0, 20, 13 and 16 samples being scored positive for antibodies against serotypes O, A, C, Asia 1, SAT 1, SAT 2 and SAT 3, respectively, while 12 anti-NSP positive samples were negative in all SPBEs (Table 2; data not shown for the testing of antibodies against serotypes A, C and Asia 1). When titrated, the few sera that were identified as positive for antibodies against serotypes A and C in the initial screening (at 1:10 dilution) had titres ≤ 40 and so were considered negative. In contrast, titres ≥ 80 were found in 5/17, 6/20, 4/13 and 3/16 of the samples titrated for antibodies against serotypes O, SAT 1, SAT 2 and SAT 3, respectively (Table 2). In summary, the positive results were obtained from 11 sera collected from 6 different herds. Six of these sera had high antibody titres against one single serotype (O: 1 sample; SAT 1: 2 samples; SAT 2: 2 samples, SAT 3: 1 sample), whereas five sera had high antibody titres against more than one of the serotypes O, SAT 1, SAT 2 and SAT 3 (Table 2).

Neutralising antibodies (as determined by VNT) were only detected against serotype O and only in three animals, while eight, six, five and six sera had inconclusive neutralizing antibody titres against O, SAT 1, SAT 2 or SAT 3, respectively, and all the other tested sera were negative (Table 2). The three VNT positive animals had SPBE antibody titres ≥ 160 and came from three different herds (H1, H14 and H19).

Diagnostic RT-qPCRs, virus isolation and antigen ELISA

In the 5′UTR RT-qPCR assay, 22 out of the 32 tested OP samples generated C_T values ranging from 22 to 39,

Table 2 Summarized results from herds with animals positive for antibodies against FMDV NSPs

Subcounties	Parishes	Herd no.	NSP ELISA Pos/tested (%)	SPBE titre				VNT titre				Serological conclusion herd-level	Cell culture BTY	Antigen ELISA on BTY harvest	3D RT - qPCR (C_T) on virus harvests	Herd diagnosis*
				O	SAT 1	SAT 2	SAT 3	O	SAT 1	SAT 2	SAT 3					
Katwe	Rwenjubu	H1	6/23 (26)	-	10	-	-	-	-	-		O				+
Kabatooro				640	320	10	40	67	-		28		CPE	-	-	
				160	-	-	-	24	-	-	-		-			
				10	20	-	-		-							
				-	10	-	-		17							
				-	10	-	-	-								
	Kijarukara	H3	3/12 (25)	10	320	10	40	-	28	-	-	(SAT 1)	-			(+)
				-	-	-	-						-			
				-	-	10	10						CPE	-	-	
	Kiganda	H7	3/5 (60)	-	-	-	-						-			+
				10	-	-	10	40	-		17		-			
				10	10	-	10	34	-		28		-			
	Top hill	H19	4/7 (57)	10	P**	-	10	-			24	O				+
				160	20	10	80	136	-	28	-	(SAT 2)	CPE	-	32	
				-	-	80	10	-	-	40						
				10	20	-	80	24	-	28	-					
	Kyakitare	H18	2/10 (20)	10	80	10	10	-	34	28		(SAT 1)	CPE	SAT 1	16	++
				10	40	40	20	-	-				CPE	SAT 1	19	
	Kiganda	H2	1/7 (14)	-	-	-	-						-			(+)
	Rwenjubu	H5	2/7 (29)	-	10	10	10		17				-			(+)
				-	-	-	-									
Nyakatonzi	Muruti	H12	5/18 (28)	-	-	-										(+)
				-	-	-	-									
				-	-	-	-									
				-	-	-	-									
				-	-	-	-									
	Muruti	H15	3/9 (33)	-	-	-	-						-			(+)
				-	10	-	-	-	17	-			-			
				40	-	-	-	-	-	-			-			

Table 2 Summarized results from herds with animals positive for antibodies against FMDV NSPs *(Continued)*

	Muruti	H14	1/5 (20)	160	160	80	20	48	24	-	-	O	CPE	-	32	+
	Kisasa	H23	4/25 (16)	160	80	20	320	24	-	-	17	(O)	CPE	-	32	+
				-	160	160	-	-	-	28		(SAT 2)	CPE	-	-	
				40	40	40	-	40	-	-	-					
				20	20	80	40	40	-	-			CPE	-	-	
	Kisasa	H22	1/6 (17)	10	20	-	10	34	-	-	28		CPE	-	-	(+)
	Kisasa	H21	1/17 (6)	-	-	-	-									(+)
	Bwanika	H11	1/13 (8)	-	-	-	-						-			(+)
No. Positive			37/247 (15)	17	20	13	16	3	0	0	0		na	2		
No. with SPBE-titre ≥ 80				5	6	4	3									

-: Negative
*: (+) only few animals with antibodies against the NSPs
+ Herds with more substantial evidence of exposure to FMDV
++ Confirmed evidence of exposure to FMDV
**: Positive in SPBE 1:10 but not titrated due to insufficient sample

of which only three samples had C_T <32 (22, 23 and 25). Ten of these 22 OP samples produced CPE when inoculated onto primary BTYcells but only two cell culture harvests (UGA/116/13 and UGA/161/13) were found positive in the 3D RT-qPCR assay (defined as positive: $C_T < 32$) and these had C_T values of 16 and 19 (indicative of high levels of FMDV RNA). Moreover, only the same two virus harvests were found positive for FMDV antigen in FMDV antigen ELISAs and were identified as serotype SAT 1 (Table 2). These two virus harvests were generated from the OP samples with the lowest C_T values in the 5′UTR RT-qPCR assay, and were both collected from herd H18. RNA extracted from cell harvests derived from one OP from each of herds H14, H19 and H23 each had a C_T value 32 in the 3D RT-qPCR, which is on the borderline of confidence in detection [46], but no FMDV could be isolated.

Herd diagnosis

There was no evidence of exposure to FMDV in ten of the 24 herds in this study (H4, H6, H8, H9, H10, H13, H16, H17, H20 and H24) (data not shown), while four herds had antibodies against FMDV NSPs only, either in one animal (H2, H11 and H21) or in five animals (H12) (Table 2). Another four herds had anti-NSP antibody seroprevalences of 17–33 % (1–3 animals) with antibodies against one or more serotypes in 1–2 of these animals (H3, H5, H15 and H22). Six herds had more substantial evidence for exposure to FMDV. This was in the form of higher seroprevalences (43–60 %) of antibodies against FMDV NSPs (H7 and H19), SPBE antibody titres ≥ 80 in more than one animal (H1, H19 and H23), neutralising antibodies in one animal (H1, H14 and H19) and isolation of FMDV from OPs (H18).

Characterisation of FMDV isolates

Sequencing revealed that the two 657 nucleotide (nt) long regions, from the 731 bp amplicons, corresponding to the VP1 coding sequences of UGA/116/13 and UGA/161/13 were identical. Alignment of these complete VP1 sequences with 18 other African FMDV isolates (Table 1) showed that they belonged to the SAT 1 topotype IV (EA-1) (see Tekleghiorghis et al. [52]), clustered together with three previous Ugandan buffalo isolates of 1970 and 2007 (UGA10/70, UGA/21/70 and UGA/1/07) and also the UGA/7/99 isolate whose species of origin was not identified (Fig. 2). The VP1 sequences of the 2013 isolates had 21 %, 20 % and 24 % nucleotide (nt) difference from these earlier buffalo isolate VP1 sequences, respectively, while their relationship with another Ugandan buffalo isolate from 1997 (UGA/1/97) and an earlier Ugandan SAT 1 cattle isolate (UGA/13/74) was even more distant (nt sequence divergences of 30 % and 31 %, respectively). However, except for the UGA/13/74 strain [topotype VII (EA-2)] and UGA/1/97 [topotype VIII (EA-3)], the various Ugandan isolates represent independent lineages within topotype IV (EA-1) (Fig. 2). The SAT 1 vaccine strain (TAN/155/71) used in Uganda belongs to a different topotype I (NWZ) and differs from the SAT 1 VP1 sequences obtained from this study by 26 % and 21 % at the nucleotide and amino acid level, respectively.

Since the VP1 sequences of the two isolates from H18 were identical, the 20 aligned SAT 1 VP1 coding sequences (Table 1) encoded 19 different amino acid sequences, each with 219 amino acid residues (Fig. 3), which were conserved at 51.3 % of the sites. Multiple amino acid substitutions were observed within the known hypervariable regions [53]. In the G-H loop, compared to the vaccine strain (TAN/155/71), residues 137 and 149–151 (the receptor binding RGD motif) remained conserved in all the 19 sequences, while multiple substitutions occurred in the section including residues 138–148 which is known to be a key antigenic region in FMDVs [53]. The seven Ugandan isolates were conserved at residues 146, 152 and 153 with each having a distinct amino acid (aa) substitution at positions 140–143. UGA/116/13 showed full aa conservation with UGA/7/99, UGA/1/07, UGA/13/74 and UGA/21/70 at positions 138, 139, 144 and 145, while the UGA/1/97 and UGA 10/70 strains had different substitutions (Fig. 3). UGA/116/13 had multiple substitutions at positions 140(N → A), 141(H → D), 142(E → Q), 143(T → A), 147(H → N) and 148(I → V) compared to the vaccine strain (TAN/155/71) and distinct substitutions in these positions were also observed in the other Ugandan isolates but without a pattern. In the H-I loop (residues 172–182), all the 19 sequences were fully conserved at positions 172, 176 and 181–182. However, there were distinct substitutions among the Ugandan isolates within this region. Near the C-terminus (residues 203–219), five positions (203, 208, 216, 218 and 219) were conserved in all the 19 isolates, while the Ugandan isolates also showed full conservation at positions 209, 210 and 213 plus almost complete conservation at positions 207, 211 and 217 (Fig. 3). The UGA/116/13 differed from the other 6 strains by having substitutions outside the G-H loop (139–153), the H-I loop (172–182) and the C-terminus (203–219) (see Fig. 3).

Herd owner replies to semi-structured questionnaires

According to the responses to questionnaires (see Additional file 1), 96 % of the herd owners grazed their herds communally inside QENP and 63 % frequently observed close contact with buffalo, especially during the dry season. Moreover, 75 % of the farmers reported that buffalo and other wildlife grazed around the cattle kraals during the night. Most farmers were aware of FMD outbreaks in their area, 58 % had experienced clinical FMD in their

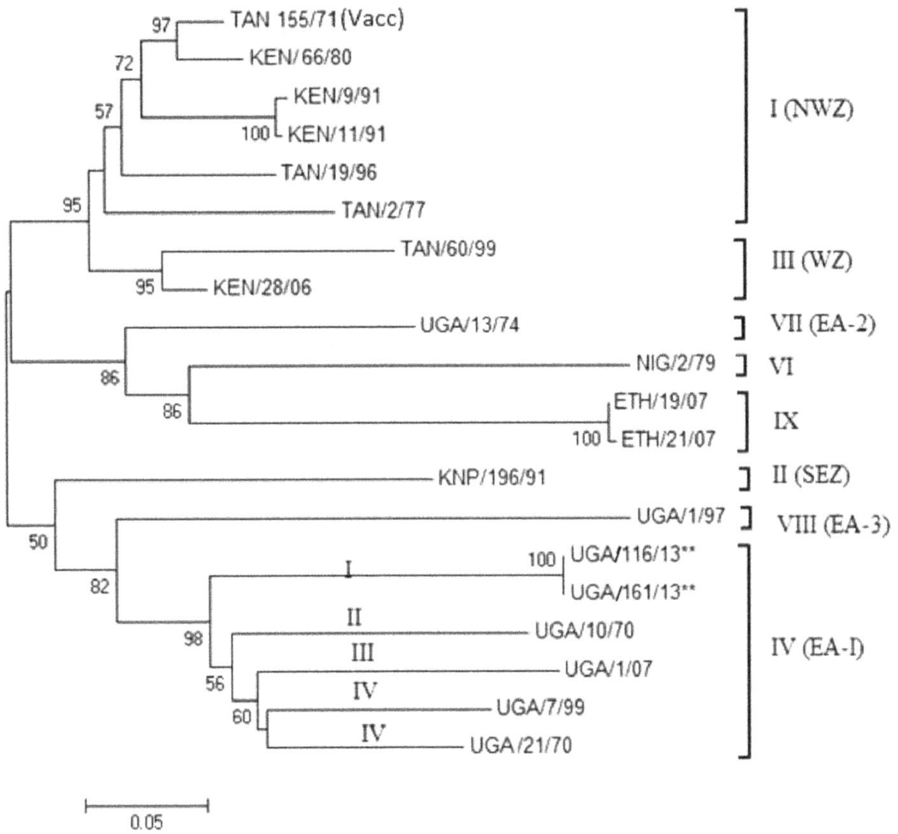

Fig. 2 A Neighbor-joining tree showing the relationships between the VP1 coding sequences (657 nt) of the two Ugandan SAT 1 isolates from this study (UGA/116/13 [KPO25678] and 161/13 [KPO 25679] (marked **)) and SAT 1 FMDV VP1 coding sequences from Uganda (UGA), Kenya (KEN), Tanzania (TAN), Ethiopia (ETH), Nigeria (NIG) and Kruger National Park (KNP) in South Africa as obtained from GenBank (http://www.ncbi.nlm.nih.gov/genbank/). Topotypes are indicated according to Tekleghiorghis et al. (2014) [49]. Bootstrap values are indicated. Scale bar indicates nucleotide substitutions per site

herds and 12.5 % had observed signs similar to clinical FMD (although not confirmed) since the last documented outbreak in 2006 (see Additional file 1). When suspected cases of FMD occurred, 63 % of the farmers reported this to the area veterinarian, 17 % drove the animals into the waters of the Albertine rift valley salt lakes, 33 % applied local herbs and 4 % treated with oxy-tetracycline sprays.

Discussion

At the QENP livestock-wildlife interface, young unvaccinated cattle from 24 herds without reports of clinical signs of FMD had an overall seroprevalence of 15 % (37/247) for antibodies against FMDV NSPs. This is higher than the 5 % seroprevalence reported in cattle herds without clinical signs in the same area in 2006 [31] but compares well with the 12 % value reported in young calves in FMD-endemic Ethiopia [41].

Evidence for prior FMDV infection varied between herds, thus evidence for exposure to FMDV was absent in ten herds, scanty in eight herds and more substantial in six herds (25 %). The observed scattered presence of antibodies does not appear to fit well with the general appreciation of the epidemiology of FMD as an efficiently spreading disease with high morbidity in affected herds and high risk of transfer to other herds through physical contact and fomites [54]. Moreover, although the farmers were well acquainted with clinical signs of FMD, a number of them would not report outbreaks, but rather used traditional control measures like application of local herbs or walking the animals through the salt lakes known to contain common salt and sodium bicarbonate [55].

There is an undefined level of trade with cattle, including young stock for fattening, coming into the area from other districts; thus individual animals with antibodies against FMDV may be explained as animals infected elsewhere and brought into the herds as replacement stock or gifts to the owners as part of local customs [32]. However, the higher antibody prevalences in H7 and H19 and the isolation of SAT 1 FMDV from OPs from two cattle in H18 support spread within these herds (originating either from within the district or from other districts); moreover, it cannot be excluded that the

```
                     10         20         30         40         50         60         70         80         90        100        110
TAN_155/71   TTSAGEGAEP VTTDASQHGG GRRTARRHHT DVSFILDRFT LVGKTVDNKL TLDLLQTKEK ALVGAILRAA TYYFSDLEVA CVGTNKWVGW TPNGAPELSE VGDNPVVFSH
UGA_161/13** .......... .......... .S.QT..Q.. ....L..... .I...KNC.. V......Q.. ........S. .......... .L.DG..A.. ......Q.TT .....F..LS
UGA/7/99     .......... .......... TS.RV..Q.. ....L..... .I...HN... V......... ........S. .......... .......... ......Q.T. ......I...
UGA/1/97     .......... .......... NA.PT..Y.. N.E.L..... .I...HN..M V..M.R.EK. ........S. .......... .....E.... V...T.DV.. .........R
UGA/1/07     .......... .....T.... HS.RT..... ....L..... .I...T...I V......R.. ........S. .......... ...N...... ......L.H. ..........
UGA_/21/70   .......... .....T.... NS.R...... ....L..... .I...K.... V......R.. ........S. .......... .......... ......Q.T. ..........
UGA/10/70    .......... ....T..... SS.R...Q.. ....L..... .I...Q.H.. V......R.. ........S. .......... .......... ......Q.R. .........R
UGA/13/74    .......... .......... ...A...Q.. ....L..... ......N... .....K.... ........S. ....A..... .....R.... L.....VPQ. ..........
NIG/2/79     ........DV ..V..TA... TQ.AT..V.. ..A.L..... .........M V..M....K. ........S. ....A..... .......... L.....VP.. ..........
KEN/28/06    .......... .......... ...A...Q.. ....L..... ......N... .......... .......... .......... .......... ........N. ..........
KNP/196/91   .......... .......... D...T..... ....L..... .....Q.... .......... .......... .......... ...D...... ........A. .........K
ETH/19/07    .........V .S...TA... N..R...V.. ..A.L..... .I....N..M V....K.... ........S. .......... .L........ L.....MPT. .........T
ETH/21/07    ...V.....V .S...TA... N..R...V.. ..A.L..... .I....N..M V....K.... ........S. .......... .L........ L.....MPT. .........T
KEN/9/91     .......... .....T.... .....Y.... .......... ...R.QN.R. .......... .......... .......... ...V....R. .......... ..........
KEN/11/91    .......... .....T.... .....Y.... .......... ...R.QN.R. .......... .......... .......... ...V....R. .......... ..........
KEN_66/80    .......... .......... .......Y.. .......... ......N... .......... .......... .......... .......... .......... .........R
TAN/60/99    ........DV ..V..AA... NQ.RT..V.. ..A.L..... .....Q...M V..M.K.... .......... .......... .......... ........N. ..........
TAN/2/77     .......... .......... .......... .......... .......... .......... ........V. .......... ...E...... .......... ..........
TAN/19/96    .......... .......... ...ATH.... ....L..... ......A... .......... .......... .......... .......... ........A. ..........

                    120        130        140        150        160        170        180        190        200        210       219
TAN_155/71   NGTTRFALPY TAPHRCLATA YNGDCKYKPN HETPRTHIRG DLATLATRIA SETHIPTTFN YGRIYTEAEV DVYVRMKRAE LYCPRPVLTH YEHQGKDRYK VALTKPAKQ
UGA_161/13** K.AA...... .....V...T .........A DQA...NV.. ......A... .QS....S.. ..Q.I.D..M .......... .......... .D.G.S.... .E.IR....
UGA/7/99     .......... .....L...V .........T EQP...N... ...V..Q... .......S.. ..Q....S.. .......... .......... .D.GD..... IE.V.....
UGA/1/97     D.A......F .....VV..S ...N...QDQ ST..L..V.. ......E... QNA....S.. ..Q....... .......... T.....L... .D.A..N... TK.VA....
UGA/1/07     .......... .....L...T .........A GQE...A... ...VI.E... .......S.. ..QL...S.. .......... ......L... .D.D...... ...VA....
UGA_/21/70   .......... .....L.... .........V GQE...N... ......E... N......S.. ..Q....... .......... ......II.. .D.N...... ...VA.E..
UGA/10/70    .D........ .....L...V .......Q.A GQP....V.. ......E... .VA....S.. ..Q....DD. .......... .......... .D.A...... .E.VA....
UGA/13/74    .........F .....V...V .........I N.DT..N... ......A.VR EQS....... ..I.L..... .......... .........T .D.ASA.... .P.VA.E..
NIG/2/79     ..V....... .....V...V ...N.R.... T.A..PT... ......A... EQA....... ..I.L..G.. .......... .....F...M .D.A.Q..R. IR.VA....
KEN/28/06    .......... .......... .......... S.A....V.. ......E... .......... .......... .......... .......... .D........ .........
KNP/196/91   GR........ .......... .........T GTA..EN... ......A... .......... ......DT.. .......... .......... .D.G.R...R T.I...V..
ETH/19/07    ..A......F .....L...Q .A......QQ P....EN... ......A..S ..S....... ..I.I..... .......... .....FL..T .D..TAE... TK.VA.E..
ETH/21/07    ..A......F .....L...Q .A......QQ P....EN... ......A..S ..S....... ..I.I..... .......... .....FL..T .D..TAE... TK.VA.E..
KEN/9/91     .......... .......... .......... T.A....... ......E... .......... ...L....D. .......... .......... .D.K.N.... .........
KEN/11/91    .......... .......... .......... T.A....... ......E... .......... ...L....D. .......... .......... .D.K.N.... .........
KEN_66/80    H......... .......... .......... ..A...N... .......... .......... .......... .......... .......... .D........ .........
TAN/60/99    .E........ .......... .......... S.A....... .FT...E... .......... .......... .......... .......... .D...R.... .........
TAN/2/77     .......... .........V .....R...T T.S....... ......E... .......... .......... .......... V......... .N........ T........
TAN/19/96    .......... .......... ....S..RSH N.E..A.... ......A... .......... .......... .......... .......... .D........ .........
```

Fig. 3 The sequence alignment for the VP1 protein of 19 SAT 1 FMD viruses. Dots indicate amino acid residues identical to the reference sequence SAT 1 TAN/155/71

infections causing antibodies in the other herds have taken place in Kasese district.

Another possibility is that some of the antibodies against FMDV observed in this study are residual maternally transferred antibodies. Since cattle in this area are likely to have their first calf at 3–4 years of age and to have several calves, it is likely that some of the dams to the sampled calf cohort (born between August 2009 and February 2011) were exposed to FMDV by infection and/or vaccination during the 2006–2007 outbreak [31, 56]. A fraction of these dams may have retained sufficient level of antibodies, especially against the NSPs, to transfer these to their offspring. Moreover, although FMD outbreaks had not been reported in the area since 2006, the District Veterinary Office noted that underreporting was suspected since quarantine restrictions due to FMD would paralyze all economic activities in the area.

Although it is not clear when, or how, some of the antibody positive animals in these herds were infected, SPBE assays showed that 11 of the 37 NSP positive samples had antibody titres ≥ 80 against one or more serotypes. Based on SPBE and VNT results from the few positive animals, it appeared that serotype O FMDV had infected some animals from H1, H14 and H19, while SAT 1 FMDV had infected some animals from H3 and possibly H18, in the latter case this was confirmed by isolation of SAT 1 FMDV from two animals. The situation was unclear in herds H19 and H23 with high SPBE antibody titres against serotypes O, SAT 1, SAT 2 and SAT 3, which could be due to the previously observed cross-reactivity between the SPBEs and also between the VNTs [31, 56]. Moreover, if animals were purchased from other districts, vaccine-derived antibodies cannot be excluded either. In accordance with previous findings in the area [31, 56], there was no conclusive serological evidence for previous infection by serotypes A, C, Asia 1 and SAT 3 in the sampled cattle, although very recently SAT 3 FMDV was isolated from an asymptomatic calf from the area [34].

The SAT 1 FMDV isolates obtained from the two healthy animals in H18 are the first reported SAT 1 isolates from Ugandan cattle since 1999 [57], while SAT 1 isolates have been obtained from buffalo in QENP in 1997 and 2007 [35, 36]. The relatively infrequent isolation of SAT 1 FMDV from outbreaks in Ugandan cattle could be the result of poor surveillance in the form of underreporting of FMD outbreaks and limited submission of samples of sufficient quality for virus isolation to the central diagnostic laboratory at the National Animal Disease Diagnostics and Epidemiology Centre (NADDEC) (Dr. Anna Rose Ademun, personal communication). Moreover, there have been limited options for typing FMDV locally in Uganda [9].

The combination of rather low C_T values (22 and 23) in the 5'UTR tests for the two H18 OP samples that yielded the SAT 1 FMDV isolates and SPBE antibody titres of 40 and 80 for antibodies against SAT 1 FMDV in sera from the same animals, indicate that these two animals were in the subacute stage of the infection. However, no clinical signs were observed during the sampling and there were no reports of clinical signs in this or in other cattle herds in the area. Moreover, the questionnaire responses indicated that the indigenous Ankole cattle from this area have less severe clinical signs of FMD than the pure exotic and crossbred cattle. Hence, these data support the notion that some of the Ugandan indigenous Long-horned Ankole cattle may go through FMDV infection with only minimal clinical signs of FMD. This is consistent with the very recent isolation of SAT 3 FMDV from an OP sample from a clinically healthy young calf in the QENP area [34] and has been previously reported for indigenous cattle in Botswana [58, 59]. If true, this notion has a bearing on the passive surveillance reporting system for FMD in Uganda that is based on clinical observations.

This study shows a considerable genetic difference between the current Ugandan SAT 1 cattle virus and the vaccine strain (TAN/155/71) that is currently used to control FMD outbreaks caused by SAT 1 FMDV in Uganda, indeed these belong to different topotypes. Thus, vaccine matching studies using the currently circulating SAT 1 strain are required. In addition, the observed differences from earlier buffalo and cattle isolates imply that different SAT 1 lineages have been in circulation in this area over the last 50 years. To verify this, more Ugandan FMDV SAT 1 isolates should be collected and characterised.

Despite the close interaction that occurs between cattle and buffalo at the QENP livestock-wildlife-interface, this study did not provide evidence to support the view that the FMD viruses circulating in cattle in this area originate from wildlife as has been observed in South Africa [60]. This could be attributed to the limited numbers of isolates from cattle and the long time-intervals between their isolations; but it also does not exclude the possibility that separate pools of viruses circulate in cattle and wildlife. The VP1 coding sequences of five of the six Ugandan SAT 1 isolates were different from those of isolates from other countries, indicating that the Ugandan SAT 1 strains may be geographically limited to Uganda as previously suggested [61].

Conclusions

Although FMD was last reported in Kasese District in 2006, evidence of infection with FMDV was found in six of 24 cattle herds from the QENP livestock-wildlife-interface. The SAT 1 FMDV isolated from one of these six herds was markedly different from the earlier buffalo isolates from the same area; thus transmission between buffalo and cattle could not be proven. The genetic difference (ca. 26 % within the VP1 coding region) between the current SAT 1 isolates and the vaccine strain used to control FMD outbreaks in the country calls for vaccine matching to ensure the effectiveness of vaccination in this region. Additional surveillance and characterization of field strains from cattle and buffalo at this livestock-wildlife interface is necessary for monitoring of emerging strains and to enhance the understanding of the role of wildlife in the epidemiology of FMD in cattle in East Africa.

Abbreviations

Amplitaq Gold: Thermostable DNA polymerase enzyme from thermophilic bacterium *Thermusaquaticus*; BLAST: Basic Local Alignment Search Tool; BOT: Botswana; bp: Base Pair; BTY: Bovine thyroid cells; cDNA: Complementary Deoxyribonucleic acid; CPE: Cytopathic effect; Ct: Cycle threshold; DNA bases used: Adenine (A), Guanine (G), Cytosine (C) and Thymine (T); DNA: Deoxyribonucleic acid; dNTP: Deoxyribonucleotide triphosphate; EA: East Africa; ELISA: Enzyme-Linked Immunosorbent Assay; FMD: Foot-and-mouth disease; FMDV: Foot-and-mouth disease Virus; G-H loop: A highly variable region within VP1 of FMDV (ca. 140–160) but which includes the highly conserved RGD motif required for receptor binding; H: Herd; MA: Massachusetts; MEGA: Molecular Evolutionary Genetic Analysis; MgCl2: Magnesium Chloride ions; MUSCLE: Multiple sequence alignment method for amino acids and nucleotides; NADDEC: National Animal Disease Diagnostics and Epidemiology Centre; NJ: Neighbor joining; NSP: Non-Structural Proteins; OD: Optical Density; ODP: Optical density percent; OP: Oro-pharyngeal fluid; PBS: Phosphate buffered saline; PCR: Polymerase chain reaction; QENP: Queen Elizabeth National Park; RLT buffer: A lysis buffer for lysing cells and tissues before RNA separation; RNA: Ribonucleic acid; RT-qPCR: Reverse transcription quantitative polymerase chain reaction; SAT: Southern African Territories; SPBE: Solid phase blocking ELISA; TAN: Tanzania; UGA: Uganda; USA: United States of America; UTR: Untranslated region; VNT: Virus neutralization test; VP: Virus protein; ZIM: Zimbabwe; 3D protein: RNA dependent RNA polymerase of FMDV.

Competing interests

The authors declare that they have no competing interests.

Author contributions

MTD, CA and KT conceived and designed the study. MTD, CA and AN did the field work and sample collection. MTD, AN, SNW and KT did the laboratory analysis. KT, GJB and SNB supervised the laboratory work. MTD was the principal writer of the manuscript and KT, GJB, CA, VBM and HRS critically revised it. All authors read and approved the final manuscript.

Acknowledgements

This work was funded by the Danish International Development Agency (DANIDA) under the Transboundary Animal Diseases in East Africa Project (TADEA, Project number: 10-006KU). We thank the Ministry of Agriculture Animal Industry and Fisheries (MAAIF) for the valuable information provided about FMD in Uganda. We are also grateful to the supervisory board at the Department of Environmental Management, College of Agricultural & Environmental Sciences, Makerere University, and to the laboratory staff at the National Veterinary Institute, Technical University of Denmark, at Lindholm and in particular to: Preben Normann, Jani Christiansen, Jane Borch and Inge Nielsen. Thanks also go to Mr Eugene Arinaitwe, Martin Esau and Simon Ruhweza at NADDEC for the field and laboratory support work.

Author details
[1]National Animal Disease Diagnostics and Epidemiology Centre, Ministry of Agriculture Animal Industry and Fisheries, P. O. Box 513, Entebbe, Uganda. [2]Department of Biotechnical and Diagnostic Sciences, College of Veterinary Medicine, Animal Resources and Biosecurity, Makerere University, P. O. Box 7062, Kampala, Uganda. [3]National Veterinary Institute, Technical University of Denmark, Lindholm, Kalvehave DK 4771, Denmark. [4]Department of Biology, University of Copenhagen, Ole Maaløes Vej 5, DK 2200 Copenhagen N, Denmark. [5]Foot-and-Mouth Disease Laboratory, Ministry of Livestock Development, P. O. Box 18021, Embakasi, Nairobi, Kenya. [6]Department of Environmental Management, College of Agricultural and Environmental Sciences, Makerere University, P. O. Box 7062, Kampala, Uganda.

References

1. Hedger RS, Condy JB, Golding SM. Infection of some species of African wild life with foot-and-mouth disease virus. J Comp Pathol. 1972;82:455–61.
2. Alexandersen S, Mowat N. Foot-and-mouth disease: host range and pathogenesis. Curr Top Microbiol Immunol. 2005;288:9–42.
3. Jamal SM, Belsham GJ. Foot-and-mouth disease: past, present and future. Vet Res. 2013;44:116–31.
4. Belsham GJ. Translation and replication of FMDV RNA. Curr Top Microbiol Immunol. 2005;288:43–70.
5. Annual OIE/FAO FMD Reference Laboratory Network Reports 2013. http://www.wrlfmd.org/ref_labs/fmd_ref_lab_reports.htm. Accessed 28 Febr 2015.
6. Sangula AK, Siegismund HR, Belsham GJ, Balinda SN, Masembe C, Muwanika VB. Low diversity of foot-and-mouth disease serotype C virus in Kenya: evidence for probable vaccine strain re-introductions in the field. Epidemiol Infect. 2010;139:189–96.
7. Vosloo W, Bastos AD, Sangare O, Hargreaves SK, Thomson GR. Review of the status and control of foot-and-mouth disease in sub-Saharan Africa. Rev Sci Tech. 2002;21:437–49.
8. Bastos AD, Anderson EC, Bengis RG, Keet DF, Winterbach HK, Thomson GR. Molecular epidemiology of SAT 3-type foot-and-mouth disease. Virus Genes. 2003;27:283–90.
9. Namatovu A, Wekesa SN, Tjornehoj K, Dhikusooka MT, Muwanika VB, Siegsmund HR, et al. Laboratory capacity for diagnosis of foot-and-mouth disease in Eastern Africa: implications for the progressive control pathway. BMC Vet Res. 2013;9:19.
10. Ahmed HA, Salem SA, Habashi AR, Arafa AA, Aggour MG, Salem GH, et al. Emergence of foot-and-mouth disease virus SAT 2 in Egypt during 2012. Transbound Emerg Dis. 2012;59:476–81.
11. Condy JB, Hedger RS, Hamblin C, Barnett IT. The duration of the foot-and-mouth disease virus carrier state in African buffalo (i) in the individual animal and (ii) in a free-living herd. Comp Immunol Microbiol Infect Dis. 1985;8:259–65.
12. Vosloo W, Bastos AD, Boshoff CI. Retrospective genetic analysis of SAT-1 type foot-and-mouth disease outbreaks in southern Africa. Arch Virol. 2006;151:285–98.
13. Dawe PS, Flanagan FO, Madekurozwa RL, Sorensen KJ, Anderson EC, Foggin CM, et al. Natural transmission of foot-and-mouth disease virus from African buffalo (*Syncerus caffer*) to cattle in a wildlife area of Zimbabwe. Vet Rec. 1994;134:230–2.
14. Thomson GR, Vosloo W, Bastos AD. Foot-and- mouth disease in wildlife. Virus Res. 2003;91:145–61.
15. Wairu BN. Observations on foot-and-fouth disease in Kenya. The Kenya Veterinarian. 1994;18:25–7.
16. Rweyemamu MM, Leforban Y. Foot-and-mouth disease and international development. Adv Virus Res. 1999;53:111–26.
17. Hedger RS, Taylor WP, Barnett IT, Riek R, Harpham D. Simultaneous vaccination of cattle against foot-and-mouth disease and rinderpest. Trop Anim Health Prod. 1986;18:21–5.
18. Rweyemamu MM. Foot-and-mouth disease control strategies in Africa. Prev Vet Med. 1984;2:329–40.
19. Bronsvoort BM, Parida S, Handel I, McFarland S, Fleming L, Hamblin P, et al. Serological survey for foot-and-mouth disease virus in wildlife in eastern Africa and estimation of test parameters of a nonstructural protein enzyme-linked immunosorbent assay for buffalo. Clin Vaccine Immunol. 2008;15:1003–11.
20. Rugadya M. Pastoralism as a conservation strategy Uganda. country report. IUCN-The World Conservation Union. 2006. http://cmsdata.iucn.org/downloads/uganda_country_study.pdf. Accessed 28 Febr 2015.
21. Bari FD, Parida S, Tekleghiorghis T, Dekker A, Sangula A, Reeve R, et al. Genetic and antigenic characterisation of serotype A FMD viruses from East Africa to select new vaccine strains. Vaccine. 2014;32:5794–800.
22. Balinda SN, Sangula AK, Heller R, Muwanika VB, Belsham GJ, Masembe C, et al. Diversity and transboundary mobility of serotype O foot-and-mouth disease virus in East Africa: implications for vaccination policies. Infect Genet Evol. 2010;10:1058–65.
23. Ndiritu CG, Ouldridge EJ, Head M, Rweyemamu MM. A serological evaluation of 1979–1982 Kenyan foot-and-mouth disease type SAT 2 viruses. J Hyg (Lond). 1983;91:336–41.
24. Balinda SN, Belsham GJ, Masembe C, Sangula AK, Siegismund HR, Muwanika VB. Molecular characterization of SAT 2 foot-and-mouth disease virus from post-outbreak slaughtered animals: implications for disease control in Uganda. Epid Infect. 2010;138:1204–10.
25. Sangula AK, Belsham GJ, Muwanika VB, Heller R, Balinda SN, Siegismund HR. Co-circulation of two extremely divergent serotype SAT 2 lineages in Kenya highlights challenges to foot-and-mouth disease control. Arch Virol. 2010;155:1625–30.
26. Muleme M, Barigye R, Khaitsa ML, Berry E, Wamono AW, Ayebazibwe C. Effectiveness of vaccines and vaccination programs for the control of foot-and-mouth disease in Uganda, 2001–2010. Trop Anim Health Prod. 2012;45:36–43.
27. Kasambula L, Belsham GJ, Siegismund HR, Muwanika VB, Ademun-Okurut AR, Masembe C. Serotype identification and VP1 coding sequence analysis of foot-and-mouth disease viruses from outbreaks in eastern and northern Uganda in 2008/9. Transbound Emerg Dis. 2012;59:323–30.
28. FAO. The Progressive Control Pathway for FMD control (PCP-FMD) Principles, Stage Descriptions and Standards. 2011. http://www.fao.org/fileadmin/user_upload/eufmd/docs/PCP/PCP_en.pdf. Accessed 28 Febr 2014.
29. FAO/OIE/AU-IBAR. GF-TADs. Workshop on the developement of a long term actionplan (roadmap) for improved surveillance and control of foot-and-mouth disease in Africa. Nairobi, Kenya. 2009. http://www.oie.int/doc/ged/D11115.PDF. Accessed 28 Febr 2015.
30. Balinda SN, Siegismund HR, Muwanika VB, Sangula AK, Masembe C, Ayebazibwe C, et al. Phylogenetic analyses of the polyprotein coding sequences of serotype O foot-and-mouth disease viruses in East Africa: evidence for interserotypic recombination. Virol J. 2010;7:199.
31. Mwiine FN, Ayebazibwe C, Olaho-Mukani W, Alexandersen S, Balinda SN, Masembe C, et al. Serotype specificity of antibodies against foot-and-mouth disease virus in cattle in selected districts in Uganda. Transbound Emerg Dis. 2010;57:365–74.
32. Namatovu A, Belsham GJ, Ayebazibwe C, Dhikusooka MT, Wekesa SN, Siegismund HR, et al. Challenges for serology-based characterization of foot-and-mouth disease outbreaks in endemic areas; Identification of two separate lineages of serotype O FMDV in Uganda in 2011. Transbound Emerg Dis. 2013. doi:10.1111/tbed.12170.
33. Namatovu A, Tjørnehøj K, Belsham G, Dhikusooka T, Wekesa S, Muwanika V, et al. Characterization of foot-and-mouth disease viruses (FMDVs) from Ugandan cattle outbreaks during 2012–2013: Evidence for circulation of multiple serotypes. PLosOne. 2015;10, e0114811.
34. Dhikusooka TM, Tjornehoj K, Ayebazibwe C, Namatovu A, Ruhweza S, Siegismund HR, et al. Foot-and-mouth disease Virus Serotype SAT 3 in Long-Horned Ankole Calf, Uganda. Emerg Infect Dis. 2015;21:111–4.
35. Kalema-Zikusoka G, Bengis RG, Michel AL, Woodford MH. A preliminary investigation of tuberculosis and other diseases in African buffalo (*Syncerus caffer*) in Queen Elizabeth National Park, Uganda. Onderstepoort J Vet Res. 2005;72:145–51.
36. Ayebazibwe C, Mwiine FN, Tjornehoj K, Balinda SN, Muwanika VB, Ademun Okurut AR, et al. The role of African buffalos (*Syncerus caffer*) in the maintenance of foot-and-mouth disease in Uganda. BMC Vet Res. 2010;6:54.
37. Ayebazibwe C, Tjornehoj K, Mwiine FN, Muwanika VB, Okurut AR, Siegismund HR, et al. Patterns, risk factors and characteristics of reported and perceived foot-and-mouth disease (FMD) in Uganda. Trop Anim Health Prod. 2010;42:1547–59.
38. Wekesa SN, Sangula AK, Belsham GJ, Tjornehoj K, Muwanika VB, Gakuya F, et al. Characterisation of recent foot-and-mouth disease viruses from African buffalo (*Syncerus caffer*) and cattle in Kenya is consistent with independent virus populations. BMC Vet Res. 2015;11:17.

39. MAAIF/UBOS, 2008. The National Livestock Census Report 2008. http://www.agriculture.go.ug/userfiles/National%20Livestock%20Census%20Report%202009.pdf. Accessed 13 Nov 2015.
40. Thrusfield M, Ortega C, de Blas I, Noordhuizen JP, Frankena K. WIN EPISCOPE 2.0 improved epidemiological software for veterinary medicine. Vet Rec. 2001;148:567–728.
41. Gelaye E, Ayelet G, Abera T, Asmare K. Seroprevalence of foot-and-mouth disease in Bench Maji Zone, Southwestern Ethiopia. J Vet Med Anim Health. 2009;1:005–10.
42. Balinda SN, Tjornehoj K, Muwanika VB, Sangula AK, Mwiine FN, Ayebazibwe C, et al. Prevalence estimates of antibodies towards foot-and-mouth disease virus in small ruminants in Uganda. Transbound Emerg Dis. 2009;56:372–1.
43. OIE. Manual of Diagnostic Tests and Vaccines for Terrestrial Animals Chapter 2.1.5. Foot-and- mouth disease. 2012. http://www.oie.int/fileadmin/Home/eng/Health_standards/tahm/2.01.05_FMD.pdf. Accessed 28 Febr 2015.
44. Reid SM, Ferris NP, Hutchings GH, Zhang Z, Belsham GJ, Alexandersen S. Detection of all seven serotypes of foot-and-mouth disease virus by real-time, fluorogenic reverse transcription polymerase chain reaction assay. J Virol Methods. 2002;105:67–80.
45. Callahan JD, Brown F, Osorio FA, Sur JH, Kramer E, Long GW, et al. Use of a portable real-time reverse transcriptase-polymerase chain reaction assay for rapid detection of foot-and-mouth disease virus. J Am Vet Med Assoc. 2002;220:1636–42.
46. Shaw AE, Reid SM, Ebert K, Hutchings GH, Ferris NP, King DP. Implementation of a one-step real-time RT-PCR protocol for diagnosis of foot-and-mouth disease. J Virol Methods. 2007;143:81–5.
47. Moss G. Nomenclature for Incompletely Specified Bases in Nucleic Acid Sequences. 1984. http://www.chem.qmul.ac.uk/iubmb/misc/naseq.html. Accessed 28 Febr 2015.
48. Wekesa SN, Sangula AK, Belsham GJ, Muwanika VB, Heller R, Balinda SN, et al. Genetic diversity of serotype A foot-and-mouth disease viruses in Kenya from 1964 to 2013; implications for control strategies in eastern Africa. Infect Genet Evol. 2014;21:408–17.
49. Tamura K, Peterson D, Peterson N, Stecher G, Nei M, Kumar S. MEGA5: Molecular Evolutionary Genetics Analysis using Maximum Likelihood, Evolutionary Distance, and Maximum Parsimony Methods. Mol Biol Evol. 2011;28:2731–9.
50. Tamura K, Nei M, Kumar S. Prospects for inferring very large phylogenies by using the neighbor-joining method. Proc Natl Acad Sci (USA). 2004;101:11030–5.
51. Tamura K, Stecher G, Peterson D, Filipski A, Kumar S. MEGA 6: Molecular Evolutionary Genetics Analysis Version 6. Mol Biol Evol. 2013;30:2725–9.
52. Tekleghiorghis T, Moormann RJM, Weerdmeester K, Dekker A. Foot-and-mouth disease transmission in Africa: Implications for control, a review. Transbound Emerg Dis. 2014; doi:10.1111/tbed.12248.
53. Strohmaier K, Franze R, Adam KH. Location and characterization of the antigenic portion of the FMDV immunizing protein. J Gen Virol. 1982;59:295–306.
54. Alexandersen S, Zhang Z, Donaldson AI, Garland AJ. The pathogenesis and diagnosis of foot-and-mouth disease. J Comp Pathol. 2003;129:1–36.
55. Kirabira JB, Kasedde H, Semukuuttu D. Towards the improvement of salt extraction at Lake Katwe. Int J Sci Tech Res. 2013;1:76–81.
56. Mwiine FN, Ayebazibwe C, Olaho Mukani W, Alexandersen S, Tjørnehøj K. Prevalence of antibodies against foot-and-mouth disease virus in cattle in Kasese and Bushenyi districts in Uganda. Int J Anim Vet Adv. 2010;2:89–96.
57. FAO. FAO World Reference Laboratory for Foot-and-Mouth Disease. Uganda. http://www.wrlfmd.org/fmd_genotyping/africa/uga.htm. Accessed 28 Febr 2015.
58. Hedger RS. The isolation and characterization of foot-and-mouth disease virus from clinically normal herds of cattle in Botswana. J Hyg (Lond). 1968;66:27–36.
59. Joris F, Caron A, Thompson PN, Dwaka R, Forgin C, d-Garine-Wichatitsky M, et al. Characteristics of foot-and-mouth diease viral strains circulating at the wildlife /livestock interface of the Great Limpopo Transfrontier Conservation Area. Transbound Emerg Dis. 2014; doi:10.1111/tbed.12231.
60. Bruckner GK, Vosloo W, Du Plessis BJ, Kloeck PE, Connoway L, Ekron MD, et al. Foot- and- mouth disease: the experience of South Africa. Rev Sci Tech. 2002;21:751–64.
61. Sahle M, Dwarka RM, Venter EH, Vosloo W. Comparison of SAT-1 foot-and-mouth disease virus isolates obtained from East Africa between 1971 and 2000 with viruses from the rest of sub-Saharan Africa. Arch Virol. 2007;152:797–804.

2

Molecular characterization of a novel Muscovy duck parvovirus isolate: evidence of recombination between classical MDPV and goose parvovirus strains

Jianye Wang[1,2*], Jueyi Ling[1,2], Zhixian Wang[1,2], Yu Huang[1,2], Jianzhong Zhu[1,2] and Guoqiang Zhu[1,2*]

Abstract

Background: Muscovy duck parvovirus (MDPV) and Goose parvovirus (GPV) are important etiological agents for Muscovy duck parvoviral disease and Derzsy's disease, respectively; both of which can cause substantial economic losses in waterfowl industry. In contrast to GPV, the complete genomic sequence data of MDPV isolates are still limited and their phylogenetic relationships largely remain unknown. In this study, the entire genome of a pathogenic MDPV strain ZW, which was isolated from a deceased Muscovy duckling in 2006 in China, was cloned, sequenced, and compared with that of other classical MDPV and GPV strains.

Results: The genome of strain ZW comprises of 5071 nucleotides; this genome was shorter than that of the pathogenic MDPV strain YY (5075 nt). All the four deleted nucleotides produced in strain ZW are located at the base-pairing positions in the palindromic stem of inverted terminal repeats (ITR) without influencing the formation of a hairpin structure. Recombination analysis revealed that strain ZW originated from genetic recombination between the classical MDPV and GPV strain. The YY strain of MDPV acts as the major parent, whereas the virulent strains YZ99–6 and B and the vaccine strain SYG61v of GPV act as the minor parents in varying degrees. Two recombination sites were detected in strain ZW, with the small recombination site surrounding the P9 promoter, and the large recombination site situated in the middle of the VP3 gene. The SYG61V strain is a vaccine strain used for preventing goose parvoviral disease. This strain was found to be solely involved in the recombination event detected in the P9 promoter region. Phylogenetic analyses between strain ZW and other classical strains of MDPV and GPV were performed. The results supported the in silico recombination analysis conclusion.

Conclusions: MDPV Strain ZW is a novel recombinant parvovirus, and the bulk of its genome originates from the classical MDPV strain. Two virulent strains and a vaccine strain of GPV were involved in the recombination process in varying degrees.

Keywords: Goose parvovirus, Muscovy duck parvovirus, Recombination, Inverted terminal repeats

Background

Muscovy duck parvovirus (MDPV) and Goose parvovirus (GPV) are etiological agents for Muscovy duck parvoviral disease and Derzsy's disease, respectively [1]. The Muscovy duck parvoviral disease, also named "three-week" disease, mainly occurs in three-week-old Muscovy ducklings; the disease is characterized by locomotor dysfunction, stunting, abnormal feather development, and death. The mortality rate of the disease ranges from 10% to 80% depending on age [2–5]. Derzsy's disease is also named "gosling plague" in China and has been primarily described by Fang in 1961; it mainly breaks out in one-month-old goslings with the mortality rate reaching as high as 90% [6–8].

In the up-to-date classification report of International Committee on Taxonomy of Viruses (ICTV), MDPV and GPV are defined as virus variants and have a

* Correspondence: wangjy@yzu.edu.cn; yzgqzhu@yzu.edu.cn
[1]College of Veterinary Medicine, Yangzhou University, 48 Wenhui East Road, 225009 Yangzhou, Jiangsu Province, People's Republic of China
Full list of author information is available at the end of the article

common species name *Anseriform dependoparvovirus* 1, which is classified into the *Dependoparvovirus* genus in the subfamily *Parvovirinae* [9]. The viral genomes are approximately 5.1-kb single-stranded DNA with equal polarities encapsidated in the viral capsids [10]. Their genomes are flanked by identical inverted terminal repeats (ITR), which consist of 456 nucleotides for MDPV, and 442 nucleotides for GPV [11, 12]. The outside portion of ITR can fold on itself to form a palindromic hairpin structure. The inside portion of ITR, also designated as the D sequence, reversely complements with the D′ sequence in the 3′ ITR, allowing the entire genomic molecule to form a larger range of palindromic structure [13]. ITR contains a terminal resolving site (TRS), Rep protein binding site (RBS), and other transcription factor binding sites, which are required for genome replication, transcription, packaging, and rescue from cloning vector [10, 14, 15].

Their genomes have two open reading frames (ORFs), whereby the genetic organization and nucleotide length are identical for both viruses [10]. The left ORF encodes the viral non-structural protein Rep, whereas the right ORF encodes the structural protein. After alternative splicing of mRNA, the larger Rep1 protein and several smaller Rep proteins are produced [16, 17]. The Rep proteins can bind to the ITR and are involved in genome replication and modulation of downstream P41 promoter [18, 19]. By alternative splicing of mRNA, usage of initiation codon, and protease cleavage, the right ORF produces three structural proteins (VP1, VP2, and VP3), which assemble the viral capsid at a ratio of 1:1:8 [20].

The virulent strain B of GPV and strain FM of MDPV share 82.2% similarity at the genome level [10]. Moreover, the two viruses share 83.0% and 81.5% homologies in Rep1 and VP1 proteins at the nucleotide level, respectively, and 90.6% and 87.6% homologies at the amino acid level, respectively [10]. Irrespective of relatively high homologies, host range difference between both viruses is obvious. MDPV only infects Muscovy ducklings and is not pathogenic to goslings, whereas GPV is pathogenic not only to goslings but also to Muscovy ducklings [1, 4].

Currently, several complete genomic data of GPV strains isolated in various places and years are available, which share high homologies (at least 93%) with each other [21, 22]. However, the complete genomic sequence data of MDPV strains are still very limited and their phylogenetic relationships largely remain unknown. Strain ZW was isolated from a deceased Muscovy duckling, which died from a disease outbreak in 2006 in Zhejiang province, China. In the course of retrospective investigation of the MDPV isolates collected from 1999 to 2006, the genome of ZW was found to possess a different restriction endonuclease digestion pattern from other MDPV isolates. In this study, the entire genome of ZW was sequenced and compared with other classical strains of MDPV and GPV. Strain ZW is a hybrid between the classical MDPV and GPV, with the bulk of its genome originating from classical MDPV, whereas the P9 promoter region and greater part of the VP3 gene from a vaccine strain and two virulent strains of GPV.

Methods

Virus propagation and purification

The viral stock of strain ZW was diluted 1:50 with sterile saline containing penicillin (2000 U/ml) and streptomycin (2000 mg/ml) and inoculated into the chorioallantoic cavity of 12-day-old susceptible embryonated Muscovy duck eggs. The procedure for inoculation of fertilized Muscovy duck eggs was approved by the Animal Care and Use Committee of Yangzhou University and performed in accordance with the "Guidelines for Experimental Animals" of the Ministry of Science and Technology (Beijing, China). No specific permits were required for these locations and activities.

The dead embryos were kept at 4 °C for 6 h and the allantoic fluids were pooled and clarified by centrifugation at 11,000×*g* for 20 min. The supernatant was further mixed with chloroform (1/3, *v*/v), shaken vigorously, and then subjected to centrifugation at 11,000×*g* for 20 min. The upper aqueous phase containing the virus was collected and pelleted by ultracentrifugation at 150,000×*g* for 3 h (SW32Ti rotor, Beckman, USA). Finally, the virus-containing pellet was re-suspended in TE buffer (50 mM Tris, 20 mM EDTA, pH 8.0) to 1/50 of the starting volume.

DNA extraction

The viral DNAs were extracted by the SDS-Proteinase K (Merck, Darmstadt, Germany) incubation method as previously described [23]. The genomic DNA was suspended in STE buffer (10 mM Tris, 1 mM EDTA, 100 mM NaCl, pH 8.0) and annealed by heating to 95 °C for 5 min, followed by slow cooling to 55 °C. The annealed double-stranded DNA of approximately 5.1 kb was examined in 0.8% agarose gel by electrophoresis.

Genome cloning and sequencing

To facilitate cloning, a pair of linker primers (5′-AGCTTCCATGGG-3′ and 5′-AATTCCCATGGA-3′) was synthesized and annealed, resulting in a linker with adhesive ends of *Hin*dIII and *Eco*RI. By inserting the linker into the plasmid pBluescript II SK (Agilent, Santa Clara, USA), the original *Eco*RV site was replaced by the *Nco*I site, thereby resulting in the plasmid pBSKN [12].

The extracted genomic DNA was digested with *Nco*I, resulting in a 0.7-kb left fragment, a 3.1-kb middle fragment, and a 1.2-kb right fragment. The digested fragments were separated by electrophoresis and purified with a gel extraction kit (Tiangen, Peiking, China). The 0.7-kb fragment containing the 5′ end ITR was ligated into the *Hin*cII-*Nco*I site of the pBSKN plasmid, thereby generating plasmid pBSKNL (Fig. 1). The middle 3.1-kb fragment was ligated into the *Nco*I site, resulting in plasmid pBSKNM. The 1.2-kb fragment containing the 3′ end ITR was ligated into the *Nco*I-*Sma*I site, generating the plasmid pBSKNR.

The cloned gene fragments were sequenced using an ABI-PRISM3730 automated sequencer and BigDye terminators v3.1 (Applied Biosystems, Foster City, USA). To overcome the difficulties in sequencing the ITRs, the plasmids were double digested with *Sph*I and *Bam*HI or *Kpn*I. The unique *Sph*I site at the loop position of the bubble region allowed us to cut the entire ITR into two halves. The resulting fragments containing half of the ITR were then subcloned into pUC18 for sequencing [24]. The sequences were assembled using SeqManII software included in the Lasergene package 5.0 (DNASTAR, Madison, USA). The complete genome sequence was submitted to GenBank.

Recombination and phylogenetic analysis

The recombination analysis software SimPlot version 3.5.1 [25] and Recombination Detection Program v.4.43 (RDP4) [26] were both used to detect possible recombinant events that occurred in strain ZW. Simplot analysis was conducted by setting the window width and the step size to 200 bp and 20 bp, respectively. The genomic sequence of strain ZW obtained in this study was used for queries, while putative parental sequences were retrieved from GenBank (Table 1). Different methods implemented in RDP4, including RDP, GENCONV, MaxChi, BootScan, SicCAN, LARD, and 3SEQ were also used to detect recombinant events under default settings for the different detection programs, likely parental isolates, and recombination break points. If a recombination event

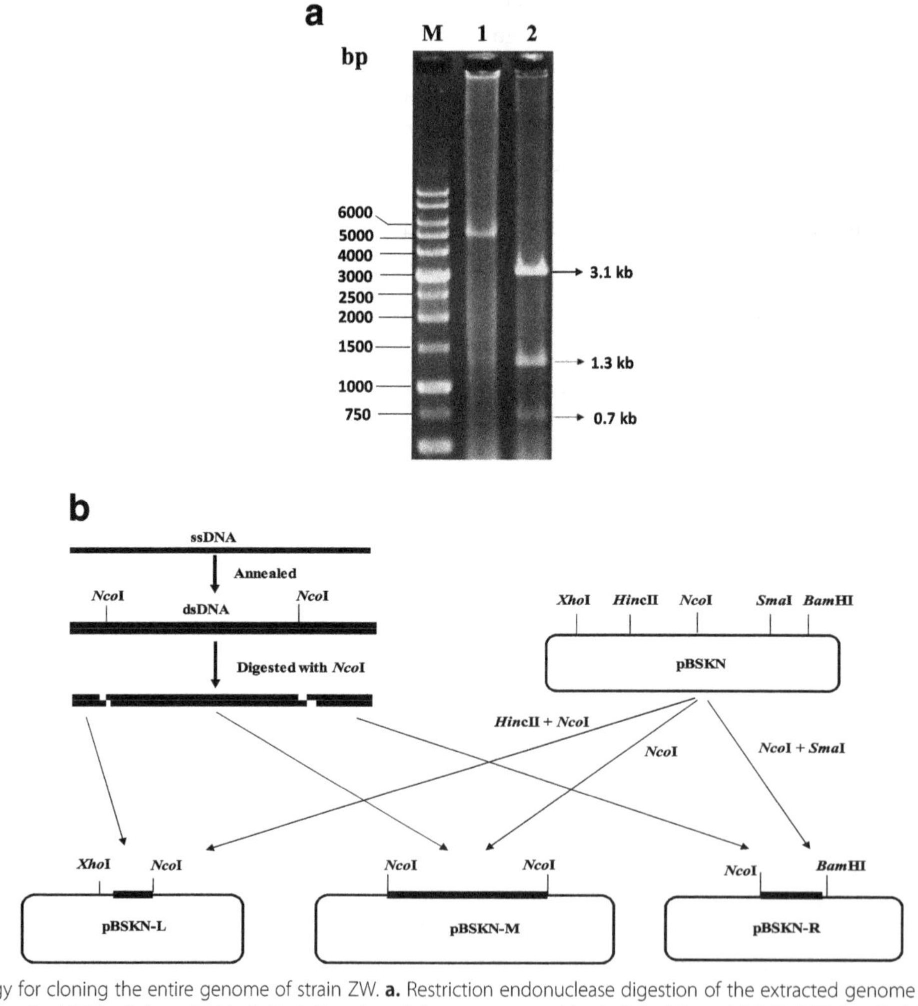

Fig. 1 The strategy for cloning the entire genome of strain ZW. **a.** Restriction endonuclease digestion of the extracted genome of strain ZW. 1. The annealed genomic dsDNA of about 5.1 kb; 2. *Nco*I digestion of the genome resulting in 3.1-, 1.3-, and 0.7-kb DNA bands; M: 1-kb DNA ladder. **b.** Schematic diagram of the experimental strategy for cloning three sub-genomic fragments of strain ZW

Table 1 Waterfowl parvovirus isolates used in this study for sequence comparison, recombination analysis, and construction of phylogenetic tree

Viral classification	Strain	Pathogenicity	Native host	Geographic origin	Collection date	GenBank accession no.
MDPV	FM	Pathogenic	Muscovy duck	France	n.a	U22967
	P	Pathogenic	Muscovy duck	China	1988	JF926697
	FZ91–30	Vaccine	Muscovy duck	China	1991	KT865605
	YY	Pathogenic	Muscovy duck	China	2000	KX000918
GPV	B	Pathogenic	Goose	Hungary	1967	U25749
	06–0329	Pathogenic	Goose	Taiwan	2006	EU583391
	82–0321	Pathogenic	Goose	Taiwan	1982	EU583390
	VG32–1	Vaccine	Goose	Germany	n.a	EU583392
	SYG61v	Vaccine	Goose	China	1961	KC996729
	LH	Pathogenic	Goose	China	2012	KM272560
	YZ99–6	Pathogenic	Goose	China	1999	KC996730
Recombinant	ZW	Pathogenic	Muscovy duck	China	2006	KY744743

n.a.: not available

was supported by at least three methods with a *P*-value $<10^{-6}$ or the recombination score is above 0.6, the recombination event is considered to be true. If the recombination score is between 0.4–0.6, the recombination event is considered to be of fair likelihood. Phylogenetic trees were constructed using the neighbor-joining method in MEGA 6.01 [27].

Agar gel precipitation test

To study the antigenic relationship between the recombinant strain ZW and the classical GPV and MDPV strains, agar gel precipitation (AGP) tests were conducted. A mouse monoclonal antibody (mAb) against GPV used in the AGP tests was developed and provided by Professor Guoxiong Dong at College of Veterinary Medicine of Yangzhou University. This mAb can specifically recognize the VP3 protein of GPV in a Western blot test [28]. A 1:20 dilution of the mAb was further diluted by two-fold series in phosphate buffered saline (pH 7.4). The viruses used as antigens in the AGP tests were concentrated by ultracentrifugation as previously described. The gel pattern consisted of a central well 3 mm in diameter containing antigen surrounded by six outer wells of the same diameter containing serially diluted mAb. All the wells were spaced 4 mm apart. Diffusion of antigen and antibody took place at 37 °C and the plates were examined for precipitin lines after approximately 24 h.

Results

Genome sequence analysis

After annealing of the single-stranded DNA, a 5.1-kb double-stranded DNA (dsDNA) was observed (Fig. 1a). The dsDNA was digested with *Nco*I, resulting in three fragments of 0.7, 1.3, and 3.1 kb. Subsequently, three sub-genomic fragments were successfully cloned into the pBSKN plasmid for sequencing (Fig. 1b). The obtained sequences were used to assemble the complete genome sequence of strain ZW.

The genome of strain ZW consists of 5071 nucleotides—four nucleotides shorter than that of the pathogenic Chinese MDPV strain YY. The ITR consists of 424 nucleotides, among which 387 nucleotides constitute the palindrome and 39 nucleotides constitute the D region (Fig. 2). The D sequence strictly complements the D′ sequence in the 3′ ITR. In comparison to strain FM and FZ91–30 of MDPV, the ITR of strain ZW produces a 14-nucleotide-pair deletions in the stem of the palindrome, which is also observed in the pathogenic strain YY of MDPV [24]. Moreover, strain ZW exhibits additional two nucleotide deletions in the palindromic stem; nevertheless, both deleted nucleotides lie at the base-pairing positions without influencing the formation of a hairpin structure. Sequence comparison of the ITRs with the pathogenic strains of MDPV and GPV showed that strain ZW shared 97.9% nucleotide similarity with the MDPV strain YY but showed lower similarities with the GPV strain LH (85.7%) and YZ99–6 (86.0%), thereby demonstrating that the ITR of strain ZW originates from the classical MDPV.

In the two open reading frames (ORFs), strain ZW shares identical genetic organization with the classical strains of MDPV and GPV. The Rep1 protein of strain ZW consists of 1884 nucleotides, coding for 627 amino acids. Homology comparison showed that the Rep1 protein of ZW displayed a higher nucleotide identity (98.0%–98.7%) with the classical MDPV strains, but a lower similarity (81.8%–83.3%) with the classical GPV strains (Table 2). The VP1 protein of ZW consists of 2199 nucleotides, coding for 732

```
                                                               61           74
FM   CTCATTGGAGGGTTCGTTCGTTCGAACCAGCCAATCAGGGGAGGGGGGAAGTGACGTAAGTTCCGGTCACGTGCTTCCGG   80
YY   -TCATTGGAGGGTTCGTTCGTTCGAACCAGCCAATCAGGGGAGGGGGGAAGTGACGTAAG--------------TTCCGG   65
ZW   -TCATTGGAGGGTTCGTTCGTTCGAACCGGCCAATCAGGGGAGGGGGGAAGTGACGTAAG--------------TTCCGG   65

FM   TCACGTGCTTCCGGTCATGTGACTTCCGGTCATGTGACTTCCGGTGACGTGTCTCCTGTCACGTGACTTCCGGTGACGCA   160
YY   TCACGTGCTTCCGGTCATGTGACTTCCGGTCACGTGACTTCCGGTGACGTGTTTCCTGTCACGTGACTTCCGGTGACGCA   145
ZW   TCACGTGCTTCCGGTCACGTG-CTTCCGGTCATGTGACTTCCGGTCACGTGTTTCCTGTCACGTGACTTCCGGTGACGCA   144

                                 ooooooooooooooooooooooooooooooooooooooooooooo
FM   CTTCCTTTGATGACGTATTTCCGGTTGTCAAGGCTGATCGGGCGCATGCGCCCGATCTGCCATGAAAATTAAACCGGAAA   240
YY   CTTCCTTTGATGACGTATTTCCGGTTGTCAAGGCTGATCGGGCGCATGCGCCCGATCTGCCATGAAAATTAAACCGGAAA   225
ZW   CTTCCTTTGATGACGTATTTCCGGTTGTCAAGGCTGATCGGGCGCATGCGCCCGATCTGCCATGAAAATTAAACCGGAAA   224

FM   TACGTCATCAAAGGAAGTGCGTCACCGGAAGTCACGTGACAGGAGACACGTCACCGGAAGTCACATGACCGGAAGTCACA   320
YY   TACGTCATCAAAGGAAGTGCGTCACCGGAAGTCACGTGACAGGAAACACGTCACCGGAAGTCACGTGACCGGAAGTCACA   305
ZW   TACGTCATCAAAGGAAGTGCGTCACCGGAAGTCACGTGACAGGAAACACGTGACCGGAAGTCACATGACCGGAAG-CACG   303

                         344          357
FM   TGACCGGAAGCACGTGACCGGAAGCACGTGACCGGAACTTACGTCACTTCCCCCCTCCCCTGATTGGCTGGTTCGAACGA   400
YY   TGACCGGAAGCACGTGACCGGAA--------------CTTACGTCACTTCCCCCCTCCCCTGATTGGCTGGTTCGAACGA   371
ZW   TGACCGGAAGCACGTGACCGGAA--------------CTTACGTCACTTCCCCCCTCCCCTGATTGGCCGGTTCGAACGA   369

                                     D sequence
FM   ACGAACCCTCCAATGAGACTCAAGGACAGCAGGACTTTTTGCGCGCCAGGAAATGGT   457
YY   ACGAACCCTCCAATGAGACTCAAGGACAGCAGGACTTTTTGCGCGCCAGGAAGTGGT   428
ZW   ACGAACCCTCCAATGAGACTCAAGGACAGCAGGACTTTTTGCGCGCCAGGAAATG     424
```

Fig. 2 Alignment of inverted terminal repeat (ITR) sequences at the 5′ terminus of the genome of strain FM, YY, and ZW of MDPV. Dashes denote nucleotide deletions. The bubble region of ITR comprises of 45 nucleotides and is indicated by open circles above the letters. The nucleotide differences between three strains are shaded grey. The nucleotides constituting the D region are italicized and underlined, which complement the D′ sequences at the 3′ ITR. The numbers above the alignment denote the nucleotide's position

amino acids. Nucleotide sequence comparison of the VP1 proteins showed that strain ZW displayed almost equal percentages of identity with the classical MDPV strains (89.0%–89.1%) and the classical GPV strains (87.9%–89.4%), whereas percentages of identity with the classical MDPV strains and the classical GPV strains are above 98.5% and 93.5%, respectively (Table 2).

The genome sequence of strain ZW was deposited in GenBank with the accession number KY744743.

Table 2 Percentages of identity of nucleotide sequences of the coding proteins Rep1 (upper right) and VP1 (lower left) between strain ZW and other classical MDPV and GPV strains

Percent identity of Rep1 (upper right); Percent identity of VP1 (lower left)

	1	2	3	4	5	6	7	8	9	10	11	12			
1		99.8	99.8	99.4	99.3	98.6	94.3	83.4	82.8	83.2	83.1	83.3	1	LH	Classical GPV
2	99.6		99.7	99.3	99.2	98.5	94.3	83.2	82.6	83.1	82.9	83.1	2	YZ99-6	
3	99.4	99.6		99.4	99.4	98.7	94.3	83.3	82.7	83.2	83.0	83.2	3	82-0321	
4	99.3	99.4	99.6		98.9	98.3	93.8	83.1	82.5	83.0	82.8	83.0	4	06-0329	
5	96.5	96.7	96.6	96.4		99.0	94.4	83.3	82.7	83.1	83.0	83.3	5	B	
6	96.1	96.3	96.2	96.0	98.7		94.5	83.4	82.7	83.1	83.0	83.3	6	VG32-1	
7	95.5	95.7	95.6	95.4	93.7	93.5		81.6	81.0	81.4	81.3	81.8	7	SYG61v	
8	80.6	80.5	80.4	80.3	81.5	81.1	79.8		98.7	99.7	99.3	98.6	8	FZ91-30	Classical MDPV
9	80.6	80.5	80.4	80.3	81.6	81.2	79.9	99.2		99.0	98.7	98.0	9	P	
10	80.6	80.6	80.5	80.4	81.8	81.4	80.0	99.5	99.3		99.6	98.9	10	YY	
11	80.6	80.6	80.5	80.4	81.5	81.1	79.8	98.7	98.5	98.8		98.7	11	FM	
12	89.3	89.4	89.3	89.1	88.8	88.5	87.9	89.0	89.1	89.1	89.1		12	ZW	
	1	2	3	4	5	6	7	8	9	10	11	12			

Recombination analysis

Two potential recombination sites that existed in Strain ZW were both detected by the Simplot and RDP software. The first recombination breakpoint in the left side of genome was generated between the YY strain of MPV and the vaccine strain SYG61v of GPV (Fig. 3). Recombination analysis executed with RDP4 showed that the breakpoint started at nucleotide position 456 and ended at position 647, with the highest probability value of RDP method reaching 10^{-49}. The major parent was strain YY, and the minor parent was SYG61v. The recombination signal extended from the interior of the 5′ ITR to the 100 nucleotides downstream of the initiation codon in Rep protein. Sequence alignment of 50 nucleotides upstream of this recombination region among YY, YZ99–6, SYG61v, and ZW clearly demonstrated that strain ZW shared 100% identity with the vaccine strain SYG61v, but had variable extents of nucleotide differences with the MDPV strain YY and the GPV strain YZ99–6 (Fig. 4), further confirming the recombination analysis result.

The second recombination breakpoint occurred in the middle of the VP3 gene. Recombination analysis using RDP4 revealed that the second recombination breakpoint started at nucleotide position 3152, which is generally situated at 120 nucleotides downstream of the initiation codon of VP3 protein, and ended at position 4278, covering a successive DNA region of approximately 1100 nucleotides in length (Fig. 3b). The YY strain of MDPV remained the major parent, whereas the two virulent strains (YZ99–6 and B) and the vaccine strain (SYG61v) of GPV acted as the minor parents with the *P*-values ranging from 10^{-88} to 10^{-4}. Furthermore, SimPlot analysis also disclosed multiple constitutive recombination signals in the VP3 gene, which were generated between strain YY and the three GPV strains YZ99–6, B, and SYG61v (Fig. 3a). The recombination events were found to mainly occur between strain YY and the virulent GPV strains, whereas only a small portion of recombination region was swapped between YY and the vaccine strain SYG61v. Therefore, locations of the putative recombination sites identified by SimPlot coincided with the recombination analysis result by RDP4.

```
          ITR←
SYG61v    TGACGTTAGGGGCTGCCCTATATAAGCCAGTAAGCTTCCGGTTTGGTTCA 490
YZ99-6    ......GCAAT..CA...............G..A..........A..... 462
YY        ..GT.CA.TCTAGGAGAG.G......GAGAGCTTT........GCA.... 474
ZW        .................................................. 472
```

Fig. 4 Alignment of partial nucleotide sequences spanning from downstream of ITR to the P9 promoter. Identical nucleotides relative to the SYG61v strain are denoted by dots. The recombinant strain ZW shares 100% nucleotide homology with the vaccine strain SYG61v

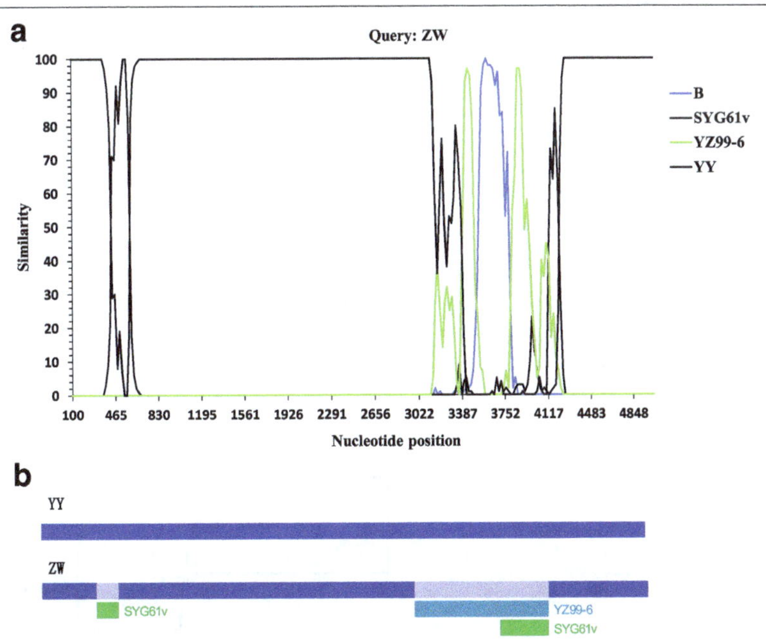

Fig. 3 Recombination analysis using Simplot 3.5.1 and RDP 3.4.1. **a.** Similarity plot analysis of full genome sequences of strain ZW, B, SYG61v, YZ99–6, and YY using Simplot. Bootscan analysis was executed with the following parameters: 1000 bootstrap replicates, sliding window of 200 bp, and step size of 20 bp. Strain ZW was used as query. **b.** Recombinant events that occurred in strain ZW were detected by RDP. The first recombination breakpoint began at nucleotide position 424 and ended at nt position 615. The second recombination breakpoint began at nucleotide position 3120 and ended at nt position 4246. In these recombinant events, strain YY is the major parent. SYG61v is the sole minor parent in the first recombinant site

Phylogenetic analysis

Based on the recombination analysis results of strain ZW, four genomic fragments were chosen to independently construct phylogenetic trees, among which three fragments are located in the non-recombination regions and one fragment encompasses the identified 1100-bp recombination region of the VP3 gene. Three non-recombination fragments included the carboxyl terminal 1774-bp fragment of the Rep1 gene (Fragment A), and the amino terminal 694-bp fragment (Fragment B) and the carboxyl terminal 405-bp fragment (Fragment C) of the VP1 gene. Moreover, Fragments B and C were adjacent to the 1100-bp recombination fragment (Fragment D).

In the phylogenetic trees constructed based on the Fragment A, B, and C, strain ZW clustered with all of the classical MDPV isolates and formed a separate branch, distinct from the branch formed by all classical GPV isolates (Figs. 5a, b, and c). In contrast, in the phylogenetic tree constructed based on the Fragment D, strain ZW clustered with the classical GPV members, and all classical MDPV isolates formed another branch (Fig. 5d). Essentially, positional alteration of strain ZW in the phylogenetic trees based on different genomic fragments is in agreement with the in silico recombination analysis result.

Antigenic analysis by AGP tests

In the AGP tests, antigens placed in the central wells were the classical GPV strain LH, the classical MDPV strain YY, and the recombinant strain ZW, respectively. A similar mAb titres with 1:160 were obviously observed when strain ZW and LH were used as the AGP antigens (Fig. 6). In contrast, in the AGP test with strain YY as the antigen, the weak precipitin lines were observed and indicated a lower mAb titre with 1:80. The AGP test results demonstrated a closer antigenic relationship between the recombinant strain ZW and the classical GPV strain, which is in agreement with the in silico recombination analysis result.

Discussion

Attenuated live viruses are involved in genetic recombination with prevailing field strains, thereby resulting in the emergence of novel variants [29, 30]. SYG61v is an attenuated vaccine strain of GPV and combined with the

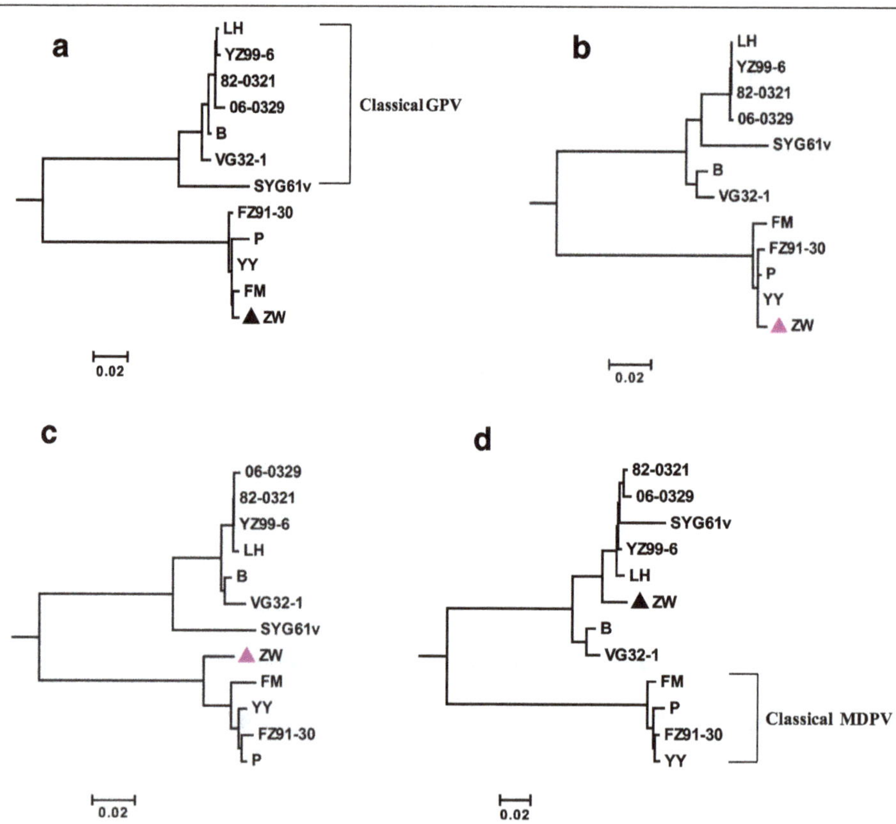

Fig. 5 Phylogenetic analysis of strain ZW and other 11 MDPV and GPV isolates. These isolates have complete Rep1 and VP1 gene sequences deposited in GenBank. The neighbor-joining method in MEGA 6.0.6 with 1000 bootstrap replications was used for construction of phylogenetic trees. Phylogenetic trees was constructed based on the C-terminal 1774-bp fragment of the Rep1 gene (**a**), the N terminal 694-bp (**b**) and the C-terminal 405-bp (**c**) fragments of the VP1 gene, and the middle 1100-bp fragment of the VP3 gene (**d**)

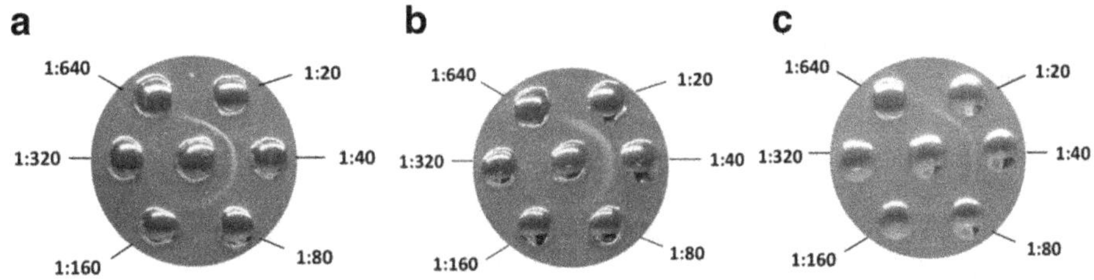

Fig. 6 Antigenic comparison between the recombinant strain ZW and the classical GPV and MDPV strains by agar gel precipitation (AGP) tests. A monoclonal antibody (mAb) against GPV was used in the AGP tests. A 1:20 dilution of this mAb was further diluted by two-fold series in phosphate buffered saline (pH 7.4) and placed in the outer wells surrounding the central well containing antigen. The classical GPV strain LH (**a**), the recombinant strain ZW (**b**), and the classical MDPV strain YY (**c**) were used as the AGP antigens, respectively

attenuated MDPV strain to prevent potential infection of either GPV or MDPV in Muscovy ducklings. However, usage of the combined vaccine also provides the chance for genetic recombination. In the present recombination analysis, we found that SYG61v not only participated in the recombination event in the P9 promoter region but was also involved in the recombination events that occurred in the VP3 gene. Remarkably, the DNA sequence in strain ZW surrounding the P9 promoter region was wholly replaced with the sequence from strain SYG61v. Considering that strain ZW itself is highly pathogenic to Muscovy ducklings, the biological purpose underlying this recombination event involving a vaccine strain remains to be investigated.

Strain B, the earliest Europe isolate of GPV, was isolated from Hungary in 1967 [8]. In this study, strain B was found to be involved as the minor parent in the recombination events that occurred in the VP3 region of strain ZW. The percentages of identity of the VP1 protein nucleotide sequences between strain B and four other Chinese virulent strains (82–0321, 06–0329, YZ99–6, and LH) ranged from 96.4% to 96.7%, whereas the same analysis among the four Chinese strains showed slightly higher percentages of identity, ranging from 99.3% to 99.6% (Table 2). Involvement of strain B in the recombination events demonstrated that GPV strains from various geographical origins collectively contributed to the generation of the recombinant strain ZW.

The VP3 gene consists of 1605 nucleotides encoding for 534 amino acids, which overlaps with the carboxyl terminus of the VP1 and VP2 proteins. As the major structural protein, the VP3 protein harbors most of the antigenic epitopes distributed on the surface of the viral capsid [10]. In this study, the VP3 gene of strain ZW incorporated approximately 1.1-kb foreign nucleotide sequence from GPV, which ultimately shaped the distinctive antigenicity of strain ZW, different from the classical strains of MDPV and GPV. In addition to the recombination events, several amino acid point mutations were also found to occur in the VP1 protein of strain ZW, all of which are specific for strain ZW and are different from those of the classical MDPV or GPV strains. Point mutations at amino acid positions 450, 485, 493, 548, and 585 were in the recombination region of the VP3 protein, whereas point mutations at positions 79 and 712 were outside of the recombination region. Therefore, the recombination and point mutations contributed to rapid evolution and increased fitness, respectively, and collectively promoted the emergence of the recombinant MDPV strain ZW.

Sequence alignment of ITR indicates the characteristic two-nucleotide deletions that occurred at the palindromic stem in the 5′ and 3′ ITR of strain ZW. ITR not only functions as an origin of genome replication, but also contains several transcription factor binding sites, including E-box, ATF/CREB, and MLTF [10, 24]. These transcription factor binding sites are densely distributed in the 200-bp stem of the palindromic structure of ITR. Although these deleted nucleotides were at the base-pairing positions and did not influence the hairpin structure formation for the remaining nucleotides, the nucleotide deletions shortened the spacing distance between adjacent transcription factors. Whether the nucleotide deletions that occurred in ITR have potential influence on the transcription efficiency and contribute to virulence of strain ZW remain to be further investigated.

Most of viral sequences used for the recombination analysis were obtained through PCR amplification [29–31]. If the PCR templates of the characterized recombinants per se were contaminated with genetic materials from multiple strains, plus degeneration of the designed primers used in PCR amplification, an inauthentic genomic sequence information will probably be generated, which would result in false conclusions in the subsequent recombination analysis. In view of this, we conducted the direct genome cloning strategy by strain ZW by restriction endonuclease digestion. Therefore, the possibility that the genomic sequence of strain ZW has been contaminated with other isolates has been excluded.

For the first time, we presented a detailed description of the genomic characteristics of the novel MDPV strain ZW and confirmed the occurrence of recombination events between GPV and MDPV. Continuous molecular epidemiological investigation should be deployed to assess the incidence of strain ZW-like recombinant viral infection in the field. In view of the widespread usage of live vaccines in the Muscovy duck flocks, direct genome cloning and sequencing against the MDPV isolates is a more reliable method than PCR amplification for acquiring accurate sequence data for recombination analysis. However, whether the traditional bi-combined vaccine currently in use can still provide robust protection for Muscovy ducklings against infection from emerging recombinant MDPV in China remains to be evaluated and clarified.

Conclusions

Strain ZW is a recombinant MDPV that produces four characteristic nucleotide deletions in the palindromic stem of ITR. Most of the genome of strain ZW, including the ITR sequence, still originates from the classical MDPV strain. Two virulent strains and a vaccine strain of GPV were involved in multiple recombination events detected in strain ZW at different levels. The attenuated vaccine strain SYG61v acted as the only minor parent, thereby contributing to the recombination event that occurred in the P9 promoter region. Considering that strain ZW emerged in 2006, we deduced that the recombinant MDPV has been co-existing with the classical MDPV strains for a long time in the field and has constantly threatened Chinese Muscovy duck industry.

Abbreviations

GPV: Goose parvovirus; ITR: Inverted terminal repeats; Kb: kilobase; MDPV: Muscovy duck parvovirus; Nt: nucleotides; ORF: Open reading frame

Acknowledgements

Not applicable.

Funding

This work was supported by the National Natural Science Foundation of China (no. 31572551, 31,172,317) and by a project funded by the Priority Academic Program Development of Jiangsu Higher Education Institutions.

Authors' contributions

JW conceived and designed the experiments. JL, ZW, and YH performed the experiments. GZ analyzed the data. JW wrote the paper. JZ and JW checked and revised the manuscript. All authors read and approved the final manuscript.

Consent for publication

Not applicable.

Competing interests

The authors declare that they have no competing interests.

Author details

[1]College of Veterinary Medicine, Yangzhou University, 48 Wenhui East Road, 225009 Yangzhou, Jiangsu Province, People's Republic of China. [2]Jiangsu Co-Innovation Center for Important Animal Infectious Diseases and Zoonoses, Yangzhou 225009, China.

References

1. Swayne DE, Glisson JR, McDougald LR, Nolan LK, Suarez DL, Nair V. Diseases of poultry (13th edition). Oxford, UK: Wiley-Blackwell Publishing Ltd; 2013. p. 444–51.
2. Chen YQ, Lin TL, Hu QL, Li YY, Zhou WM, Wu ZY. Isolation and identification of a Muscovy duckling parvovirus. Chi J Virol. 1993;9(3):228–34. (In Chinese)
3. Jestin V, Le Bras MO, Cherbonnel M, Le Gall G, Bennejean G. Mise en évidence de parvovirus (virus de la maladie de Derzsy) très pathogènes dans les élevages de canards de Barbarie. Rec Med Vet. 1991;167:849–57.
4. Glávits R, Zolnai A, Szabó É, Ivanics É, Zarka P, Mató T, Palya V. Comparative pathological studies on domestic geese (Anser Anser Domestica) and Muscovy ducks (Cairina Moschata) experimentally infected with parvovirus strains of goose and Muscovy duck origin. Acta Vet Hung. 2005;53:73–89.
5. Barnes HJ. Muscovy duck parvovirus. In: Calnek BW, Barnes HJ, Beard CW, McDougald LR, Saif YM, editors. Diseases of poultry. 10th ed. Ames, IA: Iowa State University Press; 1997. p. 1032–3.
6. Fang D, Wang Y, Zhen Y, Zhou Y, Jiang M, Dong G. Studies on the aetiology and specific control of gosling plaque. Sci Agric Sin. 1987;4:1–9. (in Chinese)
7. Fang D. Recommendation of gosling plaque. Veterinary Science in China. 1962;8:19–20. (in Chinese)
8. Derzsy D. A viral disease of goslings. I. Epidemiological, clinical, pathological and etiological studies. Acta Vet Acad Sci Hungar. 1967;17:443–8.
9. Cotmore S, Agbandje-McKenna M, Chiorini JA, Mukha DV, Pintel DJ, Qiu JM, Soderlund-Venermo M, Tattersall P, Tijssen P, Gatherer D, Davisonet AJ. The family Parvoviridae. Arch Virol. 2014;159:1239–47.
10. Zadori Z, Stefancsik R, Rauch T, Kisary J. Analysis of the complete nucleotide sequences of goose and muscovy duck parvoviruses indicates common ancestral origin with adeno-associated virus 2. Virology. 1995;212(2):562–57.
11. Wang J, Duan J, Meng X, Gong J, Jiang Z, Zhu G. Cloning of the genome of a goose parvovirus vaccine strain SYG61v and rescue of infectious virions from recombinant plasmid in embryonated goose eggs. J Virol Methods. 2014;200:41–6.
12. Wang J, Huang Y, Zhou M, Hardwidge R, Zhu G. Construction and sequencing of an infectious clone of the goose embryo-adapted Muscovy duck parvovirus vaccine strain FZ91-30. Virol J. 2016;13:104.
13. Samulski RJ, Srivastava A, Berns KI. Rescue of adeno-associated virus from recombinant plasmids: gene correction within the terminal repeats of AAV. Cell. 1983;33:135–43.
14. Snyder RO, Im DS, Muzyczka N. Evidence for covalent attachment of the adeno-associated virus (AAV) rep protein to the ends of the AAV genome. J Virol. 1990;64:6204–13.
15. Costello E, Sahli R, Hirt B, Beard P. The mismatched nucleotides in the 5'-terminal hairpin of minute virus of mice are required for efficient viral DNA replication. J Virol. 1995;69:7489–96.
16. Li L, Qiu J, Pintel DJ. The choice of translation initiation site of the rep proteins from goose parvovirus p9-generated mRNA is governed by splicing and the nature of the excised intron. J Virol. 2009;83(19):10264–8.
17. Qiu J, Cheng F, Yoto Y, Zadori Z, Pintel D. The expression strategy of goose parvovirus exhibits features of both the Dependovirus and parvovirus genera. J Virol. 2005;79(17):11035–44.
18. Legendre D, Rommelaere J. Targeting of promoters for trans activation by a carboxy-terminal domain of the NS-1 protein of the parvovirus minute virus of mice. J Virol. 1994;68:7974–85.
19. Tewary SK, Zhao H, Deng X, Qiu J, Tang L. The human parvovirus B19 non-structural protein 1 N-terminal domain specifically binds to the origin of replication in the viral DNA. Virology. 2014;449:297–303.

20. Gall-Recule GL, Jestin V. Biochemical and genomic characterization of Muscovy duck parvovirus. Arch Virol. 1994;139:121–31.
21. Shien J, Wang Y, Chen C, Shieh H, Hu C, Chang P. Identification of sequence changes in live attenuated goose parvovirus vaccine strains developed in Asia and Europe. Avian Pathol. 2008;37(5):499–505.
22. Wang J, Duan J, Zhu L, Jiang Z, Zhu G. Sequencing and generation of an infectious clone of the pathogenic goose parvovirus strain LH. Arch Virol. 2015;160(3):711–8.
23. Bossis I, Chiorini JA. Cloning of an avian adeno-assocoated virus (AAAV) and generation of recombinant AAAV particles. J Virol. 2003;77:6799–810.
24. Wang J, Huang Y, Zhou M, Zhu G. Analysis of the genome sequence of the pathogenic Muscovy duck parvovirus strain YY reveals a 14-nucleotide-pair deletion in the inverted terminal repeats. Arch Virol. 2016;161:2589–94.
25. Lole KS, Bollinger RC, Paranjape RS, Gadkari D, Kulkarni SS, Novak NG, Ingersoll R, Sheppard HW, Ray SC. Full-length human immunodeficiency virus type 1 genomes from subtype C-infected seroconverters in India, with evidence of intersubtype recombination. J Virol. 1999;73(1):152–60.
26. Martin DP, Murrell B, Golden M, Khoosal A, & Muhire B. RDP4: Detection and analysis of recombination patterns in virus genomes. Virus Evolution. 2015;1: vev003 doi: https://doi.org/10.1093/ve/vev003.
27. Tamura K, Stecher G, Peterson D, Filipski A, Kumar S. MEGA6: molecular evolutionary genetics analysis version 6.0. Mol Bio Evol. 2013;30(12):2725–9.
28. Dong G, Xinhua L, junbao L. Neutralizing monoclonal antibodies to goose parvovirus and the effect of experimental prevention and treatment for gosling plague. J Jiangsu Agric College. 1996;17(3):7–10. (in Chinese)
29. Li B, Fang L, Xu Z, Liu S, Gao J, Jiang Y, Chen H, Xiao S. Recombination in vaccine and circulating strains of porcine reproductive and respiratory syndrome viruses. Emerg Infect Dis. 2009;15:2032–5.
30. Quinteros JA, Lee S, Markham PF, Noormohammadi AH, Hartley CA, Legione AR, Coppo MC, Vaz PK, Browning GF. Full genome analysis of Australian infectious bronchitis viruses suggests frequent recombination events between vaccine strains and multiple phylogenetically distant avian coronaviruses of unknown origin. Vet Microbiol. 2016;197:27–38.
31. Moreno A, Franzo G, Massi P, Tosi G, Blanco A, Antilles N, Biarnes M, Majó N, Nofrarías M, Dolz R, Lelli D, Sozzi E, Lavazza A, Cecchinato M. A novel variant of the infectious bronchitis virus resulting from recombination events in Italy and Spain. Avian Pathol. 2017;46(1):28–35.

3

Occurrence of canine parvovirus in dogs from Henan province of China in 2009–2014

Zhanqin Zhao[1†], Huisheng Liu[1†], Ke Ding[1], Chunping Peng[1], Qiao Xue[1], Zuhua Yu[1] and Yun Xue[2*]

Abstract

Background: There is no information concerning the genotype of Canine parvovirus (CPV) currently circulating in Henan province, China. Therefore, the aim of the present study was to provide insights into the epidemiology and molecular characterization of CPV circulating in Henan province from 2009 to 2014.

Results: Nineteen thousand nine hundred seven dogs from pet hospitals in the cities of Luoyang, Anyang, Jiaozuo, Sanmenxia, Xinxiang, Zhengzhou in Henan province between 2009 and 2014 were investigated. Over the 6-year period, 1169 CPV-positive cases were identified and the morbidity of CPV infection ranged from 4.16 to 8.06 %, although morbidity was not significant ($P > 0.05$) between 2009 and 2014. Factors associated with morbidity included sampling season, dog age, breed, vaccination status, and sex. CPV co-infection with coccidium (10.00 %), canine distemper virus (4.79 %), hookworm (2.40 %), canine coronavirus (1.11 %), roundworm (1.03 %), tapeworm (0.17 %) and *Babesia* spp. (0.09 %) were observed. The new CPV-2a variant was more prevalent than the new CPV-2b variant in Henan province. CPV 2c was not observed in this study.

Conclusions: The epidemiology of CPV infection and identification of the circulating genotypes in Henan province, China from 2009 to 2014 determined that the new CPV-2a variant was more prevalent.

Keywords: Canine parvovirus, Canine distemper virus, Canine coronavirus, Parasites, Epidemiology

Background

Canine parvovirus 2 (CPV-2), a member of the genus *Protoparvovirus* within the family *Parvoviridae* (the 2014 ICTV taxonomy, website: http://ictvonline.org/virusTaxonomy.asp), is a small, highly contagious, non-enveloped icosahedral virus that causes acute gastroenteritis mainly in domestic dogs [1–5]. CPV infection is responsible for large numbers of animal deaths worldwide and one of the most dangerous infectious diseases in young puppies aged 2–6 months. The infected dogs develops acute gastroenteritis, which is characterized by vomiting, fever, diarrhoea (from mucoid to haemorrhagic), haemorrhagic enteritis, myocarditis and leucopoenia [6, 7].

CPV contains a single-stranded DNA genome of approximately 5 kb, which encodes the capsid proteins 1, 2 and 3 (VP1, VP2 and VP3, respectively). VP1 and VP2 are splice variants and mostly identical in sequence, exclusive of a 143-amino-acid (aa) N-terminal region unique to VP1, Whereas VP3 is derived from the cleavage of VP2 at the 5'-terminal region by host proteases [8]. The full-length VP2 sequence (1755 bp) encodes the major capsid protein, which is 584 aa in length and plays an important role in determining viral host ranges, tissue tropisms, and genetic and antigenic properties [9, 10]. VP2 protein had been investigated as a candidate potential vaccine antigen due to its good immunogenicity [11]. CPV-2, first identified and described in 1978 in both the United States and Australia, is closely related to feline panleukopenia virus (FPV) [12]. A few years after its emergence, the original virus type CPV-2 was replaced worldwide by three new antigenic variants (i.e., CPV-2a, CPV-2b and CPV-2c) based on aa substitutions (CPV-2a: Val-555-Ile, Asp-305-Tyr, Ala-300-Gly, Ile-101-Thr and Met-87-Leu; CPV-2b: Ile-555-Val and Asp-426-Asn; CPV-2c: Asp-426-Glu) in the VP2 gene [12–18].

* Correspondence: xueyun6688@163.com
†Equal contributors
[2]Lab of Medical Engineering, College of Medical Technology and Engineering, Henan University of Science and Technology, Luoyang, China
Full list of author information is available at the end of the article

In China, CPV infections were first described in 1982 [9]. A few years later, widespread outbreaks of canine haemorrhagic enteritis occurred throughout the country and CPV infection emerged as an important zoonosis of dogs because of the high morbidity and lethality associated with the virus [9]. Recently, different CPV genotypes were observed in Heilongjiang, Jilin, Liaoning, Shandong, Hebei, Sichuan, Shenzhen, Gansu, Beijing, and Nanjing, as well as other areas in China [19–22]. However, no previous reports included information about the prevalent genotype of CPV in Henan province.

Vaccination is considered the most effective method to control CPV infection. However, antigenic differences may decrease the effectiveness of the vaccine based on the original antigenic type [23]. Therefore, it is important to elucidate the epidemiology and molecular characterization of CPV strains currently circulating in Henan province. Hence, in this study, we investigated the epidemiology of CPV infection among domestic dogs in Henan province and the molecular characterization of CPV by polymerase chain reaction (PCR) followed by direct sequencing of isolates collected from 2009 to 2014. The findings of this study constructed a basis for the further understanding of the evolution of CPV, will help to improve measures to prevent and control the spread of CPV and to developt effective vaccines against CPV infection.

Methods

Ethics statement

All animal procedures carried out in this study were approved by the Animal Care and Use Committee of Henan University of Science and Technology. Permission to collect samples was acquired from the owner of each animal. Samples were collected by a single skilled veterinarian. No specific permissions were required for collection of field samples because they were collected from public or non-protected areas.

Samples collection

Nineteen thousand nine hundred seven dogs from pet hospitals in the cities of Luoyang, Anyang, Jiaozuo, Sanmenxia, Xinxiang, and Zhengzhou in Henan province from March 2009 to December 2014 were investigated. Among the 19,907 dogs, infections of dogs with active vomiting, fever, diarrhoea and haemorrhagic enteritis were detected using a CPV colloidal gold test strip (Bionote, Inc., Hwaseong, Gyeonggi Province, south Korea), according to the manufacturer's protocol. Suspected CPV-positive dogs were confirmed by positive results of the CPV colloidal gold test strip. Then, faecal samples from suspected CPV-positive dogs were transferred to our laboratory for detection of canine distemper virus (CDV) and canine coronavirus (CCoV) using a CDV or CCoV colloidal gold test strip (Bionote, Inc.), respectively, and for detection of coccidium, ancylostome, roundworm, tapeworm, babesiosis and nematode by microscopy [24] according to the characteristic of these parasites. Additionally, the supernatant of faecal samples emulsified in 0.1 M phosphate-buffered saline (pH 7.2) and centrifuged (10,000 g for 10 min at 4–8 °C) [8] was collected for detection of the partial VP2 gene and complete VP2 gene by PCR.

Detection of CPV genome

Viral DNA was prepared by boiling the supernatant for 10 min and chilling immediately on ice as previously described [25]. Specific primers (Table 1) for detection of the CPV genome were designed using Primer Premier 5.0 software (Premier Biosoft International, Palto Alto, CA, 85 USA) based on the conserved sequence of a previously published CPV genome sequence (GenBank accession no.: NC001539.1). The PCR reaction volume was 25 μl, which included 12.5 μl of PCR Master Mix (Sangon Biotech Company, Shanghai, China), 1 μl of each primer, 1 μl of supernatant, and 9.5 μl of ultrapure water. The PCR reaction included an initial denaturation step at 95 °C for 10 min followed by 30 cycles of 98 °C for 30 s, 55 °C for 30 s, and 72 °C for 40 s, and 72 °C for 10 min. A commercial vaccine was used as a positive control and sterile water was used as a negative control. The PCR-positive products were sent to Sangon Biotech Company for bidirectional single pass sequence analysis. The specificity of the sequences was then compared with those in the GenBank database (http://www.ncbi.nlm.nih.gov/genbank/) using the Basic Local Alignment Search Tool (www.ncbi.nlm.nih.gov/BLAST). Then, all PCR-positive sequences were aligned and three phylogenetic trees based on partial VP2 sequences were constructed by the Clustal W method using the MegAlign program (DNASTAR, Inc., Madison, WI, USA) [20].

Detection of the complete VP2 gene

Viral DNA from diverse branches was prepared as described in this study. The primers (Table 1) for detection of the complete VP2 gene were designed using Primer Premier 5.0 software based on the consensus sequence of previously published CPV genomes (GenBank accession no.: JQ268284.1). The PCR reaction volume was 25 μl, which included 12.5 μl of PCR Master Mix (Sangon Biotech Company), 1 μl of each primer, 1 μl of supernatant,

Table 1 Primers for detection of the CPV genome and complete VP2 gene

Name	Sequence (5′ → 3′)	Position (VP2)	Product (bp)
CPVF	GAATCTGCTACTCAGCCACCAAC	463–485	560
CPVR	GTGCACTATAACCAACCTCAGC	1000–1021	
VP2F	AGAGACAATCTTGCACCAAT	2768–2787	1775
VP2R	ATGTTAATATAATTTTCTAGGTGCT	4519–4543	

and 9.5 μl of ultrapure water. The PCR reaction included an initial denaturation step at 95 °C for 10 min followed by 30 cycles of 98 °C for 30 s, 48 °C for 50 s, and 72 °C for 120 s, and a final extension of 72 °C for 10 min. Sterile water was used as a negative control. The PCR positive products were sent to Sangon Biotech Company for bidirectional single pass sequence analysis. The specificity of the sequences was then compared with those in the GenBank database using BLAST algorithm.

Sequence and phylogenetic analyses

The complete VP2 nucleotide sequences and aa sequences of our samples were aligned with reference CPV sequences from different animals and areas using MegAlign sequence alignment software (DNASTAR 6.0) [26]. The phylogenetic analyses based on complete VP2 nucleotide sequences from the CPV isolates in this study and 25 reference CPV strains were conducted by the neighbour-joining method and a Kimura 2-parameter model using Molecular Evolutionary Genetics Analysis (MEGA 5.0) software [27]. The confidence level of branching in the phylogenetic tree was evaluated by the bootstrap test based on 1000 resamplings. A bootstrap value of ≥ 70 % was considered significant for phylogenetic groupings [20]. To determine the genotype of the CPV isolates in this study, the complete VP2 aa sequences were aligned with reference CPV sequences (NCBI GenBank accession no.: M38245.1, M24003.1, M74849.1, KT156832.1, KT156834.1 and KT156833.1) using the DNAMAN software package (Lynnon Biosoft, San Ramon, CA, USA) [18]. The complete VP2 DNA sequences were also submitted to the GenBank database for assignment of accession numbers.

Questionnaire survey

A questionnaire survey was created to further elucidate the epidemiology of CPV infection among domestic dogs between 2009 and 2014, as previously described with some modifications [28]. The questionnaire inquired about the followed topics: 'CPV-positive' (yes/no), 'year' (2009–2014), 'month' (spring, 3–5, summer, 6–8, autumn, 9–11, winter, 12–2), 'age' (1, 2, 3, 4, 5, 6, 6–9, 9–12, 12–36, >36 months), 'sex' (male or female), 'purebred' (yes/no), 'vaccination' (unvaccinated, intermittent vaccination: inoculation as part of an unofficial immune program, complete vaccination: inoculation as part of an official immune program), 'co-infection' (pathogen).

Statistical analysis

Statistical analysis to assess significant differences of morbidity was performed using SPSS version 17.0 software. A p-value <0.05 was considered statistically significant.

Results

Morbidity of CPV infection in dogs from Henan province

One thousand one hundred seventy eight CPV-positive cases were identified by the CPV colloidal gold test strip. PCR analysis confirmed that 1169 (99.24 %) of these cases were CPV-positive. Of the 1169 partial VP2 sequences, 33 were submitted to the NCBI Genbank database under the accession numbers KF772192–KF772224. The morbidity of CPV infection between 2009 and 2014 was 5.87 % (1169/19907). The annual morbidity rate ranged from 4.16 to 8.06 % with the highest morbidity recorded in 2009 and the lowest in 2012 (Fig. 1), but morbidity was not significant ($P > 0.05$) between March 2009 and December 2014. In addition, we observed a significant influence of age on morbidity ($P < 0.05$, Fig. 2). Morbidity was relatively high among puppies during the first 4 month of life with the highest rate occurring in the third month. Afterward, the morbidity rate gradually decreased. Seasonal morbidity ranged from 4.89 to 7.32 % with the highest during the Spring (Fig. 3). However, as a whole, differences in morbidity according to

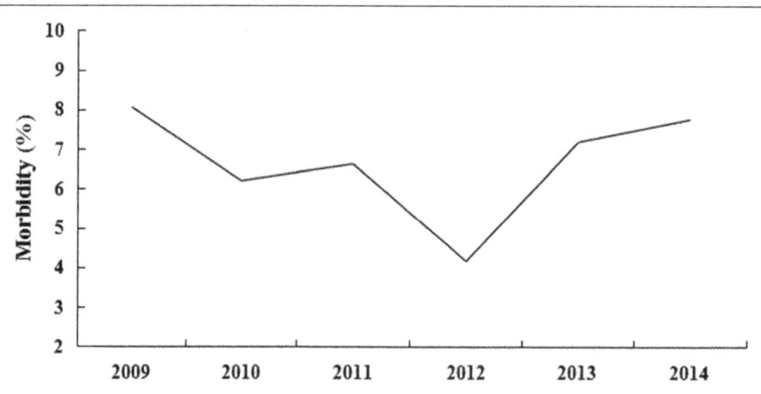

Fig. 1 Annual distribution of morbidity of CPV infection. The morbidity rates were 51/633, 142/2291, 215/3242, 322/7746, 333/4629 and 106/1366 for 2009–2014, respectively. There was no significant difference in morbidity rates between 2009 and 2014 ($P > 0.05$, χ^2 test)

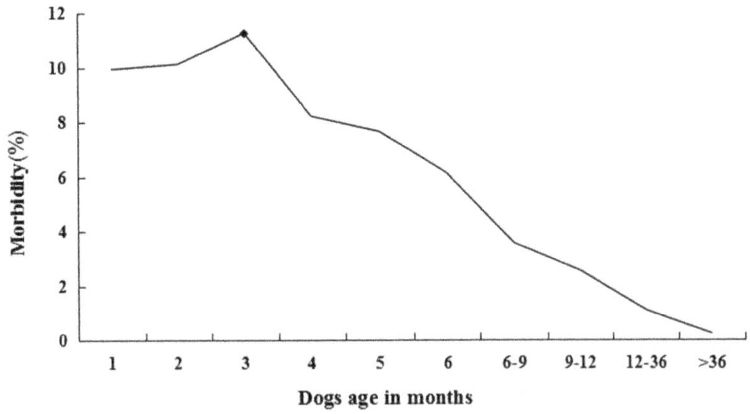

Fig. 2 Distribution of morbidity of CPV infection in relation to dog age. The incidence of morbidity at different ages was 83/836, 319/3154, 291/2584, 145/1765, 116/1516, 75/1224, 68/1916, 41/1610, 24/2210 and 7/3092, respectively. The morbidity was relatively high in the first 4 months with the highest recorded in month 3 (♦). After month 3, morbidity gradually decreased. However, as a whole, *P*-value was <0.05 for morbidity in relation to dog age. Statistical analysis was performed using the χ^2 test

season was not significant ($P > 0.05$). There was no significant difference in morbidity rates between male and female dogs (643/10937, 5.88 vs. 526/8970, 5.86 %, respectively, $P > 0.05$). The CPV-positive rate was significantly greater among purebred dogs compared to other dogs (1031/1169, 88.20 vs. 138/1169, 11.80 %, respectively, $P < 0.05$), and was highest among unvaccinated dogs (680/1169, 58.17 %), although not significantly ($P = 0.069$) as compared to intermittently vaccinated dogs (463/1169, 39.61 %), but significantly ($P < 0.05$) as compared to completely vaccinated dogs (26/1169, 2.22 %).

Co-infection

Over the 6-years period of this study, 230 (19.67 %) of 1169 CPV-positive cases were co-infected with other pathogens, such as CDV, CCoV, coccidium (*Isospora*), hookworm (*Ancylostoma*), roundworm (*Toxocara*), tapeworm (*Dipylidium*) and *Babesia spp.* at rates of 4.79 % (56/1169), 1.11 % (13/1169), 10.00 % (117/1169), 2.40 % (28/1169), 1.03 % (12/1169), 0.17 % (2/1169) and 0.09 % (1/1169), respectively. Additionally, of the 1169 CPV-positive cases, 10 were co-infected with coccidium and hookworm, five with CDV and coccidium, and four with CCoV and coccidium.

Sequence analysis

Phylogenetic trees based on 1169 partial VP2 sequences amplified using CPVF/CPVR primers were constructed, which contained seven branches. One sample was selected from each branch for amplification of the complete VP2 gene, which suggested similarity of VP2 sequences of 99 % compared to those retrieved from the GenBank database. The seven complete VP2 nucleotide sequences (NCBI GenBank accession no.: KJ438798–KJ438804) and aa sequences were analysed using DNASTAR software, which revealed 99.4–99.9 % homology of nucleotide sequences and 99.1–99.8 % homology of aa sequences among the seven isolates; 98.4–99.9 % homology of nucleotide sequences and 97.6–100.0 % homology of aa sequences with CPV isolates from other provinces in China; 98.8–99.8 % homology of nucleotide sequences and 98.1–100.0 % homology of aa sequences with CPV isolates from other countries; 98.0–98.3 % homology of nucleotide sequences and 96.8–98.0 % homology of aa sequences with the FPV isolates; <60 % homology of nucleotide and aa sequences with porcine parvovirus; and <25 % homology of nucleotide and aa sequences with goose parvovirus. Phylogenetic tree analysis based on the seven complete VP2 nucleotide sequences (Fig. 4) revealed that the seven isolates were clustered to two branches. KJ438798-Henan, KJ438799-Henan, KJ438800-Henan, KJ438802-Henan, KJ438803-Henan and KJ438804-Henan were most closely related to the isolate (JX120178) from Guangdong province, southeast China, followed by the isolate (JQ268284) from Gansu province, northwest China; KJ438801-Henan was most closely related to the isolate (JQ743897) from Heilongjiang province, northernmost China, followed by the isolate (DQ903936) from Sichuan province, southwest China.

Genotyping of CPV

Comparisons of the aa sequences among the seven isolates and the six reference strains revealed that Glu426, which is unique to strain CPV 2c, was not observed in any strain in this study. Mutations at aa 426 (N-426-D) and aa 297 (S-297-A) were found in one isolate (GenBank accession no.: KJ438800), which was typed as a new CPV-2b variant. The other isolates were typed as new CPV-2a variants due to the aa substitutions of N426 and A297 (Table 2).

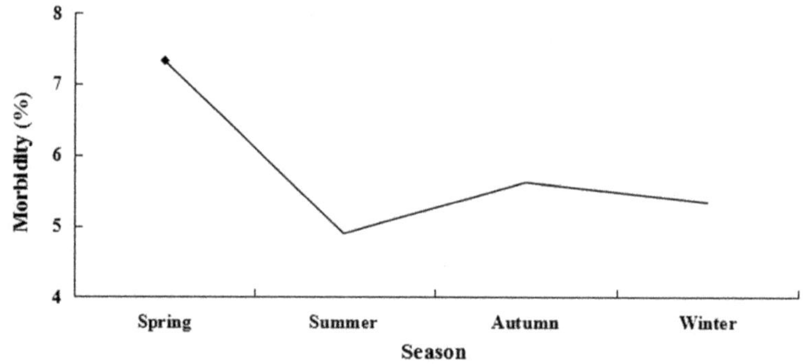

Fig. 3 Distribution of morbidity of CPV infection in relation to the season. The incidence of morbidity was 435/5946, 260/5322, 251/4465 and 223/4174 for spring, summer, autumn and winter, respectively. As a whole, the morbidity was not significant ($P > 0.05$). The highest morbidity (◆) was recorded in the spring. Statistical analysis was performed using the χ^2 test

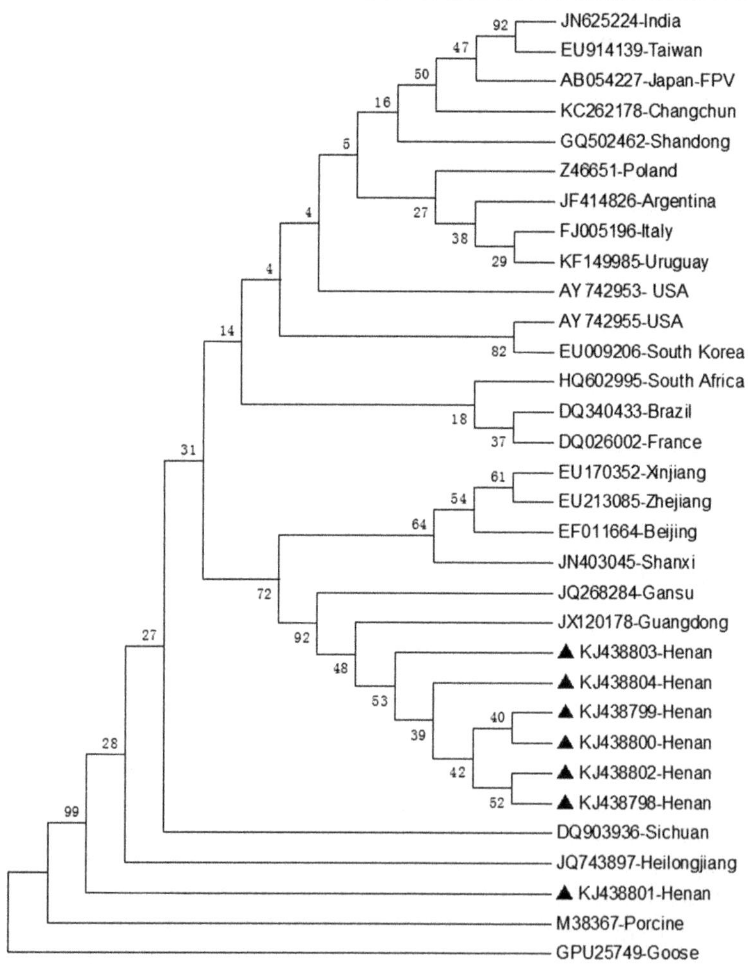

Fig. 4 A Phylogenetic tree based on VP2 gene sequences of seven CPV isolates and 25 reference CPV strains by neighbor-joining method. ▲ indicates the seven CPV isolates from Henan province, China

Table 2 Deduced amino acid variations in VP2 in the seven CPV isolates from Henan province, China

Accession no	Origin	Place of amino acid sites									Gene types
		267	297	322	324	334	341	348	426	440	
Reference											
M38245	U.S.	F	S	T	Y	A	P	S	N	T	cpv-2
M24003	U.S.	F	S	T	Y	A	P	S	N	T	cpv-2a
M74849	U.S.	F	S	T	Y	A	P	S	D	T	cpv-2b
KT156832.1	China	Y	A	T	I	A	P	S	E	T	cpv-2c
KT156834.1	China	Y	A	T	I	A	P	S	N	A	new cpv-2a
KT156833.1	China	Y	A	T	I	A	P	S	D	A	new cpv-2b
This study											
KJ438798	Henan	Y	A	-	I	G	S	-	N	A	new cpv-2a
KJ438799	Henan	Y	A	S	I	-	S	-	N	A	new cpv-2a
KJ438800	Henan	Y	A	-	I	-	-	-	D	A	new cpv-2b
KJ438801	Henan	F	A	S	I	G	-	C	N	T	new cpv-2a
KJ438802	Henan	Y	A	-	I	-	S	-	N	A	new cpv-2a
KJ438803	Henan	Y	A	-	I	-	S	-	N	A	new cpv-2a
KJ438804	Henan	Y	A	-	I	-	-	-	N	A	new cpv-2a

Identical amino acids are represented by -

Discussion

This study was the first attempt to evaluate the occurrence of CPV infection among domestic dogs between 2009 and 2014 in Henan province, China. A diagnosis of CPV infection based on clinical signs and the CPV colloidal gold test strip is rapid and often used in pet hospitals in China. Of 1178 faecal samples, 1169 (99.24 %) were CPV-positive by PCR assay, suggesting a good correlation between the antigen-detection test and molecular methods, with only nine samples being recognized as false positives. In this study, the morbidity of CPV infection was 5.87 % (1169/19907), which was lower than in recent reports from China [20, 29]. The sample size in this study was much larger than samples size described previously, thus these results should represent a more accurate estimate of morbidity of CPV infection. Additionally, the χ^2 test results showed that the morbidity of CPV infection fluctuated only slightly ($P > 0.05$) within the 6-years period of this study (2009–2014).

The results of this study showed that morbidity in the spring (months 3–5) and autumn (months 9–11) were relatively higher than observed during the other seasons, but the morbidity in Heilongjiang province differed from that reported for other provinces [29], suggesting variations in morbidity according to the season in different regions of China. In addition, our work demonstrated a clear association of CPV infection with dog age ($p < 0.05$), which in accordance with the results reported by Geng et al. [29] and Cavalli et al. [30]. Although the causes of this tendency have not yet been fully elucidated, we hypothesise that the low morbidity in dogs aged < 30 days most likely resulted from acquired maternal antibody, while the high morbidity in dogs aged 30–120 days most likely resulted from decreasing maternal antibody concentrations and stress due to weaning, and the low morbidity in dogs aged >120 days was most likely attributable to the development of adaptive immune responses [31, 32]. The finding of more male dogs in this study was consistent with those in other parts of the world, suggesting that there also is a preference of male over female dogs in Henan province [28]. Besides, to the best of our knowledge, this study is the first to report that morbidity (5.88 %) in domestic male dogs was similar to that (5.86 %) in domestic female dogs. CPV infection occurs in both unvaccinated and vaccinated dogs, in accordance with the finding of recent reports in China [29, 33]. In this study, the CPV-positive rate was highest among unvaccinated dogs, followed by intermittently vaccinated dogs and completely vaccinated dogs, suggesting that vaccines used in Henan province may play an important role in prevention and control CPV infection. These results were different from those of previous reports from other areas of China. Our work also indicated that the CPV-positive rate was higher among purebred dogs as compared to mutts. This result suggested that mutts may have greater resistance to CPV, which should be investigated in future studies.

In this study, CPV infection was identified alongside other pathogens in 230 (19.67 %) of 1169 CPV-positive samples. The pathogens that accompanied CPV were coccidium, CDV, CCoV, hookworm, roundworm, tapeworm and *Babesia spp.*, suggesting that these pathogens should be considered in vaccination programs to control

CPV outbreaks [34]. The co-infection of CPV with CDV or CCoV in this study was in agreement with previous study in China [29] and other countries [30, 35, 36]. Additionally, studies in China [37] and France [38] suggested that dogs harbouring roundworm or trichomonads were especially susceptible to CPV infection. Also, this study is the first to report the co-infection of CPV with coccidium, hookworm, tapeworm or *Babesia spp.*, and co-infection of two pathogens with CPV was also found in one sample.

Point mutations in the VP2 protein have been associated with the CPV types because the fragment encodes for at least one informative aa (residue 426) of the VP2 protein, which in used to differentiate CPV2a (Asn), CPV2b (Asp) and CPV2c (Glu) [9]. The Ser297Ala mutation was used as a marker of the new CPV-2a/2b variant [29]. CPV-2c was first identified in Jilin province, and subsequently identified in Shandong province, Heilongjiang province and Beijing [19, 29, 33]. CPV-2c was not detected in this study, while the new CPV-2a variant is more prevalent than new CPV-2b variant in Henan province. In this study, the prevalence of new CPV-2a and new CPV-2b is in agreement with most of the reports in other provinces of China [6, 8, 9, 20, 29, 33, 39, 40] and other countries [26, 41–45]. The presence of the new CPV-2a and CPV-2b variants in this study suggests that CPV-2 strains circulating in Henan province also exhibit genetic variations.

VP2 encodes a viral capsid protein that is the major structural protein of CPV-2 and is involved in the host immune response. Therefore, a small number of mutations may result in increased pathogenicity [26]. In this study, the aa sequences from the seven VP2 gene products revealed little variability at residues 322, 334 and 348, which was basically consistent with reference CPV sequences. The aa sequences from seven VP2 gene products revealed great variability at residues 267, 324, 341 and 440. Residue 267, located between loops 1 and 2 of the VP2 protein, is the main component of the antigen. However, a mutation to residue 267 may not influence the antigenicity of CPV because it is not exposed on the capsid surface, as was reported for strain CPV-2a from China and Thailand and strain CPV-2b from Vietnam [45]. Residue 324 is subject to positive selection and may influence the aa sequences at residue 323, which is known to be involved in host range via binding with the canine transferrin receptor. A mutation at residue 323 may influence interactions between residues in neighbouring loops of either the same VP2 molecule or the threefold-related VP2, thereby greatly decreasing replication in canine cells [26]. The Y-324-I mutation in CPV-2a strains has been reported in China [8, 20, 39] and other countries [43, 45]. Interestingly, variations of residue 440 (within the GH loop) occurred. Reportedly, the high substitution rate in this region is associated with the evolution of antigenic variants in circulating parvovirus types [46], such as strains CPV-2a and CPV-2b from other provinces in China [9, 29]. However, the significance of a mutation at residue 341 is unclear and warrants further investigations.

Previous reports suggested that the new CPV-2a variant was the most prevalent in China, followed by CPV-2b and CPV-2c, in accordance with the results of the present study. However, it is necessary to collect more samples form Henan province for further genotyping to improve our understanding of the evolution of CPV in China.

Conclusions

Our results disclosed novel epidemiological information of CPV infection in Henan province. VP2 sequences data revealed that the new CPV-2a variant is more prevalent than the new CPV-2b variant in Henan province. CPV-2c was not observed in this study. The findings of this study are expected to facilitate a better understanding of the current status of CPV-2 infection among dogs in China.

Abbreviations

CCoV, canine coronavirus; CDV, canine distemper virus; CPV, canine parvovirus; FPV, feline panleukopenia virus; PCR, polymerase chain reaction

Acknowledgments

We thank Jie Yang for statistical analyses and all the dog owners who participated in this study.

Funding

This study was supported by Grants from National Natural Science Foundation of China (No. 31302106) and the Research and Development Foundation of Henan University of Science and Technology (No. 2015ZDCXY04).

Authors' contributions

HSL analyzed the data and wrote the manuscript. ZQZ devised study, participated in its design. QX initiated the study and carried out collection of fecal samples. KD, YX and ZHY identified the species of parasites and amplified the PCR. CCP collected the epidemiology data. All authors read and approved the final manuscript.

Competing interests

The authors declare that they have no competing interests.

Consent for publication

Not applicable.

Author details

[1]Lab of Veterinary Microbiology, College of Animal Science and Technology, Henan University of Science and Technology, Luoyang, China. [2]Lab of Medical Engineering, College of Medical Technology and Engineering, Henan University of Science and Technology, Luoyang, China.

References

1. Gjeltema J, Murphy H, Rivera S. Clinical canine parvovirus type 2C infection in a group of Asian small-clawed otters (Aonyx cinerea). J Zoo Wildl Med. 2015;46(1):120–3.
2. Miranda C, Parrish CR, Thompson G. Canine parvovirus 2c infection in a cat with severe clinical disease. J Vet Diagn Invest. 2014;26(3):462–4.

3. Guo L, Yang SL, Chen SJ, Zhang Z, Wang C, Hou R, Ren Y, Wen X, Cao S, Guo W, Hao Z, Quan Z, Zhang M, Yan QG. Identification of canine parvovirus with the Q370R point mutation in the VP2 gene from a giant panda (Ailuropoda melanoleuca). Virol J. 2013;26(10):163.
4. Sobrino R, Arnal MC, Luco DF, Gortázar C. Prevalence of antibodies against canine distemper virus and canine parvovirus among foxes and wolves from Spain. Vet Microbiol. 2008;126(1–3):251–6.
5. Allander T, Tammi MT, Eriksson M, Bjerkner A, Tiveljung-Lindell A. Cloning of a human parvovirus by molecular screening of respiratorytract samples. Proc Natl Acad Sci. 2005;102:12891–6.
6. Zhong Z, Liang L, Zhao J, Xu X, Cao X, Liu X, Zhou Z, Ren Z, Shen L, Geng Y, Gu X, Peng G. First isolation of new canine parvovirus 2a from Tibetan mastiff and global analysis of the full-length VP2 gene of canine parvoviruses 2 in China. Int J Mol Sci. 2014;15(7):12166–87.
7. Pérez R, Calleros L, Marandino A, Sarute N, Iraola G, Grecco S, Blanc H, Vignuzzi M, Isakov O, Shomron N, Carrau L, Hernández M, Francia L, Sosa K, Tomás G, Panzera Y. Phylogenetic and genome-wide deep-sequencing analyses of canine parvovirus reveal co-infection with field variants and emergence of a recent recombinant strain. PLoS One. 2014;9(11), e111779.
8. Han SC, Guo HC, Sun SQ, Shu L, Wei YQ, Sun DH, Cao SZ, Peng GN, Liu XT. Full-length genomic characterizations of two canine parvoviruses prevalent in Northwest China. Arch Microbiol. 2015;197(4):621–6.
9. Zhao Y, Lin Y, Zeng X, Lu C, Hou J. Genotyping and pathobiologic characterization of canine parvovirus circulating in Nanjing, China. Virol J. 2013;29(10):272.
10. Ju C, Cheng Y, Ji Y, Wang Y, Sun L, Huang J. Genome sequence of canine parvovirus strain SC02/2011, isolated from a puppy with severe diarrhea in South China. J Virol. 2012;86(24):13805.
11. Feng H, Hu GQ, Wang HL, Liang M, Liang H, Guo H, Zhao P, Yang YJ, Zheng XX, Zhang ZF, Zhao YK, Gao YW, Yang ST, Xia XZ. Canine Parvovirus VP2 Protein Expressed in Silkworm Pupae Self-Assembles into Virus-Like Particles with High Immunogenicity. PLoS One. 2014;9(1), e79575.
12. Zhou P, Fu X, Yan Z, Fang B, Huang S, Fu C, Hong M, Li S. Antiviral effect of lithium chloride on infection of cells by canine parvovirus. Arch Virol. 2015; 160(11):2799–805. doi:10.1007/s00705-015-2577-x.
13. Parrish CR, O'Connell PH, Evermann JF, Carmichael LE. Natural variation of canine arvovirus. Science. 1985;230(4729):1046–8.
14. Parrish CR, Have P, Foreyt WJ, Evermann JF, Senda M, Carmichael LE. The global spread and replacement of canine parvovirus strains. J Gen Virol. 1988;69(Pt 5):1111–6.
15. Decaro N, Desario C, Addie DD, Martella V, Vieira MJ, Elia G, Zicola A, Davis C, Thompson G, Thiry E, Truyen U, Buonavoglia C. The study molecular epidemiology of canine parvovirus, Europe. Emerg Infect Dis. 2007;13(8):1222–4.
16. Decaro N, Desario C, Billi M, Mari V, Elia G, Cavalli A, Martella V, Buonavoglia C. Western European epidemiological survey for parvovirus and coronavirus infections in dogs. Vet J. 2011;187(2):195–9.
17. Calderon MG, Mattion N, Bucafusco D, Fogel F, Remorini P, La-Torre J. Molecular characterization of canine parvovirus strains in Argentina: detection of the pathogenic variant CPV2c in vaccinated dogs. J Virol Methods. 2009;159(2):141–5.
18. Perez R, Francia L, Romero V, Maya L, Lopez I, Hernandez M. First detection of canine parvovirus type 2c in South America. Vet Microbiol. 2007;124(1–2):147–52.
19. Zhao H, Wang J, Jiang Y, Cheng Y, Lin P, Zhu H, Han G, Yi L, Zhang S, Guo L, Cheng S. Typing of canine parvovirus strains circulating in north-east china. Transbound Emerg Dis. 2015. doi:10.1111/tbed.12390.
20. Xu J, Guo HC, Wei YQ, Shu L, Wang J, Li JS, Cao SZ, Sun SQ. Phylogenetic analysis of canine parvovirus isolates from Sichuan and Gansu provinces of China in 2011. Transbound Emerg Dis. 2015;62(1):91–105.
21. Wu J, Gao XT, Hou SH, Guo XY, Yang XS, Yuan WF, Xin T, Zhu HF, Jia H. Molecular epidemiological and phylogenetic analysis of canine parvovirus in domestic dogs and cats in Beijing, 2010–2013. J Vet Med Sci. 2015;77(10): 1305–10. doi:10.1292/jvms.14-0665.
22. Zhu Y, Huang Y, Wang Y, Chen K, Niu X, Luo Y, Guo X. Genome sequence of a canine parvovirus strain, cpv-s5, prevalent in Southern China. Genome Announc. 2014;2(1):e01141–13.
23. Decaro N, Desario C, Elia G, Martella V, Mari V, Lavazza A, Nardi M, Buonavoglia C. Evidence for immunisation failure in vaccinated adult dogs infected with canine parvovirus type 2c. New Microbiol. 2008;31(1):125–30.
24. Miller DL, Schrecengost J, Merrill A, Kilgo J, Ray HS, Miller KV, Baldwin CA. Hematology, parasitology, and serology of free-ranging coyotes (Canis latrans) from South Carolina. J Wildl Dis. 2009;45(3):863–9.
25. Decaro N, Elia G, Desario C, Roperto S, Martella V, Campolo M, Lorusso A, Cavalli A, Buonavoglia C. A minor groove binder probe real-time PCR assay for discrimination between type 2-based vaccines and field strains of canine parvovirus. J Virol Methods. 2006;136:65–70.
26. Lin CN, Chien CH, Chiou MT, Chueh LL, Hung MY, Hsu HS. Genetic characterization of type 2a canine parvoviruses from Taiwan reveals the emergence of an Ile324 mutation in VP2. Virol J. 2014;11:39.
27. Saitou N, Nei M. The neighbor-joining method: A new method for reconstructing phylogenetic trees. Molec Biol Evol. 1987;4(4):406–25.
28. Kitala P, McDermott J, Kyule M, Gathuma J, Perry B, Wandeler A. Dog ecology and demography information to support the planning of rabies control in Machakos District, Kenya. Acta Trop. 2001;78:217–30.
29. Geng Y, Guo D, Li C, Wang E, Wei S, Wang Z, Yao S, Zhao X, Su M, Wang X, Wang J, Wu R, Feng L, Sun D. Co-Circulation of the Rare CPV-2c with Unique Gln370Arg Substitution, New CPV-2b with Unique Thr440Ala Substitution, and New CPV-2a with High Prevalence and Variation in Heilongjiang Province, Northeast China. PLoS One. 2015;10(9), e0137288.
30. Cavalli A, Desario C, Kusi I, Mari V, Lorusso E, Cirone F, Kumbe I, Colaianni ML, Buonavoglia D, Decaro N. Detection and genetic characterization of Canine parvovirus and Canine coronavirus strains circulating in district of Tirana in Albania. J Vet Diagn Invest. 2014;26(4):563–6.
31. Pollock RV, Carmichael LE. Maternally derived immunity to canine parvovirus infection: transfer, decline, and interference with vaccination. J Am Vet Med Assoc. 1982;180(1):37–42.
32. Waner T, Naveh A, Wudovsky I, Carmichael LE. Assessment of maternal antibody decay and response to canine parvovirus vaccination using a clinic-based enzyme-linked immunosorbent assay. J Vet Diagn Invest. 1996;8(4):427–32.
33. Wang J, Lin P, Zhao H, Cheng Y, Jiang Z, Zhu H, Wu H, Cheng S. Continuing evolution of canine parvovirus in China: Isolation of novel variants with an Ala5Gly mutation in the VP2 protein. Infect Genet Evol. 2015. doi:10.1016/j. meegid.2015.12.009.
34. Park SA, Park SY, Song CS, Choi IS, Kim HY, Lee JB, Lee NH. Development of a novel vaccine against canine parvovirus infection with a clinical isolate of the type 2b strain. Clin Exp Vaccine Res. 2012;1(1):70–6.
35. Acosta-Jamett G, Surot D, Cortés M, Marambio V, Valenzuela C, Vallverdu A, Ward MP. Epidemiology of canine distemper and canine parvovirus in domestic dogs in urban and rural areas of the Araucanía region in Chile. Vet Microbiol. 2015;178(3–4):260–4.
36. Filipov C, Decaro N, Desario C, Amorisco F, Sciarretta R, Buonavoglia C. Canine parvovirus epidemiology in Bulgaria. J Vet Diagn Invest. 2011;23(1):152–4.
37. Luo HQ, Song XZ, Wang QY, Duan LC. Epidemiological investigation of canine parvovirus disease in small animal hospital in Wenzhou area. Acta Agriculturae Zhejiangensis. 2014;26(4):887–91.
38. Grellet A, Brunopolack, Feugier A, Boucraut-Baralon C, Grandjean D, Vandewynckel L, Cian A, Meloni D, Viscogliosi E. Prevalence, risk factors of infection and molecular characterization of trichomonads in puppies from French breeding kennels. Vet Parasitol. 2013;197(3–4):418–26.
39. Yi L, Tong M, Cheng Y, Song W, Cheng S. Phylogenetic analysis of canine parvovirus VP2 Gene in China. Transbound Emerg Dis. 2014. doi:10.1111/ tbed.12268.
40. Wang H, Jin H, Li Q, Zhao G, Cheng N, Feng N, Zheng X, Wang J, Zhao Y, Li L, Cao Z, Yan F, Wang L, Wang T, Gao Y, Yang S, Xia X. Isolation and sequence analysis of the complete NS1 and VP2 genes of canine parvovirus from domestic dogs in 2013 and 2014 in China. Arch Virol. 2015. doi:10.1007/s00705-015-2620-y.
41. Dogonyaro BB, Bosman AM, Sibeko KP, Venter EH, van Vuuren M. Genetic analysis of the VP2-encoding gene of canine parvovirus strains from Africa. Vet Microbiol. 2013;165(3–4):460–5.
42. Meers J, Kyaw-Tanner M, Bensink Z, Zwijnenberg R. Genetic analysis of canine parvovirus from dogs in Australia. Aust Vet J. 2007;85(10):392–6.
43. Jeoung SY, Ahn SJ, Kim D. Genetic analysis of VP2 gene of canine parvovirus isolates in Korea. Vet Med Sci. 2008;70(7):719–22.
44. Timurkan M, Oğuzoğlu T. Molecular characterization of canine parvovirus (CPV) infection in dogs in Turkey. Vet Ital. 2015;51(1):39–44.
45. Mukhopadhyay HK, Matta SL, Amsaveni S, Antony PX, Thanislass J, Pillai RM. Phylogenetic analysis of canine parvovirus partial VP2 gene in India. Virus Genes. 2014;48(1):89–95.
46. Battilani M, Ciulli S, Tisato E, Prosperi S. Genetic analysis of canine parvovirus isolates (CPV-2) from dogs in Italy. Virus Res. 2002;83(1–2):149–57.

4

Pseudorabies virus infection (Aujeszky's disease) in an Iberian lynx (*Lynx pardinus*) in Spain

A. Javier Masot[1*], María Gil[2], David Risco[3], Olga M. Jiménez[4], José I. Núñez[5] and Eloy Redondo[1]

Abstract

Background: The only natural hosts of Pseudorabies virus (PRV) are members of the family Suidae (*Sus scrofa scrofa*). In species other than suids infection is normally fatal. In these mammals, including carnivores, PRV typically causes serious neurologic disease. The endangered Iberian lynx (*Lynx pardinus*) is a wild feline endemic to south-western Europe (Iberian Peninsula). The Iberian lynx was found to be the world's most endangered felid species in 2002. In wild felines, PRV infection has only been previously reported once in a Florida panther in 1994. No seropositive lynxes have ever been found, nor has PRV been detected in dead Iberian lynxes to date.

Case presentation: We describe the first reported case of pseudorabies in an Iberian lynx (*Lynx pardinus*). Pseudorabies was diagnosed in a young wild Iberian lynx from Extremadura (SW Spain) by histopathological examination, immunohistochemistry, polymerase chain reaction (PCR) and sequence analysis. Gross lesions included alopecia of the ventral neck, bloody gastro-intestinal contents and congestion of the brain. Histopathological analysis showed a moderate nonsuppurative meningoencephalitis with diffuse areas of demyelination, necrotizing gastritis and enteritis of the small intestine. Pseudorabies virus (PRV) antigen was found in neuronal and non-neuronal cells of the brain, tonsils, and gastric glandular epithelial cells by immunohistochemical analysis. The presence of the virus in the brain was confirmed by nested PCR. The sequence analysis of the 146 bp fragment (from the viral glycoprotein B gene) showed that the amplified sequence matched (with 100% identity) the PRV genome. Furthermore, specific DNA from glycoprotein D and E encoding-genes was detected by conventional and real-time PCR, respectively, confirming the latter that this infection was produced by a wild-type PRV strain.

Conclusions: This study supports the suspicion that PRV could infect the Iberian lynx. The detection of PRV in a dead Iberian lynx suggests that the virus may have a negative impact on the survival of endangered lynxes in the wild. However, because this is the first verified instance of lynx mortality resulting from pseudorabies, its true impact on the population is unknown.

Keywords: Iberian lynx, *Lynx pardinus*, Pseudorabies virus, Aujeszky's disease, Suid Herpesvirus 1, Endangered species, Case report

Background

The Iberian lynx (*Lynx pardinus*) is an endangered wild feline endemic to the Iberian Peninsula, located in the southwest corner of Europe. The Iberian lynx population suffered a dramatic reduction in size during the 20th century [1]. From 2002 to 2015 it was considered the world's most endangered wild feline species. Recently, the Iberian lynx has been reclassified from a critically endangered to an endangered species [2]. The population was 406 at the 2015 census [3]. Iberian lynxes predominantly prey on wild rabbits (*Oryctolagus cuniculus*), although they alternatively may prey on small mammals, juvenile ungulates, partridges, other birds, reptiles and insects [4]. Moreover, Iberian lynxes occasionally consume wild boar as prey and as carrion, which puts them at risk for pseudorabies infection [5]. The species is highly solitary and territorial, although family groups

* Correspondence: jahis@unex.es
[1]Unidad de Histología y Anatomía Patológica, Departamento de Medicina Animal, Facultad de Veterinaria, Universidad de Extremadura, Avda. Universidad s.n., Cáceres 10003, Spain
Full list of author information is available at the end of the article

have occasionally been detected [6]. The Iberian lynx is found in areas of Mediterranean scrub and in habitats of open forests and thickets with high rabbit abundance [7]. The small population and low genetic diversity of the Iberian lynx make this species especially vulnerable to bacterial and viral infections. A number of infectious agents have been detected in Iberian lynxes, including a variety of feline viral and bacterial pathogens [8, 9].

The causative agent of Aujeszky's disease (AD) is Suid Herpesvirus 1 (SuHV1), which is also known as pseudorabies virus (PRV). This virus is a member of the genus *Varicellovirus* belonging to the subfamily *Alphaherpesvirinae* of the family *Herpesviridae* [10] that can infect a wide range of species, though it is does not affect the higher primates [5]. Pseudorabies is a viral disease which was first reported in dogs in 1902 [11], and is prevalent throughout the world. The only natural hosts of PRV are domestic and wild suids (*Sus scrofa scrofa*) and their hybrids [12]. Symptoms of AD depend on the age of the animal, and can include respiratory, reproductive and nervous signs [13]. PRV is a neurotropic virus which replicates in the nasopharyngeal mucosa, before taking a number of nervous pathways to reach the central nervous system (CNS). It results in a non-suppurative meningoencephalitis which is frequently fatal in piglets [14–17]. PRV seroprevalence in European wild boar varies considerably between different geographic regions. The highest seroprevalences were described in Mediterranean countries including Spain (up to 100%) [5, 12, 18–24]. In both domestic pigs and wild boar, the disease is usually subclinical because of the virus-host adaptation; however, in piglets, the infection is commonly fatal [15–17]. Like other herpesviruses, PRV usually produces latent infections in the host. PRV can infect the neurons and glial cells of apparently healthy swine over long periods. These latent infections can be reactivated, which means PRV can spread to other susceptible animals, mainly mammals, such as carnivores [14, 25], although humans seem insusceptible [26]. Species other than suids can be considered dead-end hosts because the disease is generally fatal before the virus is excreted [5]. In these mammals, including carnivores, PRV infections usually result in very severe neurological symptoms which often involve localised pruritus [26], resulting in death within hours after appearance of the first symptoms [27]. There are considerable implications for conservation, as cases have been reported in endangered carnivores such as the Florida panther [28], the wolf [25] and captive brown bears [29] after consumption of PRV-contaminated meat. No seropositive lynxes have ever been found, nor has PRV been detected in dead Iberian lynxes to date.

This article is the first reported case of pseudorabies in an Iberian lynx. We describe the second reported case of pseudorabies in a wild feline considering that PRV infection has only been previously reported once in a Florida panther in 1994 [28].

PRV infection was suspected in this lynx based on histopathological findings, and because PRV infections in wild boar are endemic in SW Spain. Infection was confirmed with immunohistochemistry, PCR, and sequence analysis.

Case presentation

The lynx that we studied was a wild ~9-month-old male, born to a healthy 3-year-old dam. It belonged to the first two litters born in Extremadura (SW Spain) after *Lynx pardinus* was re-established in this region through the LIFE+ 10NAT/ES/ 000570 project. Using camera trapping, the estimated date of its birth was established to have been between March 8 and 12, 2015.

This lynx was captured, subjected to a routine sanitary evaluation protocol, radio-collared, vaccinated against Feline Leukemia Virus (PureVax FeLV, Merial, Barcelona; Spain) and relocated back into the wild on Nov. 18, 2015. A complete blood count and plasma protein tests showed normal levels. Plasma biochemistry results were within normal ranges, although plasma concentrations of glutamyl transpeptidase and creatine phosphokinase were slightly increased. PCR tests were negative for infection with Feline Leukemia Provirus (FeLV), Feline Immunodeficiency Virus (FIV) and Canine Distemper Virus (CDV) in the blood; Feline Calicivirus (FCV) and Feline Herpesvirus (FHV1) in oropharyngeal swabs; and Feline Coronavirus (FCoV) and Feline Parvovirus (FPV) in rectal swabs. The lynx was found to be antigen-ELISA (enzyme-linked immunosorbent assay) negative for FHV1, FCoV and CDV as well as negative for FCV and FPV by fluorescent antibody testing. These tests were performed as previously described [8, 30, 31]. Finally, a blocking ELISA test (CIVTEST SUIS ADV gE, Hipra, Gerona, Spain) was used to detect the presence of serum antibodies against PRV, obtaining negative results.

The lynx was found dead on Dec 1, 2015 on private land consisting of a mixture of dense scrub and open pasture in an area known as "Hornachos-Valle del Matachel" located southwest of Badajoz (Extremadura), Spain (Latitude: 38°27′10.98″ N, Longitude: 5°54′30″W).

Post-mortem examination was carried out at the Veterinary Teaching Hospital of Extremadura (Cáceres, Spain). Upon presentation for necropsy, the lynx weighed 3,060 g, and the carcass was preserved without putrefaction changes. An X-ray examination excluded general traumatisms or the presence of shotgun wounds. Gross lesions of the lynx were minimal. In agreement with our observations, AD in many cases does not develop significant macroscopic lesions in other carnivores such as dogs and cats [32, 33] and wolves [25]. The skin of the ventral neck was denuded of hair and the radio-collar appeared torn (Fig. 1a). Intense pruritus can sometimes lead to these types of lesions due to scratching and self-mutilation as has been suggested in coyotes [34], dogs [26, 35] and cats [32]. The stomach and small intestine contained a moderate amount of partially digested blood (Fig. 1b). The large intestinal contents consisted of varying amounts of dark red to black semi-formed fecal material. The meninges were congested (Fig. 1c). These lesions are similar to those reported in the Florida panther [28], coyotes [34] and dogs [11].

Representative portions of sampled tissues were fixed in 10% neutral buffered formalin, routinely embedded in paraffin and hematoxylin and eosin (HE) stained. A histopathological analysis of the CNS showed diffuse nonsuppurative meningoencephalitis similar to that reported in domestic cats [32, 36] and other unnatural hosts such as dogs [11, 33, 35, 37], foxes [38] and coyotes [34]. Similar to that described for coyotes [34], the leptomeninges and subarachnoid space were infiltrated and expanded by slight perivascular accumulations of mononuclear cells (Fig. 2a). This meningoencephalitis was characterized by mononuclear cellular infiltrates around blood vessels (perivascular cuffs) and neuropil (Fig. 2b) composed mainly of lymphocytes, as well as multifocal to diffuse microgliosis, perineuronal glial satellitosis (Fig. 2c and d), neuronal necrosis and neuronophagia (Fig. 2d). Most neurons appeared unaffected; although within damaged brain regions, several neurons showed eosinophilic intranuclear inclusion bodies (Fig. 2e), even though eosinophilic intranuclear inclusions could be absent in the neurons of cats [39]. Diffuse areas of demyelination and malacia were observed in sections of the cerebrum and cerebellum (Fig. 2b). These lesions have been previously described in raccoons [40]. Gastrointestinal tract lesions observed in the lynx consisted of necrotizing gastritis and enteritis of the small intestine with foci of epithelial necrosis with minimal inflammatory reactions. These lesions have been reported in cats and dogs [36, 41] and in piglets [42].

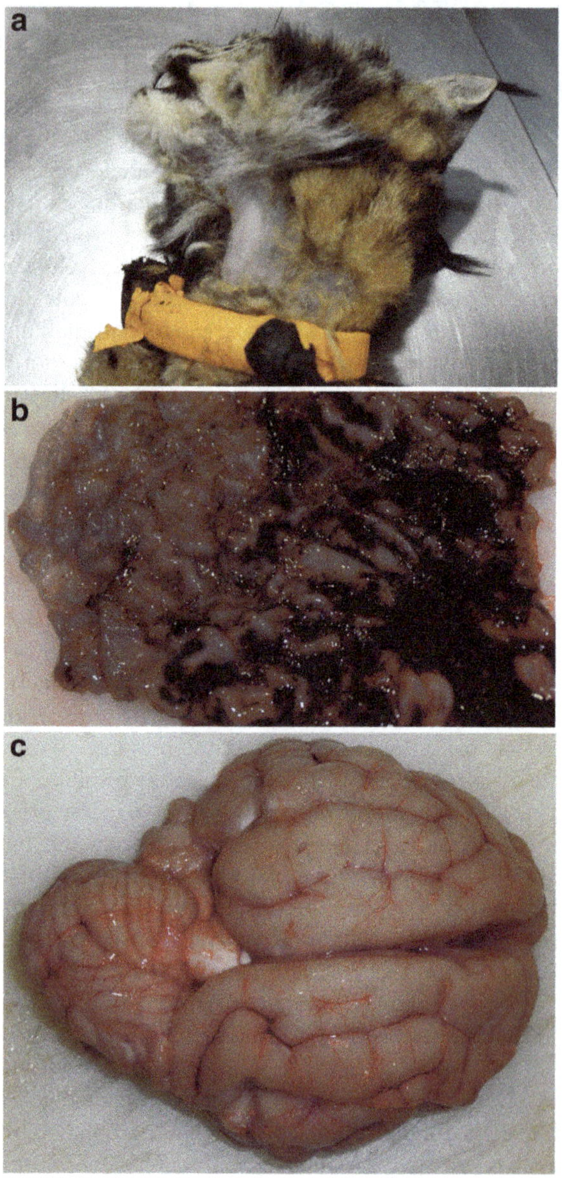

Fig. 1 Gross pathology findings. Iberian lynx. **a** Area of alopecia on the ventral neck skin. The radio-collar appears scratched. **b** Partially digested blood was present in the lumen of the stomach. **c** Congestion of the brain

PCR tests were negative for infection with FCoV (clot, spleen, mesenteric ganglia, small intestine and intestinal scraping samples), FCV (clot samples), CDV (brain tissue, clot, mesenteric ganglia and intestinal scraping samples), FPV (clot, mesenteric ganglia and intestinal scraping samples), FHV1 (clot, spleen, mesenteric ganglia, small intestine, intestinal scraping and brain tissue samples), FIV (clot and spleen samples), FeLV provirus (clot, mesenteric ganglia, intestinal scraping and brain tissue samples), *Mycoplasma haemofelis, Candidatus mycoplasma haemominutum, Candidatus mycoplasma turicensis, Anaplasma phagocytophilum, Bartonella henselae, Chlamydophila felis* [8], *Cytauxzoon felis* (clot samples) [43] and *Leptospira spp.* (kidney samples) [44]. PCR tests were positive for infection with FeLV provirus (spleen and bone marrow samples) [8] and *Pasteurella spp.* (lung samples) using PrimerDesign™ genesig Kit for Pasteurella multocida (Genesig, Chandler's Ford, United Kingdom). Toxicological analyses were negative for pesticides and other organic compounds (chloralose, barbiturates, and metaldehyde), anticoagulant rodenticides and anticholinesterase pesticides. No intestinal parasites were detected in the lynx feces.

The polymer detection method (PDM) to detect porcine PRV was carried out on deparaffinized tissue sections using an UltraVision Quanto Detection System HRP DAB (Thermo Scientific, Fremont, USA, #TL-060-

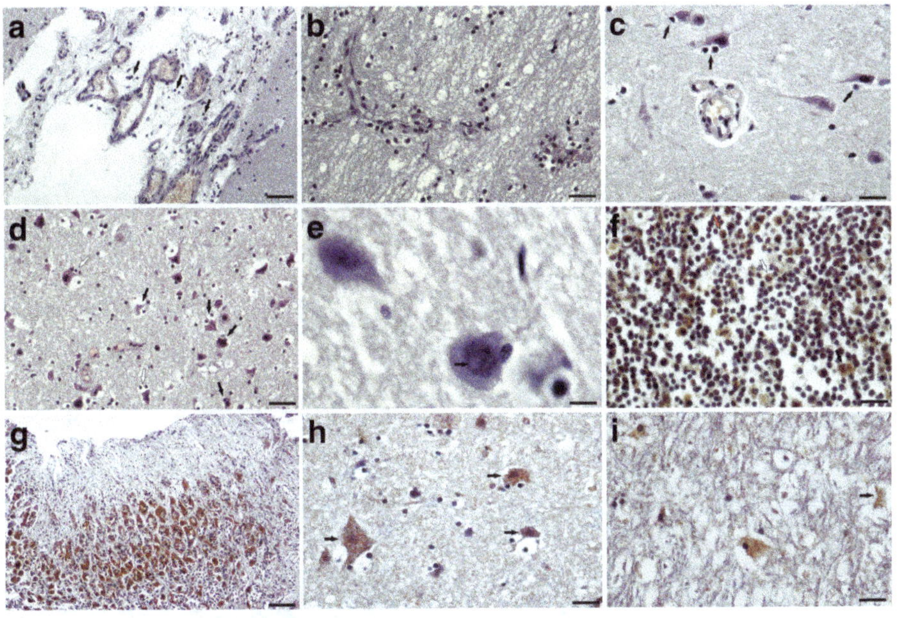

Fig. 2 Histopathology and immunohistochemistry. Iberian lynx **a** Cerebrum. The leptomeninges and subarachnoid space were infiltrated by mononuclear cells (*arrows*) HE (bar = 25 μm). **b** Cerebrum. Mononuclear cellular infiltrates around blood vessels and neuropil. Demyelination and spongiosis. HE. (bar = 35 μm). **c** Cerebrum. Glial satellitosis (*arrows*). HE. (bar = 40 μm). **d** Cerebrum. Neuronal necrosis and neuronophagia (black arrows). Satellitosis (*white arrows*). HE. (bar = 35 μm). **e** Cerebrum. Neuronal intranuclear inclusion bodies (*arrow*). HE. (bar = 50 μm). **f** Tonsils. Positive immunostaining for PRV antigen in lymphocytes (*white arrow*), plasma cells (*red arrow*) and macrophages (*black arrow*). PDM. DAB chromogen. (bar = 40 μm). **g** Stomach. PRV antigen was detected in gastric glandular epithelial cells. PDM. DAB chromogen. (bar = 35 μm). **h** Cerebrum. Immunohistochemical PRV detection in neurons (*arrows*). PDM. DAB chromogen. (bar = 40 μm). **i** Cerebellum. Immunohistochemical demonstration of PRV presence in glial cells of white matter of the cerebellum. Some cells are necrotic (*arrow*). PDM. DAB chromogen. (bar = 40 μm)

QHD) following manufacturer's directions. Primary antiserum was gE PRV-specific monoclonal antibody (Ingenasa, Madrid; Spain #M.11.ADV.B2CF2). In order to determine the specificity of the immunohistochemical reaction, primary antibody was replaced with PBS or with non-immune mouse serum (1:100). The positive control consisted of a slide containing known positive tissue (CNS of naturally PRV infected pig). Negative control slides consisted of brain sections of a PRV-free lynx. The PRV antigen was detected in the tonsils (Fig. 2f) of the Lynx. PRV has been previously detected by immunohistochemistry in the tonsils of pigs [45] and it was isolated from de tonsils of dogs [33] and racoons [40]. The replication of the virus in tonsils after its entrance via the oral route has been described in cats [32]. Positive immunostaining was also observed in numerous gastric glandular epithelial cells (Fig. 2g), consistent with that previously described in dogs [37]. The PRV antigen was found in the cytoplasm of neuronal (Fig. 2h) and non-neuronal cells (Fig. 2i) in inflamed brain areas. This localization has been described in dogs [11, 37]. Like other viruses belonging to the subfamily *Alphaherpesvirinae*, PRV first replicates in the epithelium of the mucous membranes, and then reaches the CNS via the nerve fibres that innervate the colonised tissues [46]. Specific staining was not detected in the negative control samples (Fig. 3a). The positive control, showed positive immunoreaction against the gE PRV-specific monoclonal antibody (Fig. 3b).

To assess the presence of PRV in the CNS of the affected animal, a specific nested PCR reaction (Fig. 4) designed to amplify the viral glycoprotein B gene was performed, using two pairs of primers previously described [47]. DNA from brain tissue was obtained using a commercial kit (QiAmp DNA Mini Kit®, Qiagen Ltd., Crawley, West Sussex, UK) following the manufacturer's protocol. A total of 5 μl of the extracted DNA was used as a template for the nested PCR in a 25 μl reaction mixture containing 12.5 μl of PCR Master Mix (2x) (Green Taq, Thermo Fisher Scientific, Waltham, MA, USA) and 0.2 μM of each primer. DNA was amplified using the following amplification procedure: 1 cycle at 95 °C for 3 min, 30 cycles of denaturalization (94 °C, 45 s), annealing (62 °C, 1 min) and extension (72 °C, 1 min); and a final extension at 72 °C for 10 min. The second step of the nested PCR was performed using 0.5 μl of the first PCR product as template and following the amplification procedure previously described. PCR products were separated by 2% agarose gel electrophoresis and visualized by ethidium bromide staining under UV light.

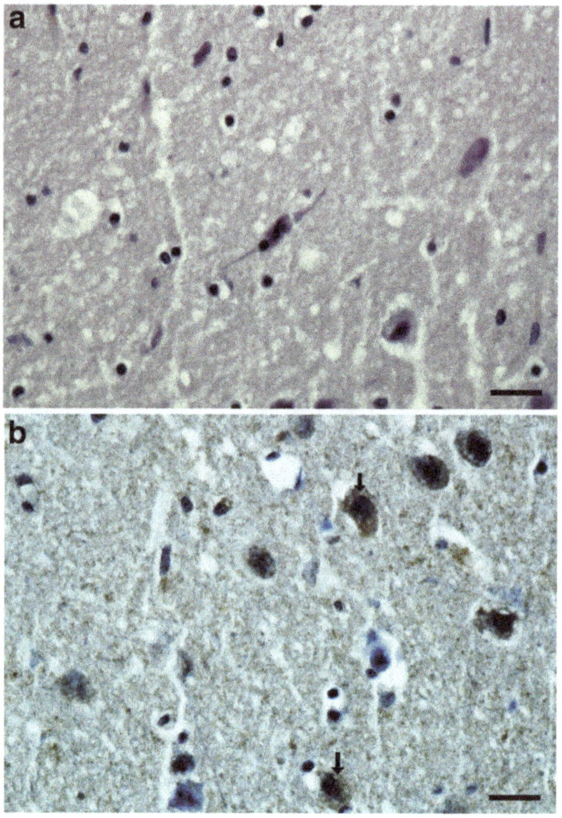

Fig. 3 Immunohistochemistry. **a** Iberian lynx. Cerebrum. Negative control for immunohistochemical PRV detection by substitution of the primary antibody with normal mouse serum (1:100). PDM. DAB chromogen. (bar = 40 μm). **b** PRV infected swine. Brain. Positive control for immunohistochemical PRV detection. PDM. DAB chromogen. (bar = 35 μm)

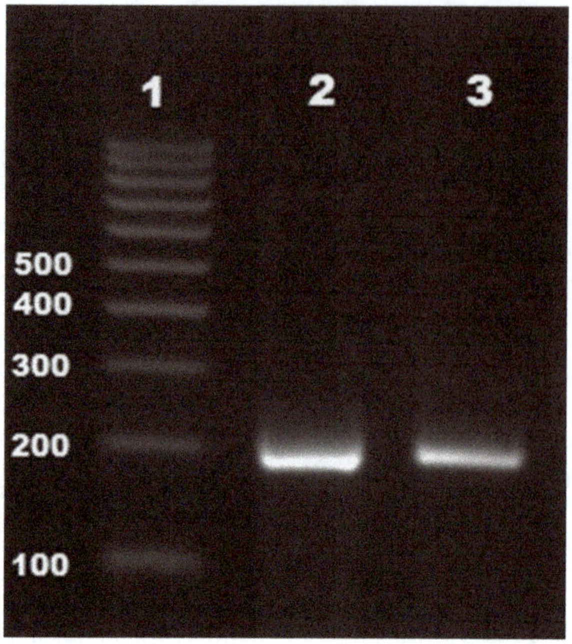

Fig. 4 Agarose gel electrophoresis of Suid Herpesvirus 1 (SuHV1) from nested PCR (gB gene) stained with ethidium bromide. Line 1: 100 bp DNA ladder. Line 2: 195 bp band obtained from a positive control of SuHV1 (strain Bartha K-61). Line 3: 195 bp band obtained from DNA extracted from brain tissue of the studied Iberian Lynx

The obtained 195 bp band was cut out of the gel, and DNA was extracted using an Ultra Clean™ GelSpin DNA Purification Kit (Mo Bio Laboratories, Inc., Carlsbad, California, 92010, USA). The 195 bp amplified product was sequenced in both directions using a BigDye Terminator v3.1 cycle sequencing kit according to the manufacturer's instructions (Applied Biosystems). Nucleotide sequences were read on a 3730xl DNA Analyzer (Applied Biosystems). After trimming sequence primers, the 146 bp sequence was initially compared with GeneBank sequences using the Basic Local Alignment Search Tool (BLAST) (http://www.ncbi.nlm.nih.gov/blast/Blast.cgi) to verify the identity of the fragment. The BLAST analysis showed that the 146 bp sequence matched with the PRV genome. The obtained sequence and PRV available sequences were aligned by Clustal Omega [48]. The alignment showed that the analyzed fragment presented 100% sequence identity with reference PRV strains such as Kaplan or Bartha. One substitution was found in strains such as NIA3 or Becker, while 2–4 substitutions were found when isolates with an Asian origin were aligned, like HUYD (DDBJ accession number KJ526432) or Rang (DDBJ accession number KP895102) isolates. An additional PCR was carried out to amplify glycoprotein D gene with primers and conditions previously described [49]. Furthermore, in order to assess whether PRV infection was produced by a wild-type or a vaccine PRV strain, a TaqMan® base real-time PCR assay for the detection of gE gene was conducted as previously described using DNA extracted from CNS as template [50]. Specific DNA from glycoprotein D and E encoding-genes was detected confirming the latter that this infection was produced by a wild-type PRV strain.

This article describes the first reported case of pseudorabies in Iberian lynxes, and it confirms that they are susceptible to PRV infection. Like other felids, PRV-infected lynxes develop lethal neurological disorders. In cats, PRV infection with brief two- to four-day incubation period, produces acute encephalitis and can cause 100% mortality in experimentally infected domestic cats [32, 51]. The cats suffer from anorexia, occasional severe itching with lesions caused by scratching and self mutilation and uncoordinated movements and paralysis [32, 51]. The outcome is invariably fatal and leads to death within 12–48 h of the first appearance of clinical signs [32]. This peracute death does not allow time for a serologic response to occur [52]. If Iberian lynxes succumb as rapidly as domestic cats, detection of the clinical phase can prove to be very difficult.

The main sources of infection for cats are uncooked pig or offal [32]. Direct spread of virus from infected to non-infected carnivores likely does not occur [34]. Wild boar are a well known reservoir for PRV and hence, may pose a risk to transmit the infection to wildlife carnivores species [25, 34]. Some authors have described recently, rates of 69.70% ELISA seropositivity and 11.30% of PRV lung infections in wild boar population throughout SW Spain [53, 54]. Wild boar are not the main component of the Iberian lynx diet; however, these animals do occasionally consume wild boar as prey and as carrion [5]. Therefore, it is conceivable that some lynxes will be exposed to PRV from the ingestion of wild boar. Indirect transmission can also occur through viral excretion by pigs, without direct contact with the pigs themselves [32]. The presence of wild boar infected with the PRV could have a negative impact on conservation of wild carnivores which consume wild boar [25] such as lynxes.

Conclusions

Our findings support the suspicion that PRV could infect the Iberian lynx [5, 22]. The detection of PRV in a dead Iberian lynx suggests that the virus may have a negative impact on the endangered lynx's survival in the wild. However, because this is the first verified instance of lynx mortality resulting from pseudorabies, its true impact on the population is unknown. A possibility for management of this species is vaccinating lynxes with an inactivated vaccine during routine captures to provide some level of immunity against this disease. This has previously been suggested for Florida panthers [28], although vaccination has not been proven efficacious. Oral vaccination of wild boar against classical swine fever virus has been shown to be successful [55], which means that oral vaccination of wild boar against PRV could be an effective strategy for protecting lynxes from the disease [25]. The effectiveness of using attenuated live vaccine for oral immunisation of wild boar against PRV has been demonstrated [56], though the safety of this technique needs to be studied in depth [25].

Abbreviations

AD: Aujeszky's disease; CDV: Canine Distemper Virus; CNS: Central nervous system; DAB: Diaminobenzidine; ELISA: Enzyme-linked immunosorbent assay; FCoV: Feline Coronavirus; FCV: Feline Calicivirus; FeLV: Feline Leukemia Virus; FHV1: Feline Herpesvirus; FIV: Feline Immunodeficiency Virus; FPV: Feline Parvovirus; HE: Hematoxylin and eosin; PCR: Polymerase chain reaction; PDM: Polymer detection method; PRV: Pseudorabies virus; SuHV1: Suid Herpesvirus 1

Acknowledgements

We thank Dr. Fernando Nájera, Julián Panadero and Ma. Jesús Palacios (Consejería de Medio Ambiente y Rural, Junta de Extremadura) for providing logistic assistance in carrying out field work and sanitary handling of lynxes and Dr. Susana Sánchez for assistance with the necropsy. The authors also greatly appreciate the help of Dr. Irene Zorrilla and the staff from the Center for Analysis and Diagnosis of Wildlife (Málaga, Spain) for performing further molecular and microbiological analyses as well as parasitological analysis. We also thank Dr. José Francisco Ruiz-Fons of the Hunting Resources Research Institute (Ciudad Real, Spain) for the serological determination of antibodies against PRV and Dr. Francisco Soler of the Veterinary Teaching Hospital of Extremadura (Cáceres, Spain) for conducting the toxicological study.

Funding

This study has been funded by the European Union (EU) through its LIFE+ project 10 NAT/ES/000570 and Junta de Extremadura with the economic support of the EU - European Regional Development Fund (ERDF). Dr. D. Risco is supported by a Torres Quevedo Grant from the Ministerio de Economía y Competitividad of Spain (PTQ14-06663).

Authors' contributions

AJM and ER carried out the necropsy, histopathology and immunohistochemistry. AJM, ER and DR were involved in the revision of literature, drafting and writing of the manuscript. MG, DR and JIN carried out the PRV detection by PCR and the sequence analysis. OMJ carried out field work, provided the case history and contributed to the necropsy. All authors read and approved the final manuscript.

Competing interests

The authors declare that they have no competing interests.

Consent for publication

Not applicable.

Author details

[1]Unidad de Histología y Anatomía Patológica, Departamento de Medicina Animal, Facultad de Veterinaria, Universidad de Extremadura, Avda. Universidad s.n., Cáceres 10003, Spain. [2]Veterinary Teaching Hospital, University of Extremadura, Cáceres, Spain. [3]Innovación en Gestión y Conservación de Ungulados S.L., Cáceres, Spain. [4]Dirección General de Medio Ambiente, Consejería de Medio Ambiente y Rural, Junta de Extremadura, Spain. [5]Institut de Recerca i Tecnologia Agroalimentàries (IRTA)-Centre de Recerca en Sanitat Animal (CReSA), UAB-IRTA, Campus de la Universitat Autònoma de Barcelona, Bellaterra, Cerdanyola del Vallès, Spain.

References

1. Rodríguez A, Delibes M. Current range and status of the Iberian Lynx (*Felis pardina* Temminck 1824) in Spain. Biol Conserv. 1992;61:189–96.
2. Hermoso V, Clavero M, Villero D, Brotons L. EU's Conservation Efforts Need More Strategic Investment to Meet Continental Commitments. Conservation Letters 2016. doi:10.1111/conl.12248.
3. Simon MA. Censo de la población de lince ibérico, año 2015. Life+ Iberlince website. 2015. www.iberlince.eu. Accessed 22 Apr 2016
4. Gil JM, Ballesteros E, Bueno JF. Feeding ecology of the Iberian lynx Lynx pardinus in eastern Sierra Morena (Southern Spain). Acta Theriolog. 2006;51:85–90.
5. Boadella M, Gortázar C, Vicente J, Ruiz-Fons F. Wild boar: an increasing concern for Aujeszky's disease control in pigs? BMC Vet Res. 2012;8:7.
6. Aldama JJ, Delibes M. Observations of feeding groups in the Spanish lynx (Felis pardina) in the Doñana National Park, SW Spain. Mammalia. 1991;55:143–7.
7. Palomares F, Delibes M, Ferrera P, Fedriani JM, Calzada J, Revilla E. Iberian lynx in a fragmented landscape: pre-dispersal, dispersal, and post-dispersal habitats. Conserv Biol. 2000;14:809–18.

8. Meli ML, Cattori V, Martínez F, López G, Vargas MA, Zorrilla I, Muñoz A, Palomares F, López-Bao JV, Pastor J, Tandon R, Willi B, Hofmann-Lehmann R, Lutz H. Feline Leukemia Virus and Other Pathogens as Important Threats to the Survival of the Critically Endangered Iberian Lynx (*Lynx pardinus*). PLoS ONE 2009. doi:10.1371/journal.pone.0004744.
9. Meli ML, Cattori V, Martínez F, López G, Vargas A, Palomares F, López-Bao JV, Hofmann-Lehmann R, Lutz H. Feline leukemia virus infection: A threat for the survival of the critically endangered Iberian lynx (*Lynx pardinus*). Vet Immunol Immunopathol. 2010;134:61–7.
10. Mettenleiter TC. Aujeszky's disease (pseudorabies) virus: The virus and molecular pathogenesis—State of the art, June 1999. Vet Res. 2000;31:99–115.
11. Quiroga MI, Nieto JM, Sur J, Osorio F. Diagnosis of Aujeszky's disease virus infection in dogs by use of immunohistochemistry and in-situ hybridization. J Vet Med. 1998;45:78–81.
12. Meier RK, Ruiz-Fons F, Ryser-Degiorgis MP. A picture of trends in Aujeszky's disease virus exposure in wild boar in the Swiss and European contexts. BMC Vet Res. 2015;11:277–85.
13. Pomeranz LE, Reynolds AE, Hengartner CJ. Molecular biology of pseudorabies virus: impact on neurovirology and veterinary medicine. Microbiol Mol Biol Rev. 2005;69:462–500.
14. Alemán N, Quiroga MI, López M, Váquez S, Guerrero F, Nieto JM. Induction and Inhibition of Apoptosis by Pseudorabies Virus in the Trigeminal Ganglion during Acute Infection of Swine. J Virol. 2001;75:469–79.
15. Card JP, Enquist LW. Neurovirulence of pseudorabies virus. Crit Rev Neurobiol. 1995;9:137–62.
16. Enquist LW. Infection of the mammalian nervous system by pseudorabies virus (PRV). Semin Virol. 1994;5:221–31.
17. Mulder WAM, Jacobs L, Priem J, Kok GL, Wagenaar F, Kimman TG, Pol JMA. Glycoprotein gE-negative pseudorabies virus has a reduced capability to infect second- and third-order neurons of the olfactory and trigeminal routes in the porcine central nervous system. J Gen Virol. 1994;75:3095–106.
18. Boadella M, Vicente J, Ruiz-Fons F, de la Fuente J, Gortazar C. Effect of culling Eurasian wild boar on the prevalence of Mycobacterium bovis and Aujeszky's disease virus. Prev Vet Med. 2012;107:214–21.
19. Ruiz-Fons F, Vicente J, Vidal D, Höfle U, Villanúa D, Gauss C, et al. Seroprevalence of six reproductive pathogens in European wild boar (Sus scrofa) from Spain: The effect on wild boar female reproductive performance. Theriogenology. 2006;65:731–43.
20. Ruiz-Fons F, Vidal D, Hofle U, Vicente J, Gortázar C. Aujeszky's disease virus infection patterns in European wild boar. Vet Microbiol. 2007;120:241–50.
21. Vicente J, León-Vizcaíno L, Gortázar C, Cubero MJ, González M, Martín-Atance P. Antibodies to selected viral and bacterial pathogens in European wild boars from southcentral Spain. J Wildl Dis. 2002;38:649–52.
22. Vicente J, Ruiz-Fons F, Vidal D, Höfle U, Acevedo P, Villanúa D, Fernández-de-Mera IG, Martín MP, Gortázar C. Serosurvey of Aujeszky's disease virus infection in European wild boar in Spain. Vet Rec. 2005;156:408–12.
23. Closa-Sebastia F, Casas-Diaz E, Cuenca R, Lavin S, Mentaberre G, Marco I. Antibodies to selected pathogens in wild boar (Sus scrofa) from Catalonia (NE Spain). Eur J Wildl Res. 2011;57:977–81.
24. Cano-Manuel FJ, López-Olvera J, Fandos P, Soriguer RC, Pérez JM, Granados JE. Long-term monitoring of ten selected pathogens in wild boar (Sus scrofa) in Sierra Nevada National Park, southern Spain. Vet Microbiol. 2014;174:148–54.
25. Verpoest S, Cay AB, Bertrand O, Saulmont M, de Regge N. Isolation and characterization of pseudorabies virus from a wolf (*Canis lupus*) from Belgium. Eur J Wildl Res. 2014;60:149–53.
26. Cramer SD, Campbell GA, Njaa BL, Morgan SE, Smith SK, McLin WR, Brodersen BW, Wise AG, Scherba G, Langohr IM, Maes RK. Pseudorabies virus infection in Oklahoma hunting dogs. J Vet Diag Invest. 2011;23:915–23.
27. Monroe WE. Clinical signs associated with pseudorabies in dogs. J Am Vet Med Assoc. 1989;195:599–602.
28. Glass CM, McLean RG, Katz JB, Maehr DS, Cropp CB, Kirk LJ, McKeirnan AJ, Evermann JF. Isolation of pseudorabies (Aujeszky's disease) virus from a Florida panther. J Wildl Dis. 1994;30:180–4.
29. Zanin E, Capua M, Casaccia C, Zuin A, Moresco A. Isolation and Characterization of Aujeszky's Disease Virus in Captive Brown Bears from Italy. J Wildl Dis. 1997;33:632–4.
30. Hofmann-Lehmann R, Fehr D, Grob M, Elgizoli M, Packer C, Martenson JS, O'Brien SJ, Lutz H. Prevalence of antibodies to feline parvovirus, calicivirus, herpesvirus, coronavirus, and immunodeficiency virus and of feline leukemia virus antigen and the interrelationship of these viral infections in free-ranging lions in east Africa. Clin Diagn Lab Immunol. 1996;3:554–62.
31. Ramsauer S, Bay G, Meli M, Hofmann-Lehmann R, Lutz H. Seroprevalence of selected infectious agents in a free-ranging, low-density lion population in the Central Kalahari Game Reserves in Botswana. Clin Vaccine Immunol. 2007;14:808–10.
32. Thiry E, Addie D, Belák S, Boucraut-Baralon C, Egberink H, Frymus T, Gruffydd-Jones T, Hartmann K, Hosie M, Lloret A, Lutz H, Marsilio F, Möstl K, Pennisi MG, Radford AD, Truyen U, Horzinek MC. Aujeszky's disease/pseudorabies in cats. ABCD guidelines on prevention and management. J Fel Med Surg. 2013;15:555–6.
33. Shell LG, Ely RW, Crandell RA. Pseudorabies in a dog. J Am Vet Med Assoc. 1981;178:1159–61.
34. Raymond JT, Gillespie RG, Woodruff M, Janovitz EB. Pseudorabies in Captive Coyotes. J Wildl Dis. 1997;33:916–8.
35. Buergelt CD, Romero CH, Chrisman CL. Pseudorabies in two dogs. Vet Med. 2000;95:439–42.
36. Hagemoser WA, Kluge JP, Hill HT. Studies on the pathogenesis of pseudorabies in domestic cats following oral inoculation. Can J Comp Med. 1980;44:192–202.
37. Schöniger S, Klose K, Werner H, Schwarz BA, Müller T, Schoon HA. Nonsuppurative Encephalitis in a Dog. Vet Pathol. 2012;49:731–43.
38. Quiroga MI, Vázquez S, López M, Guerrero F, Nieto M. Experimental Aujeszky's disease in blue foxes. J Vet. 1995;42:649–57.
39. Lulini B, Cantile C, Mandara MT, Maurella C, Loria GR, Castagnaro M, Salvadori C, Porcario C, Corona C, Perazzini AZ, Maroni A, Caramelli M, Casalone C. Neuropathology of Italian Cats in Feline Spongiform Encephalopathy Surveillance. Vet Pathol. 2008;45:626–33.
40. Thawley DG, Wright JC. Pseudorabies virus infection in raccoons: a review. J Wildl Dis. 1982;18:113–6.
41. Zhang L, Zhong C, Wang J, Lu Z, Liu L, Yang W, Lyu Y. Pathogenesis of natural and experimental Pseudorabies virus infections in dogs. Virol J. 2015;12:44–54.
42. Narita M, Kubo M, Fukusho A, Haritani M, Moriwaki M. Necrotizing enteritis in piglets associated with Aujeszky's disease virus infection. Vet Pathol. 1984;21:450–2.
43. Millán J, Naranjo V, Rodríguez A, de la Lastra JM, Mangold AJ, de la Fuente J. Prevalence of infection and 18S rRNA gene sequences of Cytauxzoon species in Iberian lynx (Lynx pardinus) in Spain. Parasitology. 2007;134:995–1001.
44. Stoddard RA, Gee JE, Wilkins PP, McCaustland K, Hoffmaster AR. Detection of pathogenic Leptospira spp. through TaqMan polymerase chain reaction targeting the LipL32 gene. Diagn Microbiol Infec Dis. 2009;64:247–55.
45. Grieco V, Gelmetti D, Finazzi G, Brocchi E, Finazzi M. Immunohistologic diagnosis of pseudorabies (Aujeszky's disease) using monoclonal antibodies. J Vet Diagn Invest. 1997;9:326–8.
46. Marcaccini A, López M, Quiroga MI, Bermúdez R, Nieto JM, Alemán N. Pseudorabies virus infection in mink: A host-specific patogénesis. Vet Immunol Immunopath. 2008;124:264–73.
47. Balasch M, Pujols J, Segalés J, Pumarola M. Aujeszky's disease (pseudorabies) virus detection in cerebrospinal fluid in experimentally infected pigs. Vet Microb. 1998;60:99–106.
48. McWilliam H, Li W, Uludag M, Squizzato S, Park YM, Buso N, Cowley AP, Lopez R. Analysis Tool Web Services from the EMBL-EBI. Nucleic Acids Res. 2013;41:W597–600.
49. Schang LM, Osorio FA. A quantitative technique for the study of the latency of Aujeszky virus. Rev Sci Tech. 1993;12:505–21.
50. Ma W, Lager KM, Richt JA, Stoffregen WC, Zhou F, Yoon KJ. Development of realtime polymerase chain reaction assays for rapid detection and differentiation of wild-type pseudorabies and gene-deleted vaccine viruses. J Vet Diagn Invest. 2008;20:440–7.
51. Horváth Z, Papp L. Clinical manifestations of Aujeszky's disease in the cat. Acta Vet Acad Sci Hung. 1967;17:48–54.
52. Hand PJ. Rabies and other viral disease of the nervous system. In: Sherding RG, editor. The cat: Diseases and clinical management. New York: Churchill Livingstone Inc; 1989. p. 379–90.
53. Risco D, Cuesta JM, Fernández P, Salguero FJ, Gonçalves P, García WL, Martínez R, Velarde R, Hermoso M, Gómez L, Hermoso J. Pathological observations of porcine respiratory disease complex (PRDC) in the wild boar (*Sus scrofa*). Europ J Wildl Res. 2015;61:669–79.
54. Risco D, Serrano E, Fernández P, Cuesta JM, Gonçalves P, García WL, Martínez R, Cerrato R, Velarde R, Gómez L, Segalés J, Hermoso J. Severity of bovine tuberculosis is associated with co-infection with common pathogens in wild boar. PLoS ONE. 2014. doi:10.1371/journal.pone.0110123.

55. Kaden V, Lange E, Fischer U, Strebelow G. Oral immunization of wild boar against classical swine fever: evaluation of the first field study in Germany. Vet Microbiol. 2000;73:239–52.
56. Maresch C, Lange E, Teifke JP, Fuchs W, Klupp B, Müller T, Mettenleiter TC, Vahlenkamp TW. Oral immunization of wild boar and domestic pigs with attenuated live vaccine protects against Pseudorabies virus infection. Vet Microbiol. 2012;161:20–5.

5

Longitudinal study of Senecavirus a shedding in sows and piglets on a single United States farm during an outbreak of vesicular disease

Steven J. P. Tousignant[1*], Laura Bruner[1], Jake Schwartz[1], Fabio Vannucci[2], Stephanie Rossow[2] and Douglas G. Marthaler[2]

Abstract

Background: The study highlights the shedding pattern of Senecavirus A (SVA) during an outbreak of vesicular disease in a sow farm from the South-central Minnesota, USA. In this study, 34 individual, mixed parity sows with clinical signs of vesicular lesions and 30 individual piglets from 15 individual litters from sows with vesicular lesions were conveniently selected for individual, longitudinal sampling. Serum, tonsil, rectal, and vesicular swabs were collected on day1 post outbreak, and then again at 1, 2, 3, 4, 6, and 9 weeks post outbreak. Samples were tested at the University of Minnesota Veterinary Diagnostic Laboratory for SVA via Real Time Polymerase Chain Reaction (RT-PCR)

Results: In sows, vesicular lesions had the highest concentration of SVA, but had the shortest duration of detection lasting only 2 weeks. Viremia was detected for 1 week post outbreak, and quickly declined thereafter. SVA was detected at approximately the same frequency for both tonsil and rectal swabs with the highest percentage of SVA positive samples detected in the first 6 weeks post outbreak. In suckling piglets, viremia quickly declined 1 week post outbreak and was prevalent in low levels during the first week after weaning (4 weeks post outbreak) and was also detected in piglets that were co-mingled from a SVA negative sow farm. Similar to sows, SVA detection on rectal and tonsil swabs in piglets lasted approximately 6 weeks post outbreak.

Conclusion: The study illustrates the variation of SVA shedding patterns in different sample types over a 9 week period in sows and piglets, and suggests the potential for viral spread between piglets at weaning.

Keywords: Swine, Senecavirus a, Seneca Valley virus, Shedding, Epidemiology, Vesicular disease, Case report

Background

Senecavirus A (SVA) or commonly known as Seneca Valley Virus belongs to the family *Pircornaviridae* and has been associated with idiopathic vesicular lesions on the snout and coronary bands in swine [3, 8]. In 2014, SVA outbreaks were reported in Brazil and subsequent SVA outbreaks occurred in the United States (US) during the 2015 [2, 4, 5, 11, 12]. While not a new virus to the US or the world, the alarmingly high rate of severe clinical disease anecdotally reported in Brazil and the US, suggests a change in the epidemiology of SVA, such as the emergence of a new variant strain [7, 8, 10]. Some swine farms report reproductive issues, and weak piglets suffering from secondary infections in the nursery [9]. Vesicular disease caused by SVA infection cannot be differentiated from other US Foreign Animal Diseases (FADs), such as foot-and-mouth disease (FMD), swine vesicular disease (SVD), vesicular stomatitis, and vesicular exanthema. Therefore, SVA has important implications in the transport and slaughter of pigs, potentially leading to significant complications with international trade.

In early September of 2015, a sow farm in South-central Minnesota, US, exhibited the sudden and dramatic onset of severe vesicular lesions in nearly 80% of all sows on the site. Due to the relative paucity of information

* Correspondence: stous@swinevetcenter.com
[1]Swine Vet Center, 1608 South Minnesota Avenue, St. Peter, MN 56082, USA
Full list of author information is available at the end of the article

regarding this virus in the field, the objectives of this study were to assess the shedding patterns of SVA in a population of sows and suckling piglets, and assess the potential spread of SVA in weaned pigs. Not only will this information provide valuable insight into the infection dynamics of SVA within a population, but it may also aid in future FADs investigations, as well as assisting in the development of better control and elimination measures of SVA in sow herds.

Methods

A farm in South central Minnesota, US, containing two geographically different sow sites (sites 1 and 2, Fig. 1) consisting of 1300 sows per site were selected for this study based on the outbreak of vesicular lesions at one of the sow sites (site 1). This farm maintains ownership of pigs throughout all life stages, and at the time of weaning, piglets are transported from sites 1 and 2 to multiple different weaned pig sites (site 3, 4, 5, and 6) within their company (Fig. 1).

Upon visual detection of vesicular lesions at site 1 (day 0 post outbreak (PO)), a FADs investigation was initiated and samples were collected by the state veterinary office and sent to the National Veterinary Services Laboratories (NVSL), the Foreign Animal Disease Diagnostic Laboratory at Plum Island Animal Disease Center and the University of Minnesota Veterinary Diagnostic Laboratory (UMNVDL). At NVSL, the samples were tested for Foot-and-Mouth Disease virus (FMDv), SVA, and Swine Vesicular Disease virus (SVDv) by real time RT-PCR. At the UMNVDL, the samples were tested for FMDv according the United States Department of Agriculture Standard Operation Procedure (SOP) titled, "Extraction of Total RNA Using a MagMax-96 Total RNA Isolation Kit for the Detection of Classical Swine Fever and Foot-and-Mouth Disease Viruses" (SOP-PVS-0004.1), which is publically available from the NVSL upon request. The detection of SVA occurred by real time Reverse Transcription Polymerase Chain Reaction (RT-PCR) using AgPath-ID One-Step RT-PCR Reagents (Thermo), forward (5′- TCTCTTGCCCTAACACTGGGG-3′) and reverse primers (5′- CTTGCCTCTAAGGACCACCACA-3′) and probe (5′- TGGCCCAAA/ZEN/GTCTCACCACT ATGATCAATG-3′) with the following thermal cycling parameters: reverse transcription, 10 min at 45 °C; Taq activation, 10 min at 95 °C; followed by 40 cycles of 15 s at 95 °C, and 45 s at 60 °C.

On the second day post visualization of vesicular disease (day 1 PO), 34 individual, mixed parity sows in gestation from site 1 were conveniently selected based on the presence of vesicular lesions on their snouts and feet. In addition, 30 mixed gender, neonatal piglets from 15-mixed parity litters showing similar clinical signs were conveniently selected and tagged at site 1 between approximately 12 and 24 h of age. Tonsil, rectal, vesicular swabs (when vesicles were present), and serum samples were collected on day 1 and then 1, 2, 3, 4, 6, and 9 weeks PO from both sows and piglets. Last samples were collected at 9 weeks PO and did not occur at weeks 5, 7, and 8 due to concerns of increased stress of the pigs due to sampling. Vesicular swab samples were not collected from the piglets since they lacked clinical vesicular lesions. At week 3 PO (at weaning), the 30 piglets from site 1 were transported to site 6 and were comingled with 30 individually identified mixed gender pigs from site 2 and sampled at 4, 6, and 9 weeks PO (Fig. 1). In addition, at day 0 PO, 10 serum samples and a single oral fluid sample were collected (from three cotton ropes hung in pens within each site) at sites 3, 4, and 5 (Fig. 1) to determine if SVA was present in earlier groups of weaned pigs from before the detection of clinical signs in the system.

Samples were refrigerated overnight and sent next day to the University of Minnesota Veterinary Diagnostic Laboratory. The RNA was extracted using previously described methods [6] for SVA by real time RT-PCR.

Results

The swine farm initially reported concerns of increased lameness in a pen of group housed replacement gilts, as well as a slight decrease in feed intake (day −2 PO). Day −1 PO, lameness and decreased feed intake was more prevalent among the rest of the sows in the herd.

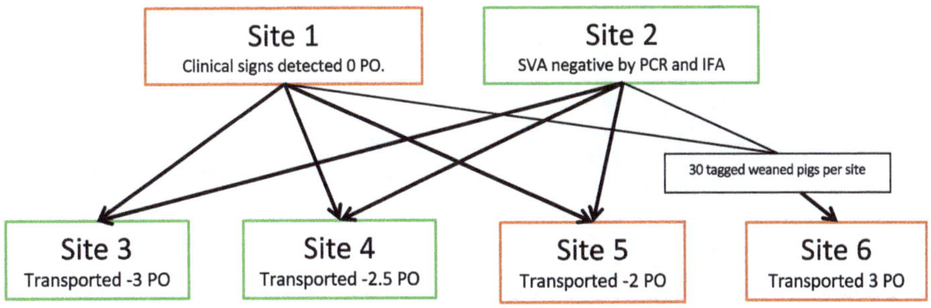

Fig. 1 Diagram of the farms (sites 1–6) involved in this study. Color of the box indicates SVA status; green is negative and red is positive. Pigs were transported at different times weeks PO

Vesicular lesions were observed on day 0 PO, consisting of un-ruptured vesicles on the snouts and feet of approximately 5–10% of the animals on site 1, and the state veterinary office was notified. By day 2 PO, nearly 80% of the animals in the herd had detectable vesicular lesions (ruptured and un-ruptured) on the snouts and feet. Lameness, lethargy, and decreased feed intake were the main clinical concerns during this time; however, by 1 week PO, there was noticeable improvement in the clinical signs within the population. At no time was fever a major concern within the herd. In farrowing, there was an increase in pre-weaning mortality from an average of 12% to a high of 22% during the first 7 days PO, and returned to average levels by 2 weeks PO. The majority of the piglet mortality was associated with dehydration due to poor milk production by the sow, and piglets being laid on, potentially due to sow lameness. No other clinical signs were detected in piglets in farrowing, and there were no detectable signs at the nursery barns at any point during or after the outbreak.

The samples collected by the state veterinary office at site 1 on the day 0 PO were negative for SVDv at NVSL while the NVSL and UMNVDL had the same results for FMDv and SVA (negative and positive, respectively). Subsequent, SVA testing only occurred at the UMNVDL through the study.

Sows displayed vesicular lesions on the snouts at day 0 PO, and SVA was present in 33 out of 34 (97%) of the vesicle swabs, with an average cycle threshold (Ct) value of 16 (range = 12–19). At 1 week PO, SVA was present in 34 out of 34 (100%) of the lesion swabs. At 2 weeks PO, most lesions had healed (only few skin tags and ruptured vesicles remained in the population), and SVA detection decreased to 12 out of 34 samples (35%). By 3 weeks PO, all of the vesicular lesions had healed, and no additional samples were collected.

Generally, viremia was detected up to 1 week PO in sows. A single positive sample was identified at 3 and 6 weeks PO (Fig. 2a). At the first sampling (day 1 PO), the Ct values from the sow serum averaged 33.1 (range = 17–36). Viremia was detected in only 7 out of 34 (20%) of the sows at 1 week PO. SVA viremia was not detected in 11 out of 34 (32%) of the sows at any point during the study. Viremia was detected in 18 out of 30 (60%) and 19 out of 30 (63%) in the suckling piglets from site 1. Additional SVA positive samples were detected at 3,

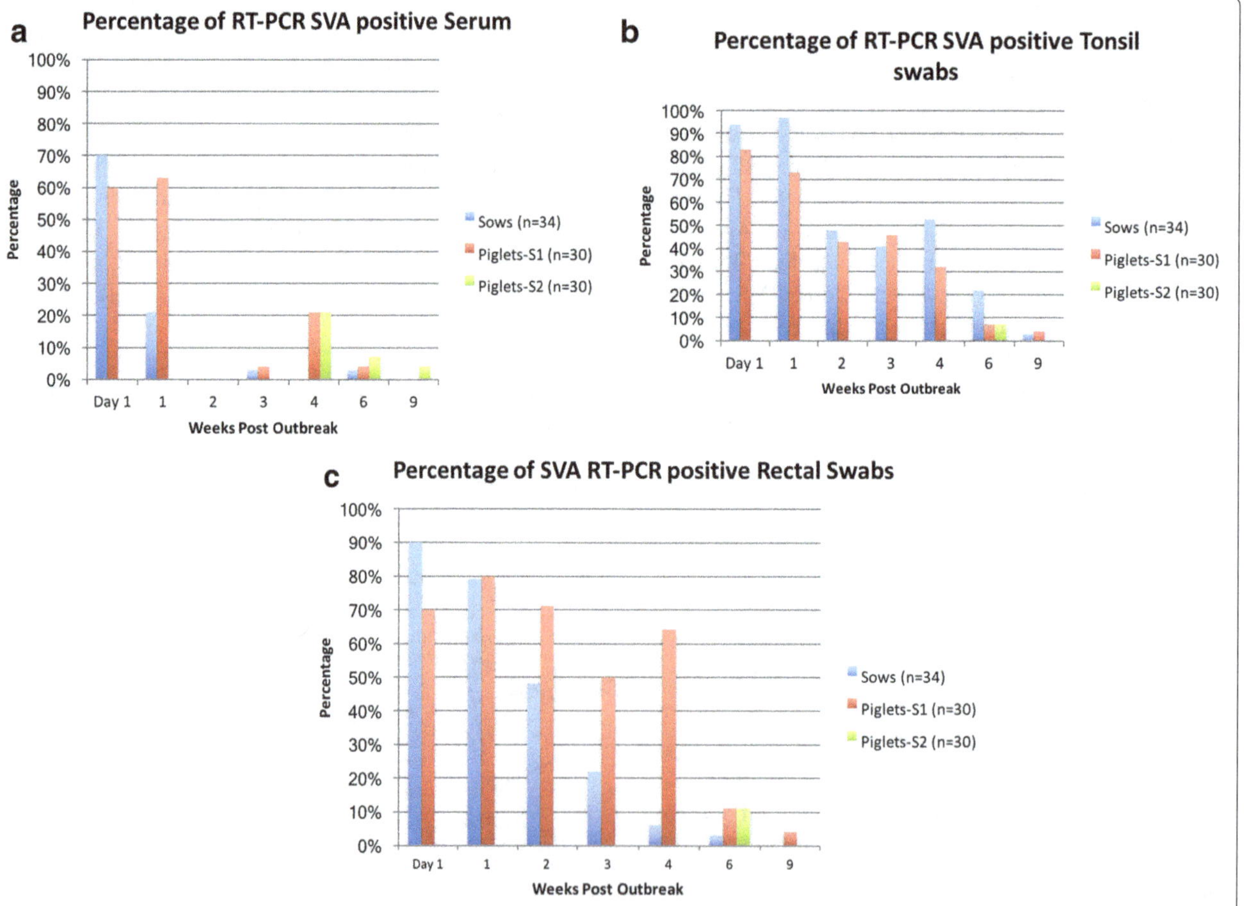

Fig. 2 Percentage of serum (**a**), tonsil swabs (**b**), and rectal swabs (**c**) positive for SVA

4, and 6 weeks PO. In suckling piglets, Ct values averaged 30.6 (range = 24–39.8). Similar to sows, viremia was not detected in 9 out of 30 (30%) of the site 1 piglets enrolled in the study. Viremia was detected in site 2 piglets at 4 (6 out of 30 (21%)), 6 (2 out of 30 (7%)), and 9 (1 out of 30 (3%)) weeks PO, with an average Ct value range of 35.7–38.0.

Tonsil swabs yielded the highest percentage of SVA detection in site 1 sows (32 out 34 (94%)) and piglets (25 out of 30 (83%))(Fig. 2b). In sows, the detection of SVA in the tonsils peaked at 1 week PO (33 out of 34 samples (97%)), with average Ct values of 24.8 (range = 20–27). In site 1 piglets, the peak shedding of SVA occurred at day 1 PO, with average Ct values of 27.1 (range = 20.3–34.6). The detection of SVA shedding decreased over time in sows and piglets, and a single sow and piglet tested positive at 9 weeks PO (Ct values of 35 and 36, respectively). SVA was only detected in 2 of the 30 piglets (7%) from site 2 at 5 weeks PO.

The peak of SVA detection from rectal swabs in sows (31 out of 34 samples (91%)) occurred at day 1 PO and continued to steadily decrease and was not detected at 9 weeks PO (Fig. 2c). In site 1 piglets, the detection of SVA peaked at 1 week PO when 27 of the 30 samples (90%) tested positive. While the detection of SVA decreased in site 1 piglets at 2 and 3 weeks PO, 19 out of 30 samples (64%) of the rectal swabs were positive at 4 weeks PO. At 6 weeks PO, the detection of SVA was same for both site 1 and 2 piglets (11%, n = 3); however, a single piglet from site 1 was still shedding SVA at 9 weeks PO.

The oral fluid and serum samples were positive for SVA from site 5, but negative from site 3 and 4. SVA was detected in 9 out of 10 (90%) of the serum samples (Ct values averaged 32.8, range = 31.8–35.9), and the single oral fluid sample had a (Ct value = 24.3), despite the fact that there were no obvious detectable clinical signs in site 5. Of importance is that site 5 appears to have received SVA positive weaned pigs from site 1 before the detection of clinical signs of decrease in feed intake and vesicular lesions.

Discussion

The study assessed the shedding pattern of SVA in sows and piglets during an outbreak on a farm in the US and investigated the spread of SVA between pigs during the post weaning period. In addition, the study suggests the spread of SVA to distant pig sites via piglets before the onset of vesicular lesions.

Fresh vesicular lesions on the sows had the greatest amounts of SVA; however, the lesions were only present for a very short period of time (2 weeks). This is important because state and federal veterinarians conducting the FAD investigations are trained to identify vesicles and collect their fluid. However, these data suggest a lower rate of detection of SVA in ruptured vesicles and dried skin tags (that are present after the first week of the outbreak) when compared to tonsil and rectal swabs, especially later in the outbreak when vesicles were no longer present. In sows, the detection of SVA in tonsil and rectal swabs was greater than 90% at 0 week PO and remained as high as 50% through 5 weeks PO, these sample types should be collected and submitted, in addition to vesicular lesion swabs and fluid (if present), as part of FAD investigations for the detection of SVA. In addition, the detection of SVA in oral fluid samples collected from site 5 and the high percentage of positive SVA tonsillar swabs suggests they may be valuable tools for the detection of SVA in pigs.

Surprisingly, SVA was detected in serum and oral fluids from site 5, which had received weaned pigs approximately −2 weeks PO, before the detection of clinical signs at site 1. Furthermore, obviously detectable clinical signs were lacking in piglets at site 5, indicating the potential to spread SVA without realization through weaned pig movements. This is a major concern for epidemiologists as well as state and federal veterinarians because the prevalence of SVA within the US swine herd could be greatly underestimated. Therefore, as part of any epidemiological investigation of SVA outbreaks (particularly on sow farms), a social network analysis, which details all pig movements to the level of the specific trailers and trucks used during the previous month should be conducted to identify the potential scope of virus spread.

Commingling of piglets at weaning is common in the US swine industry. When the piglets were commingled at week 4 PO (approximately 1 week after weaning), 12 of the 30 (40%) of the piglets sampled from sites 1 and 2 were viremic. Interestingly, site 1 and 2 piglets had the same level SVA shedding in the tonsil and rectal swabs (2 out of 30 (7%), and 3 out of 30 (10%), respectively) at 6 weeks PO. These results suggest the potential spread of SVA to site 2 piglets, and SVA may be transmitted during commingling of piglets. Therefore, caution should be exercised when considering the movement of weaned pigs during an outbreak, which includes avoiding the comingling of piglets from different sow farms.

While SVA was detected in site 2 piglets, the levels of virus were minimal in the tonsil and rectal swabs potentially implying some underlying immunity to SVA in site 2 piglets that limited viral infection and shedding. While site 2 tested negative by PCR, indicating that the herd was not infected at that time, a proper immunological assay, which may help elucidate if the herd had been infected in the past and has some level of immunity, is lacking at the time of writing this manuscript. With that in mind, immunological assays including several different

ELISA targets are currently under development at several US veterinary diagnostic laboratories [1]. In addition, these immunological assays would help to understand the prevalence of this virus in the US swine herd (in particular sow herds), which would provide better planning and allocation of resources for future SVA outbreaks that would initiate FAD investigations needed by state and federal veterinarians.

Our results suggest that SVA can be detected in a population of sows in tonsil and rectal swabs for up to 9 weeks; however, the viability of SVA at 9 weeks is currently unknown. Future studies should be developed to discern the viability of the virus from these samples, especially in the later stages of the outbreak. This information would be beneficial to veterinarians working on eliminating SVA from affected sow farms since it would dictate the duration of sow herd closure (no entry of potentially immunologically naïve animals for the duration of the shedding period) in order to elimination the virus from that population. Additionally, as part of any plan to eliminate SVA from sow farms, achieving rapid and homogeneous exposure of all animals is crucial. Therefore, studies are needed to identify the most efficient route of SVA exposure to eliminate the virus from infected sow herds.

Conclusion

In conclusion, this study highlights the detection of SVA in vesicular lesions, serum, tonsil and rectal swabs and suggests the spread of SVA between piglets during the post weaning period. In addition, this study suggests that tonsil and rectal swabs, and oral fluids may be useful for monitoring populations SVA positive animals over time.

Abbreviations

CT: Cycle threshold; FAD: Foreign Animal Disease; FMD: Foot-and-mouth disease; NVSL: National veterinary service laboratories; PO: Post outbreak; RT-PCR: Reverse Transcription Polymerase Chain Reaction; SOP: Standard operating procedure; SVA: Senecavirus A; SVD: Swine vesicular disease; US: United States

Acknowledgments

We would like to thank the following people that have contributed time, resources, thoughts and permission for this study, specifically the owner and staff of the sow farm, the veterinarians caring for the animals including, Sam Holst of the Swine Vet Center, and all the staff at the University of Minnesota Veterinary Diagnostic Laboratory, especially the Molecular Diagnostic section.

Funding

The sample collection and veterinary services were supported by the Swine Health Information Center while the University of Minnesota Veterinary Diagnostic Laboratory supported the diagnostic testing.

Authors' contributions

ST and DM contributed to study design, drafted and revised the manuscript. ST, LB and JS contributed to the study design, and oversaw data collection. FV and SR assisted with analysis and interpretation of data. All authors read and approved the final manuscript.

Consent for publication

The authors received consent from the farmer to publish this manuscript.

Competing interests

The authors declare that they have no competing interests.

Author details

[1]Swine Vet Center, 1608 South Minnesota Avenue, St. Peter, MN 56082, USA. [2]Department of Preventive Medicine, College of Veterinary Medicine, University of Minnesota, 1333 Gortner Avenue, St. Paul, MN 55106, USA.

References

1. Gimenez-Lirola LG, Rademacher C, Linhares D, Harmon K, Rotolo M, Sun Y, Baum DH, Zimmerman J, Pineyro P. Serological and molecular detection of Senecavirus a associated with an outbreak of swine idiopathic vesicular disease and neonatal mortality. J Clin Microbiol. 2016;54:2082–9.
2. Guo B, Pineyro PE, Rademacher CJ, Zheng Y, Li G, Yuan J, Hoang H, Gauger PC, Madson DM, Schwartz KJ, Canning PE, Arruda BL, Cooper VL, Baum DH, Linhares DC, Main RG, Yoon KJ. Novel Senecavirus a in swine with vesicular disease, United States, July 2015. Emerg Infect Dis. 2016;22:1325–7.
3. Hales LM, Knowles NJ, Reddy PS, Xu L, Hay C, Hallenbeck PL. Complete genome sequence analysis of Seneca Valley virus-001, a novel oncolytic picornavirus. J Gen Virol. 2008;89:1265–75.
4. Leme RA, Oliveira TE, Alfieri AF, Headley SA, Alfieri AA. Pathological, Immunohistochemical and molecular findings associated with Senecavirus A-induced lesions in neonatal piglets. J Comp Pathol. 2016;155(2-3):145–55.
5. Leme RA, Zotti E, Alcantara BK, Oliveira MV, Freitas LA, Alfieri AF, Alfieri AA. Senecavirus a: an emerging vesicular infection in Brazilian pig herds. Transbound Emerg Dis. 2015;62:603–11.
6. Marthaler D, Rossow K, Gramer M, Collins J, Goyal S, Tsunemitsu H, Kuga K, Suzuki T, Ciarlet M, Matthijnssens J. Detection of substantial porcine group B rotavirus genetic diversity in the United States, resulting in a modified classification proposal for G genotypes. Virology. 2012;433:85–96.
7. Munday BL, Ryan FB. Vesicular lesions in swine – possible association with feeding of marine products. Aust Vet J. 1982;59:193.
8. Pasma T, Davidson S, Shaw SL. Idiopathic vesicular disease in swine in Manitoba. Can Vet J. 2008;49:84–5.
9. Segales J, Barcellos D, Alfieri A, Burrough E, Marthaler D. Senecavirus A. Vet Pathol. 2017;54(1):11–21.
10. Sensi M, Catalano A, Dinaro M, Mariotti C, Panieri C, Marchi S, Costelli S. Idiopathic vesicular disease (IVD): a case report in the centre of Italy. Proc Int Pig Vet Soc 005. 2010. p46
11. Vannucci FA, Linhares DC, Barcellos DE, Lam HC, Collins J, Marthaler D. Identification and complete genome of Seneca Valley virus in vesicular fluid and sera of pigs affected with idiopathic vesicular disease. Brazil Transbound Emerg Dis. 2015;62:589–93.
12. Zhang J, Pineyro P, Chen Q, Zheng Y, Li G, Rademacher C, Derscheid R, Guo B, Yoon KJ, Madson D, Gauger P, Schwartz K, Harmon K, Linhares D, Main R. Full-length genome sequences of Senecavirus a from recent idiopathic vesicular disease outbreaks in U.S. swine. Genome Announc. 2015;3 10.1128/genomeA.01270-15

6

Prevalence and risk factors for viral exposure in rural dogs around protected areas of the Atlantic forest

Nelson Henrique de Almeida Curi[1*], Rodrigo Lima Massara[2], Ana Maria de Oliveira Paschoal[2], Amanda Soriano-Araújo[3], Zélia Inês Portela Lobato[3], Guilherme Ramos Demétrio[1], Adriano Garcia Chiarello[4] and Marcelo Passamani[1]

Abstract

Background: Despite the crucial role of domestic dogs as reservoirs for zoonosis and some of the most threatening diseases for wild carnivores such as distemper and parvovirosis, little is known about the epidemiological features and the risk factors involved in pathogen exposure of dogs that live in human/wildlife interfaces and actually contacts wildlife. Through a cross-sectional serological approach and questionnaire survey, we assessed the prevalence along with individual and environment-associated risk factors for four important viral diseases of rural dogs living in households around six Atlantic Forest fragments in southeast Brazil.

Results: Widespread exposure to canine parvovirus (97 %), canine distemper virus (15 %) and canine adenovirus (27 %) was detected, but none for canine coronavirus. Dogs from small private reserves were more exposed to parvovirus and canine distemper virus than those from larger state parks. Exposure was associated with dog sex and age, lack of health care and the number of people in the households. Remarkably, factors linked to free-ranging behaviour of dogs were associated with the exposure for all pathogens detected.

Conclusions: According to identified associations, reducing viral pathogen exposure in dogs will require inhibiting dog's movements and access to nearby forests and villages and improving veterinary assistance. Promoting dog vaccination and population control through sterilization around protected areas is also necessary. The study provides support for preventive management actions aimed to protect the health of rural dogs, and consequently of Atlantic Forest's wild carnivores.

Keywords: Atlantic Forest, *Canis familiaris*, Epidemiology, Virus exposure, Risk factor, Human/wildlife interface

Background

The domestic dog (*Canis familiaris*) is beyond question man's closest animal species, and consequently the most abundant and widespread carnivore mammal in the world. As such, it represents a conservation problem [1]. Notwithstanding the direct negative impacts on wildlife such as predation, competition and harassment [2], dogs are also the most important reservoirs of diseases that affect wild carnivore species [3]. The furthermost important diseases transmitted from dogs to wild carnivores (rabies, distemper and parvovirosis) are named as "The Big Three" due to the strongly negative impact over the latter populations [3].

Infectious disease-driven mortality is one of the major causes of population decline and extinction of wild mammal carnivores worldwide [1, 3]. It can act in conjunction with other endangerment factors, particularly when populations are small or declining due to habitat loss and fragmentation, or when spill-over occur from sympatric man-subsidized dog populations [3]. As examples, African lions (*Panthera leo*) in the Serengeti ecosystem were continuously threatened by epidemics of canine distemper acquired from dogs and other wild species [4], Ethiopian wolves (*Canis simensis*) were heavily affected by

* Correspondence: nelsoncuri@hotmail.com
[1]Postgraduate Programme in Applied Ecology, Department of Biology, Federal University of Lavras, Lavras, Brazil
Full list of author information is available at the end of the article

dog-transmitted rabies and distemper [5], and grey wolf (*Canis lupus*) populations were impacted by long-term pup mortality due to parvovirus infection [6] in North America. Although evidence on the role of domestic dogs as reservoirs of disease for wild carnivores is becoming a global pattern with other examples coming from Europe [7], Africa [8], South America [9], and Asia [10], few studies have uncovered canine disease-associated risk factors (e.g.) [9, 11], especially at wildlife/human/domestic animal interfaces, which are predicted hotspots for interspecies pathogen transmission leading to disease induced wildlife mortality and disease emergence [12]. Assessing risk factors for diseases in dog populations would, therefore, shed light on transmission and persistence patterns, being of great value for the directing of disease prevention or control efforts for domestic animals, wildlife and humans [13].

In South America, similarly to what occur in other parts of the world, recent case reports and studies revealed that dogs are sources of dangerous infectious agents such as distemper virus to wild carnivores [9, 14, 15], and that several wild carnivore populations have already been exposed to canine pathogens such as parvovirus, distemper virus, adenovirus, and *Toxoplasma gondii*, among others (e.g.) [16–19]. Fortunately, some studies were also concerned with the detection and estimation of pathogen prevalence in sympatric domestic dog populations in a conservation context (i.e. those living around protected areas) [18–23]. Dogs interact with wildlife, and the strength of such interactions is mediated by the role of the dog in the household and the level of care and nutrition given by their owners [24]. However, determinants of disease occurrence in dog populations at human-wildlife interfaces are unknown, and the assessment of risk factors and epidemiological parameters related to viral pathogen prevalence has rarely been performed in South American dog populations, except for some studies from Chile [9, 25]. These aspects have importance for disease prevention or control management because of the increasing presence of free-roaming dogs inside protected areas, enhanced dog-wildlife interaction, and the likelihood of context-dependent impact of disease circulation in different scenarios [1, 3].

Therefore, the aims of our study are to detect the presence, prevalence and risk factors associated with the exposure to viral agents relevant to carnivore conservation in populations of domestic dogs living in rural landscapes around remnants of the Atlantic Forest. This endangered biome is located in the most populous region of Brazil. Many endangered species, including carnivore mammals, depend on this highly fragmented ecosystem and occupy small areas surrounded by rural landscapes. Here, disease exposure in domestic dogs must be associated with poor management, free-roaming behaviour and other epidemiologically relevant features. A list of individual and environmental factors associated with previous exposure to viral pathogens is presented, highlighting the need for management actions for the improvement of health of dog populations and the urgent prevention of disease-induced mortality of already threatened Atlantic Forest's wild carnivores.

Methods

Ethics and consents

Sampling was performed under permission from the household head or other responsible person. Required licenses were obtained from the State Forest Institute – IEF (UC: 080/10, 081/10 and 082/10). The study was approved by the Ethics Commission on the Use of Animals of the Pontiphical Catholic University of Minas Gerais (CEUA, PUC Minas 037/2010). Regarding the collection of data from humans and households, our project was examined by the Ethics Research Committee (Comitê de Ética em Pesquisa) of the Pontiphical Catholic University of Minas Gerais (PUC-Minas). A term about the confidential character of the records was read in every household. Animal manipulation procedures adhered to the guidelines from the COBEA (Brazilian College of Animal Experimentation) and the Animal Ethics Committee of FIOCRUZ (Oswaldo Cruz Institute Foundation).

Study sites

We selected rural households located at less than two kilometres from borders of six protected areas in the remnant Atlantic Forest of the state of Minas Gerais, south-eastern Brazil. These areas were selected for the presence of a protected fragment surrounded by human-dominated agricultural matrices, and were divided for analyses into two size classes, comprising three state parks (henceforth referred as large areas): Serra do Brigadeiro (PESB, municipality of Araponga), Sete Salões (PESS, municipality of Santa Rita do Itueto), and Rio Doce (PERD, municipality of Dionísio), and three private reserves (henceforth referred as small areas): Fazenda Macedônia (RPPNFM, municipality of Ipaba), Feliciano Miguel Abdala (RPPNFMA, municipality of Caratinga), and Mata do Sossego (RPPNMS, municipality of Simonésia) (see Fig. 1 and Table 1). Several wild carnivore species were recorded in the areas, including wild canids such as the crab-eating fox (*Cerdocyon thous*) and the maned wolf (*Chrysocyon brachyurus*), felids such as the puma (*Puma concolor*) and small wild felids (*Leopardus* spp.), mustelids (*Eira barbara*, *Gallictis cuja*), and procyonids (*Nasua nasua*, *Procyon cancrivorous*). According to a concomitant camera-trap study, free-roaming domestic dogs, mostly those living in surrounding rural properties, are frequently visiting and actually occupying the interior of these areas [26]. They live as human-subsidized mixed-bred free-ranging

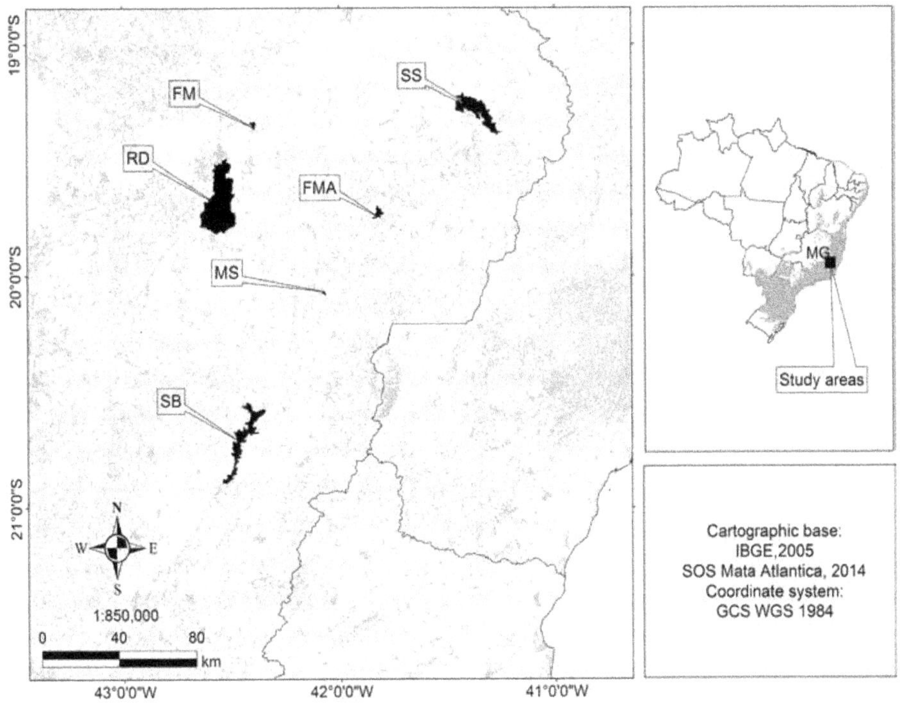

Fig. 1 Location of the study areas. SB: Serra do Brigadeiro State Park; SS: Sete Salões State Park; RD: Rio Doce State Park; FM: Fazenda Macedônia Private Reserve; FMA: Feliciano Miguel Abdala Private Reserve; MS: Mata do Sossego Private Reserve.

dog (host) populations distributed in small groups across the households and rural properties.

Questionnaire survey and blood sampling

Visits to the households, owner interviews and dog sampling were performed between January 2011 and August 2012. Every dog present at the households was aimed for data collection. Overall 320 dogs older than two months were sampled in 144 rural households. After permission from the owners, blood was collected under physical restraint from the jugular vein and a complete clinical examination of the dogs was performed by a veterinarian. A standardized questionnaire survey was administered to each owner. Factors related to animal management and behaviour that might be directly or indirectly associated with the exposure to viral agents were recorded for each household: number of dogs, mobility of dogs, access of dogs to the forest and villages, observed interactions between dogs and wildlife, recent dog disease or death, previous anti-rabies and multiple vaccination, veterinary assistance and the number of people. Individual and clinical features of dogs (sex, age, breed, sterilization, body condition, clinical alterations), which may influence behavioural patterns and pathogen exposure, were also obtained. Data were recorded in individual dog and per household files. Age of dogs was estimated through owner's information matched with dental development observation. Body condition of dogs was scored from 0

Table 1 Human and dog demographic characteristics at rural settlements around six protected areas of the Atlantic Forest of Minas Gerais State, southeast Brazil

Area (size in ha)	Distance from city (km)	Houses	Humans	Dogs	Dog:human ratio	Dogs per household
RPPNFM (3,343)	0.3	25	89	98	1.101	3.920
PESB (15,015)	3.3	31	125	86	0.688	2.774
PESS (13,370)	4.7	25	82	53	0.646	2.120
RPPNFMA (1,312)	10.5	18	53	60	1.132	3.333
RPPNMS (392)	7.7	25	102	49	0.480	1.960
PERD (36,100)	11	20	87	34	0.390	1.700
Total	-	144	538	380	0.706	2.638

(extreme emaciation) to 5 (extreme obesity). Refusals to the survey happened in six households, when the responsible person was absent.

Serological testing

Blood samples were allowed to clot for at least two hours at room temperature. Serum was extracted after centrifugation in the field, and stored at −20 °C until sent to the laboratory for antibody detection and titration through duplicated serological testing for canine parvovirus (CPV, hemagglutination inhibition, 1:20 dilution as cut-off point), canine distemper virus (CDV, serum neutralization, 1:8 dilution as cut-off point), canine coronavirus (CCV, serum neutralization, 1:2 dilution as cut-off point), and canine adenovirus type-2 (CAV, serum neutralization, 1:16 dilution as cut-off point). Cut-off points were set according to previous literature, and aimed to maximize the sensitivity of the tests [27–30]. Prevalence is referred henceforth as the proportion of animals with detectable antibodies for each pathogen and considered as an indicator of previous pathogen exposure in dogs. Titres are expressed here as the inverse of the highest positive dilution. Higher antibody titres may reflect more recent infections, larger antigenic burdens (i.e. exposure to higher viral loads) or continued exposition, but also stronger individual immune responses to exposure, which are also dependent on many factors including nutrition, stress and genetics.

Statistical analysis

Prevalence proportion ratios between grouped small versus large areas were compared through Yates-corrected chi square tests for each pathogen detected. Animals previously multiple-agent vaccination ($n = 19$) were excluded of the analysis to assess only natural viral circulation. Sex, breed, sterilization, mobility of dogs, access of dogs to the forest and villages, observed interactions between dogs and wildlife, recent dog disease or death, veterinary assistance and area size class (small and large areas) were used as binary or dummy variables. The continuous variables were age, body condition, number of dogs, and the number of people (which may act as fomites, for instance, for CDV and CPV [31, 32]) per household. Thus, fifteen variables were initially screened through univariate logistic regression tests with exposure status for each pathogen detected as the response variables.

All variables with a univariable test value of $P < 0.3$ were considered for subsequent inclusion in multivariable generalized linear mixed models (GLMM) with the exposure status for each pathogen as the response variables [33, 34]. Models were built with a manual backwards stepwise approach. Variables with lower P values were retained in the models until their exclusion resulted in a significant difference between subsequent models ($P < 0.05$). To select the best models we used the Akaike Information Criterion (AIC) values, and chose as candidate models those with $\Delta AIC < 2$ in relation to the model with lowest AIC. We accounted for site/area variation in the data by including area as a random factor in all models. Chi-square tests were performed with the software Bioestat 5.0, while logistic regressions and GLMM's were performed with the software R. We used the Strengthening the Reporting of Observational Studies in Epidemiology (STROBE) statement [35] as a guideline to report our data.

Results

Dog population and management traits

Relevant characteristics of sites, dog and human populations and the number of households sampled in each study area are described in Table 1. Males comprised 63.5 % (209/320) of dogs, thus sex ratio is male biased (1.88 males for each female). Only 21 dogs (6.5 %) are sterilized. Mixed bred dogs comprise 79.3 % (254/320) of the samples. Most dogs (78.4 %) are adult, with mean age of 3.3 years (39 months; range 3–216; mean 39.9 ± 36.05). Body condition scores are low in general (range 0.5–4, mean 2.1 ± 0.57).

Most dogs are allowed to roam freely, and only 10 % (33/320) live in restricted spaces as fenced or leashed dogs. Most dogs are reported to access near forests (249/320 or 77.8 %), and 30 % (96/320) have access to villages or small urban centres. Dog mortality or clinical disease in previous two years is reported by owners of 43 % and 31 % of dogs, respectively, but only four dogs show clinical symptoms compatible with viral disease (diarrhoea and ocular secretion) at the time of collection. Anti-rabies vaccination was performed in 85 % (261/320) of dogs, but multiple-disease vaccines (protective for the pathogens studied here) were applied in only 6 % (19/320) of dogs. Most dogs (53 %; 170/320) sampled are reported as having interacted with some wildlife species. Only 25 dogs (8 %) receive veterinary assistance throughout their lives. Most owners (63 %) feed their dogs with human leftovers, which were mostly protein-poor mixtures. Commercial dog food is provided in 39 %, and milk alone in 6 % of houses. In some households, combinations of commercial dog food plus milk (3.4 %) or leftovers (14 %) are used to feed dogs. Other items reported include milk whey and minced corn.

Prevalence and titre frequency profile

Prevalence per study area is summarized in Table 2. Almost 85 % (320 of 380) of resident dogs were sampled. Antibodies against CPV, CDV and CAV were detected with a prevalence of 97 %, 15 %, and 27.8 %, respectively. Antibodies against CCV were not detected in our samples. The three former agents were detected in all six areas, except for CDV antibodies that are absent in dogs

Table 2 Prevalence (in bold) for canine parvovirus (CPV), canine distemper virus (CDV), and canine adenovirus (CAV) in dogs sampled in the rural zone surrounding Atlantic Forest fragments in Brazil

Area	Dogs	Sampled	% sampled	CPV +	%	CDV +	%	CAV+	%
RPPNFM	98	84	85.7	83	**98.8**	25	**29.7**	28	**33.3**
PESB	86	67	77.9	65	**97.0**	11	**16.4**	15	**22.4**
PESS	53	47	88.6	47	**100**	2	**4.2**	9	**19.1**
RPPNFMA	60	49	81.6	49	**100**	0	**0**	11	**22.4**
RPPNMS	49	41	83.6	41	**100**	8	**19.5**	7	**17.1**
PERD	34	32	94.1	26	**81.2**	2	**6.2**	19	**59.3**
Total	380	320	84.2	311	**97.2**	48	**15**	89	**27.8**

from RPPNFMA. According to chi square test results, CPV is more prevalent in small areas (173/174, 99 %) than in larger areas (138/146, 94 %) ($p = 0.004$). Accordingly, more CDV positive dogs are present in small than in large areas (33/174 or 19 %, and 15/146 or 10 %, respectively; $p = 0.015$). CAV prevalence do not differ between large and smaller areas (46/174 or 26 %, and 43/146 or 29 %, respectively; $p = 0.27$).

Titre frequency distributions for the pathogens detected are depicted in Fig. 2. Most samples have high antibody titres for CPV (>160) and for CAV (>64), but for CDV most positive samples have relatively lower titres.

Risk factor analysis

Associated variables with significance values below the fixed threshold ($P < 0.3$) in the univariate screening tests are listed in Table 3. Regarding multivariable analyses, the best CAV model included sex, age of dogs, number of people, interaction with wildlife, and access to villages as significant associations. However, sex, age, number of people and access to villages were present in all candidate models. CDV best model included age of dogs, body score, access to forest and number of people per household. Age and number of people were retained in all candidate models. For CPV, four variables were retained in the best model as significantly associated with exposure: dog mobility, recent dog disease, veterinary assistance, and area size class. Mobility and veterinary assistance figured in all candidate models. Results are summarized in Table 4.

Discussion

Frequent contact with domestic dogs increases the exposure and disease risk for wild carnivores [8, 36]. Therefore, local pet management practices allowing dog's predominantly free-roaming habits, poor veterinary assistance, along with recent dog death and disease reports and the low multiple vaccination coverage detected *per se* place the wild carnivores at the study sites in a potentially dangerous scenario of disease spill over (or spillback) from dogs.

Exposure patterns and antibody titre profile

Exposure to most pathogens tested is widespread throughout the study sites, and prevalence is widespread and moderate to high, particularly for CPV. It must be noted that CDV and CPV have higher fatality rates than do CAV and CCV milder infections [31, 32, 37]. Fatality rate may impact prevalence by removing exposed individuals from the population and this can result in the low prevalence observed here, for instance, for CDV. Also, prevalence of CDV might be low in these areas because a 'wave of infection' could have passed through the area in the past, and recent circulation of this virus may not have occurred regularly [9].

Regarding antibody titre frequency and duration of immunity, mostly high levels of antibodies against CPV and CAV were found. The duration of antibodies to the viral agents studied here is longer than two years [38], and such titres may indicate that the exposure to these agents is mostly recent. However, as said before, it is not possible to accurately determine the timing of exposure from antibody titres, and our cross-sectional serological approach does not permit deeper inferences on temporal-spatial dynamics of exposure neither detects pathogen introduction or seroconversion events.

Prevalence comparisons between small and large protected areas

Proportionally more CDV and CPV-exposed dogs were found in small areas. Perhaps the reduced perimeter of these areas allows less space between properties and households, and ensures higher host densities, contact rates and exposure (including environmental) to these agents. Therefore, small areas should be prioritized in health improvement efforts for rural dogs aiming also to prevent wildlife disease-associated mortality in the Atlantic Forest, which is currently mostly composed by relatively small remnants [39].

Risk factor modelling

Of fifteen initially assessed variables, thirteen entered multivariate tests, and eleven remained as significant

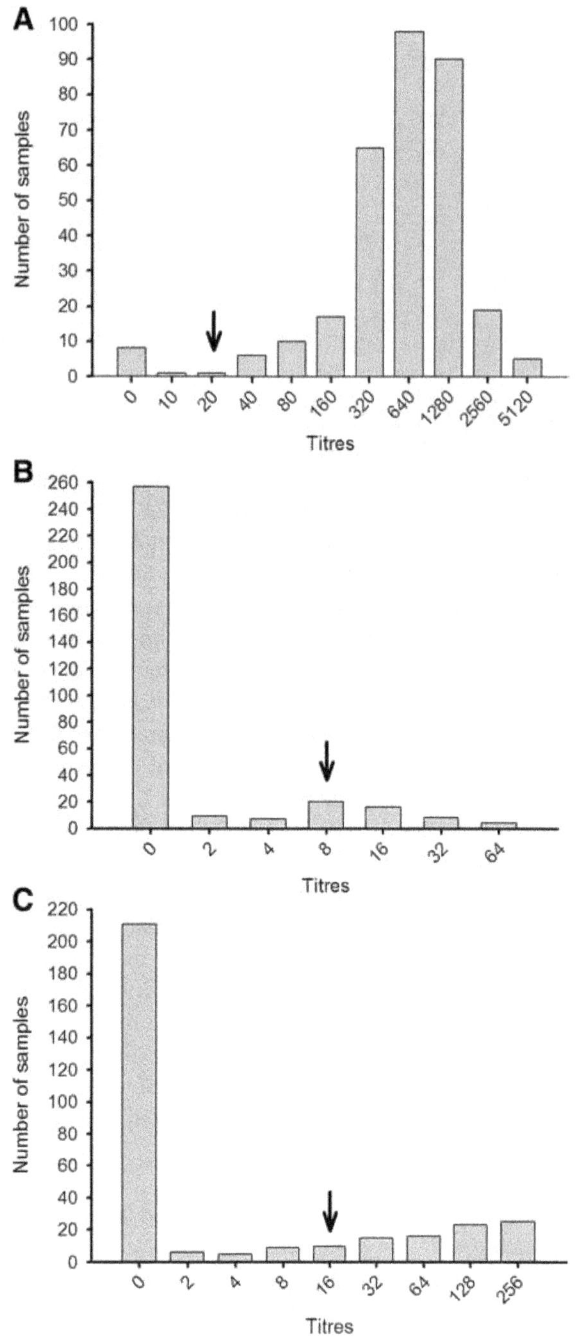

Fig. 2 Titre frequency distributions for CPV (**a**), CDV (**b**) and CAV (**c**) in domestic dogs living around protected areas of the Atlantic Forest in Minas Gerais, Brazil (2011 to 2012). Cut-off points are indicated by arrows

associations with exposure for at least one pathogen in the best models: sex, age, body score, mobility, veterinary assistance, number of people per household, interaction with wildlife, recent disease in dogs, area size class and access to villages and forests. However, one must account for associated bias due to issues with

Table 3 Univariate regression analysis results for variables associated with canine adenovirus (CAV), canine distemper virus (CDV) and canine parvovirus (CPV) status in unvaccinated dogs sampled in the rural zone surrounding Atlantic Forest fragments in Brazil

Pathogen/variables	Odds ratio	95 % CI	P value
CAV			
Sex (female)	1.617	0.927–2.90	0.09
Age	1.014	1.007–1.021	6.48×10^{-5}
Body score	1.599	1.013–2.554	0.045
Number of people	1.13	0.95–1.359	0.16
Access to villages	3.806	2.221–6.575	1.3×10^{-6}
Recent dog mortality	1.457	0.868–2.445	0.153
Interaction with wildlife	0.619	0.367–1.036	0.069
CDV			
Sex (female)	0.676	0.355–1.304	0.235
Age	1.009	1–1.016	0.024
Body score	1.756	1.001–3.11	0.05
Number of people	1.395	1.121–1.746	0.003
Number of dogs	1.120	0.996–1.252	0.048
Access to forest	3.190	1.225–10.927	0.033
Recent dog disease	1.501	0.763–2.883	0.22
Area size class	0.515	0.255–0.997	0.05
CPV			
Mobility	18.266	3.786–98.234	0.0002
Access to forest	5.092	1.09–26.42	0.036
Recent dog mortality	4.562	0.766–86.747	0.16
Recent dog disease	0.165	0.023–0.783	0.033
Interaction with wildlife	2.75	0.582–19.415	0.231
Veterinary assistance	0.076	0.015–0.41	0.001
Area size class	0.12	0.006–0.765	0.05

Only variables with significance below the threshold ($P < 0.3$) are shown

missing controls in an observational prevalence study when interpreting data for risk factor detection, and there might be biologically relevant putative causalities out of the full set of factors presented. Moreover, the statistical associations found do not necessarily imply direct causation.

Canine parvovirus

High levels of circulation indicated by the high prevalence of exposure indicate that CPV is perhaps one of the most dangerous agents in this scenario. It is one of the most commonly reported canine viral agents worldwide [3, 31], including in South American wild canids (e.g.) [16, 18, 19]. High prevalence was concomitantly observed in wild and domestic canids from two protected areas [18, 19] in the same state of the present study, although in the Cerrado Biome. CPV infection

Table 4 Generalized linear mixed modelling of factors associated with canine adenovirus (CAV), canine distemper virus (CDV) and canine parvovirus (CPV) exposure status of unvaccinated dogs sampled in the rural zone surrounding Atlantic Forest fragments, Brazil

Model	Variables	AIC	Δ AIC
CAV	Null	349.00	
Model 6	Age + city	315.73	3.71
Model 5	Age + people + city	314.46	2.44
Model 4	**Sex + age + people + city**	**312.78**	**0.76**
Model 3[a]	**Sex + age + people + city + fauna**	**312.02**	**0**
Model 2	**Sex + age + people + city + death + fauna**	**312.23**	**0.21**
Model 1	**Sex + age + score + people + city + death + fauna**	**312.98**	**0.96**
CDV	Null	241.00	
Model 7	**Age + people**	**232.13**	**1.10**
Model 6	**Age + people + forest**	**231.29**	**0.26**
Model 5[a]	**Age + score + people + forest**	**231.03**	**0**
Model 4	**Sex + age + score + people + forest**	**231.92**	**0.89**
Model 3	Sex + age + score + people + forest + size	233.69	2.66
Model 2	Sex + age + score + people + forest + sick + size	235.23	4.2
Model 1	Sex + age + score + people + dogs + forest + sick + size	237.23	6.2
CPV	Null	65.70	
Model 6	**Mob + vet**	**56.15**	**1.34**
Model 5	**Mob + sick + vet**	**54.82**	**0.2**
Model 4[a]	**Mob + sick + vet + size**	**54.80**	**0**
Model 3	Mob + forest + sick + vet + size	56.53	2.27
Model 2	Mob + forest + death + sick + vet + size	58.36	3.56
Model 1	Mob + forest + death + sick + fauna + vet + size	60.32	5.51

Models with the lowest AIC values were considered as best fit ([a]) and models with Δ AIC < 2 were considered as candidate models (in bold)
Score = body score, people = number of people, city = access to villages, death = recent dog mortality, fauna = interaction with wildlife, dogs = number of dogs, forest = access to forest, sick = recent dog disease, size = area size class, mob = mobility, vet = veterinary assistance

has proven capable to cause serious population impacts (mostly through pup mortality) in wild carnivores, for instance, grey wolves (*Canis lupus*) [6]. However, our cross-sectional approach does not distinguish epidemic from endemic states. For instance, a CDV epidemic that might blow through these mostly susceptible dog populations might also cause high dog mortality and interspecific transmission that can be dangerous for wild carnivores as well.

The modelling shows that unassisted dogs that roam freely have more chances of exposure for CPV. This is explained by higher contact rates with diseased animals and enhanced environmental exposure due to the great environmental resistance of this virus [31], therefore dog restriction must be enforced around protected areas. Dogs that never received veterinary care were also more prone to exposure, and this emphasizes the role of veterinarians in health promotion and maintenance at human/wildlife interfaces. Other factors appearing in candidate models (recent dog disease and area size class) indicate that CPV may be causing significant morbidity in the study sites, and that small reserves require priority for the control of the disease.

Canine distemper

Canine distemper is a systemic highly fatal disease, representing a major conservation concern around the globe [3, 32]. Evidence of infection in dogs is widespread in and around South American protected areas [18, 20, 22, 23]. Antibodies against distemper were already found in Brazilian wild felids and canids (e.g.)[17, 19], and there are reports of distemper-induced mortality in two Brazilian fox species, the crab-eating fox *C. thous* and the hoary fox *Lycalopex vetulus* [14, 15]. In Chile, domestic dogs have proven blamed for the transmission of CDV to wild canids [9]. However, CDV transmission may be, in some cases, predominantly maintained by wild reservoirs [4, 32, 36].

In our rural settings, age, body score, number of people in the household and access to forests were mostly associated with CDV prevalence. However, only age and the number of people appeared in all candidate models. Older animals might have had more chances of exposure events throughout their lives. However, since CDV is a highly lethal disease [32], the low prevalence and the age effect observed suggest that CDV seropositive animals may be survivors of a past wave of infection in some of the study areas. The number of people cohabiting households was positively associated with CDV seropositivity. This raises the possibility of fomite transmission, mentioned in the literature as a mode of spread of this highly infectious virus which is mainly transmitted by contact or aerosols [32]. Male dogs may be at higher risk of exposure, probably because of their more aggressive and roaming behaviours [40]. Higher body scores may also favour dog free-roaming behaviours and ensuring both exposure and antibody response to the virus, which, according to the presence of the access to forests among risk factors, might be occurring when dogs walk inside forested areas. As said before, CDV can be maintained in wild reservoir species alone [4, 36].

Canine adenovirus

Mostly unstudied, CAV is also capable to cause damage to wildlife populations [3], although its impact is still unknown. This directly transmitted virus may cause severe respiratory disease being of concern for domestic dog health, and evidence of exposure was found in many wild species [37] including in South American wild carnivores and sympatric dogs from Bolivia [16, 23] and Brazil [18, 19].

For CAV, female sex, age, number of people and access to villages entered all selected models. Females are more exposed to CAV, and this is probably related to behavioural differences, as females tend to display less roaming and aggressive behaviours [40], and thus, spend relatively more time around their homes in rural and urban settings, leading to host aggregation and enhancement of the density-dependent transmission of CAV. The explanation for increasing prevalence with age is that older dogs probably had moved more through time and faced more opportunities for contact and exposure to CAV, and this is expected since older animals tend to have more opportunities of infection when disease-induced mortality is low or infections are often fatal [40]. The association with the number of people in the households reinforces the questioning about the fomite spreading of canine viruses in rural environments. However, this is not mentioned as a CAV transmission mode [37]. The access to villages was a strongly associated factor, appearing in all candidate models. Urban settings hold higher-density dog populations [1], what enhances the maintenance and transmission of the density-dependent CAV [37]. Therefore, such freedom of rural dog movement must be prevented in order to reduce exposure and infection by CAV in near urban areas and subsequent spillover to wild species. Recently, data from the same state showed that free-roaming behaviours (e.g. hunting) are among risk factors for canine neosporosis [11]. Additionally, recent mortality in dogs may be associated with CAV infection in the study sites. Dogs with higher body scores may have survived past infection waves and sustained the mostly low antibody levels found. Interactions with wildlife may also be increasing the risk for CAV. However we cannot infer whether the main reservoirs are domestic or wild animals. Nevertheless, the free-ranging behaviour of dogs must be inhibited through fence or leash restraining in order to reduce contact rates and opportunities for general pathogen exposure and transmission in rural/wild interface areas.

Preventive aspects

Although we did not test the samples against rabies, our survey revealed that despite the apparently good previous vaccination coverage (more than 80 %), several owners reported the total absence or the periodic lack of visits of health agencies promoting vaccination against rabies in their households in some years. Canine-mediated rabies is a multi-species highly fatal disease, representing a major problem for carnivore conservation particularly in Africa [3]. In Brazil there are domestic animal rabies control programmes through vaccination since the 1980's, and reports of wildlife mortality have been attributed to the disease. Additionally, serological evidence of exposure was already found in Brazilian carnivore species [41]. Therefore, more attention should be given to rabies in wildlife-domestic animal interfaces, and the vaccination programme should be reinforced so as to continuously warrant good coverage in these areas.

In our scenario, dogs with a history of vaccination against agents other than rabies, which are not cost-free, may be an indicator of increased owner care. Better care for the dog would result in better physical and immunologic condition, and better supportive care and veterinary care in times of illness. Those healthier animals will be more likely to survive an illness, and a higher survival rate would lead to a greater proportion of seropositive dogs. Unfortunately, the mostly unvaccinated dogs in these populations may be less likely to receive a high level of owner care. Lack of owner care may result in lower probability of supportive or veterinary care when ill, and an overall decrease in animal health. Poor health and lack of veterinary care would result in a higher death rate in the result of an illness. A higher death rate would remove exposed animals from the population. Therefore, unvaccinated dogs may have less supportive care from owners, which would lead to higher death rates in the face of illness, which would lead to artificial decline in the measured population proportion of seropositives, as may be the case for CDV in this study. However, our data set does not permit such distinction, and we acknowledge the uncertainty about these relationships.

Commercial multiple vaccines against CDV, CPV, CAV, CCV and other canine pathogens are available in the region. However, owner unawareness added to the relatively prohibitive costs of vaccines, and the fact that such intervention may seem directed solely to protect the health of dogs make multiple-agent vaccination of dogs a lesser priority for the mostly low-income rural families, as shown by the low percentage of vaccinated dogs in this study. We are unaware of the use of other possible cross-reactive vaccines, such as those using adenovirus as a vector, in the area. This means that multiple vaccination have to be reinforced, even though with a more flexible and viable interval in these areas [38], if the aim is to induce protective herd immunity against other dangerous pathogens in dogs from wildlife-rich areas. Vaccination schemes for dogs around protected areas, directing to protect wild carnivore and human welfare has proven successful [42], notably with concomitant low coverage vaccination of wildlife species [5]. In our case, the dog population living in proximity of protected area borders should be targeted in comprehensive multiple-agent vaccination schemes. Vaccination of dogs can improve the collective immune status or herd immunity necessary to avoid or decrease the transmission of some agents. However, as pointed out by some authors, vaccination of naturally exposed populations may not be of great value for highly prevalent pathogens [10], and this may be the case for CPV in our study area. Nonetheless, the transmission of lower local prevalence pathogens such as CDV and CAV may be successfully limited by dog vaccination in this case. Decreasing dog numbers is also necessary to keep the population below transmission thresholds of most directly transmitted canine pathogens, and this can be achieved through sterilization and education campaigns. According to our results, prohibiting dogs from moving across the interface and spreading or acquiring pathogens is essential for disease prevention, and responsible ownership reinforcement alongside with legal penalties for irresponsible owners is highly recommended. Health monitoring should, afterwards, be continuously performed in both domestic and wildlife species, to assess the efficacy of the proposed measures.

Conclusions

This study represents the first attempt to detect pathogens of concern for carnivore conservation in dogs living in rural settlements around Atlantic forest fragments, and to reveal associated factors that can be managed to improve domestic dog's health and consequently protect wild carnivores from disease-induced population declines in these areas, even though local wildlife health status is unknown. Fortunately in this case, interventions should be directed to the human component of the system. The management involving human behaviour related to domestic animal management is more easily tractable [43] and might decrease successfully dog-to-dog and dog-to-wildlife disease transmission without relevant side effects. Some of the risk factors shown are linked to poverty, which in turn is associated with poor domestic dog health [44]. Therefore, programs involving the improvement of life quality for local human populations may warrant better domestic animal care and health. It also meets conservation goals to reduce unwanted dog-wildlife interactions such as predation, competition and harassment [1, 2]. Restriction of dog space and movements, control of the reservoir population through sterilization, and proper vaccination programmes are among required measures for the purpose. Finally, the study have generated some interesting hypothesis that can be further tested, and provided a confirmatory set of information that enhances the understanding of natural viral exposure patterns in rural (and mostly free-roaming) dog populations and of processes linked to disease transmission at human-domestic animal-wildlife interfaces.

Abbreviations

CAV: canine Adenovirus; CCV: canine Coronavirus; CDV: canine Distemper Virus; CPV: canine Parvovirus; PERD: Rio Doce State Park; PESB: Serra do Brigadeiro State Park; PESS: Sete Salões State Park; RPPNFM: Fazenda Macedônia Private Reserve; RPPNFMA: Feliciano Miguel Abdala Private Reserve; RPPNMS: Mata do Sossego Private Reserve; STROBE: strengthening the reporting of observational studies in epidemiology.

Competing interests

The authors declare that they have no competing interests.

Authors' contributions

NHAC, AGC, MP contributed to the conception, design, data collection, data analysis, drafting and writing of the manuscript. ASA and ZIPL contributed to laboratory work and drafting of the manuscript. GRD contributed for data analysis and drafting of the manuscript. AMOP and RLM contributed to the study design, data collection and manuscript drafting. All authors have read and approved the final manuscript.

Acknowledgements

The authors wish to thank IEF (State Forest Institute) for licences conceded. Especially, thanks to the household owners and the park staffs from our study areas for their hospitality and help in the field work. This work was supported by Brazilian research agencies, with scholarships from CAPES for three of the authors (NHAC, RLM and AMOP), and financial support for the field and lab work from CNPQ (472802/2010-0) and FAPEMIG (APQ-01145-10). Thanks to Jos Barlow for English revision.

Author details

[1]Postgraduate Programme in Applied Ecology, Department of Biology, Federal University of Lavras, Lavras, Brazil. [2]Postgraduate Programme in Ecology, Conservation and Management of Wildlife, Department of Biology, Institute of Biological Sciences, Federal University of Minas Gerais, Belo Horizonte, Brazil. [3]Laboratory of Viral Diseases, Department of Preventive Veterinary Medicine, School of Veterinary Medicine, Federal University of Minas Gerais, Belo Horizonte, Brazil. [4]Department of Biology, University of São Paulo, Ribeirão Preto, Brazil.

References

1. Gompper ME. Free-ranging dogs and wildlife conservation. Oxford: Oxford University Press; 2014.
2. Hughes J, Macdonald DW. A review of the interactions between free-roaming domestic dogs and wildlife. Biol Conserv. 2013;157:341–51.
3. Knobel DL, Butler JR, Lembo T, Critchlow R, Gompper ME. Dogs, disease, and wildlife. In: Gompper ME, editor. Free-ranging dogs and wildlife conservation. Oxford: Oxford University Press; 2014. p. 144–69.
4. Viana M, Cleaveland S, Matthiopoulos J, Halliday J, Packer C, Craft ME, et al. Dynamics of a morbillivirus at the domestic–wildlife interface: Canine distemper virus in domestic dogs and lions. Proc Natl Acad Sci. 2015;112:1464–9.
5. Haydon DT, Randall DA, Matthews L, Knobel DL, Tallents LA, Gravenor MB, et al. Low-coverage vaccination strategies for the conservation of endangered species. Nature. 2006;443:692–5.
6. Mech LD, Goyal SM, Paul WJ, Newton WE. Demographic effects of canine parvovirus on a free-ranging wolf population over 30 years. J Wildl Dis. 2008;44:824–36.
7. Müller A, Silva E, Santos N, Thompson G. Domestic dog origin of canine distemper virus in free-ranging wolves in Portugal as revealed by hemagglutinin gene characterization. J Wildl Dis. 2011;47:725–9.
8. Woodroffe R, Prager KC, Munson L, Conrad PA, Dubovi EJ, Mazet JA. Contact with domestic dogs increases pathogen exposure in endangered African wild dogs (*Lycaon pictus*). PLoS One. 2012;7:e30099.
9. Acosta-Jamett G, Chalmers WSK, Cunningham AA, Cleaveland S, Handel IG, Bronsvoort BM. Urban domestic dog populations as a source of canine distemper virus for wild carnivores in the Coquimbo region of Chile. Vet Microbiol. 2011;152:247–57.
10. Belsare AV, Vanak AT, Gompper ME. Epidemiology of viral pathogens of free-ranging dogs and Indian foxes in a human-dominated landscape in central India. Transbound Emerg Dis. 2014;61(s1):78–86.
11. Nogueira CI, Mesquita LP, Abreu CC, Nakagaki KYR, Seixas JN, Bezerra Jr PS, et al. Risk factors associated with seroprevalence of *Neospora caninum* in dogs from urban and rural areas of milk and coffee production in Minas Gerais state Brazil. Epidemiol Infect. 2013;141:2286–93.
12. Jones KE, Patel NG, Levy MA, Storeygard A, Balk D, Gittleman JL, et al. Global trends in emerging infectious diseases. Nature. 2008;451:990–3.
13. Cleaveland S, Meslin FX, Breiman R. Dogs can play useful role as sentinel hosts for disease. Nature. 2006;440:605.
14. Megid J, de Souza VAF, Teixeira CR, Cortez A, Amorin RL, Heinemman MB, et al. Canine distemper virus in a crab-eating fox (*Cerdocyon thous*) in Brazil: case report and phylogenetic analyses. J Wildl Dis. 2009;45:527–30.
15. Megid J, Teixeira CR, Amorin RL, Cortez A, Heinemann MB, Antunes JMAP, et al. First identification of canine distemper virus in hoary fox (*Lycalopex vetulus*): pathologic aspects and virus phylogeny. J Wildl Dis. 2010;46:303–5.
16. Fiorello CV, Noss AJ, Deem SL, Maffei L, Dubovi EJ. Serosurvey of small carnivores in the Bolivian Chaco. J Wildl Dis. 2007;43:551–7.
17. Nava AFD, Cullen Jr L, Sana DA, Nardi MS, Filho JDR, Lima TF, et al. First evidence of canine distemper in Brazilian free-ranging felids. Ecohealth. 2008;5:513–8.
18. Curi NHA, Araújo AS, Campos FS, Lobato ZIP, Gennari SM, Marvulo MFV, et al. Wild canids, domestic dogs and their pathogens in Southeast Brazil: disease threats for canid conservation. Biodiv Conserv. 2010;19:3513–24.
19. Curi NHA, Coelho CM, Malta MDCC, Magni EMV, Sábato MAL, Araújo AS, et al. Pathogens of wild maned wolves (*Chrysocyon brachyurus*) in Brazil. J Wildl Dis. 2012;48:1052–6.
20. Fiorello CV, Deem SL, Gompper ME, Dubovi EJ. Seroprevalence of pathogens in domestic carnivores on the border of Madidi National Park Bolivia. Anim Conserv. 2004;7:45–54.
21. Fiorello CV, Noss AJ, Deem SL. Demography, hunting ecology, and pathogen exposure of domestic dogs in the Isoso of Bolivia. Conserv Biol. 2006;20:762–71.
22. Whiteman CW, Matushima ER, Confalonieri UEC, Palha MDDC, Silva ADSL, Monteiro VC. Human and domestic animal populations as a potential threat to wild carnivore conservation in a fragmented landscape from the Eastern Brazilian Amazon. Biol Conserv. 2007;138:290–6.
23. Bronson E, Emmons LH, Murray S, Dubovi EJ, Deem SL. Serosurvey of pathogens in domestic dogs on the border of Noel Kempff Mercado National Park Bolivia. J Zoo Wildl Med. 2008;39:28–36.
24. Sepúlveda MA, Singer RS, Silva-Rodríguez E, Stowhas P, Pelican K. Domestic dogs in rural communities around protected areas: conservation problem or conflict solution? PLoS One. 2015;9:e86152.
25. Acosta-Jamett G, Surot D, Cortes M, Marambio V, Valenzuela C, Vallverdu A, et al. Epidemiology of canine distemper and canine parvovirus in domestic dogs in urban and rural areas of the Araucanía region in Chile. Vet Microbiol. 2015;178:260–4.
26. Paschoal AM, Massara RL, Santos JL, Chiarello AG. Is the domestic dog becoming an abundant species in the Atlantic Forest? A study case in southeastern Brazil. Mammalia. 2012;76:67–76.
27. Appel M, Robson DS. A microneutralization test for canine distemper virus. Am J Vet Res. 1973;34:1459–63.
28. Appel M, Carmichael LE, Robson DS. Canine adenovirus type-2 induced immunity to two canine adenoviruses in pups with maternal antibody. Am J Vet Res. 1975;36:1199–202.
29. Senda M, Hirayama N, Yamamoto H, Kurata K. An improved hemagglutination test for study of canine parvovirus. Vet Microbiol. 1986;12:1–6.
30. Mochizuki M, Sugiura R, Akuzawa M. Micro-neutralization test with canine coronavirus for detection of coronavirus antibodies in dogs and cats. Jpn J Vet Sci. 1987;49:563–5.
31. Steinel A, Parrish CR, Bloom ME, Truyen U. Parvovirus infections in wild carnivores. J Wildl Dis. 2001;37:594–607.
32. Deem SL, Spelman LH, Yates RA, Montali RJ. Canine distemper in terrestrial carnivores: a review. J Zoo Wildl Med. 2000;31:441–51.
33. Godsall SA, Clegg SR, Stavisky JH, Radford AD, Pinchbeck G. Epidemiology of canine parvovirus and coronavirus in dogs presented with severe diarrhoea to PDSA PetAid hospitals. Vet Rec. 2010;167:196–201.
34. Dohoo I, Martin W, Stryhn H. Veterinary epidemiologic research. Edward Island: AVC Inc., University of Prince Island; 2003.
35. von Elm E, Altman DG, Egger M, Pocock SJ, Gøtzsche PC, Vandenbroucke JP. The strengthening the reporting of observational studies in epidemiology (STROBE) statement: guidelines for reporting observational studies. Bull WHO. 2007;85:867–72.
36. Prager KC, Mazet JA, Munson L, Cleaveland S, Donnelly CA, Dubovi EJ, et al. The effect of protected areas on pathogen exposure in endangered African wild dog (*Lycaon pictus*) populations. Biol Conserv. 2012;150:15–22.
37. Buonavoglia C, Martella V. Canine respiratory viruses. Vet Res. 2007;38:355–73.
38. Schultz RD. Duration of immunity for canine and feline vaccines: a review. Vet Microbiol. 2006;117:75–9.
39. Ribeiro MC, Metzger JP, Martensen AC, Ponzoni FJ, Hirota MM. The Brazilian Atlantic Forest: how much is left, and how is the remaining forest distributed? Implications for conservation. Biol Conserv. 2009;142:1141–53.
40. Cross PC, Drewe J, Patrek V, Pearce G, Samuel MD, Delahay RJ. Wildlife population structure and parasite transmission: implications for disease management. In: Delahay RJ, Smith GC, Hutchings MR, editors. Management of disease in wild mammals. Tokio: Springer; 2009. p. 9–29.
41. Jorge RSP, Pereira MS, Morato RG, Scheffer KC, Carnieli Jr P, Ferreira F, et al. Detection of rabies virus antibodies in Brazilian free-ranging wild carnivores. J Wildl Dis. 2010;46:1310–5.
42. Cleaveland S, Kaare M, Knobel D, Laurenson MK. Canine vaccination – providing broader benefits for disease control. Vet Microbiol. 2006;117:43–50.
43. Delahay RJ, Smith GC, Hutchings MR. The science of wildlife disease management. In: Delahay RJ, Smith GC, Hutchings MR, editors. Management of disease in wild mammals. Tokio: Springer; 2009. p. 1–8.
44. Fung HL, Calzada J, Saldaña A, Santamaria AM, Pineda V, Gonzalez K, et al. Domestic dog health worsens with socio-economic deprivation of their home communities. Acta Trop. 2014;135:67–74.

7

Development and application of an indirect enzyme-linked immunosorbent assay based on recombinant capsid protein for the detection of mink circovirus infection

Junwei Ge[1,3], Xingyang Cui[1], Yunjia Shi[1], Lili Zhao[2], Chengwei Wei[1], Shanshan Wen[1], Shuang Xia[1] and Hongyan Chen[2*]

Abstract

Background: Mink circovirus (MiCV) is a newly discovered pathogen associated with mink diarrhea. The prevalence and economic importance of this virus remain poorly understood, and no specific serological assay has been developed for the diagnosis of MiCV infection.

Results: In this study, a recombinant capsid protein antigen expressed in *Escherichia coli* was utilized to establish an indirect enzyme-linked immunosorbent assay (iELISA). Results revealed that the assay had no cross-reactivity with other related pathogens, and the respective sensitivity and specificity of the proposed iELISA were 92.31% and 91.67% compared with those obtained of Western blot on 138 serum samples from minks. The correlation coefficient between iELISA and Western blot was 0.838 ($p > 0.05$). iELISA was applied to detect MiCV antibodies in 683 clinical serum samples from different farms from the major mink industry province in China, and 21 of 24 farms with 163 of 683 (23.87%) individuals were tested positive for MiCV antibodies. The positive rates of each of the 21 flocks ranged from 2.33% to 73.68%.

Conclusions: These results indicated that iELISA was a sensitive and specific method suitable for the large-scale detection of MiCV infections in mink. This study provided an effective method for the serological diagnosis and positive rate investigation of MiCV infection.

Keywords: Mink circovirus, Capsid protein, Prokaryotic expression, Indirect ELISA, Serological survey

Background

Mink circovirus (MiCV) is a newly discovered virus originally reported in 26 six- to ten-month-old minks with diarrhea from three farms in Dalian, China [1]. MiCV is a member of *Circovirus* belonging to the *Circoviridae* family. MiCVs are single-stranded circular DNA viruses with a genome of 1753 nucleotides, which contain two major open reading frames (ORF). One is ORF1, which encodes a replicase-associated protein (rep) required for viral replication. The other is ORF2, which encodes proteins that form the viral capsid (cap) and participate in host immune responses. Circoviruses have been identified in numerous species associated with various clinical disorders [2, 3], including asymptomatic infections and lethal diseases [4, 5]. Circovirus infections are also related to lymphoid depletion and immunosuppression, which likely increase the severity of secondary infection [6].

Epidemiological studies have provided evidence that MiCV is endemic in some mink farms in China [7]. However, the pathogenic role of MiCV in single or polymicrobial infections is unclear, and the prevalence and economic importance of this virus remain unknown. Therefore, a rapid and sensitive diagnosis assay or tool of the virus is essential for disease management and epidemiological surveillance.

* Correspondence: chenhongyan@caas.cn
[2]Laboratory Animal and Comparative Medicine Unit, Harbin Veterinary Research Institute, The Chinese Academy of Agricultural Sciences, No. 678 Haping Rd, Harbin 150069, China
Full list of author information is available at the end of the article

Conventional Polymerase Chain Reaction (PCR) can detect MiCV [8]. Although PCR has been used to identify MiCV infections, other methods that can detect virus-specific antibodies in serum are more convenient for large-scale epidemiological investigations. Serological methods for the identification of antibodies against MiCV infection in mink farms have yet to be reported. Antigens based on virus isolation for MiCV diagnosis have yet to be prepared because there is no report about cell system to culture MiCV.

Our study developed a sensitive, specific, and convenient indirect enzyme-linked immunosorbent assay (iELISA) utilizing the recombinant capsid protein (rCap) of MiCV expressed in *E. coli* as a coating antigen. The proposed iELISA was strongly immunoreactive to MiCV-specific serum and had no cross-reactivity with other related pathogens. This assay was validated by comparing the obtained results with those of Western blot. The applications of the proposed assay for clinical detection were also described.

Methods

Blood samples

Rehabilitation sera collected from a MiCV infection case were used as MiCV-positive mink sera. This infection caused acute gastroenteritis, and the clinical signs observed in the mink included severe diarrhea, vomiting, lethargy, anorexia, dehydration, and rough fur. Common enteric bacterial, protozoan, and viral pathogens, including *Salmonella* spp., *Clostridium* spp., *Campylobacter* spp., Shiga toxin-producing *E. coli*, enterotoxigenic *E. coli*, *Coccidium* spp., *Cryptosporidium* spp., mink aleutian disease virus (AMDV), canine distemper virus (CDV), mink enteritis virus (MEV), caliciviruses, rotaviruses, coronaviruses, and astroviruses, were excluded as causative agents, and MiCV was subsequently identified as the possible cause of the disease.

Sixty healthy minks were sampled from a MiCV-free farm to represent negative control mink sera. The MiCV-free farm was selected on the basis of prior negative testing with PCR once a year for the last 3 years.

A total of 138 serum samples were selected blindly from a pool of sera collected from healthy, diseased, or dead minks in more than 30 mink farms in Heilongjiang and submitted in 2008–2012. These samples were then tested and compared with ELISA tests. All of the serum samples were stored at −20 °C until use.

This study was performed in accordance with the recommendations in the Guide for the Care and Use of Laboratory Animals of the Ministry of Health, China. Prior to experiments, the protocol of the current study was reviewed and approved by the Institutional Animal Care and Use Committee of Northeast Agricultural University (approved protocol number 2014-SRM-24).

Expression, purification, and identification of the rCap protein

The MiCV HEB15 strain in this study was obtained previously by our team (GenBank accession No. KX268345) and used as the template in our current study. The gene encoding the Cap protein was amplified from the total viral DNA through PCR with the forward primer 5'-CGGGATCCGGCGGTTACAGATGGCG-3' and the reverse primer 5'-ACCTCGAGAGTTTGCTTTGGGA-3'. The amplified cap gene was subcloned into the *Bam*HI and *Xho*I sites of the prokaryotic expression vector pET-32a in a frame with an amino terminal six-histidine tag. Recombinant plasmids designated as pET32a–cap were transformed into *E. coli* Rossetta cells to express His-tagged rCap. pET32a–cap was sequenced with commercial primers (T7 and S tag) by Comate Biotechnology Company (Changchun, China). rCap was purified using a Ni-Agarose 6× His-tagged protein purification kit (Qiagen, German) according to the manufacturer's instructions. rCap was identified through Western blot by utilizing convalescent sera from minks infected with MiCV or healthy mink sera as primary antibodies. Horseradish peroxidase-conjugated protein A/G (Thermo Scientific) was set as a detection reagent. Similarly, rCap was also identified through Western blot analysis by applying HRP-conjugated mouse anti-His MAb (Sigma, USA) as antibodies.

Western blot analysis for the serum samples

Purified rCap protein and pET-32a vector protein as controls were separated on an SDS–polyacrylamide gel, and the samples were transferred to pure nitrocellulose blotting membranes (Pall Corporation, USA) for Western blot. These membranes were blocked with 5% skimmed milk–PBS for 2 h at 37 °C, then incubated for 2 h at 37 °C with serum samples diluted in 1:50, washed thrice with PBS–T (0.05% Tween 20 dissolved in PBS), and further incubated for 1 h with horseradish peroxidase-conjugated protein A/G. After the membranes were washed again with PBS–T, the bands were detected using DAB reagents (Biotopped, Beijing, China).

ELISA procedure

An ELISA based on a recombinant Cap antigen was conducted according to a previously published protocol [9, 10]. In brief, 96-well polystyrene immunoplates (Jet Bio-Filtration, Guangzhou, China) were coated with 100 μl of rCap protein in 0.05 M bicarbonate/carbonate buffer (pH 9.6) overnight at 4 °C. The wells were then washed thrice with PBS (pH 7.4) containing 0.05% Tween 20 (PBS–T), and the plates were blocked with 1% BSA for 1 h at 37 °C. Three additional PBS–T washes were carried out, the serum samples were diluted in PBS (pH 7.4) containing 5% skim milk, 100 μl of the diluted samples was added to the wells, and the plates were incubated for 3 h at 37 °C with each serum sample in duplicate. The plates were washed with PBS–T before the detection reagent solution (horseradish peroxidase-conjugated protein A/G) diluted at 1:10,000 in PBS was added to each well, and the plates were incubated again for 60 min at 37 °C. The plates were washed thrice, 100 μl of TMB diluted in substrate buffer was added to each well, and the plates were incubated for 30 min at 37 °C. Finally, the reactions were stopped with 2 mol/L H_2SO_4, and optical density (OD) was read at 450 nm with a microplate reader (Bio-Tek Instruments, USA).

The optimum concentrations of coating antigen, serum dilution, and horseradish peroxidase-conjugated protein A/G antibody were determined through checkerboard serial-dilution analysis.

In brief, rCap was serially diluted twofold from 4 μg/ml to 0.125 μg/ml in 0.05 mol/L Na bicarbonate/carbonate buffer. MiCV-positive and MiCV-negative control mink sera were also serially diluted twofold from 1:25–1:400 and used to optimize rCap ELISA. After the optimal antigen concentration and serum dilutions were established, checkerboard titrations were performed to identify the optimal working dilutions of the conjugate. The conjugate was added to the plate at ratios of 1:10,000, 1:20,000, 1:40,000, and 1:80,000 to determine the optimal detection antibody dilution for this ELISA. The conditions that yielded the highest OD450 ratio between positive control and negative control sera (P/N value) were considered optimal.

Determination of the cut-off value for iELISA

Negative serum control samples from 60 clinically healthy minks obtained from three farms without a history of MiCV and confirmed negative for MiCV antibodies through Western blot were diluted at the optimal dilution and assayed. The cut-off value was determined by calculating the mean OD of the negative samples in Western blot ($n = 60$) plus 3 standard deviation (SD).

Evaluation of iELISA specificity

To evaluate the potential cross-reactivity of iELISA, we used the sera from the healthy minks as negative controls and the sera extracted from minks positive to canine adenovirus type 2 (CAV-2), AMDV, MEV, pseudorabies virus (PRV) and CDV or positive to *E. coli*, *Pasteurella multocida*, and *Pseudomonas aeruginosa*. These samples were examined in terms of reactivity in iELISA and were assayed in duplicate.

Determination of the reproducibility of the assay

To determine the reproducibility of iELISA, we selected six serum samples from minks (three Western blot-positive samples and three Western blot-negative samples). To assess the intra-assay (within-plate) reproducibility, we ran six replicates of each sample on the same plate. For inter-assay (between-run) reproducibility, three replicates of each sample were run in different plates. Mean OD, SD, and coefficient of variation (CV) were calculated.

Comparison of iELISA with western blot

To investigate the specificity and sensitivity of iELISA, we examined 138 serum samples collected from minks in Heilongjiang through iELISA and Western blot and calculated the correlation between these methods.

Application of iELISA for the detection of MiCV infection

To estimate the positive rates of MiCV in the mink population, we randomly collected serum samples ($n = 683$) from 24 farms in Heilongjiang, Jilin, Shandong, Hebei, and Liaoning in China in 2014–2016. The iELISA was applied to detect these serum samples and to obtain antibody titers for any sample by serially diluting the samples in twofold.

Results

Expression and purification of rCap protein

The truncated MiCV capsid gene was amplified through PCR directly from the feces of the infected mink, and an expected band with a size of 600 bp was obtained. This gene was then cloned into the pET-32a expression vector. The construction of recombinant pET-32a-cap plasmid was confirmed through double digestion with *Bam*HI and *Xho*I and sequence analysis. The insert yielded 99% nucleotide identities with MiCV DL13 (GenBank accession no. NC_023885.1) and Hebei13 (GenBank accession no. KM586846.1). The recombinant plasmid pET-32a-cap was transformed into *E. coli* strain Rossetta (DE3). After induction, the recombinant protein (rCap) was expressed as an insoluble 44 kDa His-tagged fusion protein corresponding to the expected size. The fusion protein was purified using a Ni-NTA His Bind resin column and identified through SDS–PAGE analysis (Fig. 1). The antigenicity of the recombinant rCap protein was further confirmed through Western blot analysis involving positive serum samples and anti-His-tag monoclonal antibody (Fig. 2). The results indicated that only the 44 kDa rCap protein reacted strongly with the positive sera in Western blot, whereas the pET-32a vector protein did not react with the positive sera. The data revealed that the rCap protein exhibited a good immune reaction with a specific antibody to MiCV. This result indicated that the antigenicity of rCap protein was confirmed, and this protein antigen could be used to detect specific antibodies against MiCV. The purified rCap protein was utilized as a coating antigen in iELISA.

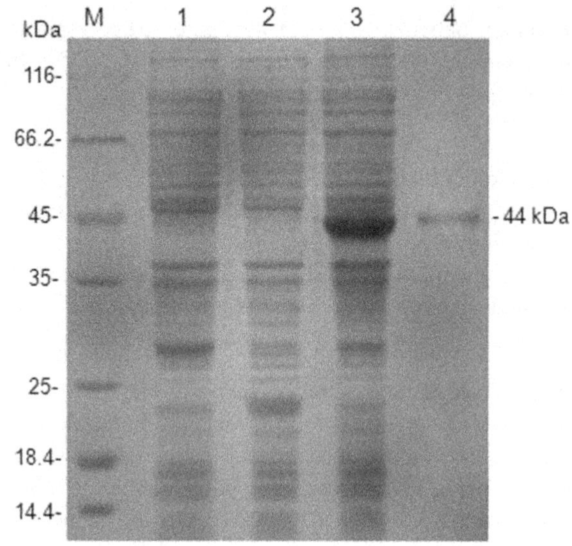

Fig. 1 SDS-PAGE analysis of the rCap fusion protein. Lane M: protein molecular weight marker; Lane 1: Rosetta control; Lane 2: pET32a vector control; Lane 3: pET32a–cap bacterial lysate; Lane 4: Purified fusion protein

Development of the rCap ELISA

Checkboard ELISAs were applied to determine the optimal coating antigen concentration and the optimal serum dilution, which were 0.5 μg/ml and 1:200, respectively (Table 1). After the optimal coating antigen concentration and the optimal serum dilution were set, other factors in rCap iELISA were optimized.

We found that 1% BSA was the optimum blocking buffer for this assay, resulting in the highest P/N value among the tested blocking solutions. The optimal working dilution of the conjugate was 1:10,000. The incubation periods for the serum samples or the detection reagents respectively set at 90 or 60 min were observed to be the optimum.

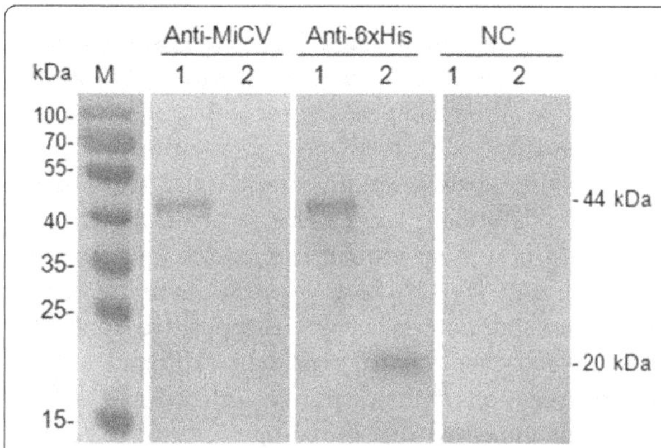

Fig. 2 Western blot was performed with MiCV positive sera (Anti-MiCV), Anti-6xHis HRP conjugated (Anti-6xHis) or MiCV negative sera control (NC). Lane M: protein molecular weight marker; Lane 1: Purified protein rCap; Lane 2: pET32a vector control

Table 1 Ratio of MiCV-positive serum to MiCV-negative serum for the optimization of assay conditions for the ELISA against recombinant rCap antigen

Serum dilution	Concentration of rCap antigen (μg/well)					
	4	2	1	0.5	0.25	0.125
1:25(+)	0.806	1.056	1.048	0.969	0.89	0.742
1:25(−)	0.108	0.166	0.16	0.153	0.133	0.104
1:50(+)	0.876	1.175	1.044	0.967	0.888	0.78
1:50(−)	0.175	0.116	0.144	0.12	0.116	0.09
1:100(+)	0.753	1.078	1.063	0.964	0.895	0.737
1:100(−)	0.096	0.121	0.129	0.1	0.114	0.089
1:200(+)	0.971	1.119	1.065	**1.004**	0.801	0.767
1:200(−)	0.113	0.127	0.15	**0.108**	0.097	0.088
1:400(+)	0.681	0.724	0.807	0.779	0.821	0.638
1:400(−)	0.094	0.068	0.111	0.083	0.083	0.068

Optimum values with the best positive-to-negative ratio are highlighted

To set a cutoff value for the rCap iELISA, 60 sera tested negative by Western blot were examined. The mean ± SD OD450 value for those sera in the rCap iELISA was 0.229561 ± 0.027542, which gave a cutoff value of 0.312 (mean + 3SD) for this assay. Therefore, serum samples with an OD450 > 0.312 in this assay were regarded as positive for MiCV.

No cross-reactions were detected by iELISA involving the antisera against the related pathogens, such as CAV-2, AMDV, MEV, PRV and CDV, *E. coli*, *P. multocida*, and *P. aeruginosa*, and the OD values ranged from 0.208 to 0.098 (Table 2). The data indicated that the developed iELISA exhibited good specificity for MiCV antibody detection.

Determination of assay reproducibility

The reproducibility of iELISA was determined by comparing CVs of each mink serum sample. The intra-assay

Table 2 Results of cross test of indirect ELISA

Serum sample	Value of OD_{450}
MiCV(+)	1.451
MiCV(−)	0.137
Blank control	0.109
AMDV	0.121
MEV	0.154
CDV	0.161
PRV	0.098
CAV-2	0.135
Escherichia coli	0.113
Pasteurella multocida	0.201
Pseudomonas aeruginosa	0.208

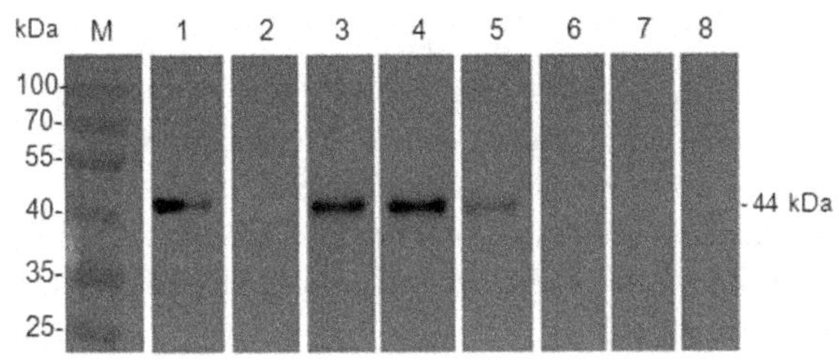

Fig. 3 Western blot analysis of the rCap fusion protein. Lane M: protein molecular weight marker; Lane 1:Positive serum control; Lane 2: Negative serum control; Lane 3: Serum 1;Lane 4: Serum 2; Lane 5: Serum 3; Lane 6: Serum 4; Lane 7: Serum 5; Lane 8: Serum 6

CVs of three serum samples and three negative serum samples determined through Western blot (Fig. 3) and iELISA ranged from 2.15% to 6.23%, with a median of 4.295%, whereas the inter-assay CV of these samples varied from 2.40% to 8.02%, with a median of 5.335%. These data demonstrated that iELISA was repeatable, yielding acceptably low variation levels (Table 3).

Comparison of iELISA with western blot

A total of 138 serum samples was investigated by iELISA, and the results were compared with those of Western blot. Of the 138 samples analyzed, 78 serum samples were detected as positive and 60 were identified as negative by Western blot. Furthermore, 77 serum samples were determined as positive and 61 samples were classified as positive by iELISA. Our findings also indicated that 72 were positive and 55 were negative by both assays. However, 11 samples presented conflicting results between the assays.

Thus, the respective sensitivity and specificity of iELISA were 92.31% and 91.67% compared with those of Western blot (Table 4). The total coincidence of iELISA and Western blot was 92.03% (Table 4). A κ coefficient of 0.838 (95% CI 0.735–0.925) was calculated between Western blot and iELISA. According to the criteria by Landis and Koch [11], this finding indicated an excellent agreement between iELISA and Western blot.

Application of iELISA for the detection of MiCV infection

To evaluate iELISA, we detected the antibodies against MiCV in the sera obtained from the minks from Shandong, Hebei, Heilongjiang, Jilin, Liaoning provinces in China by using the proposed technique (Fig. 4). Our results are shown in Table 5. Overall, the positive rate of MiCV-specific antibodies was 23.87% (163/683) in mink farms, and these sera were found positive by iELISA with an OD range of 0.313–2.256 (mean 0.413; S.D. 0.111). Of these, 21 of 24 farms with 163 of 683 (23.87%) individuals were tested positive for MiCV antibodies. The positive rates for each of the 21 flocks ranged from 2.33% to 73.68% (Table 5). The positive rates of MiCV in different mink farms were 13.04% in Heilongjiang Province, 27.87% in Jilin Province, 25.00% in Liaoning Province, 33.81% in Hebei Province, and 26.79% in Shandong Province (Table 5).

Three positive samples and three negative samples were selected as examples to be used in iELISA to determine the titer for the serum samples. In Fig. 5, the antibody titer of the three positive (samples JL1, HL36 and HB45) samples was 1:800, 1:400 and 1:400, respectively, by the serial dilution of sera.

Discussion

This study aimed to develop iELISA based on recombinant antigen for the detection of anti-MiCV antibodies in minks.

Cap is the only structural protein of circovirus and is the major immunogenic protein produced in circovirus-infected animals [12, 13]. Cap is the only structural protein of circovirus and is the major immunogenic protein produced in circovirus-infected animals. It had a large number of arginine residues concentrated at the N-terminus, which can inhibits the mRNA translation. As such, this protein is a major viral target, it plays a critical role in virus antigenic and useful tool for epidemiological surveys. Using recombinant capsid protein to develop ELISA method for the detection of circovirus like PCV2 and DuCV have been confirmed [9, 14–17]. Wang et al. reports that PCV2 can infect mink [18].

Table 3 Repeatability and reproducibility analysis of indirect ELISA

Sample	Intra-assay(OD450)						Inter-assay(OD450)					
	1	2	3	Mean	SD	CV%	1	2	3	Mean	SD	CV%
1	0.382	0.401	0.432	0.405	0.025	6.23	0.386	0.413	0.411	0.403	0.015	3.73
2	0.641	0.664	0.594	0.633	0.036	5.64	0.604	0.656	0.693	0.651	0.045	6.87
3	0.471	0.487	0.468	0.475	0.010	2.15	0.459	0.466	0.481	0.469	0.011	2.40
4	0.282	0.271	0.256	0.270	0.013	4.84	0.248	0.281	0.243	0.257	0.021	8.02
5	0.244	0.261	0.252	0.252	0.009	3.37	0.253	0.258	0.225	0.245	0.018	7.25
6	0.180	0.194	0.188	0.187	0.007	3.75	0.182	0.195	0.194	0.190	0.007	3.80

Table 4 Comparison of the ELISA and Western blot test

ELISA results	Western blot results Positive	Negative	Total
Positive	72	5	77
Negative	6	55	61
Total	78	60	138
Total (% coincidence)	92.31(72/78)	91.67(55/60)	92.03(127/138)

The amino acid sequences of Cap, especially in the first 40 amino acid residues of the N-terminal regions, in PCV2 are highly homologous to those of MiCV. To avoid the possible cross-reaction of the two viruses in future detections, we deleted the first 40 amino acid residues of the N-terminal regions, which unlikely affect protein antigenicity [9, 19].

In this study, the truncated Cap gene was cloned and the corresponding protein was expressed in *E. coli* because bacterial expression systems are more convenient. Using the purified recombinant Cap as a diagnostic antigen, we developed specific and sensitive iELISA to identify MiCV infection. Our data also demonstrated the specificity of this antigen, which does not react with antibodies directed against CAV-2, AMDV, MEV, PRV and CDV, *E. coli*, *P. multocida*, and *P. aeruginosa*.

In our experiments, goat anti-feline IgG secondary antibodies (Thermo Scientific) were selected and used as a secondary antibody. Checkboard ELISAs were also utilized to determine the following optimal working conditions: coating antigen concentration, 0.05 μg/ml; serum dilution, 1:200; detection antibody dilution, 1:20,000; blocking buffer, 5% skimmed milk; and incubation periods for the serum samples or the secondary antibodies, 90 and 60 min, respectively. The assay cut-off value based on the Western blot negative sera was defined as 0.08. After we compared the results of iELISA with those of Western blot, we found a coincidence of 83% between these methods. Therefore, we chose horseradish peroxidase-conjugated protein A/G as a detection reagent in rCap iELISA.

To date, no standard methods are available. As such, we compared the specificity and sensitivity of the newly developed iELISA in detecting MiCV-specific antibodies with Western blot. The data from rCap ELISA were consistent with the detection results from Western blot, with a relative sensitivity of 92.31% and a specificity of 91.67%. A kappa of 0.838 was statistically obtained to verify the concordance between iELISA and Western blot, resulting in an excellent agreement between these assays. According to the criteria by Landis and Koch [11], this finding suggested an excellent agreement between iELISA and Western blot.

We used the developed iELISA in this study to detect MiCV antibodies in clinical serum samples conducted in 24 farms and to understand the MiCV infection of large-scale mink farms in China.

The results indicated that most of the farms, except two farms, were MiCV seropositive. The total positive rate of MiCV antibodies was 23.87% in different minks. There are some differences in the prevalence of the MiCV infection in different provinces, and also obvious differences in the positive rate in different farms in the same area, such as the positive rate of MiCV antibodies in minks in Shandong was significantly higher than that of other minks in Heilongjiang.

Wang et al. applied PCR to detect 185 mink samples collected from Shandong, Hebei, and Liaoning provinces in September 2013 to September 2014 [8]. They obtained 101 positive samples, and the positive rate was 54.6%. The highest positive rate was 63.2% in Hebei, followed by 54% and 44.4% in Liaoning and Shandong, respectively.

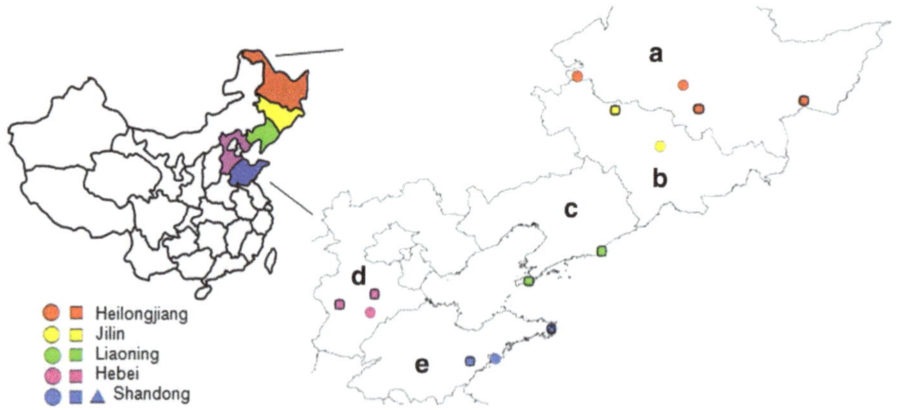

Fig. 4 Geographical distribution of the sampled mink farms. The area covers 5 provinces in China: (**a**) Heilongjiang, (**b**) Jilin, (**c**) Liaoning, (**d**) Hebei, and (**e**) Shandong. The farms are marked with circles, squares, and triangles

Table 5 Detection of MiCV-specific antibody in sera from breeder minks

Province	Farm	Number positive/number tested	Positive rate(%)
Heilongjiang	1	7/62	11.29
	2	9/31	29.03
	3	0/34	0
	4	6/23	47.83
	5	0/21	0
	6	5/36	13.89
Shandong	1	1/43	2.33
	2	13/29	44.83
	3	14/19	73.68
	4	11/31	35.48
	5	4/30	13.33
	6	2/16	12.50
Hebei	1	16/39	41.03
	2	6/33	18.18
	3	9/27	33.33
	4	14/22	63.64
	5	2/18	11.11
Liaoning	1	14/26	53.85
	2	0/17	0
	3	7/33	21.21
	4	6/32	18.75
Jilin	1	14/32	45.16
	2	1/12	8.33
	3	2/17	11.76
Total		163/683	23.87

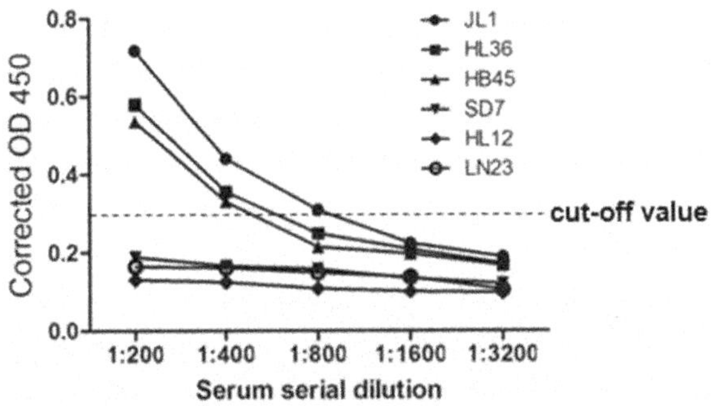

Fig. 5 Anti-MiCV antibody titres in positive and negative mink serum samples. Positive and negative mink serum samples were prepared in dilutions of 1:200, 1:400, 1:800, 1:1600 and 1:3200 used in an ELISA assay. The cut-off value cutoff was determined by counting the mean OD value of the ELISA negative samples plus 3 standard deviation (SD)

These results suggested that MiCV infections are probably epidemic in Heilongjiang, Jilin, Shandong, Hebei, and Liaoning provinces in China. The harmful effects of this virus on mink farm production should be further investigated.

Conclusions

MiCV infection has become common in major mink culture regions in China. rCap may be a useful antigen for the serodiagnosis of MiCV. iELISA with high levels of sensitivity, specificity, and reproducibility was developed successfully for the detection of antibodies to MiCV. The assay shows potential for the serological diagnosis of MiCV infection, large-scale serological surveys, and antibody titer monitoring.

Abbreviations

AMDV: Mink aleutian disease virus; CAV-2: Canine adenovirus type 2; CDV: Canine distemper virus; CV: Coefficient of variation; iELISA: Indirect enzyme-linked immunosorbent assay; MEV: Mink enteritis virus; MiCV: Mink circovirus; ORF: Open reading frames; PCR: Polymerase chain reaction; PRV: Pseudorabies virus;; rCap: Recombinant capsid protein; SD: Standard deviation

Acknowledgments

We would like to thank Xuwei Qin, Dr. Wanzhe Yuan, Yadong Sun, and Dr. Jianke Wang for helping with sample collection. We would like to thank the owners who provided access to the animals examined in this study.

Funding

This research was supported by the Natural Science Foundation of Heilongjiang Province (LC2015006), National Natural Science Foundation of China (31101845) and State Key Laboratory of Veterinary Biotechnology Foundation (SKLVBF201611).

Authors' contributions

Conceived and designed the experiments: JG HC. Performed the experiments: XC JG YS SW LZ. Analyzed the data: JG XC LZ. Contributed reagents/materials/analysis tools: LZ CW SX. Wrote the paper: JG XC. All authors read and approved the final manuscript.

Ethics approval

This study was performed in accordance with the recommendations in the Guide for the Care and Use of Laboratory Animals of the Ministry of Health, China. Prior to experiments, the protocol of the current study was reviewed and approved by the Institutional Animal Care and Use Committee of Northeast Agricultural University (approved protocol number 2014-SRM-24). Samples were collected only from animals for laboratory analyses, avoiding unnecessary pain and suffering of the animals. The owners gave their written consent for sample collection, and the locations where we sampled are not privately owned or protected in any way. The studies did not involve endangered or protected species.

Consent for publication

Not applicable.

Competing interests

The authors declare that they have no competing interests.

Author details
[1]College of Veterinary Medicine, Northeast Agricultural University, Harbin 150030, China. [2]Laboratory Animal and Comparative Medicine Unit, Harbin Veterinary Research Institute, The Chinese Academy of Agricultural Sciences, No. 678 Haping Rd, Harbin 150069, China. [3]Northeastern Science Inspection Station, China Ministry of Agriculture Key Laboratory of Animal Pathogen Biology, Harbin 150030, China.

References

1. Lian H, Liu Y, Li N, Wang Y, Zhang S, Hu R. Novel circovirus from mink, China. Emerg Infect Dis. 2014;20(9):1548.
2. Decaro N, Martella V, Desario C, Lanave G, Circella E, Cavalli A, Elia G, Camero M, Buonavoglia C. Genomic characterization of a circovirus associated with fatal hemorrhagic enteritis in dog, Italy. PLoS One. 2014;9(8):e105909.
3. Segalés J. Porcine circovirus type 2 (PCV2) infections: clinical signs, pathology and laboratory diagnosis. Virus Res. 2012;164(1):10–9.
4. Todd D. Avian circovirus diseases: lessons for the study of PMWS. Vet Microbiol. 2004;98(2):169–74.
5. Kiupel M, Stevenson GW, Galbreath EJ, North A, HogenEsch H, Mittal SK. Porcine circovirus type 2 (PCV2) causes apoptosis in experimentally inoculated BALB/c mice. BMC Vet Res. 2005;1(1):7.
6. Todd D. Circoviruses: immunosuppressive threats to avian species: a review. Avian Pathology. 2000;29(5):373–94.
7. Yu-ying W, Ye L, Hai L. Molecular epidemiology of mink circovirus. Chinese. J Vet Med. 2015;51(5):6–8.
8. Wang Y, Liu Y, Lian H, Li N, PCR A. Method for detection of mink circivirus. Chinese. J Vet Sci. 2015a;35:1774–6.
9. Liu S-N, Zhang X-X, Zou J-F, Xie Z-J, Zhu Y-L, Zhao Q, Zhou E-M, Jiang S-J. Development of an indirect ELISA for the detection of duck circovirus infection in duck flocks. Vet Microbiol. 2010;145(1):41–6.
10. Wen L-B, Wen S-F, He K-W. Development and application of an indirect enzyme-linked immunosorbent assay using recombinant truncated cap protein for the diagnosis of porcine circovirus-like virus P1. BMC Vet Res. 2016;12(1):12.
11. Landis JR, Koch GG. An application of hierarchical kappa-type statistics in the assessment of majority agreement among multiple observers. Biometrics. 1977:363–74.
12. Segalés J. Best practice and future challenges for vaccination against porcine circovirus type 2. Expert review of vaccines. 2015;14(3):473–87.
13. Song Y, Jin M, Zhang S, Xu X, Xiao S, Cao S, Chen H. Generation and immunogenicity of a recombinant pseudorabies virus expressing cap protein of porcine circovirus type 2. Vet Microbiol. 2007;119(2):97–104.
14. Jin Q, Yang J, Lu Q, Guo J, Deng R, Wang Y, Wang S, Wang S, Chen W, Zhi Y. Development of an immunochromatographic strip for the detection of antibodies against porcine circovirus-2. J Vet Diagn Investig. 2012;24(6): 1151–7.
15. Sun S-Q, Guo H-C, Sun D-H, Yin S-H, Shang Y-J, Cai X-P, Liu X-T. Development and validation of an ELISA using a protein encoded by ORF2 antigenic domain of porcine circovirus type 2. Virol J. 2010;7(1):274.
16. Yang C, Xu Y, Jia R, Li P, Zhang L, Wang M, Zhu D, Chen S, Liu M, Yin Z. Prokaryotic expression of a codon-optimized capsid gene from duck circovirus and its application to an indirect ELISA. J Virol Methods. 2017;247:1–5.
17. Okda F, Liu X, Singrey A, Clement T, Nelson J, Christopher-Hennings J, Nelson EA, Lawson S. Development of an indirect ELISA, blocking ELISA, fluorescent microsphere immunoassay and fluorescent focus neutralization assay for serologic evaluation of exposure to north American strains of porcine epidemic diarrhea virus. BMC Vet Res. 2015;11(1):180.
18. Wang G-S, Sun N, Tian F-L, Wen Y-J, Xu C, Li J, Chen Q, Wang J-B. Genetic analysis of porcine circovirus type 2 from dead minks. J Gen Virol. 2016;97(9):2316–22.
19. Heath L, Williamson A-L, Rybicki EP. The capsid protein of beak and feather disease virus binds to the viral DNA and is responsible for transporting the replication-associated protein into the nucleus. J Virol. 2006;80(14):7219–25.

8

First recorded case of paramyxovirus infection introduced into a healthy snake collection in Croatia

Jelena Prpic[1*], Tomislav Keros[1], Maja Lang Balija[2,3], Dubravko Forcic[2,3] and Lorena Jemersic[1]

Abstract

Background: In the present study, we describe the first paramyxovirus infection in a snake collection in Croatia caused by an introduction of new snakes that were not previously tested and didn't show any signs of disease.

Case presentation: In less than a month after introduction into a healthy colony, new snakes began to show respiratory symptoms (i.e. mouth opening, wheezing, etc.) and died within a month and a half after antibiotic therapy was applied. The same symptoms and a high mortality rate were then observed in in-contact snakes from other collections belonging to different snake families.

Conclusions: Two entries of new snakes in different time periods were recorded and recognized as possible sources of infection. We stress the need for veterinary health control and monitoring of snakes prior to transportation as well as implementing obligatory quarantine measures to minimize the risk of infection among newly established snake groups.

Keywords: Snake, Paramyxovirus, Nested RT-PCR, Phylogenetic characterization, Infection, Croatia

Background

Paramyxoviruses (PMV) are negative sensed single stranded RNA viruses with a helical nucleocapsid packaged in a pleomorphic envelope and are classified as members of the *Paramyxoviridae* family, genus *Ferlavirus* [5, 6, 11]. According to studies based on partial sequences of L, HN, and U genes [1, 11, 3], members of the genus *Ferlavirus* are grouped into three subgroups, subgroups A, B and C. There are numerous reports of *Ferlavirus* isolation worldwide from zoological and private collections. Up to now, the occurrence of PMVs has been detected in several snake (sub) families: *Colubridae, Elapidae, Viperidae, Crotalidae, Boidae* and *Pythonidae* [4, 7, 9, 11]. The purchase and introduction of new reptiles into an established collection is of high risk in regards to disease spread and manifestation as well as a probable cause of a higher mortality rate. It has been demonstrated that viral infections such as inclusion body disease (IBD) and PMV [12], as well as some bacterial infections, represent a significant risk when latently infected snakes are introduced into healthy snake collections [13].

The objective of this study was to detect PMV RNA in samples derived during 2015 from a collection of exotic snakes showing signs of disease. Furthermore, sequencing of a highly conserved fragment within PMV L-gene region was performed to define the genetic heterogeneity of the virus isolates and to compare the sequences with previously described ones from the GenBank. The aim was to retroactively define the probable sources of infection. In consensus with earlier publications [8, 10] we used a nested RT-PCR protocol targeting the L-gene [2] as the most sensitive method currently available for basic diagnostics of PMV infection.

Case presentation

In less than a month after introduction of *Dendroaspis jamesoni jamesoni* (purchased from a private keeper from the Czech Republic in September 2014) into a healthy colony, the mamba began to show respiratory symptoms (i.e. mouth opening, wheezing, etc.) and died within a month and a half after antibiotic therapy (Marbocyl for 10 days) was applied. The same symptoms and a high mortality rate were then observed in other

* Correspondence: balatinec@veinst.hr
[1]Croatian Veterinary Institute, Savska cesta 143, 10 000 Zagreb, Croatia
Full list of author information is available at the end of the article

snakes from collections belonging to different snake families. In February 2015 the breeder purchased new snakes and introduced them into the collection. One pair (male and female) of *Dendroaspis viridis* (caught in the wild in Ghana) was purchased from a private keeper from the Czech Republic, whereas snakes *Bitis nasicornis* were purchased from Poland. *Dendroaspis viridis* didn't show any respiratory symptoms but was in a poor condition and died within a month and a half. The snake owner noticed the same clinical signs and a high mortality rate in other snakes from his collection belonging to different snake families. Autopsy showed signs of fibrotic pneumonia.

Lung tissue (CRO-PMV-1 to CRO-PMV-6 and CRO-PMV-12) and tracheal and cloacal swab samples (CRO-PMV-7 to CRO-PMV-11) were collected (Table 1). Approximately, 0.1 g of lung samples were homogenized in 1 mL of phosphate-buffered saline (PBS; pH 7.4) and then vortexed for 1 min and centrifuged for 15 min at 1000 × *g*. Tracheal and cloacal swabs were taken by moistened cotton-tipped sterile swabs and sterile MEM-H from the snakes that began to show the signs of disease. After filtration (0.45 μm), swab samples were inoculated into a Vero cell culture and propagated for up to two passages. Vero cell culture was maintained in minimal essential medium with Hank's salts (MEM-H), supplemented with 10% foetal calf serum (FCS) and 50 mg/ml neomycin and the incubation was carried out at 32 ° C in a medium with added 2% FCS until a cytopathic effect was observed. An amount of 100 μL of each homogenized lung supernatant, swab sample and cell culture sample was used for viral RNA purification using iPrep Total RNA Kit (Invitrogen, USA) according to the manufacturer's instructions.

The amplification of PMV L-gene fragments was adopted from previously published methodology [2]. One-step reverse transcription PCR and nested PCR assays for the amplification of 627-bp and 566-bp long products of L-gene, respectively, were performed using SuperScript III One-Step RT-PCR with PlatinumTaq (Invitrogen, USA) and PlatinumBlue PCR SuperMix (Invitrogen, USA) using primer pairs and the amplification procedure described by Ahne et al. [2]. PCR products were separated by agarose gel electrophoresis in a 1.5% agarose gel stained with ethidium bromide and visualized by UV transillumination. Twelve gel purified PCR amplicons (Wizard SV gel and PCR Clean up system, Promega, USA) derived from 10 snakes were sequenced directly (Macrogen Inc., Amsterdam, The Netherlands). To determine the phylogenetic grouping of the obtained sequences (GenBank KU207735 to KU207746) the prototype PMV sequences [11] were retrieved from GenBank. Also, similar sequences obtained using BLAST algorithm (http://www.ncbi.nlm.nih.gov) were included in the study. Sequences were aligned using ClustalX, version 2.0 [16] and analyzed by MEGA 5 [15].

Discussion

The amplification of PMV L-gene region from all samples (CRO-PMV-1 to CRO-PMV-12) resulted in clear PCR products with the expected molecular size. The phylogenetic relationship analysis of the obtained sequences showed that all analyzed PMV sequences grouped into group B (Fig. 1) of the proposed genus *Ferlavirus* [11]. Sequences

Table 1 Animals used in the study

Host	Origin of snakes	Sample/time of death	Label
Crotalus m. molossus	Imported in September 2014 from Germany	Lung tissue March 2015	CRO-PMV-1
Crotalus m. molossus	Imported in September 2014 from Germany	Lung tissue August 2015	CRO-PMV-2
Crotalus m. pyrrus	Imported in 2013 from Germany	Lung tissue August 2015	CRO-PMV-5
Dendroaspis viridis	Imported in February 2015 from Czech Republic	Lung tissue April 2015	CRO-PMV-3
Dendroaspis j. jamesoni	Imported in September 2014 from Czech Republic	Lung tissue April 2015	CRO-PMV-4
Bitis atropos	Imported in 2012 from South Africa	Lung tissue September 2015	CRO-PMV-6
Bitis nasicornis	Imported in February 2015 from Poland	Lung tissue August 2015	CRO-PMV-12
Morelia viridis	Imported in 2009 from Croatia	Tracheal/ cloacal swab October 2015	CRO-PMV-7 CRO-PMV-8
Crotalus l. klauberi	Imported in 2014 from Austria	Tracheal/ cloacal swab October 2015.	CRO-PMV-9 CRO-PMV-10
Aspidites melanocephala	Imported in 2011 from Germany	Tracheal swab Still alive	CRO-PMV-11

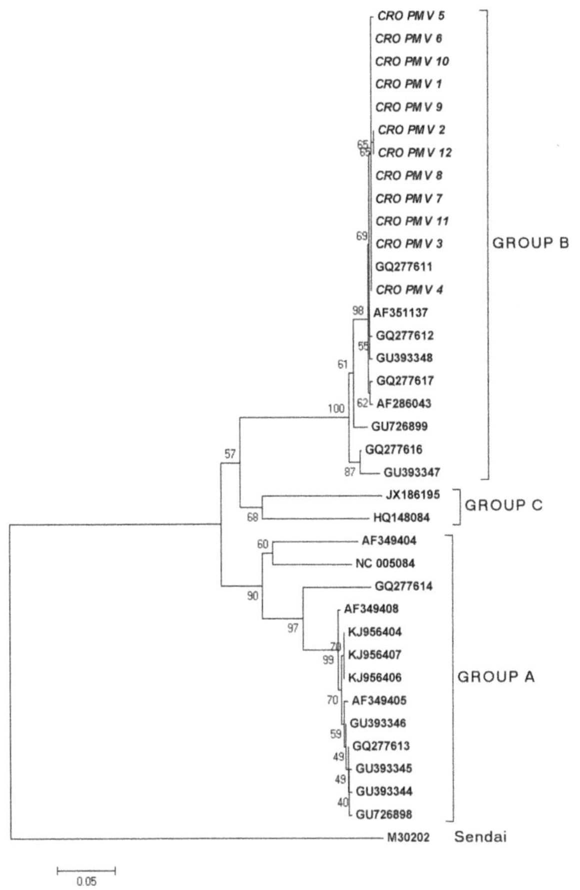

Fig. 1 Neighbor-joining phylogenetic tree obtained by the analysis of the partial L-gene region of PMV strains derived from snake (bold, italic) samples in Croatia. Genetic distances were calculated using the Kimura two-parameter method. Genotype reference sequences (bold) were adopted from Papp et al., [11]. Bootstrap values are presented next to tree nodes. The bar represents 0.05 nucleotide substitution per site

CRO-PMV-1, CRO-PMV-3, CRO-PMV-4 and CRO-PMV-6 to CRO-PMV-11 were found to be 100% identical among themselves in the 443 nt L-gene region, while sequences CRO-PMV-2, CRO-PMV-12 and CRO-PMV-5 differed from these sequences in one nucleotide on positions 241 and 413, respectively. Nucleotide differences in 443 nt long region coding for 143 aa long polypeptide caused differences in aa composition (aa position 81 and 138). The valine replacement by the phenylalanine residue at position 81 of the 143 aa long L-polypeptide doesn't show any effect on protein structure and function, since both of these amino acids are hydrophobic. However, the replacement of hydrophilic glutamine by the basic arginine residue at position 138 could have an impact on viral characteristics, as has been observed in Newcastle disease virus when the replacement of glutamine by the arginine residue in F protein reduced viral replication and attenuated the virus pathogenicity [14].

All Croatian PMV isolates showed high nucleotide identity with sequences of PMV isolates from Germany (GQ277611, AF351137, GQ277612, GU393348 and GQ277617) and Austria (AF286043).

According to the data gained, there are two possible sources of infection. The first source of infection was *Dendroaspis jamesoni jamesoni* (CRO-PMV-4) imported from the Czech Republic in September 2014. The disease spread to *Crotalus molosus molosus* (CRO-PMV 1). Virus sequences isolated from these snakes are mutually identical. The second sources of infection were *Dendroaspis viridis* (CRO-PMV-3) and *Bitis nasicornis* (CRO-PMV-12) that were introduced into the collection in February 2015. We can presume that the disease spread from *Bitis nasicornis* (CRO-PMV-12) to *Crotalus molosus molosus* (CRO-PMV-2) since the virus sequences isolated from these snakes are mutually identical. However, the source of infection for the strain isolated from *Crotalus molosus Pyrrus* (CRO-PMV-5) could not be identified. We presume that point mutations could be initiated by multiple passages in vivo originating from previously introduced clusters since this snake was in the colony since 2013. The passages in Vero cells couldn't be responsible for the observed mutations, since the sequences from swab samples and cell culture supernatants were 100% identical.

Conclusions

Our results imply that the infection was introduced into the healthy collection by new snakes that were not previously tested or showing signs of disease. Since no vaccine is presently commercially available, basic veterinary health checks and quarantine measures are of great importance to minimize the risk of infection among newly established snake groups.

Acknowledgements

The authors are grateful to Mr. Neven Vrbanic for providing the experimental samples and for excellent technical assistance in handling snakes.

Authors' contributions

JP made substantial contributions to conception and design, acquisition of data, analysis and interpretation of data. TK, DF, MLB, LJ have been involved in drafting the manuscript or revising it critically for important intellectual content. All authors read and approved the final manuscript.

Competing interests

The authors declare that they have no competing interests.

Consent for publication

Not applicable.

Author details

[1]Croatian Veterinary Institute, Savska cesta 143, 10 000 Zagreb, Croatia. [2]Centre for Research and Knowledge Transfer in Biotechnology, University of Zagreb, Rockefellerova 10, 10 000 Zagreb, Croatia. [3]Center of Excellence for Viral Immunology and Vaccines, CERVirVac, Zagreb, Croatia.

References

1. Abbas MD, Marschang RE, Schmidt V, Kasper A, Papp T. A unique novel reptilian paramyxovirus, four atadenovirus types and a reovirus identified in a concurrent infection of a corn snake (Pantherophis guttatus) collection in Germany. Vet Microbiol. 2011;150:70–9.
2. Ahne W, Batts WN, Kurath G, Winton JR. Comparative sequence analyses of sixteen reptilian paramyxoviruses. Virus Res. 1999;63:65–74.
3. Franke J, Essbauer S, Ahne W, Blahak S. Identification and molecular characterization of 18 paramyxoviruses isolated from snakes. Virus Res. 2001;80:67–74.
4. Hyndman TH, Shilton CM, Marschang RE. Paramyxoviruses in reptiles: A review. Vet Microbiol. 2013;165:200–13.
5. Kurath G, Batts WN, Ahne W, Winton JR. Complete genome sequence of Fer-de-Lance virus reveals a novel gene in reptilian paramyxoviruses. J Virol. 2004;78:2045–56.
6. Kurath G. https://talk.ictvonline.org/files/ictv_official_taxonomy_updates_since_the_8th_report/m/vertebrate-official/4161?Redirected=true. Accesed 3 Apr 17.
7. Manvell R, Geach M, Lewis J. Isolation of ophidian paramyxovirus type 7 from a reticulated python in the UK. Vet Rec. 2000;147:696.
8. Marschang RE, Papp T, Frost JW. Comparison of paramyxovirus isolates from snakes, lizards and a tortoise. Virus Res. 2009;144:272–9.
9. Oros J, Torrent A, Castro P, Deniz S, Casal A, Jacobson E, Homer B. Ophidian paramyxovirus in snakes in the Canary Islands: An Immunohistochemical Study. Vet Rec. 2001;149:21–3.
10. Papp T, Pees M, Schmidt V, Marschang RE. RT-PCR diagnosis followed by sequence characterization of paramyxovirus infections in clinical samples from snakes reveals concurrent infections within populations and/or individuals. Vet Microbiol. 2010;144:466–72.
11. Papp T, Gál J, Abbas MD, Marschang RE, Farkas FL. A novel type of paramyxovirus found in Hungary in a masked water snake (*Homalopsis buccata*) with pneumonia supports the suggested new taxonomy within the Ferlavirus genus. Vet Microbiol. 2013;162:195–200.
12. Pasmans F, Blahak S, Martel A, Pantchev N. Introducing reptiles into a captive collection: the role of the veterinarian. Vet J. 2008;175:53–68.
13. Pees M, Schmidt V, Marschang RE, Heckers KO, Krautwald-Junghanns ME. Pevalence of viral infections in captive collections of boid snakes in Germany. Vet Rec. 2010;166:422–5.
14. Samal S, Kumar S, Khattar SK, Samal SK. A single amino acid change, Q114R, in the cleveage-site sequence of Newcastle disease virus fusion protein attenuates viral replication and pathogenicity. J Gen Virol. 2011;92:2333–8.
15. Tamura K, Peterson D, Peterson N, Stecher G, Nei M, Kumar S. MEGA5: molecular evolutionary genetics analysis using maximum likelihood, evolutionary distance, and maximum parsimony methods. Mol Biol Evol. 2011;28:2731–9.
16. Thompson JD, Gibson TJ, Plewniak F, Jeanmougin F, Higgins DG. The CLUSTAL X windows interface: flexible strategies for multiple sequence alignment aided by quality analysis tools. Nucleic Acids Res. 1997;25:4876–82.

9

Infectious keratoconjunctivitis in semi-domesticated Eurasian tundra reindeer (*Rangifer tarandus tarandus*): microbiological study of clinically affected and unaffected animals with special reference to cervid herpesvirus 2

Javier Sánchez Romano[1,7*], Torill Mørk[2], Sauli Laaksonen[3], Erik Ågren[4], Ingebjørg H. Nymo[1,5], Marianne Sunde[6] and Morten Tryland[1*]

Abstract

Background: Infectious keratoconjunctivitis (IKC) is one of the most common ocular diseases in ruminants worldwide. In addition to keratitis and conjunctivitis, animals with IKC can develop uveitis, corneal ulcer, and in severe cases, blindness. The bacteria *Moraxella* spp. has been described as the primary causative agent of infectious bovine keratoconjunctivitis (IBK) in cattle (*Bos taurus*), while *Chlamydia* spp. and *Mycoplasma conjunctivae* are considered the main causative agents of IKC in sheep (*Ovis aries*). Previous studies indicated cervid herpesvirus 2 (CvHV2) as the primary causative agent of IKC in semi-domesticated reindeer (*Rangifer tarandus tarandus*). The aim of the study was to investigate the presence and prevalence of potential pathogens for IKC in reindeer, and compare the ocular microbiota of animals with IKC, with apparently healthy animals.

Results: Semi-domesticated reindeer ($n = 341$), with ($n = 108$) or without ($n = 113$) ocular clinical signs, or with no information on clinical status ($n = 120$), were sampled in Norway, Sweden and Finland in 2010–2014. Seroprevalence was 37.4% for alphaherpesvirus (95/254), 3.8% for gammaherpesvirus (8/211) and 7.1% for pestivirus (15/211) (ELISA). PCR analyses of conjunctival swab samples revealed a prevalence of 28.5% for CvHV2 (57/200), 11.9% for *Chlamydiaceae* (16/135) and 1.0% for *M. conjunctivae* (2/197). Bacteriological cultivation of 202 conjunctival swab samples revealed bacterial growth from 75.2% of the samples, with *Moraxella* spp. being isolated from 21.6% (11/51) of the animals with and 5.6% (5/84) without ocular clinical signs. A significant association ($p < 0.001$) existed between the presence of clinical signs of IKC and CvHV2 DNA in the affected eyes, an association that was not present for other microorganisms.

Conclusions: These results support the hypothesis that CvHV2 is the primary agent of IKC in semi-domesticated reindeer in Fennoscandia, with *Moraxella bovoculi* being a secondary candidate, since it was isolated in two different outbreaks of IKC. Further studies should be carried out to better understand the infection biology and the pathogenesis of IKC in reindeer.

Keywords: Alphaherpesvirus, Gammaherpesvirus, Pestivirus, Bacteria, Eye disease, IKC, Microbiology, Reindeer

* Correspondence: javier.s.romano@uit.no; morten.tryland@uit.no
[1]Department of Arctic and Marine Biology, Arctic Infection Biology, UiT – The Arctic University of Norway, Stakkevollveien 23, 9010 Tromsø, Norway
Full list of author information is available at the end of the article

Background

Infectious keratoconjunctivitis (IKC) is a severe transmissible ocular disease, which affects many ruminant species worldwide, including reindeer (*Rangifer tarandus*). In cattle (*Bos taurus*), infectious bovine keratoconjunctivitis (IBK) is considered the most important eye disease worldwide [1], and the bacterium *Moraxella bovis* is considered as the main causative agent [2]. However, IBK is regarded as a multifactorial disease, to which also other bacteria, viruses and environmental factors can play a role [3, 4]. In sheep (*Ovis aries*) and goats (*Capra aegagrus hircus*), bacteria from the family *Chlamydiaceae* can be involved in the development of IKC [5]. In sheep in Norway, *Mycoplasma conjunctivae* and possibly *Moraxella (Branhamella) ovis* are considered primary causative agents [6]. IKC has also been described in several wildlife species [7, 8], e.g. chamois (*Rupicapra rupicapra*) [9, 10], alpine ibex (*Capra ibex*) [9] and moose (*Alces alces*) [11]. Many attempts have been made to isolate bacteria from ruminants during outbreaks of IKC, although it is not always obvious if the bacteria isolated have been the responsible pathogen, or if they rather represented opportunistic or environmental bacteria. It has been shown that many different species of bacteria can be cultured from the eyes of apparently healthy ruminants, with no associated clinical signs. Rehbinder and Glatthard [12] indicated that several bacterial species could be cultured from the eyes of 86% of clinically healthy and 90% of diseased reindeer. Barber et al. [13] and Egwu et al. [14] also found this to be true in most clinically unaffected cows ($n = 261$; Scotland, UK) and 97.5% of sheep ($n = 480$; England, UK), respectively.

IKC is a rather common disease in reindeer which usually affects individual animals or small groups, particularly calves and young animals, but the disease may also appear as regular outbreaks, affecting tens or hundreds of animals in a herd, and having major impact on animal welfare and reindeer herding economy [15]. An illustrated questionnaire distributed to reindeer herders in Norway and Sweden revealed that 55.0% of the responding herders (35/63) had observed clinical signs similar to IKC the previous year (2010) [16]. This disease has been described in reindeer for more than 100 years [17]. IKC in reindeer is considered a multi-factorial disease. Many types of bacteria have been isolated from reindeer with IKC, such as *Moraxella bovoculi*, *Moraxella ovis*, *Escherichia coli*, *Listeria monocytogenes* or *Staphylococcus* sp. [18–20], which all may play a role in the development of the disease. However, from an outbreak of IKC in reindeer it was concluded that Cervid herpesvirus 2 (CvHV2) was the causative and transmissible agent, accompanied by secondary opportunistic bacterial infections [15] and it has recently been shown experimentally that CvHV2, alone and in combination with Moraxella bovoculi, was able to cause clinical sympotms characteristic for IKC in reindeer [21].

Other viruses may be relevant in ocular diseases, such as gammaherpesvirus and pestivirus. Antibodies against a virus from the subfamily *Gammaherpesvirinae* were detected in semi-domesticated reindeer in Finnmark County, Norway, with a prevalence of 3.5% in 2013 [22], and the presence of a novel gammaherpesvirus was also found to be circulating among semi-domesticated reindeer in Norway [23]. Other viruses in this subfamily are associated with malignant catarrhal fever (MCF) in different wild and domestic ruminant species, which may cause keratoconjunctivitis, with ocular discharge and panophthalmitis, as seen in cattle [24, 25], or ocular discharge, keratitis and conjunctival hyphema, as observed in American Bison (*Bison bison*) [26]. Serological screenings have demonstrated that pestivirus infections are enzootic in semi-domesticated reindeer in Norway [27, 28] and Sweden [29] and the susceptibility of these animals to bovine viral diarrhea virus infection (BVDV; family *Flaviviridae*, genus *Pestivirus*) has been experimentally demonstrated [30]. A pestivirus (V60-Krefeld; Reindeer-1), genetically related to border disease virus (BDV), was isolated from a captive reindeer in Duisburg Zoo (Germany) [31]. However, pestivirus has not yet been isolated from wild or semi-domesticated reindeer [32]. Some ocular signs, including ocular discharge, conjunctivitis and hemorrhages in the sclera and palpebral conjunctiva, have been reported in cattle infected with BVDV [33], but the possible association between pestivirus infection and IKC in reindeer is not known.

Environmental factors, such as stress, dust, or UV light have also been proposed to contribute to the development of the disease [15, 34–36]. According to the questionnaire survey, IKC in reindeer is most often seen during September to November in connection with the collection, transport and handling of reindeer, which also coincides with the period when animals are observed more carefully and closely, and also when animals are more stressed [16].

Methods

The aim of the study was to investigate the presence and prevalence of potential pathogens for IKC in reindeer, and to compare the ocular microbiota of animals with IKC, to that of apparently healthy animals.

Sampling of reindeer

Semi-domesticated reindeer ($n = 341$) were sampled in Norway ($n = 171$), Sweden ($n = 139$) and Finland ($n = 31$) (Fig. 1) in the period 2010–2014, either during herd gatherings (live animals, $n = 143$) or from slaughterhouses (dead animals, $n = 198$).

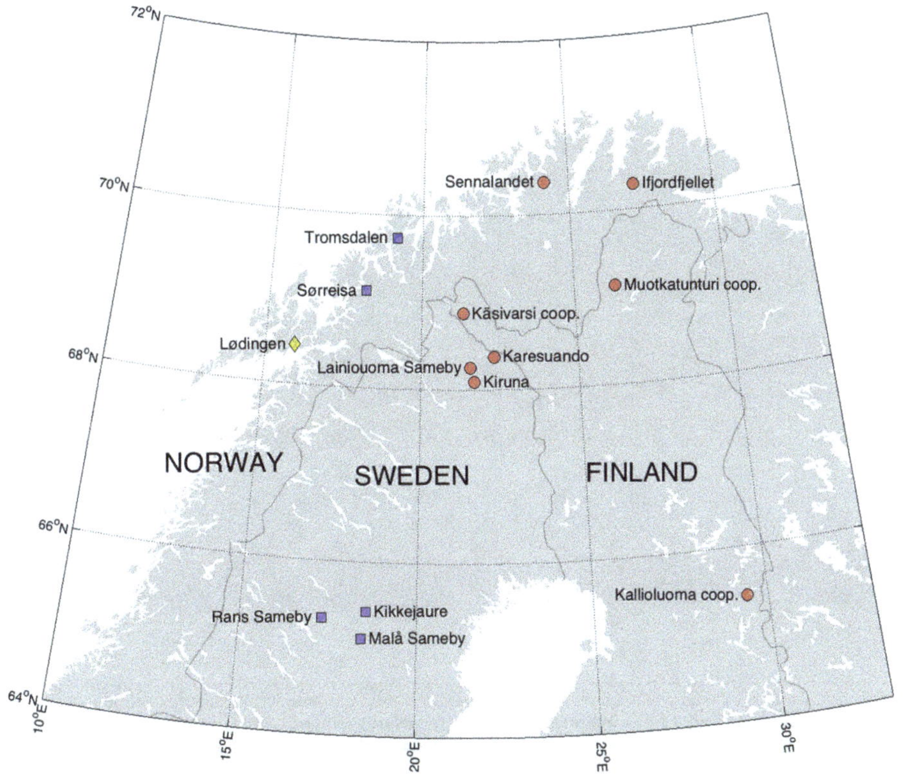

Fig. 1 Distribution of sampling sites of semi-domesticated reindeer ($n = 332$) with names of the administrative units (siida, sameby and cooperatives, in Norway, Sweden and Finland, respectively), indicating sampling of live animals (blue squares), slaughtered animals (red circles) or both live and slaughtered animals (yellow diamond)

In both cases, reindeer with clinical signs of IKC were prioritized for sampling when observed. In total, 108 animals had clinical signs related to IKC, 113 did not show such signs, and for 120 animals, information on clinical signs was not available (Table 1).

The age of the animals was determined by reindeer owners. Animals born in the previous calving season and therefore under 1 year of age were registered as calves ($n = 192$). Animals born in previous calving seasons were registered as adults ($n = 75$), and for 74 animals, age-class information was not available.

For the animals with clinical information available, severity of the ocular disease was scored from 0 to 2, with 0 for asymptomatic animals, 1 for animals with increased lacrimation and/or mild conjunctivitis or 2 for animals with moderate to severe clinical signs of IKC, including corneal and periorbital oedema, conjunctivitis, keratitis, pus with or without blood in the eye or its surrounding area, corneal ulcus or collapse and fibrosis of the eye.

Blood samples were collected from the jugular vein in blood tubes with and without K2EDTA (BD Vacutainer®; BD, Plymouth, UK), using a venoject needle (Terumo, Leuven, Belgium) for live animals, or by collecting blood directly into open tubes during bleeding of slaughtered animals. Tubes were centrifuged for 10 min at 3.000 g to prepare serum or plasma and were then stored at −20 °C until analysis.

Swab samples for virology (Applimed SA, Châtel-St-Denis, Switzerland) were inserted into the conjunctival fornix, rubbed gently against the conjunctival mucosa and placed in sterile cryotubes with 800 µl of Eagle's Minimum Essential Medium (EMEM) with antibiotics (final concentrations of 100 IU/ml of penicillin, 100 µg/ml of streptomycin, 50 µg/ml of gentamicin and 2.5 µg/ml amphotericin B) and stored at −80 °C until analysis.

Swab samples for bacteriology were obtained from the conjunctival fornix as described for the virology swabs and placed in Amies transport medium with charcoal (Transwab® Amies Charcoal Transport; MWE, Wiltshire, England), transported unfrozen to the laboratory and cultured within 2–9 days after sampling, depending on transport time to the laboratory.

When the reindeer was sampled both for virology and bacteriology, the bacteriology swab was obtained immediately after the virology swab and from the same eye.

Serology

Serum samples were tested for the presence of antibodies against alphaherpesvirus with a commercial

Table 1 Semi-domesticated reindeer sampled in 2010–2014 in Norway, Sweden and Finland

		Reindeer (all ages) sampled[1]					Reindeer calves (≤1 year old) sampled					Reindeer adults (>1 year old) sampled				
		Ocular clinical signs [b]					Ocular clinical signs [b]					Ocular clinical signs [b]				
Country	Location	Total	0	1	2	NR	Total	0	1	2	NR	Total	0	1	2	NR
Norway	Ifjordfjellet	28	-	2	-	26	9	-	1	-	8	12	-	1	-	11
	Lødingen	49	20	-	-	29	-	-	-	-	-	20	20	-	-	-
	Sennalandet	23	-	2	-	21	6	-	-	-	6	12	-	-	-	12
	Sørreisa	35	9	10	16	-	26	5	8	13	-	9	4	2	3	-
	Tromsdalen	36	30	6	-	-	27	27	-	-	-	9	3	6	-	-
Sweden	Karesuando	34	16	7	11	-	34	16	7	11	-	-	-	-	-	-
	Kiruna	20	8	12	-	-	20	8	12	-	-	-	-	-	-	-
	Kikkejaure	32	2	1	5	24	-	-	-	-	-	-	-	-	-	-
	Lainiouoma Sameby	33	-	21	12	-	27	-	20	7	-	6	-	1	5	-
	Malå Sameby	5	-	-	-	5	2	-	-	-	2	3	-	-	-	3
	Rans Sameby	15	-	-	-	15	10	-	-	-	10	4	-	-	-	4
Finland	Kallioluoma cooperation	10	9	-	1	-	10	9	-	1	-	-	-	-	-	-
	Käsivarsi cooperation	11	9	1	1	-	11	9	1	1	-	-	-	-	-	-
	Muotkatunturi cooperation	10	10	-	-	-	10	10	-	-	-	-	-	-	-	-
		341	113	62	46	120	192	84	49	33	26	75	27	10	8	30

[a]The number of reindeer (all ages) sampled includes animals from which the age information was unavailable, together with the number of calves and adults.
[b]The severity of the ocular disease was scored with 0 for asymptomatic animals, 1 for animals with increased lacrimation and/or mild conjunctivitis or 2 for animals with moderate to severe clinical signs of IKC. Animals from which information was not registered were placed in column NR

BoHV1 blocking enzyme-linked immunosorbent assay (bELISA) kit (LSI, Lissieu, France) previously validated for the testing of reindeer serum samples for CvHV2 specific antibodies [37]. Positive and negative controls for cattle provided in the bELISA kit were included on each plate.

A direct competition ELISA (cELISA) for the detection of antibodies against the MCFV group [38] was performed to detect the presence of gammaherpesvirus antibodies in reindeer serum as previously described [22].

A serological screening was also carried out for the detection of antibodies against pestivirus using a commercial bELISA kit for the detection of BVDV antibodies in cattle (SERELISA™ BVD p80 Ab Mono blocking; Synbiotics Europe SAS, Lyon, France), which has been previously evaluated for testing reindeer serum samples [39].

Polymerase chain reaction analysis

DNA was extracted from swab samples with a QIAamp DNA MiniKit (Qiagen, Hilden, Germany) following the manufacturer's instructions. Different subsets of reindeer samples were analyzed for the presence of DNA specific to CvHV2 ($n = 200$), *Chlamydiaceae* ($n = 135$) or *M. conjunctivae* ($n = 197$) depending on the availability of DNA extracted from the swab samples.

A nested pan-alphaherpesvirus PCR targeting the UL27 gene encoding glycoprotein B (gB) of CvHV2 was performed as described by Ros and Bèlak [40] for CvHV2 (strain Salla82, Finland; Ek-Kommonen et al. [41], initially named rangiferine herpesvirus 1), in a subset of samples (n = 200). DNA extracted from purified CvHV2 was used as positive control and diethylpryocarbonate (DEPC) water was used as negative control.

One hundred and thirty-five ($n = 135$) samples were analyzed (National Veterinary Institute, Sweden) by a TaqMan real-time PCR specific for members of the family *Chlamydiaceae*, targeting the 23S rRNA operon [42]. The cut-off value was set at $C_t > 38$, so every sample with a threshold cycle (C_t) below that was considered positive for the presence of *Chlamydiaceae* DNA.

A specific PCR assay based on unique sequences of the *LppS* gene [43] was used for detection of *Mycoplasma* spp. in a subset of samples ($n = 197$). DNA purified from *M. conjunctivae* strain HRC/581 originating from sheep (ATCC 25834; NCTC 10147) was used as positive control [44], while DEPC water was used as negative control.

Amplified DNA products were separated by agarose gel (1.0%) electrophoresis and stained with ethidium bromide. Amplicons similar to the expected size (139 bp for *M. conjunctivae* and 294 bp for CvHV2) were purified and sequenced. Consensus amplicon sequences were assembled with the Chromas pro software (version 1.7.7, Technelysium Pty Ltd., South Brisbane, QLD, Australia) and blasted in GenBank (NCBI, USA) for confirmation and comparison to available matching sequences of CvHV2 or *M. conjunctivae.*

Bacteriological investigation

Swab samples from the conjunctiva of the most affected eye in animals with clinical signs of IKC, and one of the eyes when sampling apparently healthy animals were cultivated on two 5.0% sheep blood agar plates, incubated aerobically and anaerobically, and on one lactose-saccharose-bromothymol blue agar plate (equal to MacConkey agar) incubated aerobically. All plates were incubated at 37 °C and inspected after 24 and 48 h. Bacterial growth was categorized as rich, moderate, or poor. Dominant colonies or colonies suspected as relevant, were subcultured for purity and characterized (morphology, Gram staining, catalase, oxidase). API® strips (bioMérieux, Marcy l'Etoile, France) were used for bacterial identification. If identification to species level was not successful, isolates were characterized by 16S ribosomal RNA (16S rRNA) gene sequencing. The proximal part of the 16S rRNA gene was amplified and sequenced using the MicroSeq® 500 16S rRNA Bacterial Identification Kits (Applied Biosystems, Foster City, CA, USA). The sequencing reactions were run on a capillary sequencer 3130xl Genetic Analyzer (Applied Biosystems Life Technologies, Thermo Fisher Scientific Inc., Waltham, MA). Sequences were analyzed using the CLC bio Combined Workbench (CLC bio, QIAGEN, Aarhus, Denmark) or the BioEdit program (http://www.mbio.ncsu.edu/bioedit/bioedit.html) and homology search was performed using NCBI GeneBlast2 program.

Statistical analysis

All statistical analysis was performed using SYSTAT 13 for Windows, using Fisher's exact test. Differences were considered significant when $p < 0.05$.

Results

Serology

Seroprevalence of antibodies against alphaherpesvirus was 79.5% (31/39) in adults and 24% (31/129) in calves. For calves, the seroprevalence increased with increasing severity of clinical signs, while for adults, no such difference was present and the seroprevalence was 66.7–100% regardless of the clinical score (Figs. 2 & 4).

There was a statistically significant and positive association between the presence of clinical signs of IKC and the presence of antibodies against alphaherpesvirus in calves ($p = 0.006$). No association was found for adults ($p = 0.682$) or for the whole sample set when age class was not specified ($p = 0.143$).

Eight out of 211 animals (3.8%) were seropositive for the presence of antibodies against gammaherpesvirus. Among animals with known clinical status ($n = 140$), it was not possible to establish an association between the presence of antibodies against gammaherpesvirus and the presence of clinical signs of IKC ($p = 0.257$), a lack of association that persisted also when addressing calves ($p = 0.394$) or adults ($p = 0.312$) separately.

The presence of antibodies against pestivirus could not be associated with the presence of clinical signs of IKC, either when analyzing calves and adults together ($n = 140$; $p = 0.761$), or among just calves ($p = 1.000$). Since all seropositive animals were calves no such calculation was possible for adults as a separate category. If animals without known clinical information were included ($n = 211$), 15 reindeer had antibodies against pestivirus (7.1%). Six additional animals were classified as doubtful in the ELISA, retested with the same results, and subsequently excluded from our statistical analysis.

In total, 202 animals were screened for the presence of antibodies against all the three viruses (Table 2). Among them, ten animals had antibodies against pestivirus and

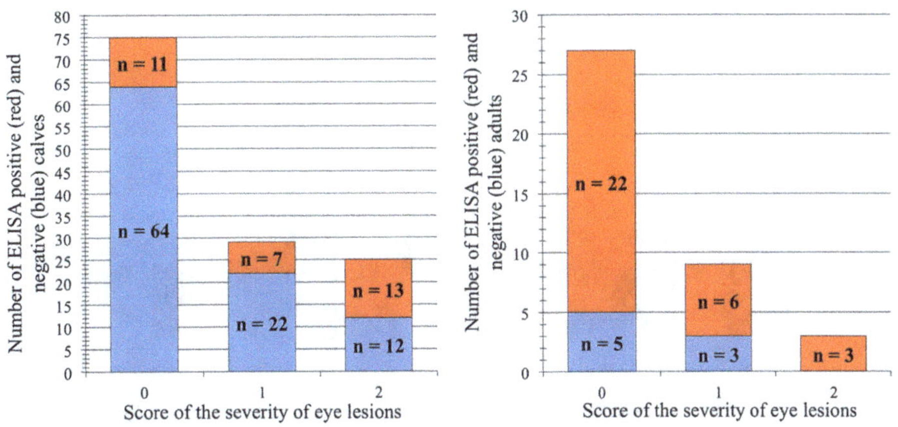

Fig. 2 Alphaherpesvirus seroprevalence among reindeer without eye lesions (0), with mild (1), or moderate/severe (2) eye lesions presented as seronegative (blue) and seropositive (red) comparing calves (left) and adults (right)

Table 2 Semi-domesticated reindeer screened by ELISA ($n = 202$) for antibodies against alphaherpes-, gammaherpes- and pestivirus

	Ocular clinical signs [a]			
	0	1	2	Not registered
Alphaherpesvirus	29 / 89 (32.6)	7 / 24 (29.2)	16 / 27 (59.3)	10 / 62 (16.1)
Gammaherpesvirus	3 / 89 (3.4)	2 / 24 (8.3)	2 / 27 (7.4)	1 / 62 (1.6)
Pestivirus	7 / 86[b] (8.1)	4 / 24 (16.7)	1 / 27 (3.7)	3 / 59[b] (5.1)
Gammaherpesvirus and Alphaherpesvirus	1 / 3	1 / 2	2 / 2	0 / 1
Pestivirus and Alphaherpesvirus	6 / 7	4 / 4	0 / 1	0 / 3

Results are presented as positive/screened (%). No individuals were seropositive for both gammaherpes- and pestivirus, nor for the combination of all the three viruses

[a]The severity of the ocular disease was scored with 0 for asymptomatic animals, 1 for animals with increased lacrimation and/or mild conjunctivitis or 2 for animals with moderate to severe clinical signs of IKC

[b]Three samples were considered doubtful and run twice with the same result and therefore excluded from the analysis

alphaherpesvirus, while four had antibodies against gamma- and alphaherpesvirus. None of the animals were seropositive for both pestivirus and gammaherpesvirus, or for all the three viruses. Among the pestivirus seropositive animals, 66.7% (10/15) were also seropositive to alphaherpesvirus, with a statistical significant association between the presence of antibodies against alphaherpesvirus and pestivirus ($p = 0.003$). This association did not exist in any of the other combinations of antibodies.

Cervid herpesvirus 2 detection

The CvHV2 PCR results showed a positive significant association between the presence of CvHV2 DNA in the conjunctival swab samples and the severity of the clinical signs of IKC. This association was valid both for the total number of animals independently of age-class ($p < 0.001$) and also for calves ($p = 0.002$) and adults ($p = 0.022$) as separate groups (Figs. 3 & 4). Nine out of 59 of the asymptomatic animals (15.3%) had CvHV2 DNA in their eyes.

Chlamydiacea detection

DNA specific for *Chlamydiacea* was detected in 16 of 135 animals (11.9%), eight with and eight without clinical signs of IKC. No statistical association could be established ($p = 1.000$) between the presence of clinical signs of IKC and the detection of bacteria from the family *Chlamydiacea*.

Mycoplasma conjunctivae detection

DNA specific for *M. conjunctivae* was detected in 2 of 197 individuals (1.0%). No link between the presence of clinical signs and *M. conjunctivae* could be established ($p = 1.000$).

Bacteriological investigations

A total of 202 animals, one eye from each, were sampled for bacteriology. Bacteria were cultivated from the conjunctiva of 152 reindeer, of which 35 presented clinical signs of IKC, 52 did not show signs of IKC, and the clinical status was unknown for 65 individuals. In animals from which clinical information was not available, bacteria such as *Acinetobacter* spp. ($n = 13$), *Aeromonas hydrophila* ($n = 5$), *Escherichia coli* ($n = 9$), *Micrococcus lylae* ($n = 8$) and *Staphylococcus* spp. ($n = 3$) were the major findings.

Bacteria from the genus *Moraxella* were isolated from 11 of the 51 animals showing signs of IKC (21.6%) and

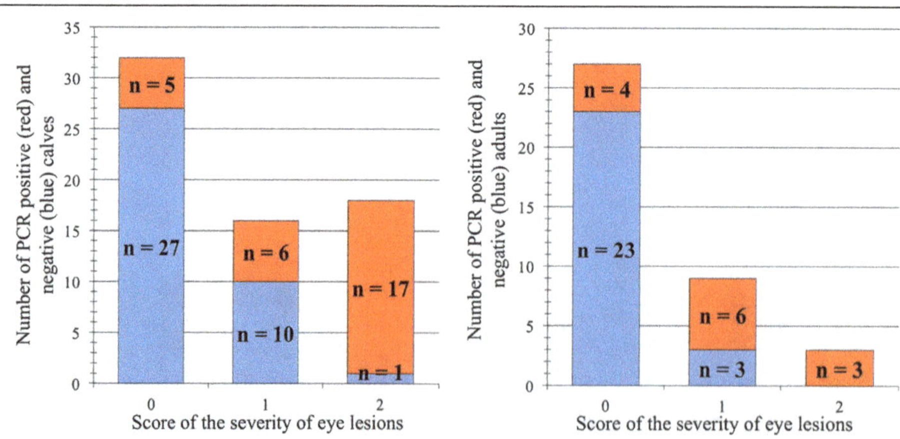

Fig. 3 Alphaherpesvirus PCR results (eye swab) among reindeer without eye lesions (0), with mild (1), or moderate/severe (2) eye lesions presented as PCR negative (blue) and PCR positive (red) comparing calves (left) and adults (right)

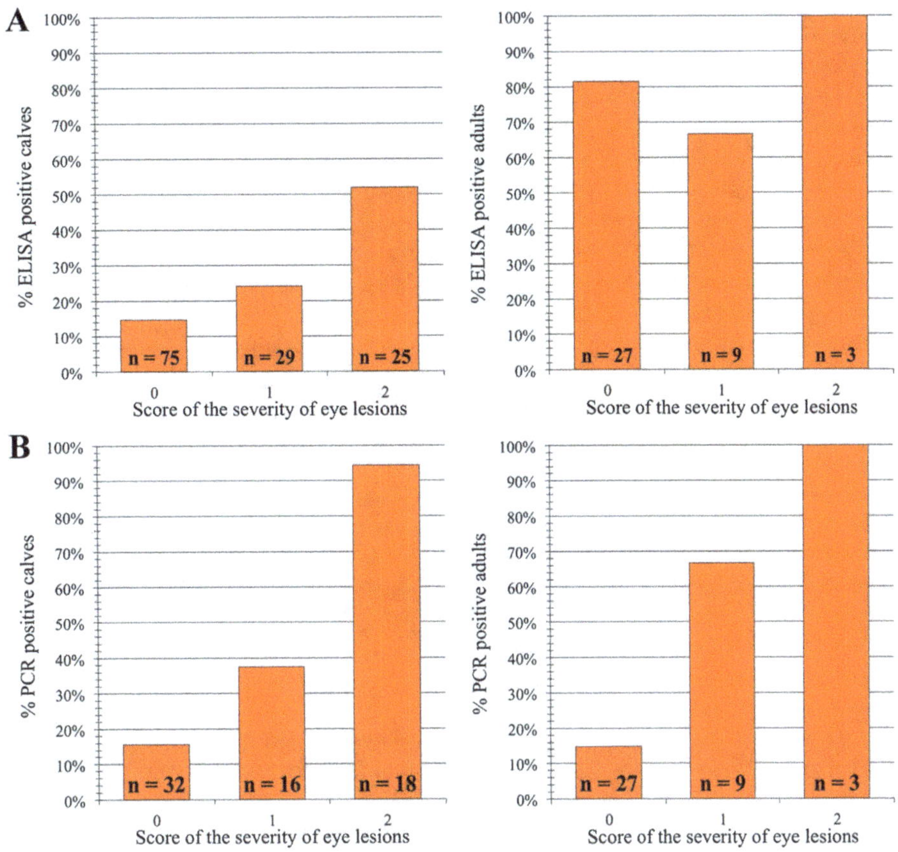

Fig. 4 Alphaherpesvirus seroprevalence (**a**) and alphaherpesvirus PCR results (eye swab) (**b**) among reindeer without eye lesions (0), with mild (1), or moderate/severe (2) eye lesions presented as percentage comparing calves (left) and adults (right)

from 5 out of 84 with no signs (5.6%). Seven of the 11 isolates were identified at species level as *M. bovoculi*.

One of the *M. bovoculi* isolates was cultured from the eye swab from one reindeer with mild signs of IKC in Ifjordfjellet (Finmark County, Norway) (Fig. 1). All other *Moraxella* spp. isolates were obtained from two herds with active IKC outbreaks. However, no significant differences were found between the presence of *Moraxella* spp. in reindeer with IKC and reindeer without IKC ($p = 0.148$).

Several species of bacteria were isolated from the eyes of symptomatic and non-symptomatic animals (Fig. 5), but statistical association between the presence of any of these bacteria and clinical signs of IKC could not be established. For 52 of the reindeer (25.7%, one conjunctival swab from each animal obtained for bacteriology), the cultivation results were not conclusive due to poor bacterial growth or the absence of a dominant species, i.e. nonspecific mixed culture.

Discussion

There was a positive correlation between the presence of antibodies against alphaherpesvirus and the presence of clinical signs of IKC in calves ($p < 0.001$), but not in adults ($p = 0.417$). Calves had higher scores of IKC clinical signs and seemed to be suffering more acute forms of the disease as compared to older animals, most likely due to the lack of previous exposures to the virus and therefore absence of immunity during the establishment of the infection. The higher seroprevalence of antibodies against alphaherpesvirus in adults as compared to calves was expected, since alphaherpesviruses produce lifelong infections [45], which is also in line with previous findings [46].

Adult animals that were previously exposed and infected could be carrying a latent infection without showing clinical signs at the time of sampling. Reactivation from this latency stage will stimulate a quick onset of the immune response protecting the animals from developing disease.

The detection of CvHV2 DNA in eye swabs by PCR and the prevalence of PCR positive individuals, which increased with the severity of the clinical signs of IKC (Fig. 3), supports the hypothesis that CvHV2 is a primary agent in the development of IKC in reindeer [15]. CvHV2 DNA was also amplified by PCR from the eyes of 15.3% of the apparently healthy reindeer. These

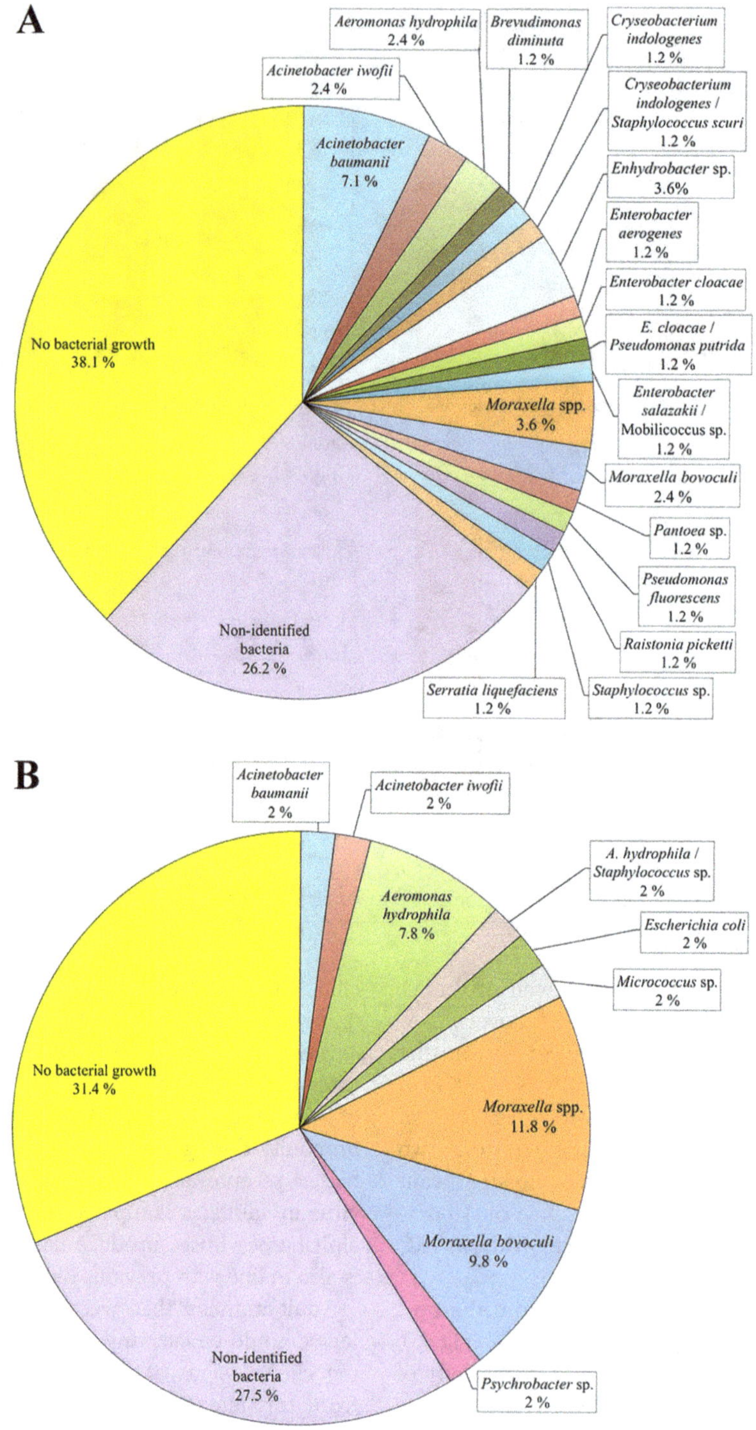

Fig. 5 Bacterial species that dominated the culture plates inoculated with swab samples from eyes of semi-domesticated Eurasian reindeer (*Rangifer tarandus tarandus*) without (**a**) and with (**b**) clinical signs of infectious keratoconjunctivitis (IKC), including the percentage of swabs from which the bacteria were isolated

asymptomatic animals may have been sampled during the incubation period of the disease or the virus may have been replicating in the conjunctival mucosa without producing clinical IKC signs.

It was not possible to detect CvHV2 DNA from 12 animals with mild and one with severe signs of IKC. The signs included in the first category are defined as non-specific signs associated to IKC, such as increased lacrimation and mild conjunctivitis, which can have a non-infectious cause such as dust, dirt, allergies or minor trauma. In a natural outbreak of IKC in reindeer, the virus was most often detected and isolated at higher titers, from animals with mild or early stage signs of IKC and only from a few animals with severe signs. It was hypothesized that the peak of viral replication and shedding occurred at earlier stages, whereas secondary bacterial infections were dominant in later stages of the disease [15, 21]. It is also possible that the virus, during the late stages of IKC, is entering the latency stage, shutting down the active replication cycle and the shedding of progeny virus.

The statistical analysis of our data supports these observations. There was a strong association between the presence of CvHV2 DNA in the eye of the animals and the presence of clinical signs ($p < 0.001$). These results indicate that during an acute CvHV2 infection, with active replication of the virus in the conjunctival mucosa, clinical signs characteristic of IKC may develop.

Interestingly, all CvHV2 seropositive calves were also positive for the presence of CvHV2 DNA in their eyes (12/12). The ratio of PCR-positive animals also positive for the presence of antibodies against CvHV2 increased with the development of more severe clinical signs of IKC (Score 0 = 0% (0/5), Score 1 = 16,7% (1/6), Score 2 = 64,7% (11/17)). Those results support the hypothesis of CvHV2 infected calves seroconverting in later stages of the disease. Seronegative calves with positive PCR results ($n = 16$) might still be in the window period of the disease, in which the animals have been infected, but it is not possible to detect antibodies.

Despite serological screenings reporting antibodies against both pestivirus and gammaherpesvirus in reindeer in Fennoscandia [22, 27], little information is available about their pathogenic potential related to eye disease. The lack of association between the presence of antibodies against pestivirus and gammaherpesvirus and the presence of clinical signs of IKC indicated that these viruses do not contribute to the development of IKC in reindeer. However, it has been speculated that there might be an interaction between pestivirus and alphaherpesvirus in reindeer, in the way that infection with one of the viruses increases the chances of infection by the second virus [29]. The statistical association between the presence of antibodies against pestivirus and alphaherpesvirus in our study could reinforce this hypothesis ($p = 0.003$). Interestingly, all animals that were seropositive to both alphaherpes- and pestivirus ($n = 10$) were sampled from the same herd and period, which could also means that the animals in that herd were managed differently, increasing the possibility of exposure to the pestivirus.

Bacteria belonging to the genus *Moraxella* were isolated from the eyes of eleven animals with, and five animals without clinical signs of IKC. Seven of these isolates were characterized as *M. bovoculi*. Together with *M. bovis*, *M. bovoculi* has been identified as a causative agent of IBK in cattle [47, 48], but a randomized blinded challenge study suggested that *M. bovoculi* was not causally related with IBK in this species [49].

A statistically significant association did not exist between the isolation of *Moraxella* spp. and the presence clinical signs of IKC in reindeer ($p = 0.461$). However, fifteen of the samples from which *Moraxella* spp. were cultivated were obtained during two different IKC outbreaks, in Sørreisa (Norway) and Karesuando (Sweden), supporting the hypothesis of a biological significance of *Moraxella* spp. in the development of IKC in reindeer.

Dickey et al. [50] showed that there are large genomic differences between *Moraxella bovoculi* isolates from IBK affected cattle and asymptomatic animals. These results open the possibility to the presence of different strains of *Moraxella bovoculi* with different pathogenic potential. Therefore, further genomic investigations should be carried out in order to identify if pathogenic characteristics are present in the *Moraxella* spp. isolated from the eyes of apparently healthy and diseased semi-domesticated reindeer.

DNA specific for *Chlamydiacea* and *M. conjunctivae*, both known to be involved in IKC and eye infections in other host species, was detected in a few reindeer samples, both from animals with or without clinical signs of IKC. However, the lack of association between the presence of *Chlamydiacea* or *M. conjunctivae* DNA and the presence of clinical signs of IKC may suggest that these bacteria are not essential to the pathogenesis of IKC in reindeer.

A great variety of other bacteria were isolated from the eyes of both healthy and IKC affected animals (Fig. 5), including some potentially pathogenic bacteria (e.g. *Pseudomonas* spp. or *Staphylococcus* spp. [51, 52]), but also several bacterial species that do not have any known importance in veterinary medicine, most likely representing contamination from the environment (i.e. dust, soil, feces etc.). However, no significant association could be identified between the presence of any of the isolated bacteria and the presence of clinical signs of IKC, which may suggest that none of these bacteria have a significant importance for the development of IKC in reindeer. Bacteria did not grow in 24.8% of the cultured plates, a percentage that seems higher than those reported in other ruminant species [13, 14]. This increment could be attributed to the somewhat long (2–9 days) transport time for some samples to the laboratory which may in some cases have reduced the survival of bacteria in the samples prior to cultivation, or simply reflect a different environment (i.e. free ranging animals as opposed to livestock).

Some species of bacteria might require the presence of damage of the mucosal membrane to be able to establish an infection, as occurs with the cytopathic effect (CPE) produced by CvHV2 during its lytic cycle. A depression of the cell-mediated immunity due to virus-induced lymphocytolysis after infection with BoHV1 has been described [53], and it is relevant to think that CvHV2, a close relative to BoHV1, could produce a similar effect on the reindeer's immune system, favoring the establishment of secondary bacterial infections. On the other hand, the possible role of bacterial infection as a trigger for the reactivation of latent CvHV2 cannot be discarded either. Bovine Herpesvirus 4 (BoHV4) can enter a lytic replication cycle from latency after endometrial infection with *E. coli*, causing uterine disease in cattle [54]. However, BoHV4 belongs to the subfamily *Gammaherpesvirinae*, and whether this finding can be applied to CvHV2 or any other ruminant alphaherpesviruses remains unclear and should be studied in further detail.

Conclusions

Among the microorganism identified in this study, CvHV2 is the most plausible candidate as the causative agent of IKC in semi-domesticated reindeer, and pestivirus and gammaherpesvirus may be discarded as primary causative agents of IKC in reindeer. The isolation of *M. bovoculi* during two different outbreaks of IKC makes this bacterial species an alternative candidate as a possible primary agent of this disease, or maybe more likely, as a secondary and opportunistic pathogen, following a CvHV2 infection as is probably the case for other bacterial species identified in this study. Further studies should be carried out to better understand the infection biology and the pathogenesis of IKC in reindeer.

Abbreviations

16S rRNA: 16S ribosomal RNA; BDV: Border disease virus; bELISA: Blocking enzyme-linked immunosorbent assay; BoHV1: Bovine Herpesvirus 1; BoHV4: Bovine Herpesvirus 4; BVDV: Bovine viral diarrhea virus; cELISA: Competitive enzyme-linked immunosorbent assay; CPE: Cytopathic effect; C_t: Threshold cycle; CvHV2: Cervid Herpesvirus 2; DEPC: Diethylpryocarbonate; EMEM: Eagle's Minimum Essential Medium; gB: Glycoprotein B; IBK: Infectious bovine keratoconjunctivitis; IKC: Infectious keratoconjunctivitis; MCF: Malignant catarrhal fever; MCFV: Malignant catarrhal fever virus; PCR: Polymerase chain reaction

Acknowledgements

Thanks to Eva Marie Breines and Ellinor Hareide (UiT – The Arctic University of Norway, Tromsø, Norway) for laboratory analyses, to Karin Elisabeth Holmgren (Norwegian Veterinary Institute, Tromsø, Norway) for contributing to the bacteriology work, to Nina Marcin and Tone Lille-Mæhlum for contributing to selected analyses, and to Emily E. Magnusson (UiT – The Arctic University of Norway, Tromsø, Norway) for language corrections. We also acknowledge Dr. Hong Li (Animal Disease Research Unit, United States Department of Agriculture-Agricultural Research Service, USA) for providing reagents for the gammaherpesvirus ELISA, to Dr. Branko Kokotovic (Technical University of Denmark) for providing the Mycoplasma conjunctivae positive control, as well as reindeer herders and abattoir staff, for their interest and patience during sampling.

Funding

This study was funded by Reindriftens Utviklingsfond (RUF) and Nordic Council of Ministers. The role of the funding bodies was to provide funding as an indirect support to reindeer herders to find new knowledge with regards to the causative agents of an important reindeer disease.

Authors' contributions

JSR analyzed samples, organized the dataset, conducted statistics and wrote the first draft of the manuscript. MT secured funding for the study and organized the sampling. MT, SL, EÅ, IHN and JSR contributed to the sampling of animals. TM and MS conducted the bacteriology. All authors contributed to the writing and accepted the final version of the manuscript.

Consent for publication

Not applicable.

Competing interests

The authors declare that they have no competing interests.

Author details

[1]Department of Arctic and Marine Biology, Arctic Infection Biology, UiT – The Arctic University of Norway, Stakkevollveien 23, 9010 Tromsø, Norway. [2]Norwegian Veterinary Institute, Stakkevollveien 23, 9010 Tromsø, Norway. [3]Department of Veterinary Biosciences, Faculty of Veterinary Medicine, University of Helsinki, Helsinki, Finland. [4]Department of Pathology and Wildlife Diseases, Swedish National Veterinary Institute, 751 89 Uppsala, Sweden. [5]Norwegian Veterinary Institute, Stakkevollveien 23, 9010 Tromsø, Norway. [6]Norwegian Veterinary Institute, Ullevålsveien 68, 0454 Oslo, Norway. [7]UiT – Arctic University of Norway, Arctic Infection Biology, Stakkevollveien 23, 9010 Tromsø, Norway.

References

1. Postma GC, Carfagnini JC, Minatel L. *Moraxella bovis* pathogenicity: an update. Comp Immunol Microbiol Infect Dis. 2008;31(6):449–58.
2. Henson JB, Grumbles LC. Infectious bovine keratoconjunctivitis. I. Etiology. Am J Vet Res. 1960;21:761–6.
3. Angelos JA. *Moraxella bovoculi* and infectious bovine Keratoconjunctivitis: cause or coincidence? Vet Clin N Am Food Anim Pract. 2010;26(1):73–8.
4. Zbrun MV, Zielinski GC, Piscitelli HC, Descarga C, Urbani LA. Dynamics of *Moraxella bovis* infection and humoral immune response to bovine herpes virus type 1 during a natural outbreak of infectious bovine keratoconjunctivitis in beef calves. J Vet Sci. 2011;12(4):347–52.
5. Constable PD, Gay CC, Hinchcliff KW, Radostits OM. Veterinary medicine : a textbook of the diseases of cattle, horses, sheep, pigs and goats. 10th ed., Saunders, Edinburgh. 2007.
6. Åkerstedt J, Hofshagen M. Bacteriological investigation of infectious Keratoconjunctivitis in Norwegian sheep. Acta Vet Scand. 2004;45(1):19–26.
7. Gortázar C, Fernández-De-Luco D, Frölich K. Keratoconjunctivitis in a free-ranging red deer (*Cervus elaphus*) population in Spain. Eur J Wildl Res. 1998;44(4):257–61.
8. Meagher M, Quinn WJ, Stackhouse L. Chlamydial-caused infectious keratoconjunctivitis in bighorn sheep of Yellowstone National Park. J Wildl Dis. 1992;28(2):171–6.
9. Giacometti M, Janovsky M, Belloy L, Frey J. Infectious keratoconjunctivitis of ibex, chamois and other *Caprinae*. Rev Sci Tech Off Int Epizoot. 2002;21(2):335–45.
10. Marco I, Mentaberre G, Ballesteros C, Bischof DF, Lavín S, Vilei EM. First report of *Mycoplasma conjunctivae* from wild *Caprinae* with infectious keratoconjunctivitis in the Pyrenees (NE Spain). J Wildl Dis. 2009;45(1):238–41.
11. Dubay SA, Williams ES, Mills K, Boerger-Fields AM. Association of *Moraxella ovis* with keratoconjunctivitis in mule deer and moose in Wyoming. J Wildl Dis. 2000;36(2):241–7.

12. Rehbinder C, Glatthard V. Keratitis in reindeer: relation to bacterial infections. Acta Vet Scand. 1986;18:56–64.
13. Barber DM, Jones GE, Wood A. Microbial flora of the eye of cattle. Vet Rec. 1986;118:204–6.
14. Egwu GO, Faull WB, Bradbury JM, Clarkson MJ. Ovine infectious keratoconjunctivitis: a microbiological study of clinically unaffected and affected sheep's eyes with special reference to *Mycoplasma conjunctivae*. The Veterinary record. 1989;125(10):253–6.
15. Tryland M, das Neves CG, Sunde M, Mørk T. Cervid herpesvirus 2, the primary agent in an outbreak of infectious keratoconjunctivitis in semidomesticated reindeer. J Clin Microbiol. 2009;47(11):3707–13.
16. Tryland M, Stubsjøen SM, Ågren E, Johansen B, Kielland C. Herding conditions related to infectious keratoconjunctivitis in semi-domesticated reindeer: a questionnaire-based survey among reindeer herders. Acta Vet Scand. 2016;58:22.
17. Bergman A. Contagious keratitis in reindeer. Scand Vet. 1912;2:145–77.
18. Aschfalk A, Kemper N, Höller C. Bacteria of pathogenic importance in faeces from cadavers of free-ranging or corralled semi-domesticated reindeer in northern Norway. Vet Res Commun. 2003;27(2):93–100.
19. Laaksonen S. Tunne poro - poron sairaudet ja terveydenhuolto. In: The diseases and health care of reindeer. Riga, Latvia: Livonia print, in press; 2016.
20. Oksanen A, Laaksonen S, Hirvelä-Koski V. Silmätulehdus nietosten keskellä porotarhassa. [pink-eye in a winter-corralled reindeer herd.]. Suomen Eläinlääkärilehti. 1996;102:138–41.
21. Tryland M, Sánchez Romano J, Marcin N, Nymo IH, Josefsen TD, Sørensen KK, Mørk T. Cervid herpesvirus 2 and not Moraxella bovoculi caused keratoconjunctivitis in experimentally inoculated semi-domesticated Eurasian tundra reindeer. Acta Vet Scand. 2017;59(1):23.
22. das Neves CG, Ihlebæk HM, Skjerve E, Hemmingsen W, Li H, Tryland M. Gammaherpesvirus infection in semidomesticated reindeer (*Rangifer tarandus tarandus*): a cross-sectional, serologic study in northern Norway. J Wildl Dis. 2013;49(2):261–9.
23. das Neves CG, Tryland M, Li H. Identification of a putative new gammaherpesvirus in reindeer (*Rangifer tarandus tarandus*) in Norway. In: 4th ESVV Herpesvirus Symposium. Zurich, Switzerland: European Society of Veterinary Virology; 2013. p. P31.
24. Knowles DP. Chapter 9 - Herpesvirales. In: MacLachlan NJ, Duvobi EJ (4th edition) Fenner's veterinary virology. Academic press, San Diego. 2011.
25. Van Metre D, Tennant BC, Whitlock RH. Infectious diseases of the gastrointestinal tract. In: divers TJ, peck SF, editors. (1st edition) diseases of dairy cattle. St Louis: Saunders Elsevier; 2008.
26. O'Toole D, Li H. The pathology of malignant catarrhal fever, with an emphasis on ovine herpesvirus 2. Veterinary Pathology Online. 2014;51(2):437–52.
27. Lillehaug A, Vikøren T, Larsen I-L, Akerstedt J, Tharaldsen J, Handeland K. Antibodies to ruminant alpha-herpesviruses and pestiviruses in Norwegian cervids. J Wildl Dis. 2003;39(4):779–86.
28. Tryland M, Mørk T, Ryeng KA, Sørensen KK. Evidence of parapox-, alphaherpes- and pestivirus infections in carcasses of semi-domesticated reindeer (*Rangifer tarandus tarandus*) from Finnmark, Norway. Rangifer. 2005;25-2:75–83.
29. Kautto AH, Alenius S, Mossing T, Becher P, Belák S, Larska M. Pestivirus and alphaherpesvirus infections in Swedish reindeer (*Rangifer tarandus tarandus L.*). Vet Microbiol. 2012;156(1–2):64–71.
30. Morton JK, Evermann JF, Dieterich RA. Experimental infection of reindeer with bovine viral diarrhea virus. Rangifer. 1990;10(2):75–7.
31. Becher P, Orlich M, Kosmidou A, König M, Baroth M, Thiel HJ. Genetic diversity of Pestiviruses: identification of novel groups and implications for classification. Virology. 1999;262(1):64–71.
32. Larska M. Pestivirus infection in reindeer (*Rangifer tarandus*). Front Microbiol. 2015;6:1187.
33. Bielefeldt-Ohmann H. The pathologies of bovine viral diarrhea virus infection. A window on the pathogenesis. The veterinary clinics of North America food animal. Practice. 1995;11(3):447–76.
34. Dubay SA, Williams ES, Mills K, Boerger-Fields AM. Bacteria and nematodes in the conjunctiva of mule deer from Wyoming and Utah. J Wildl Dis. 2000;36(4):783–7.
35. Nayar PS, Saunders JR. Infectious bovine keratoconjunctivitis I. Experimental production. Canadian Journal of Comparative Medicine. 1975;39(1):22–31.
36. Rehbinder C, Nilsson A. An outbreak of kerato-conjunctivitis among corralled, supplementary fed, semidomestic reindeer [*Rangifer tarandus*] calves. Rangifer. 1995;15(1):9–14.
37. das Neves CG, Roger M, Yoccoz NG, Rimstad E, Tryland M. Evaluation of three commercial bovine ELISA kits for detection of antibodies against Alphaherpesviruses in reindeer (*Rangifer tarandus tarandus*). Acta Vet Scand. 2009;51:9.
38. Li H, McGuire TC, Müller-Doblies UU, Crawford TB. A simpler, more sensitive competitive inhibition enzyme-linked immunosorbent assay for detection of antibody to malignant catarrhal fever viruses. Journal of veterinary diagnostic investigation : official publication of the American Association of Veterinary Laboratory Diagnosticians, Inc. 2001;13(4):361.
39. Nymo IH, Poulain VM. Pestivirusinfeksjon hos semi-domestisert rein i Finnmark. In: 18th Nordic section meeting. Svalbard, Norway: Nordic wildlife disease association; 2007.
40. Ros C, Belák S. Studies of genetic relationships between bovine, caprine, Cervine, and Rangiferine Alphaherpesviruses and improved molecular methods for virus detection and identification. J Clin Microbiol. 1986;37(5):1247–53.
41. Ek-Kommonen C, Pelkonen S, Nettleton PF. Isolation of a herpesvirus serologically related to bovine herpesvirus 1 from a reindeer (*Rangifer tarandus*). Acta Vet Scand. 1986;27(2):299–301.
42. Everett KD, Hornung LJ, Andersen AA. Rapid detection of the *Chlamydiaceae* and other families in the order Chlamydiales: three PCR tests. J Clin Microbiol. 1999;37(3):575–80.
43. Belloy L, Vilei EM, Giacometti M, Frey J. Characterization of LppS, an adhesin of *Mycoplasma conjunctivae*. Microbiology. 2003;149:185–93.
44. Barile MF, Del Giudice RA, Tully JG. Isolation and characterization of *Mycoplasma conjunctivae* sp. n. From sheep and goats with Keratoconjunctivitis. Infect Immun. 1972;5:70–6.
45. Pellett PR, Roizman B (2007) The family Herpesviridae: a brief introduction. In: Knipe DM, Howley PM (5th edition) fields virology. Volume 2. Lippincott Williams & Wilkins, Pennsylvania.
46. das Neves CG, Thiry J, Skjerve E, Yoccoz NG, Rimstad E, Thiry E, Tryland M. Alphaherpesvirus infections in semidomesticated reindeer: a cross-sectional serological study. Rangifer. 2009;18(3):262–9.
47. Angelos JA, Spinks PQ, Ball LM, George LW. *Moraxella bovoculi* sp. nov., isolated from calves with infectious bovine keratoconjunctivitis. Int J Syst Evol Microbiol. 2007;57(4):789–95.
48. Galvão KN, Angelos JA. Ulcerative blepharitis and conjunctivitis in adult dairy cows and association with *Moraxella bovoculi*. The Canadian Veterinary Journal. 2010;51(4):400–2.
49. Gould S, Dewell R, Tofflemire K, Whitley RD, Millman ST, Opriessnig T, Rosenbusch R, Trujillo J, O'Connor AM. Randomized blinded challenge study to assess association between *Moraxella bovoculi* and infectious bovine Keratoconjunctivitis in dairy calves. Vet Microbiol. 2013;164(1–2):108–15.
50. Dickey AM, Loy JD, Bono JL, Smith TPL, Apley MD, Lubbers BV, DeDonder KD, Capik SF, Larson RL, White BJ, Blom J, Chitko-McKown CG, Clawson ML. Large genomic differences between Moraxella bovoculi isolates acquired from the eyes of cattle with infectious bovine keratoconjunctivitis versus the deep nasopharynx of asymptomatic cattle. Vet Res. 2016;47(1):31.
51. Garrity GM, Bergey DH (2001) Bergey's manual of systematic bacteriology. 2nd Edition. Springer, New York.
52. Quinn PJ, Markey BK, Leonard FC, FitzPatrick ES, Fanning S, Hartigan PJ (2011) Veterinary microbiology and microbial disease, 2nd Edition. Wiley-Blackwell, Portland.
53. Griebel PJ, Ohmann HB, Lawman MJP, Babiuk LA. The interaction between bovine herpesvirus type 1 and activated bovine T lymphocytes. J Gen Virol. 1990;71(2):369–77.
54. Donofrio G, Ravanetti L, Cavirani S, Herath S, Capocefalo A, Sheldon IM. Bacterial infection of endometrial stromal cells influences bovine herpesvirus 4 immediate early gene activation: a new insight into bacterial and viral interaction for uterine disease. Reproduction. 2008;136(3):361–6.

10

Surviving and fatal Elephant Endotheliotropic Herpesvirus-1A infections in juvenile Asian elephants – lessons learned and recommendations on anti-herpesviral therapy

Akbar Dastjerdi[1*†], Katharina Seilern-Moy[1,2†], Karin Darpel[2], Falko Steinbach[1,2] and Fieke Molenaar[3]

Abstract

Background: Elephant Endotheliotropic Herpesviruses (EEHVs) can cause acute haemorrhagic disease in young Asian elephants (*Elephas maximus*) and clinical EEHV infections account for the majority of their fatalities. The anti-herpesviral drug famciclovir (FCV) has been used routinely to treat viraemic at-risk elephants, but thus far without proven efficacy. This paper presents clinical and virological investigations of two EEHV-1A infected elephants treated with FCV, and discusses anti-herpesvirus therapies of viraemic elephants.

Cases presentations: Two 1.5 year old male Asian elephants at a zoological collection in the UK developed clinical EEHV-1A infections. Case 1 showed signs of myalgia for the duration of 24 hours before returning back to normal. EEHV-1A DNAemia was confirmed on the day of clinical signs and continued to be present for 18 days in total. Trunk shedding of the virus commenced 10 days after detection of initial DNAemia. Case 2 tested positive for EEHV-1A DNAemia in a routine blood screening sample in the absence of clinical signs. The blood viral load increased exponentially leading up to fatal clinical disease seven days after initial detection of DNAemia. Both calves were treated with 15 mg/kg FCV per rectum on detection of DNAemia and penciclovir, the FCV metabolite, could be detected in the blood at assumed therapeutic levels. The early indicators for clinical disease were a marked absolute and relative drop in white blood cells, particularly monocytes prior to the detection of viraemia. The most prognostic haematological parameter at later stages of the disease was the platelet count showing a continuous sharp decline throughout, followed by a dramatic drop at the time of death.

Conclusions: The EEHV-1A viraemic animals investigated here further highlight the ongoing threat posed by these viruses to juvenile Asian elephants. The findings call into question the efficacy of rectal FCV in clinical cases and direct towards the use of alternative anti-herpesvirus drugs and complementary treatments such as plasma infusions if no improvement in either viral load or the above-mentioned blood parameters are observed in the initial days of viraemia despite anti-herpesvirus therapy.

Keywords: EEHV-1, elephantid herpesvirus, EEHV-haemorrhagic disease, EEHV-HD, famciclovir, ganciclovir

Abbreviations: BID, Bis in die (twice a day); DNA, Deoxyribonucleic acid; EDTA, Ethylenediaminetetraacetic acid; HPLC, High performance liquid chromatography; i/v, Intravenous; PBS, Phosphate buffered saline; PCR, Polymerase chain reaction; qPCR, Quantitative PCR; TID, Ter in die (thrice a day)

* Correspondence: akbar.dastjerdi@apha.gsi.gov.uk
†Equal contributors
[1]Animal and Plant Health Agency-Weybridge, New Haw, Addlestone, Surrey KT15 3NB, UK
Full list of author information is available at the end of the article

Background

Elephant Endotheliotropic Herpesviruses (EEHVs) or Elephantid Herpesviruses (ElHVs) belong to the genus *Proboscivirus* of the family *Herpesviridae* [1, 2] and fall into 7 genotypes [3–9]. Phylogenetically, the viruses are most closely, although distantly, related to human cytomegalovirus (HCMV) and three human *Roseolo* viruses (human herpesvirus-6A, -6B, and -7), all members of the subfamily *Betaherpesvirinae* [1].

EEHVs, in particular EEHV-1, are the cause of acute haemorrhagic disease (EEHV-HD) in young Asian elephants (*Elephas maximus*), and clinical EEHV infections account for most of the fatalities in juvenile Asian elephants, both in their natural habitat and in captivity [7–13]. EEHV-1 induced acute haemorrhagic disease is manifested initially by sudden onset of non-specific clinical signs, which often develop into haemorrhagic disease and sudden death within 1 to 7 days [9, 12]. It has also been documented that EEHV viraemia is detectable at least several days before the onset of clinical signs [13, 14]. To enable early therapeutic intervention in response to detection of EEHV viraemia, some zoological collections have implemented regular blood sampling and laboratory testing of juvenile Asian elephants.

Conferring from herpesviruses' properties, it could be assumed that once an elephant is infected it remains a latent carrier for life. Screenings of elephant herds have revealed widespread prevalence of the viruses and their periodical reactivation and shedding through biological fluids, especially trunk secretions [13–19]. Routes of EEHVs transmission to naïve individuals are still unclear, however, considering other herpesviruses' transmission routes, contact with infected bodily secretions is a very likely possibility and vertical transmission cannot be excluded.

EEHVs, similar to viruses in the subfamily *Alphaherpesvirinae* and *Gammaherpesvirinae*, comprise of a genome with a thymidine kinase (TK) and a serine/threonine protein kinase (PK) [7, 20], which encode enzymes crucial for processing many anti-herpesviral prodrugs into their active derivatives. Based on approaches in treatment of other herpesviruses with TK and PK genes, three nucleoside analogues [famciclovir (FCV) and more recently ganciclovir (GCV) and aciclovir (ACV)] have been administered to treat viraemic elephant calves, with the aim to avert progression to clinical disease, but as yet without proven clinical efficacy. It is known that several elephant calves have survived laboratory confirmed EEHV infections. These elephant calves were treated with FCV at doses of 5.5-8.0 mg/kg twice daily (BID) rectally [9, 18, 19, 21–24] or with GCV at 5 mg/kg BID intravenously followed by oral administration [14, 25]. One elephant calf with advanced EEHV-1 clinical signs has been treated successfully with ACV at 12mg/kg BID intravenously for 15 days along with penicillin G and supportive treatment including vitamin C, physiological saline and 5 % Dextrose [26]. Apart from the latter case, it seems likely that many of surviving elephant calves represent relatively mild cases, in view of length of time taken to reach the highest viral load, level of viraemia at this point and recovery of blood parameters. It is therefore likely that these affected individuals might have recovered without drug intervention [9].

FCV, chemically known as 2-[2-(2-amino-9H-purin-9-yl)ethyl]-1,3-propanediol diacetate, is a synthetic acyclic guanosine analogue that is rapidly de-acetylated and oxidized in the body to its metabolite penciclovir (PCV). Activation of PCV requires phosphorylation in the virally infected cells by viral and cellular kinases. The drug has a half-life of approximately three hours and its catabolite is excreted renally [27]. PCV interacts with herpesvirus DNA polymerase, the enzyme responsible for creating DNA molecules through assembly of nucleotides (building blocks of DNA), and thus terminates DNA synthesis. A recent study showed that when administered to healthy young Asian elephants both orally or per rectum, FCV is absorbed and metabolised to PCV with plasma levels considered therapeutic in humans [27, 28]. ACV, another guanosine analogue with a biological half-life of 2-4 hours, is still used widely for the treatment and prevention of clinical Herpes Simplex Virus (HSV) and Varicella Zoster Virus (VZV) diseases in humans. Activation of ACV within cells via the viral and cellular kinases yields ACV–triphosphate, which interacts adversely with herpesvirus DNA synthesis [29]. GCV is another guanosine analogue that is activated via viral and cellular kinases. Its oral prodrug valganciclovir (VGCV) is the most commonly prescribed drug for the prevention and therapy of HCMV in immunocompromised patients [29].

This paper describes the investigations into two EEHV-1A viraemic elephants from a UK zoological collection that were both treated with FCV. It also discusses findings of the investigations in relation to anti-herpes viral therapies in EEHV viraemic elephants.

Case presentations

Virus screening

Blood samples of EDTA whole blood and blood swabs were collected under trained behaviour from an ear vein after aseptic preparation of the medial aspect of the ear pinna. For EDTA whole blood samples, the animal was placed in lateral recumbency and the lowermost ear was sampled, using a standard 21G 1-inch needle and a Vacutainer® blood collection system. For blood swabs, a dry 6-inch foam tipped swab (Sigma Aldrich, UK) was used for collection of a drop of blood after puncture of an ear vein with an insulin needle, with the elephant in standing position. Blood samples were kept at room temperature before being shipped to the laboratory, where they were stored at 4–8 °C until being processed. Under trained behaviour, conjunctival swabs and trunk swabs were collected. Conjunctival swabs were collected using a sterile dry swab for each eye, running these on the inside of the lower palpebra. Trunk secretions from the mucosa of each naris were collected on a dry 6-inch foam tipped swab at a depth of approximately 8–10 cm, under trained behaviour, and stored at −20 °C prior to further testing. Blood smears were made of freshly collected EDTA blood samples, air dried and stained with Diff-Quick (LabPak, UK) for an in-house relative white blood cell (WBC) differential count.

Nucleic acid was extracted from 140 µl EDTA whole blood using the QIAamp® Viral RNA Mini kit (Qiagen, UK) according to the manufacturer's protocol. For blood swabs, 560 µl buffer AVL from the kit were directly added to the foam tipped swabs, left for 15 minutes at room temperature, vortexed and spun briefly, and processed as per the manufacturer's instructions. To process trunk swab samples for nucleic acid extraction, 300 µl PBS and 6–8 glass beads (3 mm in diameter) were added to the swab inside a 2 ml Eppendorf tube, vortexed briefly and incubated for 30 minutes at room temperature. The tube content was then vortexed and nucleic acid was extracted following the EDTA whole blood protocol using 140 µl of the cleared suspension.

The qPCR used in this study was performed as described [16] using the QuantiFast® Pathogen PCR + IC kit (Qiagen). Briefly, 2 µl extracted DNA was added to 0.1 µl each forward and reverse primer (100 pmol/µl), 0.05 µl hydrolysis probe (100 pmol/µl), 5 µl 5× QuantiFast Pathogen Master Mix, 0.5 µl 50× High-ROX Dye solution, and 17.25 µl RNase-Free Water. The qPCR was performed on a MX3005P machine (Agilent Technologies, UK) using the cycling conditions of one cycle of 95 °C for five minutes followed by 45 cycles of 95 °C for 15 seconds, 60 °C for 30 seconds, and signal acquisition at the end of each cycle. The conventional PCRs were carried out as described [30] using several primer pairs to amplify partial sequences of polymerase (POL), glycoprotein L (gL) and gM genes.

The DNA standard used was a HPLC purified 100 bases synthetic oligonucleotide (Eurofins Genomics, UK), identical to the sequence of the qPCR target, diluted to provide serial copy numbers from 10^6 to 10^1 copies per PCR test. The synthetic oligonucleotide dilutions were run in triplicate in the PCRs to create a standard curve for EEHV genome quantification.

Supportive therapy and drug administration

Rectal fluids were provided after manual removal of all faeces from the rectum. Several litres of hand-warm water were then deposited into the distal colon at approximately one meter depth, through a standard garden hose pipe. Intravenous (i/v) access was acquired after antiseptic preparation of the medial aspect of the ear pinna, using an 18G 2.5-inch indwelling catheter (Milacath®, Mila International, USA) in an ear vein. The catheter was secured using Durapore® tape and superglue. Standard giving sets were used for i/v fluids and filtered giving sets for the administration of blood and blood components (Baxter, UK). Plasma was collected from adult herdmates under trained behaviour, in lateral recumbency from either an ear vein or a medial hind leg vein, in one litre citrate blood collection bags (Crusse, Denmark), stored for a minimum of eight hours at 5 °C and separated using manual pressure. The plasma was then stored at 5 °C and warmed to room temperature prior to administration.

Anti-herpes viral treatment consisted of either FCV or GCV. FCV (Novartis Pharmaceuticals, UK) 250 and/or 500 mg tablets were crushed using a pestle and mortar and suspended in hand warm water. Using a 60 ml syringe and a meter long tube, the suspension was administered in the distal colon after removal of all faeces as described above. GCV (Cymevene® 500 mg, Roche, UK) was diluted in one litre of physiological saline attached to a giving set and an i/v catheter, and administered slowly over a period of one hour.

For measurement of plasma levels of GCV and PCV, the FCV metabolite, whole blood samples obtained approximately 6-10 hours following drugs administration, were centrifuged at 800 × g for 10 minutes and plasma was collected and stored at −20 °C for later analysis. Plasma samples were analysed at the College of Veterinary Medicine, University of Tennessee, USA using a reverse phase HPLC method with solid phase extraction (SPE). The compounds were separated on an Atlantis T3 (4.6 × 250 mm) column with a mobile phase of 10 mM ammonium phosphate pH 2.9 and acetonitrile (95:5). The flow rate was 1.2 ml/min and fluorescence was measured at excitation 253 nm and emission 360 nm. Standard curves for plasma analysis were prepared by fortifying untreated, pooled elephant plasma with the drug to produce a linear concentration range of 10-5000 ng/ml. Average recovery was 100 % while intra and inter-assay variability ranged from 0.5 to 5.1 %. The lower limit of quantification was 10 ng/ml.

Case 1

In 2013, 1.5 year old male Asian elephant calf 'Scott' was presented with unwillingness to bend either foreleg, swinging both legs forward when walking. Its ears were drooping, the head was down and the calf was off solid food. An EDTA whole blood sample taken on the day tested qPCR positive for EEHV-1 DNA. Prior to this event, routine blood samples and trunk swabs tested negative for EEHV-1. Using a qPCR assay, the blood viral load was determined as $8.16*10^3$ viral genome copies (vgc)/ml (Fig. 1). Genomic analysis of this EEHV-1 by sequencing of PCR amplicons of partial viral POL, gL and gM genes identified the virus as EEHV-1A genotype. The sequences comparison with those of two EEHV-1A fatalities in 2009 (Riddle and Betts) at the collection revealed several nucleotide substitutions in the POL, gL and gM gene segments, indicating a genomically different virus from those in Riddle and Betts (Fig. 2).

Treatment with 15 mg/kg FCV three times daily (TID) per rectum was instigated eight hours after these initial clinical signs. The first two treatments, six hours apart, consisted of ground FCV tablets suspended in ultrasound gel (Healthlife®, Barclays-Swan Ltd, UK); however, most of the drug was expelled at the next defaecation. Twelve hours after the initial presentation, the calf started to voluntarily bend his right foreleg again, and by the next morning, despite some stiffness in the shoulders, the legs were in normal use and its appetite had returned. The dose of FCV was therefore reduced to 12 mg/kg TID (Day 1); this time dissolved in hand warm water and placed 1.5 meters deep into the rectum. All clinical signs were resolved by Day 2, when the blood viral load peaked at $3.61*10^4$ vgc/ml, after which it started to decrease gradually. The FCV dose was further reduced to 8 mg/kg BID on Day 7. Full haematology at this point showed a relatively low monocyte count ($5.94*10^9$/L, 26 % of WBC), but was normal (51 % of WBC) when tested three weeks later (Table 1a). No virus was detectable in the blood from Day 18 onwards (Fig. 1), and FCV treatment ceased on Day 21. Viral DNA excretion through eye (data not shown) and trunk secretions commenced on Day 10 and continued for at least two months, with a peak at around Day 48 of $4.66*10^3$ vgc/test reaction. No further samples were tested beyond Day 57.

As a pre-emptive measure, the calf's two siblings, a 3-year old male and a 4-year old female, were treated simultaneously with 12 mg/kg FCV TID from Day 0 to Day 6, which was tapered to 8 mg/kg BID from Day 7 to Day 12, after which treatment ceased. Neither sibling was positive for EEHV-1 DNA in blood or bodily secretions throughout this period.

Plasma PCV levels, measured at trough levels 8-10 hours following the latest FCV administrations in both Case 1 (Fig. 3) and its male sibling (data not shown), ranged between 68 and 934 ng/ml. Levels measured at the dosing regimens of 15 mg/kg TID and 12 mg/kg TID reached values considered therapeutic in humans with genital herpes (>100 ng/ml) [27].

Case 2

In 2015, a blood swab collected during routine weekly sampling of 1.5 year old male calf 'Max' tested positive for EEHV-1 DNA by qPCR. This result was confirmed by a subsequent EDTA whole blood sample that tested qPCR positive at $5.0*10^2$ vgc/ml of blood. At this point monocytes were abundant ($12.46*10^9$/L, 54 % of WBC) and the platelet count was $950*10^9$/L. (Table 1b, Day -33). A follow-up blood sample four days later was EEHV-1 DNA negative by qPCR and the calf remained negative on four subsequent blood swabs taken during a three-week period. On week 4 and one day prior to the calf being diagnosed again with EEHV-1 DNAemia the calf was presented with a swollen right temporal gland, which was painful on palpation and from which purulent discharge could be expressed. The gland was treated with pevidine (Sanofi, UK) flushes and topical amoxicillin/clavulanic acid application following bacteriological culture and sensitivity testing. After this positive EEHV

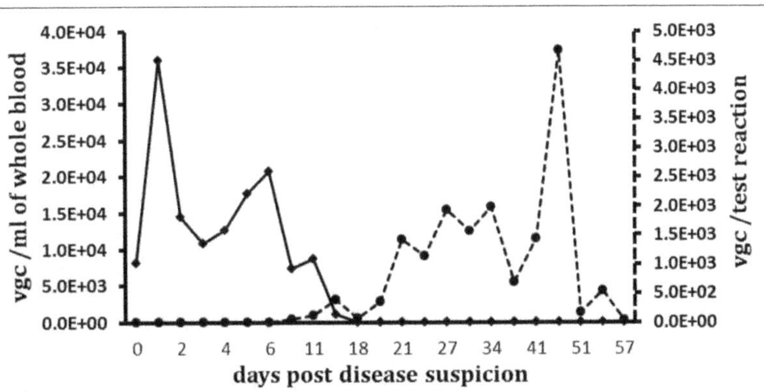

Fig. 1 EEHV-1A DNA levels in blood and trunk secretions of Case 1. Clinical suspicion of EEHV infection was confirmed by detection of EEHV-1A DNA in blood. The animal showed clinical signs suggestive of active EEHV-1A infection on Day 0 and Day 1. EEHV-1A DNA load in EDTA whole blood (solid line) and trunk secretions (dashed line) was measured using a qPCR

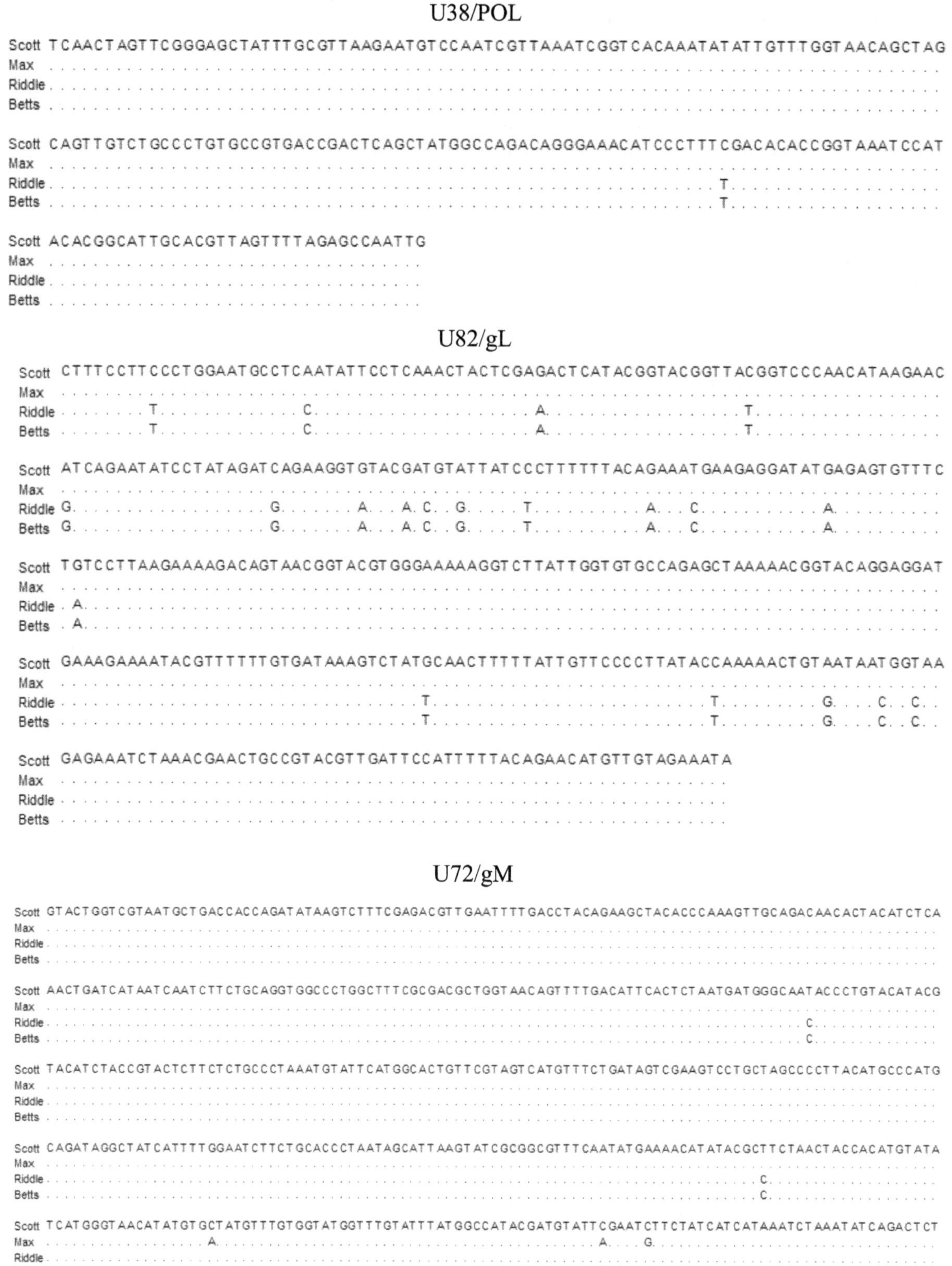

Fig. 2 Nucleotide sequence comparison of the EEHV-1A detected. Partial nucleotide sequences of DNA polymerase [U38/POL (194 bp)], glycoprotein L [U82/gL (381 bp)] and glycoprotein M [U72/gM (500 bp)] from Case 1 and Case 2 were compared with those of two previous EEHV-1A fatalities (Riddle and Betts) from the same zoological collection. Sequences were aligned using the MegAlign 13 software of the DNASTAR Lasergene 13 package (DNASTAR Inc. Madison, USA). Identical nucleotides to those of Case 1 are denoted by dots in the alignments

Table 1 Haematological parameters of Case 1 and Case 2 measured during clinical EEHV-1A infection

A

Days	WBC (*10e9/L)	Neutrophils (*10e9/L)	Lymphocytes (*10e9/L)	Monocytes (*10e9/L)	Eosinophils (*10e9/L)	Basophils (*10e9/L)
7	22.85	7.77	8.91	5.94 (26 %)	0.23	0
23	13.69	5.75	2.87	6.16 (45 %)	0	0
213	15.91	4.61	5.73	5.25 (33 %)	0.32	0
Physiological mean (% of WBC)	15.51	3.77 (25.5 %)	5.02 (23.65 %)	6.46 (50 %)	0.24 (1.55 %)	0.02 (0.10 %)

Days	RBC (*10e12/L)	HGB (g/dL)	HCT (%)	MCV (fL)	MCH (pg)	MCHV (g/dL)	RDW (%)	PLT (*10e9/L)	PCV (%)
7	3.54	13.4	37.7	107	37.8	35.5	14.3	**470**	36
23	5.06	19.2	55.1	109	37.9	34.8	14.5	968	55
213	3.62	13.3	39.2	108	36.8	33.9	13.9	996	37
Physiological (mean)	3.55	14.28	40.60	114.25	40.19	35.17	14.33	617.65	40.80

B

Days	EEHV-1A (vgc/ml)	WBC (*10e9/L)	Neutrophils (*10e9/L)	Lymphocytes (*10e9/L)	Monocytes (*10e9/L)	Eosinophils (*10e9/L)	Basophils (*10e9/L)
-33	5.0×10^2	**23.08**	4.62	**5.77**	**12.46 (54 %)**	0	0
-29	ND	**25.34**	4.56	**7.6**	**13.18 (52) %**	0	0
-5	1.2×10^5	**6.18**	3.46	**1.85**	**0.8 (13 %)**	0.06	0
-3	2.7×10^6	**7.35**	5.22	**1.32**	**0.81 (11 %)**	0	0
0	7.2×10^6	**13.25**	8.22	**2.65**	**2.25 (17 %)**	0.13	0
1	1.9×10^7	**12.925**	7.565	**2**	**2.975 (23 %)**	0	0.195
Physiological mean (% of WBC)		15.51	3.77 (25.5 %)	5.02 (23.65 %)	6.46 (50 %)	0.24 (1.55 %)	0.02 (0.10 %)

Days	RBC (*10e12/L)	HGB (g/dL)	HCT (%)	MCV (fL)	MCH (pg)	MCHV (g/dL)	RDW (%)	PLT (*10e9/L)	PCV (%)
-33	3.65	14.6	43.2	118.3	39.9	33.7	13.9	**950**	42
-29	3.58	14.5	41.4	115.5	40.4	35	38.1	**760**	38
-5	3.48	14.2	41.8	120.4	41	34	14	**560**	37
-3	3.36	14.2	38.4	114.4	42.4	37.1	13.7	**183**	38
0	2.89	12.4	32.9	113.7	42.9	37.8	13.8	**98**	34
1	3.07	12.95	35.05	114.2	42.2	36.9	13.6	**13**	36.5
Physiological mean	3.55	14.28	40.60	114.25	40.19	35.17	14.33	617.65	40.80

The haematological parameters for Case 1 (A) were only available for Days 7, 23 and 213 following suspicion of clinical EEHV-1A infection. The haematological parameters and viral load for Case 2 (B) were measured on several occasions from 33 days prior to the observation of signs indicative of clinical EEHV-1A infection (Day 0) to the Day 1 when the elephant succumbed to the infection at midnight. Normal platelet range of live juveniles in the collection was established, during a period of seven months from 20 blood samples of the elephants, to be at 372-878*10e9/L (mean of 625*10e9/L). The rest of the physiological parameters were from 24 measurements from four individuals under eight years of age (age range at time of sampling: 1.5-7y). Parameter values with a substantial change are highlighted in bold. Percentages of monocytes in the white blood cells are also given in the table

vgc/ml, viral genome copies per millilitre of EDTA whole blood; WBC, white blood cell count; RBC, red blood cell count; HGB, haemoglobin; HCT, haematocrit; MCV, mean cell volume; MCH, mean corpuscular haemoglobin; MCHV, mean corpuscular haemoglobin volume; RDW, red blood cell distribution width; PLT, platelet count; PCV, packed cell volume; ND, not detected

qPCR result from a blood swab, an EDTA whole blood sample also tested positive, with a viral load of $1.2*10^5$ vgc/ml, the monocyte count had markedly reduced to $0.8*10^9$/L (13 % of WBC) and the platelet count almost halved to $560*10^9$ /L, in the absence of clinical signs (Day -5). PCR results for this sample became available two days after the actual sampling date and treatment was immediately instigated at 15 mg/kg FCV TID per rectum. Blood samples were then taken regularly for EEHV-1 qPCR, viral quantification and haematology.

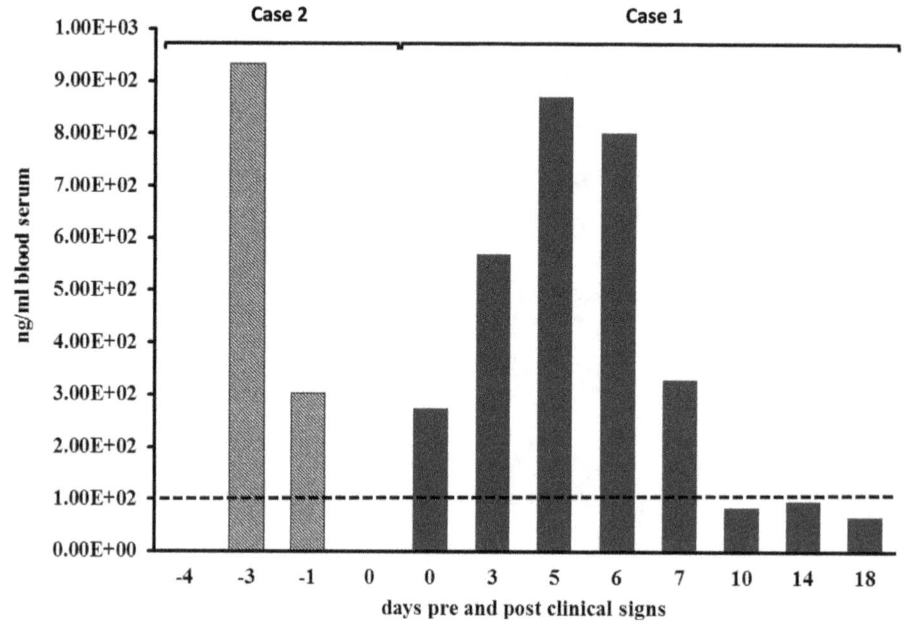

Fig. 3 Penciclovir, the metabolite of famciclovir, plasma levels in 2 juvenile Asian elephants with EEHV-1A DNAemia. Famciclovir (FCV) was rectally administered in Case 1 at 15 mg/kg twice daily (BID) on observation of clinical signs indicative of EEHV-1A infection (Day 0) and continued at the same dose rate until Day 1, when it was reduced to 12 mg/kg thrice daily (TID). This was followed by further reduction on Day 3 to 8 mg/kg BID and continued unchanged until Day 18. In Case 2 FCV was administered at 15 mg/kg TID for two days following the detection of EEHV-1A DNA in the blood (Day -5), five days prior to observation of EEHV-1A clinical signs, and continued at the same dosage till the last dose of FCV at 9:00 am on Day 0; blood was only collected at 17:00 pm on that day. The death of Case 2 was at midnight on Day 1; seven days after first detection of EEHV-1 DNA in the blood. Dashed line indicates the minimum level of PCV considered therapeutic in humans with genital herpes (>100 ng/ml) [27]

Genomic analysis of this EEHV-1 by sequencing of PCR amplicons of partial viral POL, gL and gM genes identified the virus as EEHV-1A genotype. However, comparing these nucleotide sequences to those of Case 1, it was revealed that the virus was genomically slightly different, but both cases were more dissimilar to Riddle and Betts (Fig. 2). Nucleotide sequences of the partial segments of the three genes for Riddle and Betts were identical. This was not unexpected as the two fatalities occurred within two weeks of each other, but longer sequence reads would be necessary to verify this further.

Viral load increased exponentially as time progressed, during which the monocyte count stabilised around $2.54*10^9$/L (17 % of WBC), but platelet counts showed a continuous decline (Table 1b). Lymphocyte count has also shown substantial reduction on the detection of DNAemia, but other haematological parameters such as neutrophil and basophil counts remained unchanged. PCV plasma levels as high as 934 ng/ml were attained during the first days of treatment (Fig. 3). Five days into the DNAemia, the calf started to show signs of lethargy. At this point, PCV plasma levels had dropped to 303 ng/ml, about a third of its previous peak.

The decision was made to start i/v fluids, consisting of Harmann's (15 ml/kg/h, Vetivex 11, Dechra, UK) supplemented with Duphalyte (1 ml/kg BW, Pfizer, UK), and complement the treatment from solely FCV per rectum to i/v plasma and GCV. The calf first displayed clinical signs of haemorrhagic disease six days into the DNAemia: oedema of the head and ventral abdomen, tongue petechiae and progressive signs of cyanosis. The platelet count had also reduced drastically at this point to $98*10^9$/L and viral load had increased to $7.2*10^6$ vgc/ml of blood. Intravenous cannulas were in place in both ears for administration of 1 ml/kg plasma TID, fluids and antibiotics (2 mg/kg marbofloxacin, Marbocyl®, Vetoquinol). Due to logistics, GCV (5 mg/ml) could not be administered until 16:00h that day, but achieved plasma levels of 2529 ng/ml following i/v injection. Clinical signs progressed despite treatment and the platelet count further reduced to $13*10^9$/L and viral load increased to $1.9*10^7$ vgc/ml of blood. The calf subsequently died at midnight, just into the next day as a result of hypoxaemia and hypovolaemia.

Discussion

The early clinical signs of EEHV-HD are non-pathognomonic and often manifested as lethargy, anorexia and lameness. As a consequence of generalized capillary endothelial cell damage, these early clinical signs are likely to be followed by more severe and generally terminal signs [5, 8, 12]. Routine blood testing of at-risk Asian elephants for EEHV viraemia has been suggested as part of a monitoring scheme to predict and potentially prevent fatal disease, as the viral DNA can be detected at least several days prior to any clinical signs [13, 14]. This routine monitoring was proven to be valuable in this study, where Case 2 continuous EEHV-1 DNAemia was detected five days prior to the earliest clinical signs, although unfortunately this early initiated treatment was not able to prevent fatality.

In addition to detection and quantification of viral DNA through real-time qPCR, drop in the monocyte/neutrophil ratio, and absolute reduction of the platelet count, make both the monocytes and platelets the most useful prognostic haematological parameters of EEHV-HD, although the exact physiological process for these changes is as yet unknown. It is possible that the monocytes are subjected to immediate assault of the virus [19], and that the viral damage to the endothelial cells beyond the adaptive nature of the host response leads to the development of disseminated intravascular coagulation (DIC) and hence critical loss of platelets. In Case 2, the platelet count showed a gradual decline well before the fatal progressive viraemia, reaching a dangerously low level before death. Archived data from three previous EEHV fatalities at the same collection show a similar critically low platelet count following clinical EEHV-1 manifestation (Table 2). Similar findings have also been recently reported from Asian elephants affected by EEHV-1B, 4 and 5 viraemia [13, 18, 19]. It is noteworthy that mean haematological parameters vary substantially in Asian elephants' blood, e.g. a reported range of 80-975*10^9/L for platelets [31–35]. Monocytes are usually the most abundant white blood cells in the majority of juveniles. In these cases, the relative drop of monocytes, compared to neutrophils, in the early stages of the disease could easily be identified on straightforward in-house white blood cell differentials. There are, however, individuals in which the monocytes are on average less abundant and hence this early indicator will be less beneficial in these cases. It is therefore advisable to establish individual baselines for at least the abovementioned haematological parameters for each at-risk elephant in advance, and that clinicians familiarise themselves with in-house blood smear differentials.

Monitoring kinetics of EEHV-1A load in the two elephants revealed rapid increase in viral load in the elephant that succumbed to the disease (Case 2) despite continuous anti-herpesviral treatment up to the EEHV-1 clinical signs. From at least three days prior to onset of clinical signs, PCV reached plasma levels suggested as therapeutic for treatment of diseases caused by alphaherpesviruses infections in humans [27], but here it had failed to control virus replication as the virus load continued to increase. Considering the approximate three hour half-life

Table 2 Haematological parameters of three additional fatal cases of EEHV-1A and EEHV-1B infections from the same zoological collection

Animals (date of sampling)	Virus type	WBC (*10e9/L)	Neutrophils (*10e9/L)	Lymphocytes (*10e9/L)	Monocytes (*10e9/L)	Eosinophils (*10e9/L)	Basophils (*10e9/L)		
Emilia									
(18/12/2006)	EEHV-1B	17	11.85	3.21	**1.9 (11.2 %)**	0.03	0.02		
Riddle									
(01/05/2009)	EEHV-1A	**2.71**	1.49	**0.84**	**0.27 (10 %)**	0	0		
Betts									
(15/05/2009)	EEHV-1A	**5.1**	3.11	**1.02**	**0.97 (19 %)**	0	0		
Physiological mean (% of WBC)		15.51	3.77 (25.5 %)	5.02 (23.65 %)	6.46 (50 %)	0.24 (1.55 %)	0.02 (0.10 %)		
Animals (date of sampling)	RBC (*10e12/L)	HGB (g/dL)	HCT (%)	MCV (fL)	MCH (pg)	MCHV (g/dL)	RDW (%)	PLT (*10e9/L)	PCV (%)
Emilia									
(18/12/2006)	3.05	12.8	39.2	122	42	34.4	15.7	**34.6**	NA
Riddle									
(01/05/2009)	3.55	13	37.7	106	36.7	34.6	17.4	**25.6**	35
Betts									
(15/05/2009)	3.16	12.9	55.1	112	40.8	36.5	17.3	**71.5**	NA
Physiological (mean)	3.55	14.28	40.60	114.25	40.19	35.17	14.33	617.65	40.80

Blood samples were taken following the observation of EEHV-1 infection clinical signs. WBC, lymphocyte, monocyte and platelet counts (highlighted in bold) consistently show substantial drop from their physiological level in the two fatalities caused by EEHV-1A. Percentages of monocytes in the white blood cells are also given in the table

WBC, white blood cell count; RBC, red blood cell count; HGB, haemoglobin; MCV, mean cell volume; MCH, mean corpuscular haemoglobin; MCHV, mean corpuscular haemoglobin volume; RDW, red blood cell distribution width; PLT, platelet count; PCV, packed cell volume; NA, not available

of PCV [27], the peak levels could have been up to three times higher than measured, as blood samples were taken 6-8 hours following the FCV administration.

The efficacy of FCV treatment to curb progression to EEHV-HD in clinical EEHV has always been debatable, as compromised cellular function at enteric level could affect absorption. This was indicated by the measured PCV level in Case 2, which dropped remarkably 48 hours prior to the onset of outwardly visible clinical signs. Factors such as drug expulsion and individual differences in drug metabolism are also considered possible causes of this drop [24]. These findings therefore favour those anti-herpesviral drugs that could be administered intravenously, to bypass the intestinal absorption step. Additionally, the available sequences for EEHV TK and PK have only 25 % amino acid identity with their orthologues in HSV and HCMV, target viruses for these drugs [9] and indirect surrogate in vitro assays have shown mild sensitivity for only the PK against PCV [36].

Taking into account the EEHV viraemia sequel following FCV administration in current and previous studies, the efficacy of FCV remains doubtful. Therefore the use of other, i/v administered and potentially more effective, anti- herpesviral therapies should be explored, especially in cases where pre-EEHV-HD viraemia, established through routine blood PCR monitoring, does not appear to be affected by FCV within the first days of treatment. In the absence of comprehensive data on a highly effective and safe anti-herpesviral drug, alternative drugs at present could include i/v administered nucleoside analogues such as GCV and ACV. The second-line drugs could be the pyrophosphate analogue foscarnet and the nucleotide analogue cidofovir, but these drugs all have their own safety issues. The most common adverse effect during GCV therapy in humans has been haematological toxicity, but this appears to be readily reversible on discontinuation of the drug [37]. It should also be noted that ACV is a hundred times more potent than FCV in inhibiting herpesviruses replication, but it suffers from a shorter half-life and intracellular concentration [38]. This drug has been recommended for clinical situations in humans where a rapid decrease in viral load is desirable, and could be of similar therapeutic value in EEHV clinical infections. The renal toxicity of the drug should also be considered in its therapy. Frequent measurement of EEHV load in blood samples is therefore of paramount value to establish the efficacy of ongoing therapy.

Complementary therapies that are likely to be of value include supportive therapies e.g. maintaining hydration and actions to prevent DIC and shock, such as i/v plasma administration from EEHV antibody positive adult donors, as a source of both antibodies and platelets, and a broad spectrum antibiotic to combat potential concurrent bacterial infections that might possibly be at the root of triggering the viral replication, predisposing to the infection or arise as a secondary infection.

Intravenous access appears to be of significant value for supportive treatment and anti-viral drug administration, and is straightforward in trained elephants that are used to being handled. The EEHV Advisory Group convened to debate this in 2014 and currently recommends minimum standards of care for all at-risk elephants irrespective of management systems, which include a section on Calf Training for intravenous access (www.eehvinfo.org). In elephants that have not attained this stage of training at the time of infection, repeated standing sedations using butorphanol and detomidine are possible, as used successfully in other institutions (Lauren Howard, personal communication).

As far as antibodies are concerned, Case 1 had been positive on an indirect ELISA for glycoprotein B (gB) about 9 months prior to the clinical signs and survived the viraemia [17]. On the other hand, Case 2 was also highly positive on the same gB ELISA (van den Doel, pers. communication) at the time of EEHV infection, but succumbed to the virus. For other closely related betaherpesvirus infections (e.g. HCMV), antibodies to the gB protein seemed to enhance protection by curbing at least the dissemination of the virus in the blood [29]. However, considering the fatality in Case 2 despite high anti-gB antibody, sole measurement of gB antibody may not be an indicator of protection against EEHV, as it is currently unknown which viral proteins are targeted by neutralising antibodies. The possibility also exists that early IgG antibodies to EEHV show a low avidity for the antigen and hence an avidity test is required to determine the value of antibodies against EEHV [39]. Also, in the view that herpesviruses (EEHVs and elephant gamma herpesviruses [EGHVs]) are ubiquitous in Asian elephant populations, the notion that the above mentioned ELISA is cross reactive with gB of similar viruses or other unknown agents cannot be excluded [9].

In this study, a detectable EEHV-1 DNAemia was correlated with the disease symptoms only when the blood viral load was at around $8.16*10^3$ vgc/ml of blood for Case 1 and $7.2*10^6$ vgc/ml for Case 2. A previous report states that a threshold of around $1.0*10^4$ vgc/ml of blood had coincided with apparent illness [14]. Clinical signs appeared at a much higher viral load in Case 2, emphasising a daily rapid increase in viral load as a more favourable determinant of initiating anti-herpesviral therapy, its success and disease prognosis. Our results also further endorse that DNAemia precedes virus shedding in trunk secretions of EEHV-1A infected animals, similar to those reported previously [13, 14, 18, 19]. Although there is no evidence that infectious particles are shed at a level sufficient to infect an in-contact animal, the potential risk these carrier elephants may pose following a clinical EEHV case should be considered.

Conclusions

The EEHV viraemic cases investigated here further highlight the ongoing threat posed by the virus to the juvenile Asian elephants, potentially leading to gradual disappearance of their free-living population and an inability to maintain a viable captive population to safeguard the species from extinction. Therefore, effective control of future EEHV infections is fundamental to improve the survival rate of affected animals. Routine EEHV testing combined with viral quantification, WBC, monocyte and platelet counts following confirmed DNAemia in at-risk elephants should deliver an early warning of the clinical disease and prognosis, providing enough time to evaluate treatment opportunities to avert a fatal outcome. This investigation further questions the efficacy of the rectally administered FCV in controlling the viraemia and urges towards the exploration of alternative therapies. These therapies could include preferably i/v administered anti-herpes viral drugs, complementary plasma transfusions and antibiotics against potential secondary infections.

Acknowledgements

We are grateful to Nic Masters, Jo Dodds and Karla Berry for veterinary support and to Lee Sambrook and his excellent team of elephant keepers for sample collection, which has made this study possible. We also thank Dr. Sherry Cox at the College of Veterinary Medicine, the University of Tennessee, USA for the penciclovir and ganciclovir measurements. Provision of the gB ELISA results by Petra van den Doel from Erasmus Medical Center, The Netherlands is highly appreciated. Many thanks also to Christopher Finnegan, APHA for performing some of the qPCRs. The funding bodies played no role in the design of this study, analysis and interpretation of data; in the writing of the manuscript; or in the decision to submit the manuscript for publication.

Funding

Funding for this work was partly provided by the Zoological Society of London, Chester Zoo and Rotterdam Zoo.

Authors' contribution

KSM performed the laboratory investigation. FM undertook the clinical work on the elephants. AD, KSM and FM led the manuscript preparation. KSM, AD, FM, KD, FS contributed to the interrogation of results and manuscript preparation. All authors read and approved the final manuscript.

Competing interests

The author(s) declare that they have no competing interests.

Author details

[1]Animal and Plant Health Agency-Weybridge, New Haw, Addlestone, Surrey KT15 3NB, UK. [2]School of Veterinary Medicine, Faculty of Health and Medical Sciences, University of Surrey, Guildford GU2 7XH, UK. [3]ZSL Whipsnade Zoo, Dunstable, Bedfordshire LU6 2LF, UK.

References

1. Davison AJ, Eberle R, Ehlers B, Hayward GS, McGeoch DJ, Minson AC, et al. The order Herpesvirales. Archives of Virology. 2009;154:171–7.
2. Richman LK, Hayward GS. Elephant herpesviruses. In: Fowler ME, Miller RE, editors. Zoo and wild animal medicine. 7th ed. 2012. p. 496–502.
3. Richman LK, Montali RJ, Garber RL, Kennedy MA, Lehnhardt J, Hildebrandt T, et al. Novel endotheliotropic herpesviruses fatal for Asian and African elephants. Science. 1999;283:1171–6.
4. Fickel J, Richmann LK, Montali RJ, Schaftenaar W, Goritz F, Hildebrandt TB, et al. A variant of the endotheliotrophic herpesvirus in Asian elephants (*Elephas maximus*) in European zoos. Vet Microbiol. 2001;82:2001.
5. Garner MM, Helmick K, Ochsenreiter J, Richman LK, Latimer E, Wise AG, et al. Clinico-pathological features of fatal disease attributed to new variants of endotheliotropic herpesvirus in two Asian elephants (*Elephas maximus*). Vet Pathol. 2009;46:97–104.
6. Latimer E, Zong JC, Heaggans SY, Richman LK, Hayward GS. Detection and evaluation of novel herpesviruses in routine and pathological samples from Asian and African elephants: identification of two new probosciviruses (EEHV5 and EEHV6) and two new gammaherpesviruses (EGHV3B and EGHV5). Vet Microbiol. 2011;147(1-2):28–41.
7. Wilkie GS, Davidson AJ, Wason M, Kerr K, Sanderson S, Bouts T, et al. Complete genome sequences of elephant endotheliotropic herpesviruses 1A and 1B determined directly from fatal cases. J Virol. 2013;87(12):6700–12.
8. Wilkie GS, Davidson AJ, Kerr K, Stidworthy MF, Redrobe S, Steinbach F, et al. First fatality associated with elephant endotheliotropic herpesvirus 5 in an Asian elephant: Pathological findings and complete viral genome sequence. Sci Rep. 2014;4:6299.
9. Long SY, Latimer EM, Hayward GS. Review of elephant endotheliotropic herpesviruses and acute haemorrhagic disease. ILAR J. 2015;56(3):283–96.
10. Zachariah A, Zong JC, Long SY, Latimer EM, Heaggans SY, Richman LK, et al. Fatal herpesvirus haemorrhagic disease in wild and orphan Asian elephants in Southern India. J Wildl Dis. 2013;49(2):381–93.
11. Zong JC, Latimer E, Heaggans SY, Richman LK, Hayward GS. Pathogenesis and molecular epidemiology of fatal elephant endotheliotropic disease associated with the expanding *Proboscivirus* genus of the *Betaherpesvirinae*. Orlando: International Elephant Conservation and Research Symposium; 2007. p. 23–35.
12. Richman LK, Montali RJ, Cambre RC, Schmitt D, Hardy D, Hildebrandt TB, et al. Clinical and pathological findings of a newly recognised disease of elephants caused by endotheliotropic herpesviruses. J Wildlife Dis. 2000;36:1–12.
13. Atkins L, Zong JC, Tan J, Mejia A, Heaggans SY, Nofs SA, et al. Elephant endotheliotropic herpesvirus 5, a newly recognized elephant herpesvirus associated with clinical and subclinical infections in captive Asian elephants (*Elephas maximus*). J Zoo Wildl Med. 2013;44(1):136–43.
14. Stanton JJ, Zong JC, Eng C, Howard L, Flanagan J, Stevens M, et al. Kinetics of viral loads and genotypic analysis of elephant endotheliotropic herpesvirus-1 infection in captive Asian elephants (*Elephas maximus*). J Zoo Wildlife Med. 2013;44(1):42–54.
15. Stanton JJ, Zong JC, Latimer E, Tan J, Herron A, Hayward GS, et al. Detection of pathogenic elephant endotheliotropic herpesvirus in routine trunk washes from healthy adult Asian elephants (*Elephas maximus*) by use of real-time quantitative polymerase chain reaction assay. Am J Vet Res. 2010;71:925–33.
16. Hardman K, Dastjerdi A, Gurrala R, Routh A, Banks M, Steinbach F, et al. Detection of elephant endotheliotropic herpesvirus type 1 in asymptomatic elephants using TaqMan real-time PCR. Vet Rec. 2012;170(8):205.
17. van den Doel P, Prieto VR, van Rossum-Fikkert SE, Schaftenaar W, Latimer E, Howard L, et al. A novel antigen capture ELISA for the specific detection of IgG antibodies to elephant endotheliotropic herpesvirus. BMC Vet Res. 2015;11:203.
18. Fuery A, Tan J, Peng R, Flanagan JP, Tocidlowski ME, Howard LL, Ling PD. Clinical infection of two captive Asian elephants (*Elephas maximus*) with elephant endotheliotropic herpesvirus 1B. J Zoo Wildl Med. 2016;47(1):319–24.
19. Fuery A, Browning GR, Tan J, Long S, Hayward GS, Cox SK, et al. Clinical infection of captive Asian elephants (*Elephas maximus*) with elephant endotheliotropic herpesvirus 4. J Zoo Wildl Med. 2016;47(1):311–8.
20. Ehlers B, Dural G, Marschall M, Schregel V, Goltz M, Hentschke J. Endotheliotropic elephant herpesvirus, the first betaherpesvirus with a thymidine kinase gene. J Gen Virol. 2006;87:2781–9.
21. Schmitt DL, Hardy DA, Montali RJ, Richman LK, Lindsay WA, Isaza R, et al. Use of famciclovir for the treatment of endotheliotropic herpesvirus infections in Asian elephants (*Elephas maximus*). J Zoo Wildl Med. 2000;31:518–22.

22. Schaftenaar W, Mensink JMCH, de Boer AM, Hildebrandt TB, Fickel J. Successful treatment of a subadult Asian elephant bull (*Elephas maximus*) infected with the endotheliotropic elephant herpes virus. Proceedings. 40th Int Symp Dis Zoo Wild Anim 2001, 141–146.
23. Tocidlowski ME, Marin M, Flanagan JP, Howard LL. Medical monitoring and treatment of clinical EEHV viraemia in juvenile Asian elephants (*Elephas maximus*) at the Houston zoo. Proceedings. 10th International Elephant Endotheliotropic Herpesvirus (EEHV) Workshop 2015, Houston, USA. Page 38
24. Howard LL, Cox S. Penciclovir levels in Asian elephants undergoing famciclovir treatment for clinical EEHV viremia at the Houston Zoo. Proceedings. 10th International Elephant Endotheliotropic Herpesvirus (EEHV) Workshop 2015, Houston, USA. Pages 33-34
25. Padilla, LR. Use of ganciclovir in Asian elephants for treatment of EEHV infection. Proceedings. 10th International Elephant Endotheliotropic Herpesvirus (EEHV) Workshop 2015, Houston, USA. Page 32
26. Boonprasert K, Mahasawangku1 S, Angkawanish T, Jansittiwej S, Langkaphin W, Sombutputorn P, et al. Endotheliotropic herpesvirus treatments in a wild orphan baby Asian elephant (*Elephas maximus*). Proceedings. 10th International Elephant Endotheliotropic Herpesvirus (EEHV) Workshop 2015, Houston, USA. Page 35
27. Gill KS, Wood MJ. The clinical pharmacokinetics of famciclovir. Clin Pharmacokinet. 1996;31:1–8.
28. Brock AP, Isaza R, Hunter RP, Richman LK, Montali RJ, Schmitt DL, et al. Estimates of the pharmacokinetics of famciclovir and its active metabolite penciclovir in young Asian elephants (*Elephas maximus*). Am J Vet Res. 2010;73(12):1996–9.
29. Field HJ, Vere Hodge RA. Recent developments in anti-herpesvirus drugs. Br Med Bull. 2013;106:213–49.
30. Seilern-Moy K, Darpel K, Steinbach F, Dastjerdi A. Distribution and load of elephant endotheliotropic herpesviruses in tissues from associated fatalities of Asian elephants. Virus Res. 2016;220:91–6.
31. Silva ID, Kuruwita VY. Haematology, plasma, and serum biochemistry values in domesticated elephants (*Elephas maximus ceylonicus*) in Sri Lanka. Gajah. 1994;12:47.
32. Niemuller C, Gentry PA, Liptrap RM. Longitudinal study of haematological and biochemical constituents in blood of the Asian elephants (*Elephas maximus*). Comp Biochem Physiol. 1990;96A:131–4.
33. Lewis JH. Comparative haematology: Studies on elephants, *Elephas maximus*. Comp Biochem Physiol. 1974;49A:175–81.
34. Brown IRF, White PT. Elephant blood haematology and chemistry. Comp Biochem Physiol. 1980;65B:1–12.
35. Wiedner E. Proboscidea. In: Fowler's zoo and wildlife medicine, 8th Edition, Eds Fowler ME & Miller RE. 2015, 524
36. Ackermann M, Schetle N. In vitro investigation into antiviral efficacy and EEHV. Proceedings. 10th International Elephant Endotheliotropic Herpesvirus (EEHV) Workshop 2015, Houston, USA. Pages 31
37. Markham A, Faulds D. Ganciclovir. An update of its therapeutic use in cytomegalovirus infection. Drugs. 1994;48(3):455–84.
38. Cassady KA, Whitely RJ. New therapeutic approaches to the alphaherpesvirus infections. J Antimicrob Chemother. 1997;39(2):119–28.
39. Prince HE, Lapé-Nixon M. Role of cytomegalovirus (CMV) IgG avidity testing in diagnosing primary CMV infection during pregnancy. Clin Vaccine Immunol. 2014;21(10):1377–84.

11

Development and application of an indirect enzyme-linked immunosorbent assay using recombinant truncated Cap protein for the diagnosis of porcine circovirus-like virus P1

Li-bin Wen[1,2,3*†], Shi-fu Wen[1,2,3†] and Kong-wang He[1,2,3]

Abstract

Background: Porcine circovirus-like virus P1 is a newly discovered virus. To date, there has been no specific serological assay for use in the diagnosis of P1 infection.

Results: Because P1 has high homology to porcine circovirus type 2 (PCV2) at the nucleotide level, the C-terminal portion of the capsid protein (amino acids 73–114), a discriminative antigen, was expressed in a prokaryotic expression system. The recombinant product (rctCap), composed of three identical repeated domains, was shown to be strongly immunoreactive to P1-specific serum. This assay was validated by comparison with an indirect immunofluorescence assay (IFA). The diagnostic sensitivity and specificity of the rctCap enzyme-linked immunosorbent assay (ELISA) developed in this study are 93.6 % and 98.3 %, respectively, compared with the results from IFAs on 450 sera samples from pigs.

Conclusions: The indirect ELISA that we developed with rctCap, the recombinant capsid fragment containing the 217–342 nt repeat domain, was sensitive, specific, and suitable for the large-scale detection of P1 infections in swine.

Keywords: Porcine circovirus-like virus P1, ORF1 protein, ELISA, Swine farms

Background

Porcine circovirus (PCV) is a nonenveloped, single-stranded, DNA virus with a circular genome of approximately 1.7 kb, belonging to the family *Circoviridae*. Porcine circovirus type 1 (PCV1) was first isolated as a nonpathogenic contaminant virus in a porcine kidney cell line [1], whereas porcine circovirus type 2 (PCV2) is recognized as a causative agent of postweaning multisystemic wasting syndrome (PMWS) [2], a multifactorial swine disease first identified in Canada in 1991 [3]. PCV2 has since been reported in most pig-producing countries worldwide, including China [4–6]. The PCV2 genome contains three major open reading frames (ORFs): ORF1, ORF2, and ORF3 [7–9]. ORF1 encodes the 35.7-kDa Rep proteins, which are essential for viral DNA replication [10]; ORF2 encodes the 30-kDa structural capsid protein involved in the host immune response [11]; and the ORF3 protein is involved in PCV2-induced host cell apoptosis [12].

Porcine circovirus-like virus P1 was recently identified and has the smallest genome of all DNA viruses (648 nucleotides), which is highly homologous to that of PCV2. Like the PCVs, P1 has a single-stranded circular DNA genome. P1 is thought to be a recombinant virus formed between PCV2 and another virus [13], and it similarly contains three major ORFs: ORF1, ORF2, and ORF3. Recently, we reported that ORF1 of P1 encodes a major structural protein of approximately 12.5 kDa. This protein reacts strongly with serum from P1-infected swine, suggesting its possible utility in diagnostic assays

* Correspondence: wlbwh@hotmail.com
†Equal contributors
[1]Institute of Veterinary Medicine, Jiangsu Academy of Agricultural Sciences, Nanjing 210014, China
[2]Key Laboratory of Veterinary Biological Engineering and Technology, Ministry of Agriculture, Nanjing 210014, China
Full list of author information is available at the end of the article

[14]. A comparison of the deduced N-terminal amino acid sequence of P1 ORF1 revealed that it has a high homology with the N-terminal domain of PCV2 ORF2. However, they only share a low amino acid sequence homology in the C-terminal region because there has been a frameshift in the P1 ORF1.

Epidemiological studies have confirmed that the P1 virus is endemic on pig farms in China [15]. In vivo studies have shown that P1 infects pigs and the infected animals show the clinical signs of PMWS [16].

To determine the prevalence of P1 infection and to clarify how PMWS develops, specific tools for antibody detection are essential. Testing for P1 antibodies in sera is currently performed with indirect immunofluorescence assays (IFAs) or immunoperoxidase monolayer assays (IPMAs) [16]. However, these assays are very time-consuming, whereas enzyme-linked immunosorbent assays (ELISAs) can be automated and are more convenient. Notably, two antigenic epitopes of the P1 capsid (Cap) protein have been identified at amino acid residues 6–18 and 80–92. A peptide antibody derived from the immunorelevant 6–18 epitope was used in our previous investigations [17]. However, the resulting test was not specific for P1 because there is a slight amount of antigenic cross-reactivity between PCV2 and P1. A 2014 report demonstrated that a peptide antibody test using the 80–92 epitope was highly specific for P1. Therefore, we used this epitope to establish methods for the specific serological detection of P1 [17]. A recombinant C-terminally truncated capsid protein (rctCap) of P1, expressed in an *Escherichia coli* system, was used as an antigen to develop an indirect ELISA.

The objectives of the present study were to establish and validate a diagnostic indirect ELISA for the serological detection of anti–P1 serum antibodies.

Methods

Ethics statement

This study was approved by the Committee on the Ethics of Animal Experiments of the Institute of Veterinary Medicine, Jiangsu Academy of Agricultural Sciences (JAAS no 20100604) (Nanjing, China).

Expression, purification, and identification of the rctCap protein

To construct a plasmid expressing rctCap, genomic DNA was obtained from P1-infected porcine kidney epithelial (PK15) cells and used as the template for polymerase chain reaction (PCR). To obtain the target gene, ORF1 without the N-terminal 216-nucleotides (nt), three pairs of primers (Table 1) were designed according to the published genome sequence of P1 strain JSNJ (GenBank: KJ612072).

The PCR product generated using the A1 and A2 primer pair was doubly digested with *Nco*I and *Eco*RI and cloned into the prokaryotic expression vector pET-28a (+) (Invitrogen, CA, USA). The resulting recombinant expression plasmid, pET28a-mono-ORF1 was ligated to the PCR product generated with the B1 and B2 primer pair and doubly digested with *Eco*RI and *Sac*I. The PCR product generated using the C1 and C2 primer pair was then digested with the *Sac*I and *Hind*III endonucleases and transferred into the above construct, resulting in the recombinant expression plasmid, pET28a-bi-ORF1. The pET28a-tri-ORF1 plasmid was then constructed similarly and used to transform competent *E. coli* DH5α cells (Fig. 1). Clones containing the recombinant plasmid were identified with restriction enzyme digestion and DNA sequencing (GenScript Corporation, China).

The rctCap plasmid has three tandem repeats, each encoding 42 amino acids. The three central repeats are identical except for a few linker amino acids.

To express the cloned gene, competent *E. coli* BL21-(DE3) cells (TransGen Biotech, China) were transformed with pET28a-tri-ORF1. Alternately, these cells were transformed with plasmid pET-28a (+) as a control. Single-positive clones of the transformed cells were grown in Luria-Bertani medium containing 80 μg/ml kanamycin at 37 °C (with shaking) to an optical density at 600 nm (OD_{600}) of about 0.4–0.6. Protein expressin was induced in these cells by the addition of isopropyl

Table 1 Sequences of primers used for the PCRs

Primers	Sequences (5′-3′)	Underlined restriction site
A1	TTATCCATGGGCCACCACCACCACCACCACACTACTCCTCCCGCCAT ACAAT	*Nco*I
A2	GCCGAATTCGCCAAAGCTGATTCTT	*Eco*RI
B1	ATGAATTCACTACTCCTCCCGCCATAC	*Eco*RI
B2	TTGGAGCTCGCCAAAGCTGATTCCT	*Sac*I
C1	ATAGAGCTCACTACTCCTCCCGCCATACAAT	*Sac*I
C2	CGAAGCTTATTAGCCAAAGCTGATTCCTTTTGTT	*Hind* III

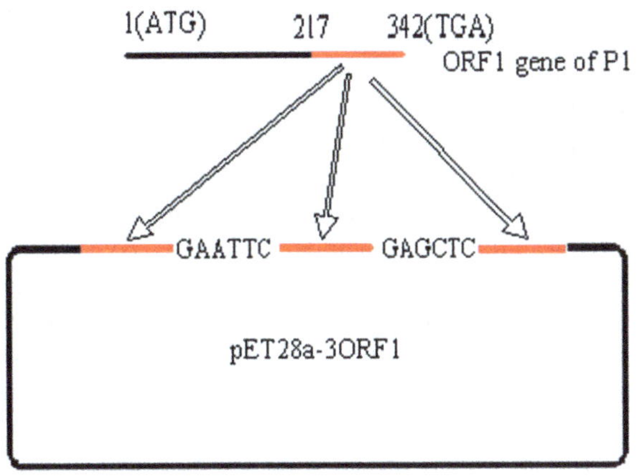

Fig. 1 Construction of the rctCap expression plasmid. A schematic diagram showing the construction of the rctCap expression plasmid used in this study. The fragments of identical sequence are marked in red

β-D-1-thiogalactoside (IPTG) to a final concentration of 1 mM for 6–8 h at 37 °C. The bacteria were pelleted and resuspended in phosphate-buffered saline (PBS), and then lysed with sonication on ice. The sonicated cells were centrifuged at 10,000 × g for 30 min at 4 °C and the precipitate was resuspended and purified by Ni^{2+}-NTA agarose (Qiagen, Germany), according to the manufacturer's instructions. The eluates containing the rctCap protein were pooled and dialyzed against 0.01 M PBS (pH 7.2). The purified proteins were analyzed with sodium dodecyl sulfate–polyacrylamide gel electrophoresis (SDS-PAGE) and transferred electrophoretically to a nitrocellulose membrane. The membrane was blocked with blocking buffer (Tris-buffered saline containing 0.1 % Tween-20 and 2 % skim milk powder) overnight at 4 °C and then incubated with rabbit anti-P1 antibody (diluted 1:200) raised against the synthetic peptide CSPNPSPTTPVTSH. Horseradish peroxidase (HRP)-conjugated goat anti-rabbit IgG antibody (1:3000) (Boster Biological Technology, Wuhan, China) was used as the secondary antibody. Immunoreactivity was visualized with diaminobenzidine (Boster Biological Technology).

The concentration of the purified rctCap protein was determined with the Bradford method using bovine serum albumin (BSA, Sigma-Aldrich, St. Louis, MO, USA) as the standard, and the purified rctCap protein was stored at −70 °C until use in later assays.

ELISA procedure

High-binding 96-well microtiter plates (Greiner BioOne, USA) were coated with 100 μl of rctCap protein in 0.05 M bicarbonate/carbonate buffer (pH 9.6) overnight at 4 °C. After three washes in PBS (pH 7.4) containing 0.05 % Tween 20 (PBS-T), the plates were blocked with 1 % BSA for 1 h at 37 °C. Serum samples were diluted in PBS (pH 7.4) containing 5 % dry milk, 100 μl of the diluted samples were added to the wells, and the plates were incubated for 1.5 h at 37 °C. The plates were then washed five times with PBS-T and incubated for 45 min at 37 °C with 100 μl of diluted HRP-conjugated goat anti-swine IgG antibody (KPL, Gaithersburg, MD). The plates were then washed four times, and the colorimetric reaction was developed with 50 μl of Tetramethylbenzidine Liquid Substrate (Sigma-Aldrich) for 10 min at 37 °C. The color reaction was stopped by the addition of 50 μl of 1 M H_2SO_4, and the OD_{450} was measured with a microplate reader (Bio-Tek Instruments, USA).

Based on the procedure described above, the optimal antigen concentration and serum dilution were determined with a checkerboard serum dilution analysis. In brief, the rctCap protein was serially diluted 2-fold from 5.24 μg/ml to 0.33 μg/ml. Additionally, P1-positive swine sera and P1 seronegative control swine sera were also subjected to a similar serial 2-fold dilution from 1:25 −1:800 for use in the optimization of the rctCap ELISA. After the optimal antigen and antiserum dilutions were established, the HRP-labeled goat anti-swine IgG antibody was added to the plate at dilutions of 1:5000, 1:10,000, 1:20,000, and 1:40,000 to determine the optimal detection antibody dilution for this ELISA. The conditions that gave the highest positive control OD_{450}/negative control OD_{450} (P/N) ratio and had an OD_{450} value close to 1.0 for positive serum were considered to be the optimal working conditions.

Determination of the negative–positive cut-off

Nine hundred swine serum samples were collected sequentially from P1-free pigs that tested negative both for P1 antibodies via IFA and for P1 nucleic acids via PCR assays. These samples were used to set the negative–positive cut-off value for the rctCap ELISA. The mean S/P ratio (x) and standard deviation (SD) were calculated, and the cut-off value was calculated as x + (3 × SD).

Evaluation of assay performance

To evalute the negative–positive cut-off value for this assay, 450 serum samples from farm pigs were tested in duplicate with the newly developed rctCap ELISA. The diagnostic accuracy of this ELISA was determined by calculating the diagnostic sensitivity and specificity of the test. IFA was used as the reference method to classify the samples as positive or negative. The sensitivity and specificity of the rctCap ELISA were determined as follows: sensitivity = (TP/[TP + FN]) × 100, and specificity = (TN/[TN + FP]) × 100, where TP, FN, TN and FP indicate the true-positive, false-negative, true-negative, and false-positive, respectively.

To detect the specificity of the rctCap ELISA, seropositive sera for PCV2, classical swine fever virus

(CSFV), porcine parvovirus (PPV), porcine pseudorabies virus (PRV), or porcine reproductive and respiratory syndrome virus (PRRSV) were tested with the rctCap ELISA. Each sample was tested in triplicate, and the S/P ratios were calculated.

Determination of assay reproducibility

To determine the reproducibility of the rctCap ELISA, six serum samples from farm pigs (three IFA-postitve samples and three IFA-negative samples) were selected for use in the reproducibility experiments. We ran four replicates of each serum sample on the same plate to assess the intra-assay (within-plate) reproducibility, and we ran five replicates of each sample on different plates to assess the inter-assay (between-run) reproducibility.

The results were used to calculate the mean S/P ratios and coefficients of variation (CV).

IFA

Confluent PK15 cell monolayers, either untransfected or transfected with an infectious molecular clone of the P1 virus, in 96-well plates (Costar, Corning, NY, USA) were fixed in methanol-acetone for 15 min at −20 °C, and the plate was then washed three times with PBS (pH 7.2). Serum samples (50 μl) diluted 1:20 in PBST were added to the plates and incubated for 1 h at 37 °C. After three washes with PBST, fluorescein-conjugated anti-swine IgG antibody (KPL), diluted 1:100, was added and the samples were incubated for 30 min at 37 °C. Fluorescence was observed with an inverted fluorescence microscope (Olympus, Japan).

Serum samples

A serological study was performed to estimate the seroprevalence of P1 in the swine population. Serum samples ($n = 1135$) were collected randomly from 11 herds with or without PMWS in the Jiangsu, Anhui, Shandong, and Zhejiang Provinces and Shanghai Municipality, China in 2008–2011. The origins of the serum samples were as follows: 86 and 70 serum samples were from farm A and farm B in Jiangsu Province, respectively; 72, 86, and 54 serum samples were from farm C, farm D, and farm E in Anhui Province, respectively; 42 and 106 serum samples were from farm F, and farm G in Shandong Province, respectively; 90 serum samples were from farm H in Shanghai Municipality; and 55, 69, and 405 serum samples were from farm I, farm J, and farm K in Zhejiang Province, respectively. The 405 serum samples from farm K in Zhejiang Province were obtained from different animal growth stages: suckling piglets (0–5 weeks, 140 sera), nursing pigs (8–13 weeks, 145 sera), fattening pigs (18–19 weeks, 60 sera), sows (45 sera), and breeding boar (15 sera).

Results

Cloning, expression and purification of the rctCap protein

The truncated ORF1 was amplified with PCR and used with the appropriate primers to construct the recombinant truncated ORF1 fragment, which is composed of three repeated identical domains. The result was cloned into the pET-28a (+) vector, from which recombinant proteins were expressed as histidine (His) fusion proteins. After IPTG induction, the recombinant *E. coli* carrying the pET-28a-tri-ORF1 cassette expressed a 14.7-kDa protein, which corresponded to the expected size of the rctCap protein (containing an N-terminal peptide of six histidines). The recombinant protein was expressed as inclusion bodies in *E. coli*, and its size was confirmed with SDS-PAGE. *E.coli* carrying the recombinant plasmid were lysed with lysozyme (final concentration, 1 mg/ml) and sonication. The rctCap protein was purified from the lysate by using affinity chromatography. Most of the rctCap protein was eluted from a Ni^{2+}-NTA affinity column. The purified protein was separated with SDS-PAGE and blotted onto a nitrocellulose membrane for immunodetection. The SDS-PAGE analysis of the eluted fractions revealed that the protein was purified as

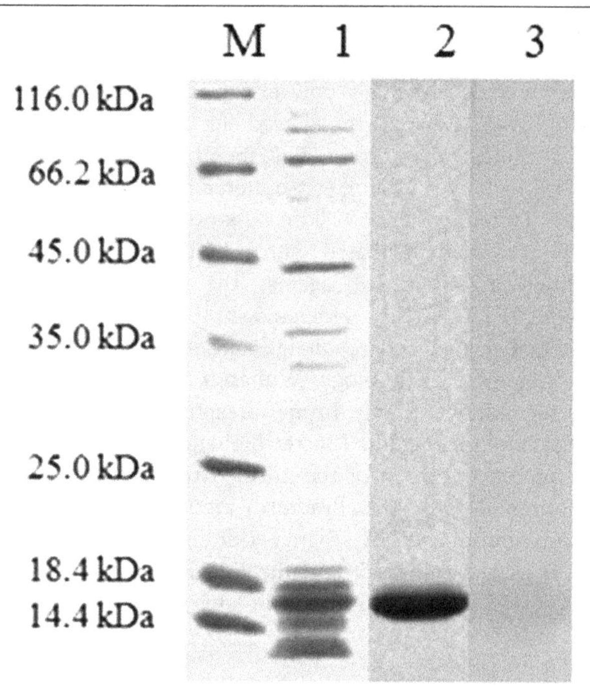

Fig. 2 Identification of the rctCap protein with SDS-PAGE and western blotting. M: protein molecular weight marker; 1: IPTG-induced cell lysate; 2: rctCap protein purified with a Ni^{2+}-NTA affinity chromatography column; 3: the purified rctCap protein reacted strongly with rabbit anti-P1 polyclonal antibody detected with HRP- conjugated goat anti-rabbit antibody as the secondary antibody

a single 15-kDa band. The reactivity of the rctCap protein to rabbit anti-P1 serum was observed with a western blotting assay (Fig. 2). These results confirm that this antigen can be used to detect specific antibodies directed against P1.

Optimization of the rctCap ELISA

We used checkboard ELISAs to determine the optimal antigen concentration and the serum sample dilution, which were set at 2.62 μg/ml and 1:100, respectively, based on the criteria that under these conditions the OD_{450} value for positive serum was close to 1.0 and the P/N value was highest. After these conditions were met, other factors in the rctCap ELISA were optimized. We found that 1 % BSA was the best blocking solution for this assay., giving the highest P/N value, compared with the other tested blocking solutions The optimal dilution of the conjugate was 1:5000. When the optimal exposure time for the serum samples or detection antibody was investigated, incubation for 90 min or 45 min, respectively, was shown to be best.

Reproducibility of the rctCap ELISA

The intra-assay and inter-assay reproducibility of the rctCap ELISA were determined by comparing the S/P ratios for each farm pig serum sample tested in triplicate. The intra-assay CVs of three serum samples that had been determined as P1 seropositive by IFA (IFA-positive) in the rctCap ELISA ranged from 1.5–3.3 %. The inter-assay CVs for IFA-positive serum samples in the rctCap ELISA ranged from 2.91–7.61 % (Table 2). The rctCap ELISA also showed good repeatability with three pig sera that had been determined as P1 seronegative by IFA (IFA-negative), as indicated by the low variability among the three replicates of identical samples. These data show that this assay is repeatable, yielding acceptably low levels of variation.

Determination of the negative–positive cut-off

To set a negative–positive cut-off value for the rctCap ELISA, 900 presumed P1 seronegative farm swine sera collected from normal uninfected pigs were examined. The mean ± SD OD_{450} value for the normal pig sera in the rctCap ELISA was 0.21008 ± 0.04484, which gave a negative–positive cut-off S/P value of approximately 0.345 (mean + 3SD) for this assay. Therefore, serum samples with an $OD_{450} > 0.345$ in this assay were regarded as seropositive for P1.

Table 2 Repeatability of the rctCap ELISA for IFA-positive serum samples of farm pig sera

Repeatability	Intra-assay			Inter-assay		
1	1.162	1.040	1.233	0.878	1.113	1.134
2	1.135	1.079	1.191	0.913	1.220	1.088
3	1.121	1.066	1.164	0.934	1.231	1.261
4	1.137	1.008	1.252	0.886	1.019	1.146
5	-	-	-	0.872	1.178	1.053
CV	1.50 %	3.00 %	3.30 %	2.91 %	7 .61 %	6.95 %

Specificity of the rctCap ELISA

The specificity of the rctCap ELISA was determined by testing the reactivity of 10 samples each of PPV, CSFV, PRV, PRRSV, or PCV2-positive sera, which came from the commercial ELISA kit. The results show that the mean OD_{450} values for the sera, described above were 0.193, 0.131, 0.185, 0.178, and 0.206, respectively. Therefore, based on our defined negative–positive cut-off value of $OD_{450} > 0.345$, none of these antisera was detected as P1 seropositive by the rctCap ELISA. These findings confirm that the rctCap antigen is specific for antibodies directed against P1.

Validation of the rctCap ELISA

Of the 1135 swine serum samples described above, 450 randomly selected samples were assessed with both the rctCap ELISA and IFA. Of these, IFA found 162 samples as P1 seropositive and 288 samples as P1 seronegative, while evaluation with the rctCap ELISA at a cutoff value of 0.345 found 156 samples as P1 seropositive and 294 samples as P1 seronegative. When the samples were judged by both methods, 151 were considered P1 seropositive and 283 were considered P1 seronegative. Comparatively, five samples assessed as P1 seropositive by the rctCap ELISA were assessed as P1 seronegative by the IFA, and 11 samples determined as P1 seronegative by the rctCap ELISA were assessed as P1 seropositive by the IFA (Table 3). The sensitivity and specificity of the rctCap ELISA were 93.6 % and 98.3 %, respectively, based on the assumption that the IFA, considered the gold standard for P1 antibody detection, was 100 % accurate. The rate of accordbetween these two methods was 96.4 %.

Results for farm pig serum samples assessed by the rctCap ELISA

The results for the 1135 farm pig serum samples tested with the rntCAP ELISA are presented in Table 4. Of these, 352 samples were positive and 783 samples were

Table 3 Comparison of the rctCAP ELISA with IFA for 450 farm pig serum samples

IIF results	ELISA results		
	Positive	Negative	Total
Positive	151	11	162
Negative	5	283	288
Total	156	294	450

Table 4 Prevalence of antibodies to P1 by ELISA in swine serum samples obtained from Jiangsu, Anhui, Shandong, Shanghai and Zhejiang

Farms	Jiangsu		Anhui			Shandong		Shanghai	Zhejiang		
	A	B	C	D	E	F	G	H	I	J	K
No. of sera tested	86	70	72	86	54	42	106	90	55	69	405
No. of sera positive	3	51	14	7	19	35	32	13	0	22	156
% sera positive	3.5	72.9	19.4	8.1	35.2	83.3	30.2	14.4	0	31.9	38.5

negative for anti-P1 antibodies. The seroprevalence of P1 in farm K in Zhejiang Province was 48.6 % for suckling piglets, 34.5 % for nursing pigs, 18.3 % for fattening pigs, 53.3 % for sows, and 20 % for breeding boars (Table 5).

Discussion

The increasing incidence of PMWS on pig farms has become a real threat to the global swine industry. Because P1 is associated with PMWS [16], detecting P1 in pig herds is essential for the control of this syndrome. Therefore P1-specific diagnostic tools are required to clarify the course of infection. To date, only PCR, IFA, and IPMA assay are used to detect P1 infection.

IFA is considered to be a sensitive method for detecting P1, but it requires virus-infected cells as well as experienced technicians to examine the stained plates, and it is laborious and time-consuming. Therefore, IFA is not suitable for large-scale surveys. The purpose of this study was to develop an indirect ELISA to detect antibodies specific for P1.

The N-terminal region of Cap contains one potential epitope shared by PCV2 and P1. Therefore, to avoid complications from antigenic cross-reactivity, we did not use the full-length Cap protein in this assay. The C-terminal 42 amino acids of Cap are unique to P1 and can be used to differentiate between antibodies directed against PCV2 and those directed against P1. However, because the conserved C-terminal region is very small, we constructed a plasmid containing three tandem repeats, each encoding the same 42 amino acids. Each 42-amino acid repeat was separated by 6 nt of a restriction enzyme recognition site, which created a two amino-acid linker between repeats. The plasmid was also constructed in frame with an N-terminal peptide of six histidines, which allowed the expressed capsid protein to be purified easily with chromatography. A strong specific signal was observed via western blotting, confirming that the truncated protein did not destroy the C-terminal epitope.

Table 5 Anti-P1 antibodies in different categories of pigs from Hangzhou pig farm K

	suckling piglets	nursing pigs	fattening pigs	sows	breeding boar
No. of sera tested	140	145	60	45	15
No. of sera positive	68	50	11	24	3
% sera positive	48.6	34.5	18.3	53.3	20

We compared the newly developed indirect ELISA for detecting P1-specific antibodies with an IFA. The data from the rctCap ELISA agreed quite well with the data from the IFA, with a relative sensitivity of 93.6 % and a specificity of 98.3 %.

There is high homology between the amino acid sequences of ORF2 of PCV2 and ORF1 of P1, especially in the N-terminal regions. Therefore, to determine the usefulness of the rctCap ELISA for P1, we had to evaluate its specificity against PCV2. Our results confirm that the rctCap ELISA does not react with antibodies directed against PCV2. Our data also demonstrate the specificity of this assay, which does not detect antibodies directed against PPV, CSFV, PRV, or PRRSV.

Epidemiological studies of P1 infections conducted on 11 farms in China showed that all of the herds were P1 seropositive, except for one, irrespective of the presence or absence of clinical signs of PMWS. A high P1 seroprevalence was observed in suckling piglets and sows (48.6 % and 53.3 %, respectively).

Conclusions

The rctCap ELISA described in this study can be used for the detection of antibodies directed against P1, and this assay is highly sensitive, specific, and widely applicable to screening large numbers of serum samples. This report is the first to demonstrate different P1 serological profiles of pigs at different stages in herds with or without clinical signs of PMWS. However, further serological surveys are required to determine the dynamics of P1 infection in herds and the relationship of P1 to PMWS.

Competing interests

The authors declare that they have no competing interests.

Authors' contributions

LW and SW carried out the experiments and wrote the manuscript. KH designed the experiments. All authors read and approved the final manuscript.

Acknowledgements

This study was funded by the National Natural Science Foundation of China (31272574, 30972184) and Fund for Independent Innovation of Agricultural Sciences in Jiangsu province CX(14)2045.

Author details

[1]Institute of Veterinary Medicine, Jiangsu Academy of Agricultural Sciences, Nanjing 210014, China. [2]Key Laboratory of Veterinary Biological Engineering and Technology, Ministry of Agriculture, Nanjing 210014, China. [3]National Center for Engineering Research of Veterinary Bio-products, Nanjing 210014, China.

References

1. Tischer I, Gelderblom H, Vettermann W, Koch MA. A very small porcine virus with circular single-stranded DNA. Nature. 1982;295:64–6.
2. Allan GM, McNeilly F, Kennedy S, Daft B, Clarke EG, Ellis JA, et al. Isolation of porcine circovirus-like viruses from pigs with a wasting disease in the USA and Europe. J Vet Diagn Invest. 1998;10:3–10.
3. Clark EG: Post-weaning multisystemic wasting syndrome. In: Proceedings of the American Association of Swine Practitioners, Quebec City: American Association of Swine Practitioners, Perry, IA; 1997. pp. 499–501.
4. Allan GM, Ellis JA. Porcine circoviruses: a review. J Vet Diagn Invest. 2000;12:3–14.
5. Segales J, Domingo M. Postweaning multisystemic wasting syndrome (PMWS) in pigs. A review. Vet Quarterly. 2002;24:109–24.
6. Wen L, Guo X, Yang H. Genotyping of porcine circovirus type 2 from a variety of clinical conditions in China. Vet Microbiol. 2005;110:141–6.
7. Hamel AL, Lin LL, Nayar GP. Nucleotide sequence of porcine circovirus associated with postweaning multisystemic wasting syndrome in pigs. J Virol. 1998;72:5262–7.
8. Meehan BM, McNeilly F, Todd D, Kennedy S, Jewhurst VA, Ellis JA, et al. Characterization of novel circovirus DNAs associated with wasting syndromes in pigs. J Gen Virol. 1998;79:2171–9.
9. Morozov I, Sirinarumitr T, Sorden SD, Halbur PG, Morgan MK, Yoon KJ, et al. Detection of a novel strain of porcine circovirus in pigs with postweaning multisystemic wasting syndrome. J Clin Microbiol. 1998;36:2535–41.
10. Mankertz A, Mankertz J, Wolf K, Buhk H. Identification of a protein essential for replication of porcine circovirus. J Gen Virol. 1998;79:381–4.
11. Nawagitgul P, Morozov I, Bolin SR, Harms PA, Sorden SD, Paul PS. Open reading frame 2 of porcine circovirus type 2 encodes a major capsid protein. J Gen Virol. 2000;81:2281–7.
12. Liu J, Chen I, Kwang J. Characterization of a previously unidentified viral protein in porcine circovirus type 2-infected cells and its role in virus-induced apoptosis. J Virol. 2005;79:8262–74.
13. Wen L, He K, Yu Z, Mao A, Ni Y, Zhang X, et al. Complete Genome Sequence of a Novel Porcine Circovirus-Like Agent. J Virol. 2012;86:639.
14. Wen L, Wang F, He K, Li B, Wang X, Guo R, et al. Transcriptional analysis of porcine circovirus-like virus P1. BMC Vet Res. 2014;10:287–94.
15. Wen L, He K, Yang H, Yu Z, Mao A, Zhong S, et al. Prevalence of porcine circovirus-like agent P1 in Jiangsu, China. Virol J. 2011;8:543–7.
16. Wen L, He K, Xiao Q, Yu Z, Mao A, Ni Y, et al. A novel porcine circovirus-like agent P1 is associated with wasting syndromes in pigs. PLoS One. 2012;7(8):e41565.
17. Wen L, Wang F, He K, Ni Y, Zhang X, Guo R, et al. The establishment of immunlchemistry test based on a synthetic peptide antibody for the detection of a porcine circovirus-like virus P1. Agri Sci Technol. 2014;15(2):187–90.

12

Molecular analysis of carnivore Protoparvovirus detected in white blood cells of naturally infected cats

Andrea Balboni[1], Francesca Bassi[1], Stefano De Arcangeli[1], Rosanna Zobba[2], Carla Dedola[2], Alberto Alberti[2] and Mara Battilani[1*]

Abstract

Background: Cats are susceptible to feline panleukopenia virus (FPV) and canine parvovirus (CPV) variants 2a, 2b and 2c. Detection of FPV and CPV variants in apparently healthy cats and their persistence in white blood cells (WBC) and other tissues when neutralising antibodies are simultaneously present, suggest that parvovirus may persist long-term in the tissues of cats post-infection without causing clinical signs. The aim of this study was to screen a population of 54 cats from Sardinia (Italy) for the presence of both FPV and CPV DNA within buffy coat samples using polymerase chain reaction (PCR). The DNA viral load, genetic diversity, phylogeny and antibody titres against parvoviruses were investigated in the positive cats.

Results: Carnivore protoparvovirus 1 DNA was detected in nine cats (16.7%). Viral DNA was reassembled to FPV in four cats and to CPV (CPV-2b and 2c) in four cats; one subject showed an unusually high genetic complexity with mixed infection involving FPV and CPV-2c. Antibodies against parvovirus were detected in all subjects which tested positive to DNA parvoviruses.

Conclusions: The identification of FPV and CPV DNA in the WBC of asymptomatic cats, despite the presence of specific antibodies against parvoviruses, and the high genetic heterogeneity detected in one sample, confirmed the relevant epidemiological role of cats in parvovirus infection.

Keywords: Canine parvovirus, Cat, Coinfection, Feline panleukopenia virus, White blood cells, PCR

Background

Parvoviruses are non-enveloped single-stranded DNA viruses which infect a wide range of mammalian species, including several members of the order *Carnivora*. The Carnivore protoparvovirus 1, belonging to genus *Protoparvovirus*, family *Parvoviridae*, subfamily *Parvovirinae*, includes several closely related autonomous viruses causing a range of serious conditions, especially in young animals: feline panleukopenia virus (FPV, the prototype virus of the former carnivore parvovirus), canine parvovirus (CPV), mink enteritis virus (MEV), and raccoon parvovirus (RaPV) [1].

Feline panleukopenia virus has been known to be a cause of disease in cats since the beginning of the twentieth century, although there are other similar parvovirus species affecting cats, such as MEV and CPV. Natural infections in cats with CPV have been reported but FPV remains the most prevalent parvovirus causing disease in cats [2–4]. Since cats are susceptible to FPV and CPV 2a, 2b, 2c variants, superinfection and co-infection with multiple parvovirus strains associated with high viral genetic heterogeneity can occur with relatively high frequency in feline hosts [3, 5–7].

Parvoviruses commonly cause acute infection with high levels of viral shedding which generally ceases within 1–2 weeks post-infection, after the development of high titres of virus-neutralising antibody [8, 9]. Nevertheless, parvoviruses can be detected in faeces forup to 6 weeks after recovery, depending on the sensitivity of

* Correspondence: mara.battilani@unibo.it
[1]Department of Veterinary Medical Sciences, Alma Mater Studiorum - University of Bologna, Via Tolara di Sopra 50, 40064 Ozzano dell'Emilia, BO, Italy
Full list of author information is available at the end of the article

the diagnostic method used [10]. Cats experimentally infected with FPV shed the virus in both urine and faeces up to day 41–42 post-infection with parvovirus persisting in the lungs and kidneys for more than 50 weeks in cats which have recovered [11]. The detection of FPV and CPV variants in apparently healthy cats suggests that parvovirus infection may be common in some populations of clinically normal cats, and that asymptomatic cats may be able to shed parvovirus for prolonged periods of time [12–14]. Furthermore, the ability of FPV and CPV to persist in the peripheral blood mononuclear cells (PBMC) of cats irrespective of the presence of neutralising antibodies [13–17] and the presence of parvoviral DNA in the bone marrow of healthy cats [18], suggests that parvovirus may persist long term in the tissues of cats post-infection without causing clinical signs.

The aim of this study was to screen a population of 54 cats from Sardinia (Italy) for the presence of both FPV and CPV DNA within buffy coat samples. The DNA viral load, genetic diversity, phylogeny and antibody titres against parvoviruses were investigated in the cats testing positive to DNA parvoviruses.

Methods

Study design and sampling

This was a retrospective study, carried out on stored blood samples taken for routine diagnostic investigations undertaken at the Department of Veterinary Medicine, University of Sassari - UNISS (Sassari, NO Sardinia, Italy). Buffy coats from cats sampled between October 2011 and March 2012 were tested for the presence of feline and canine parvovirus DNA using real-time polymerase chain reaction (PCR). The partial VP2 gene of the viruses identified was sequenced and used for statistical analyses and phylogenetic comparisons. In addition, the sera of the cats which were positive to DNA parvoviruses were tested for the parvovirus antibody using the haemagglutination inhibition (HI) assay. Samples of owned or stray cats with different life-style conditions (indoor or outdoor, living alone or in community) were tested to evaluate different exposure to parvoviruses. Date of sampling, gender, age, breed, habitat and the clinical symptoms of the 54 cats sampled are reported in Table 1. According to these data, the animals were divided into two groups called A and B. The cats included in Groups A were predominantly healthy cats from four multi-cat households. The cats in Group B were sampled in the Emergency Room of the Veterinary Teaching Hospital of the Department of Veterinary Medicine (UNISS) and were predominantly stray cats showing different clinical signs (sick cats). Twenty-two of the 54 (40.7%) cats were clinically normal; 26/54 (48.1%) showed clinical signs attributable to various diseases; 3/54 (5.6%) showed gastrointestinal signs, such as vomiting and diarrhoea compatible with parvovirus infection; clinical status was unavailable for 3/54 (5.6%) cats. The vaccination status of the cats included in the study was unknown, although it was hypothesised that the stray cats were unvaccinated.

Anti-coagulated peripheral blood samples in ethylenediaminetetraacetic acid (EDTA) and coagulated blood for serology were collected from each cat. The blood samples were stored a + 4 °C and sera at – 20 °C until use.

DNA extraction

Buffy coat-containing mononuclear cells was isolated from 3 ml of EDTA anti-coagulated peripheral blood samples using Histopaque-1077 (Sigma Aldrich, St. Louis, Mo, USA). The DNA was extracted using the DNeasy Blood and tissue Kit (QIAGEN, Hilden, Germany), according to the manufacturer's instructions. The extracted DNA was eluted in 100 μl of ultrapure RNasi and DNasi free water, and was stored at – 20 °C after analysis.

Detection of parvovirus infection using SYBR green real-time PCR

Parvovirus screening was carried out using real-time PCR using two conserved primers (A-for and B-rev, Table 2) targeting a 99 bp fragment of the VP2 gene. Quantitative PCR (qPCR) was carried out using SYBR Premix Ex Taq II (Takara Bio inc., Shiga, Japan) and the Rotor-Gene 3000 system (Corbett Research, Mortlake, NSW, Australia). The fluorescence signal was acquired on the FAM channel (multi-channel machine, source, 470 nm; detector, 510 nm; gain set to 5) with a fluorescence reading taken at the end of each elongation step. Each run consisted of an initial incubation in order to activate the hot-start DNA polymerase at 95 °C for 30 s followed by 40 cycles of denaturation at 95 °C for 10 s, annealing at 60 °C for 20 s and polymerisation at 72 °C for 30 s. During the melt cycle, the temperature was increased by increments of 1 ° C from 65 °C to 95 °C. A pCR 4 plasmid (Invitrogen, Carlsbad, California, USA) containing one copy of the VP2 target sequence was produced as the external standard for the construction of the assay standard curve for quantitative analysis. Duplicates of six 10-fold dilutions of the standard plasmid, duplicates of the buffy coat DNA extracts of the cats sampled and a no template control were simultaneously analysed. Specimens were considered positive if the fluorescence curve in the amplification plot showed an exponential increase, and if a specific melting peak was observed. Copies of viral DNA were expressed per microlitre of DNA extract.

Molecular characterisation of viral sequences

Amplification and sequencing of the VP2 gene

In order to differentiate between FPV and CPV variants 2a, 2b and 2c, a fragment of the VP2 gene coding for critical amino acid residues 297, 300, 305, 323 and 426

Table 1 Characteristics of the 54 cats sampled

Cat	Date of sampling	Group	Breed	Gender	Age	Clinical signs	Habitat
01	06/10/2011	B	Mixed	MaN	2Y	Lethargy, dyspnoea, weight loss	Outdoor
02	11/10/2011	B	Mixed	MaN	3Y	Icterus, weight loss, CRF	Indoor
03	13/10/2011	B	Mixed	Fe	6Y	None	Outdoor
04	12/10/2011	A	Siamese	Fe	10Y	None	Outdoor
05	12/10/2011	A	Siamese	Ma	4Y	None	Outdoor
06	13/10/2011	A	Mixed	Ma	ND	None	ND
07	13/10/2011	A	Mixed	ND	ND	None	ND
08	13/10/2011	A	Mixed	ND	ND	None	ND
09	20/10/2012	B	Mixed	Fe	8M	Limb fracture	Outdoor
10	25/10/2011	B	Mixed	FeS	15Y	Vomit	Indoor
11	27/10/2011	A	Mixed	FeS	10Y	None	Outdoor
12	27/10/2011	A	Mixed	MaN	4Y	None	Outdoor
13	03/11/2011	A	Mixed	Fe	7Y	None	Outdoor
14	08/11/2011	B	Mixed	Fe	3Y	Vomit, diarrhoea	Indoor
15	20/09/2011	A	Mixed	Fe		ND	Outdoor
16	10/11/2011	A	Mixed	Ma	6Y	Respiratory signs	Outdoor
17	10/11/2011	A	Mixed	Fe	6Y	Respiratory signs	Outdoor
18	10/11/2011	A	Mixed	Fe	5Y	None	Outdoor
19	17/11/2011	A	Mixed	Fe	5Y	None	Outdoor
20	12/10/2011	A	Mixed	Ma	2Y	Stunted growth, respiratory signs	Outdoor
21	11/10/2011	A	Mixed	Ma	3Y	None	Outdoor
22	22/11/2011	A	Mixed	Fe	6Y	None	Outdoor
23	13/12/2011	A	ND	ND	ND	ND	ND
24	11/10/2011	B	Mixed	Ma	2Y	Trauma	Indoor
25	12/01/2011	B	Mixed	Ma	3Y	Horner syndrome, intracranial mass	Outdoor
26	24/01/2012	B	Mixed	MaN	4Y	None	Indoor
27	30/01/2012	B	Persian	Fe	ND	Behavioural disorders, Inappetence	Indoor
28	30/01/2012	B	Mixed	MaN	6Y	Anorexia, weight loss, third eyelid ptosis	Outdoor
29	09/02/2012	B	Mixed	Ma	12Y	Vomit, diarrhoea	Indoor
30	13/02/2012	B	Mixed	Fe	7Y	Multiple fractures	Outdoor
31	17/02/2012	A	Mixed	Ma	ND	None	ND
32	21/02/2012	A	Mixed	FeS	5Y	Icterus	Outdoor
33	21/02/2012	A	Mixed	Ma	3Y	None	Outdoor
34	27/02/2012	B	Mixed	MaN	7Y	Skin lesions, anorexia, anaemia, weight loss	Indoor
35	28/02/2012	B	Mixed	FeS	2Y	EG	Indoor
36	07/03/2012	B	Mixed	FeS	2Y	Alopecia and crusts in the ears, nose and limbs.	Indoor
37	08/03/2012	B	Mixed	MaN	5Y	Gingival lesions, mucocutaneous MCT	Indoor
38	09/03/2012	B	Mixed	FeS	1Y	Itching without skin lesions.	Outdoor
39	09/03/2012	B	Mixed	FeS	13Y	Breast neoformations	Indoor
40	01/12/2011	B	Mixed	FeS	6Y	SCC in the ears, nose and eyes	Outdoor
41	29/11/2011	B	Mixed	MaN	15Y	CRF	Indoor
42	13/03/2012	A	Mixed	Fe	8Y	None	ND
43	12/03/2012	A	Mixed	Fe	10Y	Skin lesions	Outdoor
44	13/03/2012	A	Mixed	Ma	7Y	None	ND
45	12/03/2012	A	Mixed	Ma	7Y	None	ND
46	12/03/2012	A	Mixed	Fe	6Y	None	ND
47	14/03/2012	B	Mixed	Fe	7Y	Blindness	Outdoor
48	14/03/2012	B	Mixed	Fe	5Y	Dysuria, hematuria	Outdoor
49	15/03/2012	B	Mixed	MaN	ND	Strangury, dysuria	Indoor
50	21/03/2012	B	Mixed	MaN	9Y	EG, unilateral otitis	Indoor
52	26/03/2012	A	Mixed	Fe	2Y	Skin lesions	Outdoor
54	23/03/2012	B	Mixed	Ma	ND	ND	Indoor
55	27/03/2012	A	ND	Ma	ND	None	Outdoor
56	27/03/2012	B	ND	ND	ND	None	Indoor

Ma male, *Fe* female, *MaN* male neutered, *FeS* female spayed, *Y* Years, *M* months, *CRF* chronic renal failure, *MCT* mast cell tumors, *SCC* Squamous cell carcinoma, *EG* Eosinophilic granuloma, *ND* Not determined
In grey: cats which tested positive for FPV or CPV

Table 2 Primers used

	Primer name	Primer sequence	Nucleotide position	Fragment amplified
Real Time-PCR	A-for	5'-AGCTACTATTATGAGACCAGCTGAG-3'	3767–3791	A-B: 99 bp
	B-rev	5'- CCTGCTGCAATAGGTGTTTTAA-3'	3844–3865	
Hemi-nested-PCR	C-for (P3[b])	5'-CCATTTCTAAATTCTTTG –3'	3651–3668	C-D: 881 bp
	D-rev (VPrev[a])	5'-TTTCTAGGTGCTAGTTGAG –3'	4513–4531	
	E-rev (P4[b])	5'-AAGTCAGTATCAAATTCTT –3'	4201–4219	C-E: 569 bp

The primer positions refer to the nucleotide sequence of FPV reference strain CU-4 (GenBank accession number M38246). [41][a], [42][b]

affecting the biological and antigenic proprieties was amplified and sequenced for each virus identified using real-time PCR. A hemi-nested PCR assay was developed by using three conserved primers (C-for, D-rev and E-rev, Table 2) for this purpose. Both PCR reactions were carried out using *Taq* DNA Polymerase (QIAGEN, Hilden, Germany) producing DNA fragments of 881 bp and 569 bp in length for the first and the second reaction, respectively. The temperature cycling protocol of the first amplification consisted of 94 °C for 5 min, 45 cycles with 1 cycle at 94 °C for 30 s, at 48 °C for 1 min, and at 72 °C for 1 min, followed by a final elongation at 72 °C for 10 min. In the second amplification, the PCR conditions were 94 °C for 5 min, 35 cycles with 1 cycle at 94 °C for 30 s, at 49 °C for 1 min, and at 72 °C for 45 s, followed by a final elongation at 72 °C for 10 min. In both PCR reactions, FPV 1033/09 [3] was used as a positive control while ultrapure water was used in each experiment to avoid false positive results. The nucleotide sequences were obtained using both forward and reverse primers.

Direct sequencing of the PCR products of one virus identified (number 41/2011) showed an unusually high number of ambiguities, suggesting a mixed viral population. Therefore, the amplification product was cloned into the pCR 4/TOPO vector using the TOPO cloning kit (Invitrogen, Carlsbad, CA, USA), and was transformed into *Escherichia coli* DH5α-competent cells according to the manufacturer's protocol. Ten recombinant clones were sequenced using both forward and reverse primers.

Sequence data

The nucleotide sequences obtained were assembled and translated into amino acid sequences using BioEdit sequence alignment editor version 7.2.5 [19]. The VP2 assembled nucleotide sequences were aligned with reference sequences of feline and canine parvoviruses available in the GenBank (http://www.ncbi.nlm.nih.gov/genbank), including the modified live FPV vaccine strains available, using the ClustalW method implemented with BioEdit software.

A variety of statistical analyses aiming to investigate nucleotide diversity, sequence variability and natural selection were carried out on the sequence data set using DnaSP package version 5.10.01 [20]. Statistical analysis was carried out on the subpopulations, grouping the sequence data in the FPV, CPV and 41/2011 (all clones of sample 41/2011) clusters.

The following parameters were estimated for each cluster: total number of mutations (η), nucleotide diversity (π) and its standard error, total number of synonymous differences (SynDif), and total number of non-synonymous differences (NSynDif). Mutation frequency (total number of changes/total number of bases sequenced) and the percentage of mutated clones were used as indicators of genetic diversity of the viral population of virus 41/2011.

Phylogenetic relationships among the viruses detected and the parvovirus reference sequences were evaluated using MEGA version 7.0.20 [21]. The best-fit model of nucleotide substitution was determined using the Find Best DNA/Protein Model function implemented in MEGA, and the Tamura 3-parameter model was found to be optimal for all the sequence data (including reference strains). Phylogenetic trees were constructed using the Maximum Likelihood method, and bootstrap values were determined by 1000 replicates to assess the confidence level of each branch pattern.

Nucleotide sequence accession numbers

The nucleotide sequences obtained in this study have been submitted to the GenBank under accession numbers KT151621 to KT151638.

Assessment of antibody titre by haemagglutination inhibition test

The parvovirus antibody titre was investigated using the haemagglutination inhibition (HI) test in the sera of the cats which tested positive to parvovirus DNA by direct molecular diagnosis. A CPV-2b isolate (number 115/2010), recovered from the faeces of a dog with non-fatal enteritis, and isolated by the authors on the Crandell Rees feline-kidney (CRFK, cell line was obtained from the Biobanking of Veterinary Resources of the Istituto Zooprofilattico Sperimentale della Lombardia e dell'Emilia Romagna IZSLER "Bruno Ubertini" http://www.ibv-r.org/Services/CellCultures.aspx) cell line, was used as the viral antigen. This strain was used in HI experiments because there are no significant differences in serum titres inhibiting the haemagglutination reaction when cats are infected by FPV or CPV, if CPV is used as an antigen [22]. To calculate 8 haemagglutinating units (HAU) of the viral antigen, a haemagglutination (HA) assay was carried out on the CPV-2b isolate following procedures described previously by Carmichael et al. [22]. Porcine erythrocytes were washed three times in Bis-Tris Buffered Saline (BTBS, pH 6.2 at 4 °C) and suspended into 0.5% (*v*/v) BTBS containing 1% bovine serum albumin. To reveal the haemagglutination of both viruses, the test was conducted at a pH of 6–6.8 and was incubated at 4 °C [23, 24].

The HI tests were carried out as previously reported by Senda et al. [25]. All sera were tested in duplicate on two different plates; two-fold dilutions of a commercial canine hyperimmune serum raised against canine distemper, canine hepatitis and canine parvovirosis (Stagloban, ATI, Ozzano Emilia, BO, Italy), was used as positive controls.

For all sera, the mean value of the results from the duplicate HI tests was calculated. If the mean value of the result from one sera was included between two successive dilutions, the lower titre was reported. Cats with an HI titre ≥1:8 were considered positive and cats with an HI titre ≥1:80 were considered to be protected from infection.

Results

Detection of parvovirus in buffy-coat samples

The buffy coat DNA extracts of 54 cats were tested in duplicate for the presence of parvovirus using a SYBR Green real-time PCR assay which showed a limit of detection of 1 copy of the VP2 target DNA per microlitre of extract. Nine (16.7%) of the cats sampled tested positive: 18/2011, 21/2011, 22/2011, 38/2012, 41/2011, 46/2012, 52/2012, 55/2012 and 56/2012. Positive cats were detected in both groups A and B. Six positive cats were clinically normal (6 out of 22 clinically normal cats, 27.3%) and three showed clinical signs of various diseases (3 out of 26 cats with clinical signs of various diseases, 11.5%) (Table 1); no cat with gastrointestinal signs tested positive for parvovirus DNA. In the positive samples, the amount of viral DNA ranged from orders of magnitude 10^0 to 10^2 copies of DNA/μl of extract.

A melting curve analysis showed a solitary peak between 81.8° and 82 °C for standard plasmid dilutions and between 81° and 82 °C for each positive cat sample.

Molecular characterisation of viral sequences

The nucleotide sequences of the partial VP2 gene obtained from positive samples were 532 bp in length (177 amino acid codons), and corresponded to residue 295–471 of the FPV reference strain CU-4 (GenBank accession number M38246). Nucleotide sequences of the VP2 partial gene were also obtained for ten recombinant clones of sample 41/2011, numbered from C01 to C10, respectively.

Analysis of the deduced amino acid residues at critical positions allowed the identification of the following carnivore protoparvoviruses: FPV (viruses 21/2011, 22/2011, 38/2012, 52/2012 and clones C01, C02, C03, C05, C06, C07, C08 and C10); CPV-2b (viruses 18/2011, 55/2012 and 56/2012) and CPV-2c (virus 46/2012 and clones C04 and C09). Six main viral populations were detected in cat 41/2011: clones C02, C05, C06, C07 and C10 resembled the predominant FPV circulating in the sampling area; clone C01 was an FPV which showed a change located in residue 312 (Lys → Arg); clone C03 was an FPV which displayed two coding changes in Thr391-to-Ala and Pro461-to-Ser; C04 was a CPV-2c with an amino acid change located at position 437 (Gly → Arg); C09 was a typical CPV-2c and clone 41/2011-C08 displayed amino acids identical to FPV in residues 297, 300, 305 and 323 while it showed glutamic acid typical of CPV-2c in position 426. The predicted amino acid sequence changes are summarised in Table 3.

Several synonymous and non-synonymous substitutions were detected by comparing the sequences as reported in Table 4. Feline panleukopenia viruses showed a total number of mutations slightly higher than CPV viruses, although synonymous changes predominated in the FPV sequences while non-synonymous changes were prevalent in the CPV viruses. Sample 41/2011 showed high genetic complexity generated within the host, and its sequence variability was higher than the variability of the other sequence data analysed as was seen by the values of parameter π. The non-synonymous fraction was greater for sample 41/2011, indicating clear prevalence of the number of non-synonymous mutations in the sample: 10 non-synonymous mutations out of a total of 15 mutations. The proportion of mutated viral clones was 60% for sample 41/2011 and the mutation frequency was on the order of 2.8×10^{-3} (Table 4).

Unrooted phylogenetic trees constructed from alignments of the nucleotide sequences obtained in this study with additional reference sequences showed two main clusters referable to FPV and CPV. The sequence of clone 41/2011-C08 formed a monophyletic branch inside the FPV clade (Fig. 1). Nucleotide sequences of the modified live FPV vaccine strains available from GenBank were distinguishable from all the FPV and CPV sequences obtained in this study, and direct relationships between them were not evident from the phylogenetic tree.

Haemagglutination inhibition test

The HI titres obtained are reported in Table 5. All the cats which tested positive for parvovirus DNA were also positive for antibodies against parvoviruses; cats 22/2011 and 55/2012 showed a titre higher than 1:80.

Table 3 Change of amino acids to VP2 partial protein

SAMPLES	GROUP	297	300	305	312	323	359	371	375	391	418	426	437	461	TYPE
FPV[a]		Ser	Ala	Asp	Lys	Asp	Ala	Ala	Asp	Thr	Ile	Asn	Gly	Pro	
CPV-2[b]		-	-	-	-	Asn	-	-	Asn	-	-	-	-	-	
CPV-2a[c]		-	Gly	Tyr	-	Asn	-	-	-	-	-	-	-	-	
CPV-2b[d]		-	Gly	Tyr	-	Asn	-	-	-	-	-	Asp	-	-	
CPV-2a[e]		Ala	Gly	Tyr	-	Asn	-	-	-	-	-	-	-	-	
CPV-2b[f]		-	Gly	Tyr	-	Asn	-	-	-	-	-	Asp	-	-	
CPV-2c[g]		Ala	Gly	Tyr	-	Asn	-	-	-	-	-	Glu	-	-	
18/2011	A	Ala	Gly	Tyr	-	Asn	-	Gly	-	-	Thr	Asp	-	-	CPV-2b
21/2011	A	-	-	-	-	-	Gly	-	-	-	-	-	-	-	FPV
22/2011	A	-	-	-	-	-	-	-	-	-	-	-	-	-	FPV
38/2012	B	-	-	-	-	-	-	-	-	-	-	-	-	-	FPV
46/2012	A	Ala	Gly	Tyr	-	Asn	-	-	-	-	-	Glu	-	-	CPV-2c
52/2012	A	-	-	-	-	-	-	-	-	-	-	-	-	-	FPV
55/2012	A	Ala	Gly	Tyr	-	Asn		Gly	-	-	Thr	Asp	-	-	CPV-2b
56/2012	B	Ala	Gly	Tyr	-	Asn	-	Gly	-	-	Thr	Asp	-	-	CPV-2b
41/2011-C01	B	-	-	-	Arg	-	-	-	-	-	-	-	-	-	FPV
41/2011-C02	B	-	-	-	-	-	-	-	-	-	-	-	-	-	FPV
41/2011-C03	B	-	-	-	-	-	-	-	-	Ala	-	-	-	Ser	FPV
41/2011-C04	B	Ala	Gly	Tyr	-	Asn	-	-	-	-	-	Glu	Arg	-	CPV-2c
41/2011-C05	B	-	-	-	-	-	-	-	-	-	-	-	-	-	FPV
41/2011-C06	B	-	-	-	-	-	-	-	-	-	-	-	-	-	FPV
41/2011-C07	B	-	-	-	-	-	-	-	-	-	-	-	-	-	FPV
41/2011-C08	B	-	-	-	-	-	-	-	-	-	-	Glu	-	-	FPV
41/2011-C09	B	Ala	Gly	Tyr	-	Asn	-	-	-	-	-	Glu	-	-	CPV-2c
41/2011-C10	B	-	-	-	-	-	-	-	-	-	-	-	-	-	FPV

The host-specific amino acids which differentiate FPV and CPV are represented by grey dashes
Deduced amino acid sequences of the VP2 gene were obtained from GenBank
[a]Prototype FPV: strain FPV-b (M38246)
[b]Prototype CPV type 2: strain CPV-b (M38245)
[c]Prototype CPV type 2a: strain CPV-15 (M24003)
[d]Prototype CPV type 2b: strain CPV-39 (M74849)
[e]Reference strain CPV type 2a: CPV-677 (AF306445)
[f]Reference strain CPV type 2b: CPV-637 (AF306450)
[g]Reference strain CPV type 2c: CPV-695 (AF01519)

Discussion

The present study screened the occurrence of parvovirus DNA and the feline host-immune status in a cat population. Asymptomatic and symptomatic cats sampled in Sardinia (Italy) during 2011–2012 were tested for the presence of both FPV and CPV DNA in WBC using qPCR, and the partial VP2 gene of the viruses identified was characterised. Parvoviruses have commonly been titrated in the faeces of infected animals, insofar as the viruses shed in faeces reflect virus replication; the Authors chose to analyse the WBC for the presence of viral DNA as, in addition to the intestinal crypt cells, bone marrow and other lymphoid tissues are also a major target for parvoviruses in both dogs and cats [9]. Furthermore, since parvovirus can frequently be isolated in infected cats, even in the presence of high virus-neutralising antibodies [15, 17], antibody titres against parvovirus were established in the sera of positive cats using an HI assay.

Nine (16.7%) out of a total of 54 cats tested positive for parvovirus DNA with viral DNA quantities ranging from 10^0 to 10^2 copies/μl of extract, demonstrating that the viral genome was detectable, although at low levels, in the WBC of a relatively large number of cats. All the cats which tested positive for parvovirus DNA had

Table 4 Statistical analysis of the sequence data set

Sample	η^b	π^c	*SynDif*[d]	*NSynDif*[e]	% Mutated clones	Total mutations/bases sequenced	Mutation frequency
FPV ($n^a = 4$)	6	0.00627 (SE 0.00149)	5	1	-	-	-
CPV ($n = 4$)	4	0.00376 (SE 0.00199)	1	3	-	-	-
41/2011 ($n = 10$)	15	0.01032 (SE 0.00281)	5	10	60 (6/10)	15/5320	2.8×10^{-3}

Summaries of sample sequence variability and quasispecies variation in the viral populations detected within cat 41/2011
[a]n: sample size
[b]η: total number of mutations
[c]π: nucleotide diversity
[d]*SynDif*: total number of synonymous differences
[e]*NSynDif*: total number of non-synonymous differences

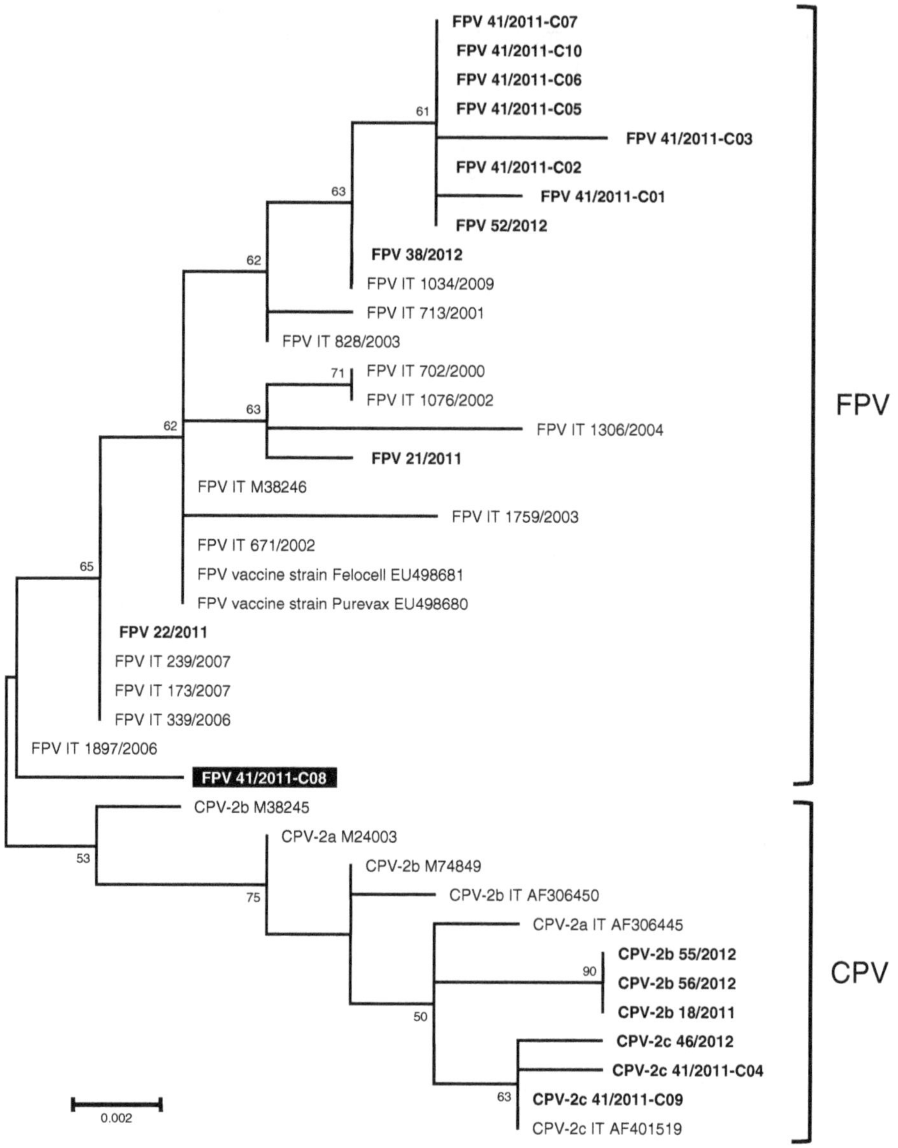

Fig. 1 Unrooted phylogenetic tree. The phylogenetic tree was constructed with the nucleotide sequences of the partial VP2 gene generated in this study and with feline and canine parvovirus reference sequences available on the GenBank nucleotide database or analysed by the authors in a previous study (Battilani et al., [3]). Bootstrap values greater than 50%, calculated on 1000 replicates, are indicated on the respective branches. The feline and canine parvoviruses identified in Italy not detected in this study but included in the phylogenetic analysis are designated by IT. In bold: Nucleotide sequences generated in this study. Underlined: clone 41/2011-C8

antibodies against parvoviruses. Positive cats included healthy and diseased cats. Although sick cats had a potentially greater probability of being persistently infected, none of the samples from cats showing signs of gastroenteritis tested positive.

The presence of FPV and CPV DNA in the faecal and peripheral blood samples of healthy cats has previously been reported [3, 12, 15–17], raising important questions regarding the role of cats in the epidemiology of parvoviruses. In our study, the absence of clinical signs consistent with parvovirosis in the cats which tested positive, together with the low amount of viral DNA detected, suggested that the infection was asymptomatic or that residual viral DNA remains in the organism after recovery from acute infection. Furthermore, the detection of parvoviral DNA in WBC reveals the presence of the virus in the bone marrow or in other lymphoid tissues which might reflect chronic or latent infection. The detection of CPV DNA in apparently healthy domestic cats confirmed a previous survey in which a high prevalence (37%) of CPV in apparently healthy domestic cats living in rescue shelters was identified [14]. Canine parvovirus-like DNA was also detected in the tissues of wildlife carnivores which had no

Table 5 The HI titre of cats which were positive in Real-time PCR

Sample	HI titre
18/2011	1:32
21/2011	1:32
22/2011	1:256
38/2012	1:16
41/2011	1:64
46/2012	1:32
52/2012	1:32
55/2012	1:256
56/2012	1:16
Stagloban	1:256

clinical signs of active infection and, therefore, it was likely that this virus caused latent or persistent infection not only in domestic cats [26]. Animal parvoviruses, such as Rodent protoparvovirus and Aleutian mink disease parvovirus, have been shown to persist in their host [27, 28]. Persistence is a common feature also for human parvovirus B19 (B19V) infection [29]: B19V parvoviral DNA has been documented in a wide range of tissues and the bone marrow of asymptomatic adults, although the majority of people harbour parvoviral DNA in a form which does not actively replicate [30, 31].

Of the nine cats testing positive for parvovirus DNA, four showed FPV DNA, four CPV DNA (three CPV-2b and one CPV-2c), and cat 41/2011 showed unusually high genetic diversity and evidenced DNA belonging to two species of parvovirus in the same patient.

The pathogenicity of CPV variants for cats is not fully understood. Some studies have suggested that CPV had the same pathogenic potential as FPV in cats [3, 32–35]; in other studies, clinical signs were not observed in infected animals, with the exception of transient leukopenia [36, 37]. These results led to the speculation that CPV, compared to FPV, can most frequently cause asymptomatic and persistent infection in cats, even if additional studies are clearly needed to fully understand the potential of cats as CPV carriers. In our study, an equivalent prevalence of FPV and CPV was found in the samples examined; this result might be related to the type of cat population sampled, which consisted mainly of healthy cats and cats showing clinical signs not related to parvovirosis. Alternatively, it could be due to the biological matrix analysed since parvoviruses have commonly been investigated in the faeces of infected animals; instead, in our survey the WBC were analysed.

The rates of variation of the FPV and CPV nucleotide sequences analysed in this study were similar, although genetic diversity in the FPV sequences was generated primarily by synonymous mutations which did not result in amino acid substitutions. This result was congruent with the evolutive behaviour of FPV which, since its emergence in 1920, has not undergone significant changes in antigenic and biological properties. Feline panleukopenia virus varied at a slow rate by random genetic drift and it maintained host-specificity [38]. Instead, in the CPV sequence data set, non-synonymous mutations were predominant. This finding is compatible with the pattern of evolution observed for CPV. Since its emergence in the late 1970s, CPV evolution has been driven by strong positive selection, giving rise to new antigenic variants which have replaced the original type [38].

An unusual genetic complexity was reported for sample 41/2011, with six different viral DNAs ascribable to two distinct species of parvovirus, FPV and CPV type 2c. Although co-infection by more than one parvovirus species is a rare event, it has already been described in a cat simultaneously infected by FPV and CPV-2a [7].

Carnivore protoparvoviruses show an estimated annual substitution rate on the order of 10^{-4} to 10^{-5} whereas the mutation frequency detected in sample 41/2011 was on the order of 2.8×10^{-3}, a value which determines the quasispecies distribution in RNA virus populations. Carnivore parvoviruses are very prone to genetic evolution, showing substitution rates similar to those of RNA viruses, with values of approximately 10^{-4} substitutions per site per year. This result, together with the detection of CPV-2c, which has already been reported in multiple infections of high genetic complexity [3, 5, 39], confirmed that co-infection with different species of parvovirus in feline hosts led to a high genetic variability and to the potential emergence of new viruses [3].

The presence of distinctive mutations between the FPV DNA sequences detected and the sequences of modified live FPV vaccine strains available, together with the lack of information regarding the vaccination history of the cats sampled, allowed the Authors to exclude the possibility that DNA from vaccine strains was detected and did not allow speculation regarding the persistence of modified live vaccine strains in the cats sampled. However, viraemia persisting up to 24 days post vaccination has been reported in dogs vaccinated with modified live canine parvovirus [40].

Conclusions

Additional studies are required to investigate the nature and clinical significance of the presence of parvovirus DNA in the WBC of healthy cats and the potential of cats as parvovirus carriers. Ideally, faeces for the examination of shedding should also be included in the sampling; viral isolation could be useful for testing viral vitality, and reverse transcription-PCR assay targeting viral mRNA could be carried out to determine if there is active replication.

Abbreviations
BTBS: Bis-Tris Buffered Saline; CPV: Canine parvovirus; CRFK: Crandell feline kidney; EDTA: Ethylenediaminetetraacetic acid; FPV: Feline panleukopenia virus; HA: Haemagglutination assay; HAU: Haemagglutinating units; HI: Haemagglutination inhibition; MEV: Mink enteritis virus; PCR: Polymerase chain reaction; qPCR: Quantitative PCR; RaPV: Raccoon parvovirus; TAE: Tris-acetate-EDTA; VP2: Viral protein 2; WBC: Whole blood cells

Acknowledgements
None.

Funding
This research received no grant from any funding agency in the public or commercial sectors.

Authors' contributions
MB and AA designed the study. RZ and CD collected the blood samples and the background information on the samples. Preparation of buffy coat and DNA extraction was performed by AA. The PCR and VP sequencing was carried out by AA, FB and SDA under the supervision of MB. AB analysed the sequence data and drafted the manuscript. MB critically revised the manuscript for important intellectual content. All the authors read the manuscript and approved the final version.

Consent for publication
Not applicable.

Competing interests
The authors declare that they have no competing interests.

Author details
[1]Department of Veterinary Medical Sciences, Alma Mater Studiorum - University of Bologna, Via Tolara di Sopra 50, 40064 Ozzano dell'Emilia, BO, Italy. [2]Department of Veterinary Medicine, University of Sassari, Via Vienna, 2, Sassari 07100, Italy.

References
1. International Committee on Taxonomy of Viruses ICTV. http://ictvonline.org/virustaxonomy.asp. Accessed 23 Mar 2017.
2. Decaro N, Desario C, Miccolupo A, Campolo M, Parisi A, Martella V, Amorisco F, Lucente MS, Lavazza A, Buonavoglia C. Genetic analysis of feline panleukopenia viruses from cats with gastroenteritis. J Gen Virol. 2008;89:2290–8.
3. Battilani M, Balboni A, Ustulin M, Giunti M, Scagliarini A, Prosperi S. Genetic complexity and multiple infections with more parvovirus species in naturally infected cats. Vet Res. 2011;42:43.
4. Miranda C, Vieira MJ, Silva E, Carvalheira J, Parrish CR, Thompson G. Genetic analysis of feline Panleukopenia virus full-length VP2 gene in domestic cats between 2006-2008 and 2012-2014, Portugal. Transbound Emerg Dis. 2016. https://doi.org/10.1111/tbed.12483.
5. Battilani M, Scagliarini A, Ciulli S, Morganti L, Prosperi S. High genetic diversity of the VP2 gene of a canine parvovirus strain detected in a domestic cat. Virology. 2006;352:22–6.
6. Hoelzer K, Shackelton LA, Holmes EC, Parrish CR. Within-host genetic diversity of endemic and emerging parvoviruses of dogs and cats. J Virol. 2008;82:11096–105.
7. Battilani M, Balboni A, Giunti M, Prosperi S. Co-infection with feline and canine parvovirus in a cat. Vet Ital. 2013;49:127–9.
8. Greene CE. Canine parvovirus enteritis. In: Greene CE, editor. Infectious diseases of the dog and the cat. 4th ed. USA: Elsevier; 2012. p. 67–75.
9. Greene CE. Feline parvovirus infection. In: Greene CE, editor. Infectious diseases of the dog and the cat. 4th ed. USA: Elsevier; 2012. p. 80–8.
10. Decaro N, Buonavoglia C. Canine parvovirus post-vaccination shedding: interference with diagnostic assays and correlation with host immune status. Vet J. 2017;221:23–4.
11. Csiza CK, Scott FW, de Lahunta A, Gillespie JH. Immune carrier state of feline panleukopenia virus-infected cats. Am J Vet Res. 1971;32:419–26.
12. Mochizuki M, Harasawa R, Nakatani H. Antigenic and genomic variabilities among recently prevalent parvoviruses of canine and feline origin in Japan. Vet Microbiol. 1993a;38:1–10.
13. Ikeda Y, Nakamura K, Miyazawa T, Takahashi E, Mochizuki M. Feline host range of canine parvovirus: recent emergence of new antigenic types in cats. Emerg Infect Dis. 2002;8:341–6.
14. Clegg SR, Coyne KP, Dawson S, Spibey N, Gaskell RM, Radford AD. Canine parvovirus in asymptomatic feline carriers. Vet Microbiol. 2012;157:78–85.
15. Miyazawa T, Ikeda Y, Nakamura K, Naito R, Mochizuki M, Tohya Y, Vu D, Mikami T, Takahashi E. Isolation of feline parvovirus from peripheral blood mononuclear cells of cats in northern Vietnam. Microbiol Immunol. 1999;43:609–12.
16. Ikeda Y, Mochizuki M, Naito R, Nakamura K, Miyazawa T, Mikami T, Takahashi E. Predominance of canine parvovirus (CPV) in unvaccinated cat populations and emergence of new antigenic types of CPVs in cats. Virology. 2000;278:13–9.
17. Nakamura K, Ikeda Y, Miyazawa T, Tohya Y, Takahashi E, Mochizuki M. Characterisation of cross-reactivity of virus neutralising antibodies induced by feline panleukopenia virus and canine parvoviruses. Res Vet Sci. 2001a;71:219–22.
18. Haynes SM, Holloway SA. Identification of parvovirus in the bone marrow of eight cats. Aust Vet J. 2012;90:136–9.
19. Hall TA. BioEdit: a user-friendly biological sequence alignment editor and analysis program for windows 95/98/NT. Nucl acids Symp Ser. 1999;41:95–8.
20. Librado P, Rozas J. DnaSP v5: a software for comprehensive analysis of DNA polymorphism data. Bioinformatics. 2009;25:1451–2.
21. Kumar S, Stecher G, Tamura K. MEGA7: molecular evolutionary genetics analysis version 7.0 for bigger datasets. Mol Biol Evol. 2016;33:1870–4.
22. Carmichael LE, Joubert JC, Pollock RV. Hemagglutination by canine parvovirus: serologic studies and diagnostic applications. Am J Vet Res. 1980;41:784–91.
23. Senda M, Hirayama N, Ito O, Yamamoto H. Canine parvovirus: strain difference in haemaglutination activity and antigenicity. J Gen Virol. 1988;69:349–54.
24. Garcia Rde C, de Castro TX, de Miranda SC, Lopes G Jr, de Lima M, Labarthe NV, Leite JP. Characterization of parvoviruses from domestic cats in Brazil. J Vet Diagn Investig. 2011;23:951–5.
25. Senda M, Hirayama N, Yamamoto H, Kurata K. An improved hemagglutination test for study of canine parvovirus. Vet Microbiol. 1986;12:1–6.
26. Allison AB, Kohler DJ, Ortega A, Hoover EA, Grove DM, Holmes EC, Parrish CR. Host-specific parvovirus evolution in nature is recapitulated by in vitro adaptation to different carnivore species. PLoS Pathog. 2014; 10:e1004475.
27. Best SM, Bloom ME. Pathogenesis of Aleutian mink disease parvovirus and similarities to B19 infection. J Vet Med B Infect Dis Vet Public Health. 2005;52:331–4.
28. Janus LM, Mähler M, Köhl W, Smoczek A, Hedrich HJ, Bleich A. Minute Virus of mice: antibody response, viral shedding, and persistence of viral DNA in multiple strains of mice. Comp Med. 2008;58:360–8.
29. Soderlund-Venermo M, Hokynar K, Nieminen J, Rautakorpi H, Hedman K. Persistence of human parvovirus B19 in human tissues. Pathol Biol. 2002;50:307–16.
30. Cassinotti P, Burtonboy G, Fopp M, Siegel G. Evidence for persistence of human parvovirus B19 DNA in bone marrow. J Med Virol. 1997;53:229–32.
31. Corcioli F, Zakrzewska K, Rinieri A, Fanci R, Innocenti M, Civinini R, De Giorgi V, Di Lollo S, Azzi A. Tissue persistence of parvovirus B19 genotypes in asymptomatic persons. J Med Virol. 2008;80:2005–11.
32. Mochizuki M, Horiuchi M, Hiragi H, San Gabriel MC, Yasuda N, Uno T. Isolation of canine parvovirus from a cat manifesting clinical signs of feline panleukopenia. J Clin Microbiol. 1996;34:2101–5.
33. Truyen U, Platzer G, Parrish CR. Antigenic type distribution among canine parvoviruses in dogs and cats in Germany. Vet Rec. 1996;138:365–6.

Isolation of canine parvovirus from a cat manifesting clinical signs of feline panleukopenia. J Clin Microbiol. 1996;34:2101–5.

33. Truyen U, Platzer G, Parrish CR. Antigenic type distribution among canine parvoviruses in dogs and cats in Germany. Vet Rec. 1996;138:365–6.
34. Decaro N, Buonavoglia D, Desario C, Amorisco F, Colaianni ML, Parisi A, Terio V, Elia G, Lucente MS, Cavalli A, Martella V, Buonavoglia C. Characterisation of canine parvovirus strains isolated from cats with feline panleukopenia. Res Vet Sci. 2010;89:275–8.
35. Decaro N, Desario C, Billi M, Mari V, Elia G, Cavalli A, Martella V, Buonavoglia C. Western European epidemiological survey for parvovirus and coronavirus infections in dogs. Vet J. 2011;187:195–9.
36. Chalmers WS, Truyen U, Greenwood NM, Baxendale W. Efficacy of feline panleucopenia vaccine to prevent infection with an isolate of CPV2b obtained from a cat. Vet Microbiol. 1999;69:41–5.
37. Nakamura K, Sakamoto M, Ikeda Y, Sato E, Kawakami K, Miyazawa T, Tohya Y, Takahashi E, Mikami T, Mochizuki M. Pathogenic potential of canine parvovirus types 2a and 2c in domestic cats. Clin Diagn Lab Immunol. 2001b;8(3):663–8.
38. Shackelton LA, Parrish CR, Truyen U, Holmes EC. High rate of viral evolution associated with the emergence of carnivore parvovirus. Proc Natl Acad Sci U S A. 2005;102:379–84.
39. Battilani M, Gallina L, Vaccari F, Morganti L. Co-infection with multiple variants of canine parvovirus type 2 (CPV-2). Vet Res Commun. 2007;31(Suppl 1):209–12.
40. Decaro N, Crescenzo G, Desario C, Cavalli A, Losurdo M, Colaianni ML, Ventrella G, Rizzi S, Aulicino S, Lucente MS, Buonavoglia C. Long-term viremia and fecal shedding in pups after modified-live canine parvovirus vaccination. Vaccine. 2014;32:3850–3.
41. Mochizuki M, San Gabriel MC, Nakatani H, Yoshida M, Harasawa R. Comparison of polymerase chain reaction with virus isolation and haemagglutination assays for the detection of canine parvoviruses in faecal specimens. Res Vet Sci. 1993b;55:60–3.
42. Battilani M, Scagliarini A, Tisato E, Turilli C, Jacoboni I, Casadio R, Prosperi S. Analysis of canine parvovirus sequences from wolves and dogs isolated in Italy. J Gen Virol. 2001;82:1555–60.

13

Recombinase polymerase amplification assay for rapid detection of lumpy skin disease virus

Mohamed A. Shalaby[1], Ayman El-Deeb[1], Mohamed El-Tholoth[2], Donata Hoffmann[3], Claus-Peter Czerny[4], Frank T. Hufert[5], Manfred Weidmann[6] and Ahmed Abd El Wahed[4*]

Abstract

Background: Lumpy skin disease virus (LSDV) is a *Capripoxvirus* infecting cattle and Buffalos. Lumpy skin disease (LSD) leads to significant economic losses due to hide damage, reduction of milk production, mastitis, infertility and mortalities (10 %). Early detection of the virus is crucial to start appropriate outbreak control measures. Veterinarians rely on the presence of the characteristic clinical signs of LSD. Laboratory diagnostics including virus isolation, sequencing and real-time polymerase chain reaction (PCR) are performed at well-equipped laboratories. In this study, a portable, simple, and rapid recombinase polymerase amplification (RPA) assay for the detection of LSDV-genome for the use on farms was developed.

Results: The LSDV RPA assay was performed at 42 °C and detected down to 179 DNA copies/reaction in a maximum of 15 min. Unspecific amplification was observed with neither LSDV-negative samples (n = 12) nor nucleic acid preparations from orf virus, bovine papular stomatitis virus, cowpoxvirus, Peste des petits ruminants and Blue tongue virus (serotypes 1, 6 and 8). The clinical sensitivity of the LSDV RPA assay matched 100 % (n = 22) to real-time PCR results. In addition, the LSDV RPA assay detected sheep and goat poxviruses.

Conclusion: The LSDV RPA assay is a rapid and sensitive test that could be implemented in field or at quarantine stations for the identification of LSDV infected case.

Keywords: Lumpy skin disease virus, Recombinase polymerase amplification assay, Point of need test, Cattle

Background

Lumpy skin disease (LSD) affects primarily cattle and occasionally buffalo [1, 2]. It causes pyrexia, generalized skin and pox lesions of internal organs, as well as generalized lymphadenopathy [3, 4]. The disease exists in three forms, acute, subacute or unapparent [5]. LSD is caused by an enveloped double-stranded DNA virus called LSD virus (LSDV), which together with sheep poxvirus (SPV) and goat poxvirus (GPV) constitutes the genus *Capripoxvirus* of the *Chordopoxvirinae* subfamily of the *Poxviridae* family [6, 7].

The origin of LSDV is unknown. It was reported for the first time in Zambia in 1929 as a hypersensitivity reaction of cattle to insect bites [8, 9]. In Egypt, LSDV was first reported in Suez and Ismailia Governorates in May and October 1988 and thereafter spread throughout Egypt leading to 50,000 infected cattle and 1,449 mortalities in 1998 [10, 11]. During epizootics LSDV is mainly transmitted mechanically by blood feeding insects e.g. *Aedes aegypti* [12]. Due to the rapid spread of LSDV and the severe economic losses caused, the Office International des Epizooties (OIE) includes LSDV in the listed notifiable disease of cattle [13].

Diagnosis of LSD depends initially on clinical signs. Definite diagnosis can be performed *via* virus isolation, electron microscopy, identification of antigen by immunofluorescence, serum neutralization, agar gel precipitation, antigen capture ELISA and Dot ELISA [3, 14]. In addition, conventional and real-time polymerase chain reactions (PCR) for the detection of the

* Correspondence: abdelwahed@gwdg.de
[4]Division of Microbiology and Animal Hygiene, Department of Animal Sciences, Faculty of Agriculture Sciences, Georg-August-University, 37077 Goettingen, Germany
Full list of author information is available at the end of the article

LSDV have been described [3, 15–18]. All the above-mentioned methods are not suitable for screening cattle under field conditions or at quarantine stations, as they require highly skilled staff and a well-equipped laboratory. Simple, portable, and rapid tests to detect LSDV at the point of need could improve initiation of control measures as early as possible. This study describes the development and evaluation of a real-time RPA assay for the detection of LSDV genome.

Methods

DNA molecular standards

To produce a molecular LSDV DNA standard, a 910 nt fragment of the G-protein-coupled chemokine receptor (GPCR) gene (6981-7891 of the Genbank accession number: AF325528.1) of the LSDV reference strain (Neethling strain provided by the Pirbright Institute to the Friedrich-Loeffler-Institute, Greifswald-Insel Riems, Germany) was amplified using the in-house designed forward primer (FP): 5′-CATAGTCGATATCCCACATT G-3′, the reverse primer (RP): 5′- GCTAATACTACCA GCACTAC-3′ and the Taq DNA Polymerase (5 PRIME GmbH, Hilden, Germany). The PCR temperature profile was as follows: initial activation at 95 °C/3 min, 30 cycles of 94 °C/60 s, 55 °C/60 s and 72 °C/60 s and a final extension step of 72 °C/5 min. The amplified fragment was ligated into pCR®II using the TA-cloning kit dual promoter and transformed into One shot® chemically competent *E.coli* (Invitrogen, Darmstadt, Germany). Purified plasmids were verified by sequencing (Seqlab, Goettingen, Germany). The plasmid was linearized using the FastDigest HindIII (Fisher Scientific GmbH, Schwerte, Germany). The number of DNA molecules per microliter was measured by the Quant-iT™ PicoGreen® dsDNA Assay Kit (Fisher Scientific GmbH, Schwerte, Germany). Then the DNA standard was diluted to achieve a concentration range of 10^7–10^1 DNA molecules/µl. The standard was tested by applying primers and a modified probe (FP, 5′-GATAGTATCGCTAAACAATGG-3; RP, 5′-ATCCAAACCACCATACTAAG-3′; P, 5′-FAM-AC CTAGCTGTAGTTCACCCAGTAAA-TAMRA-3′) of a published real-time PCR protocol [16] using the Light Cycler 2.0 and the FastStart DNA Master HybProbe kit (Roche, Manheim, Germany).

LSDV RPA oligonucleotides and conditions

RPA primers and exo probe (Fig. 1) were synthesized by TIB MOLBIOL (Berlin, Germany). The LSDV RPA was performed in a 50 µl volume using the TwistAmp™ exo lyophilized kit (TwistDx, Cambridge, UK), using 420 nM RPA primers and 120 nM RPA exo-probe, 29.5 µl of rehydration buffer, 12.2 of molecular biology grade water. A mastermix was added directly to the lyophilized pellet provided in the tubes of a 8-tubes strip. Thereafter, 2.5 µl of Mg acetate (1 mM) were added to each lid. Finally, one microliter of DNA template was added to the pellet. The tube was closed, centrifuged, mixed well and centrifuged again before placed into the tubescanner (Twista, TwistDx, Cambridge, UK) for 15 min at 42 °C. After 230 s, the strip was retrieved, vortexed, centrifuged and placed again into the tubescanner (Twista, TwistDx, Cambridge, UK). The fluorescence signal was measured each 20 s using the FAM channel. In each run positive and negative controls were included. A combined threshold and 1st derivative analysis was used for signal interpretation. Samples produced an exponential amplification curve above the threshold of the negative control were consider positive.

LSDV assay cross reactivity

The Friedrich-Loeffler-Institute, Greifswald-Insel Riems, Germany provided reference nucleic acids for LSDV, SPV, GPV, orf virus, bovine papular stomatitis virus, cowpoxvirus, Peste des petits ruminants and Blue tongue virus (serotypes 1, 6 and 8) (Table 1). All samples contained a high concentration of viral nucleic acid as determined by the respective real-time PCRs recommended by the OIE (CT: 12-20).

Clinical sensitivity and specificity of the LSDV RPA assay

Twenty-two skin nodules of suspected LSDV-infected cattle were collected during the summer of 2012 in Dakahlia Governorate, Egypt. Diseased cattle exhibited either localized or generalized multiple skin nodules with or without systemic signs.

DNA was extracted from the twenty-two skin nodules and twelve skin samples from apparently healthy cows using QIAamp DNA Mini Kit (Qiagen, Hilden, Germany). All samples were screened simultaneously by the LSDV RPA assay and real-time PCR as

```
                                    Consensus
CRATARTATMGCTAAACAATGGAGT-77-GATGAGTATYGATAGATAYCTAGCTRTAGYTYACCCAGTAAAATCAATDHC-5-GGACAAAACRATAYGGAATTGTACTTAG
CGATAGTATCGCTAAACAATGGAGT
                             GATGAGTATCGATAGANANCNAGCTGTAGTTCACCCAGTAAAATCAATGCC
                                                                                    GGACAAAACGATATGGAATTGTACTTAG
    Forward primer                                  exo-probe                                  Reverse primer
```

Fig. 1 Alignment of the LSDV RPA primers and exo-probe sequences with the consensus sequence of 132 *capripoxviruses* GPCR genes downloaded from Genbank (Geneious® 6.1.5, Biomatters Limited, New Zealand). Mismatches are indicated in bold and underlined. NNN are sites of the quencher and flurupohore in following order (BHQ1-dT) (Tetrahydrofuran) (FAM-dT). R is A or G; Y, C or T; M, A or C; D, A or G or T; H, A or C or T

Table 1 List of reference viral strains

Virus	Strain	Reference
Lumpy skin disease virus	Neethling strain	[40]
Sheep poxvirus	Russia	NA
Goat poxvirus	Indian	NA
Cowpoxvirus	2	[41]
Orf Virus	Burgheßler	[42]
Bovine papular stomatitis virus	M1	[43]
Peste de petite Ruminant Virus	lineage IV_Kurdistan2011	[44]
Blue tongue virus	Serotypes 1, 6 and 8	[45]

NA is non-applicable

described above. The real time PCR CT values for these samples ranged from CT 18 to 35 (Additional file 1: Table S1).

Statistical methods

For the determination of the LSDV RPA assay analytical sensitivity by the molecular DNA standard, a semi-log regression analysis (PRISM, Graphpad Software Inc., San Diego, California) and a probit analysis (STATISTICA, StatSoft, Hamburg, Germany) were performed by plotting the RPA threshold time against the number of molecules detected. Clinical sensitivity and specificity values were calculated using standard formulas.

Results

The LSDV GPCR gene plasmid standard was used to determine the analytical sensitivity of the assay using a dilution range between 10^7–10^1/μl (Fig. 2). The LSDV RPA assay was performed eight times on the molecular standard, in which 10^7–10^3 DNA molecules were detected in 8/8 runs, 10^2, 7/8 and 10^1, 2/8 (Fig. 3a, Additional file 2: Table S2). Due to the inconsistency in the results, a probit regression analysis was applied, in which the sensitivity in 95 % of cases was determined at 179 DNA molecules/reaction (Fig. 3b). While the real-time PCR analytical sensitivity was 37 DNA copies/reaction [16].

The LSDV RPA assay showed no cross detection with orf virus, bovine papular stomatitis virus, cowpoxvirus, Peste des petits ruminants and Blue tongue virus (serotypes 1, 6 and 8) genome. SPV and GPV, however, were detected by the LSDV RPA assay as well. The LSDV RPA assay was validated using 12 negative skin samples and 22 LSDV positive skin nodule samples. In comparison to real-time PCR, clinical sensitivity and specificity of the LSDV RPA assay was 100 % (Additional file 1: Table S1).

Discussion

Veterinarians rely mainly on the appearance of clinical signs for LSD diagnosis [8]. Establishment of a rapid diagnostic test to identify early stages of an LSD outbreak would allow rapid execution of control measures.

The developed LSDV RPA assay was highly sensitive (179 DNA copies detected/reaction) and rapid (total time: 2–15 min). In addition, we were able to obtain the same clinical sensitivity and specificity as the well-established real-time PCR assay [16] when testing 22 skin samples. The RPA assay is a technique for the isothermal amplification of DNA using enzymes and proteins to replace the repetitive cycles of three temperatures used for PCR [19]. Thus, RPA can be operated by portable more simple heating and detection devices instead of using thermal cycler devices. Moreover, RPA reagents are cold chain independent [20–22], which make them ideal for point of need testing.

The LSDV RPA exo-probe was designed to detect LSDV by placing two mismatches to the sequences of SPV and GPV at its 3′ prime end (Fig. 1 and Additional file 3: Figure S1) as well as the primers amplified 186 of the most variable gene in the *capripoxviruses*, GPCR

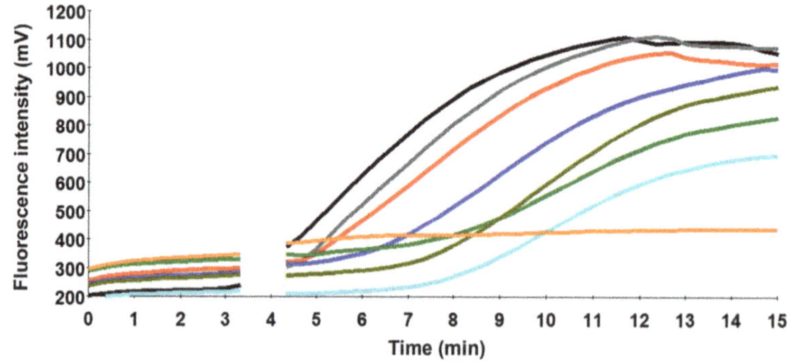

Fig. 2 The results layout of one LSDV RPA assay run. Fluorescence development over time using a dilution range of 10^7–10^1 molecules/μl of the DNA molecular standard (Graph generated by ESEquant tubescanner software). 10^7 represented by black line; 10^6, gray; 10^5, red; 10^4, blue; 10^3, green; 10^2, cyan; 10^1, dark khaki; negative control, orange. The LSDV RPA assay detected down to 10 DNA molecules/reaction. After 230 s, the strip was taken out of the tubescanner for mixing, therefore, no fluorescence signals were recorded

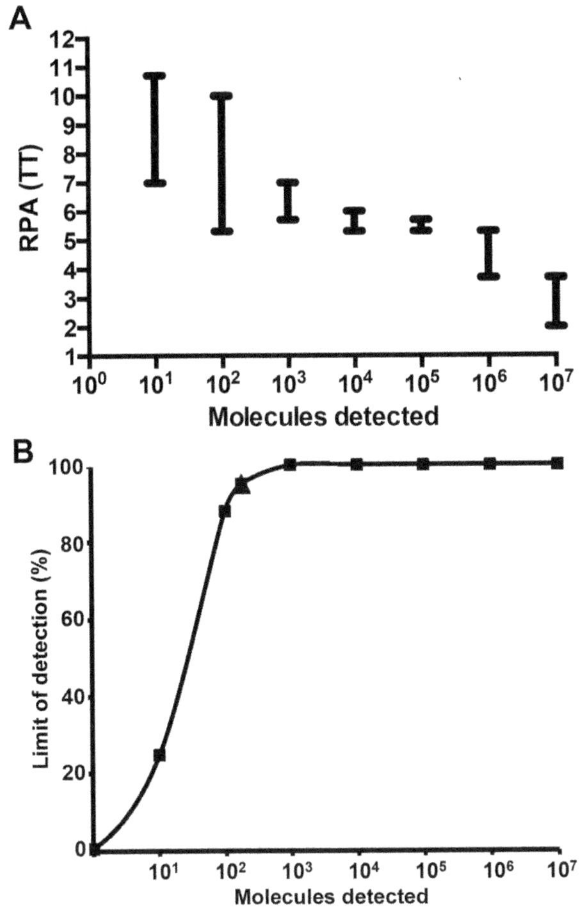

Fig. 3 Performance of the LSDV RPA assay using data set of eight RPA assay runs. **a** Semi-logarithmic regression (**b**) Probit regression analysis. The LSDV RPA assay yielded results between 2–12 min. The results of the 10^7–10^3 were consistence, therefore no error bars was included (**a**). The limit of detection (179 DNA molecules) at 95 % probability was is depicted by a triangle (**b**)

gene [23, 24]. Nevertheless, SPV and GPV were detected. This might be due to the fact that the length (48–52 bp) of the RPA exo probe compensates for the presence of nucleotide mismatches [25, 26]. Also, the position of mismatches appear not to affect RPA oligonucleotide binding [27], but have a great influence on the PCR primes and probe [28]. However, the assay will be also useful for detecting SPV and GPV, unfortunately, no clinical samples were available to validate the assay for both viruses.

Several conventional and real-time PCRs have been established to identify the *capripoxviruses* [18, 29–34], but none are able to distinguish between various species [35]. One PCR assay was established for the differentiation between these viruses; however, many GPVs were identified as SPV [16]. This is due to the high homology of up to 96 % between the members of this genus [23], which also affected the LSDV RPA assay. The OIE recommends sequencing and phylogenetic analysis to differentiate between LSDV, SPV and GPV. For a point of need field test the LSDV-RPA described here can still be of help as SPV and GPV are not known to infect cattle and using it on cattle samples, therefore, provides the specificity needed especially as the panel of other cattle infecting viruses tested all scored negative in the cross detection assessment.

Several loop-mediated isothermal amplification (LAMP) assays have been established to identify *capripoxviruses* [36–38]. The design of LAMP assays requires four to six oligonucleotides and a minimum of four binding sites. The LAMP results can be read by naked eye, if turbidity read out is used [39] after about 60 min. In contrast, the RPA assay developed here was very fast (15 min) and required two primers and one probe.

Conclusion

In conclusion, LSDV RPA yielded similar results as the corresponding real-time PCR assay, but RPA was quicker and much easier to handle. Furthermore, combination with a simple extraction method will allow its employment at low resource settings, quarantine stations or farms.

Additional files

Additional file 1: Table S1. Screening 22 skin nodules samples with real-time PCR and RPA assays. (DOCX 57 kb)

Additional file 2: Table S2. Reproducibility of LSDV RPA assay using data sets of eight RPA assay runs using the DNA molecular standards. 10^7–10^3 DNA molecules were detected 8 out of 8 runs; 10^2, 7/8 and 10^1, 2/8. (DOCX 54 kb)

Additional file 3: Figure S1. Mapping 132 nucleotide sequences derived by BLAST nucleotide search to the LSDV RPA amplicon as well as RPA primers and probe. The alignment was performed by using Geneious (V: 9.0.5. Biomatters Limited. New Zealand). The Genbank accession number and name were given. Grey represents the identical sequence. A. C. G. T were highlighted in red. violet. yellow. green. respectively. whenever a mismatch to the LSDV RPA amplicon was recorded. (DOCX 515 kb)

Abbreviations

FP: Forward primer; GPCR: G-protein-coupled chemokine receptor; GPV: Goat poxvirus; LAMP: Loop-mediated isothermal amplification; LSD: Lumpy skin disease; LSDV: Lumpy skin disease virus; n: Number; OIE: Office International des Epizooties; PCR: Polymerase chain reaction; RP: Reverse primer; RPA: Recombinase polymerase amplification; SPV: Sheep poxvirus

Acknowledgement

Not applicable.

Funding

The study was funded by Alexander von Humboldt foundation (project ID: 3.4 - Fokoop-DEU/1144102). The funding agency has no role in the design of the study and collection, analysis, and interpretation of data and in writing the manuscript.

Authors' contributions

Conceived and designed the experiments: MAS, FTH, MW & AAEW. Performed the experiments: MAS; AED; MET, DH, AAEW. Data analysis: MAS, AED, MET, DH, CPC, FTH, MW & AAEW. Drafted the manuscript: MW & AAEW. Critical revision: MAS, AED, MET, DH, CPC, FTH, MW & AAEW. All authors read and approved the final manuscript.

Competing interests

The authors declare that they have no competing interests.

Consent for publication

Non-applicable.

Author details

[1]Virology Department, Faculty of Veterinary Medicine, Cairo University, 12211 Giza, Egypt. [2]Virology Department, Faculty of Veterinary Medicine, Mansoura University, 35516 Mansoura, Egypt. [3]Institute of Diagnostic Virology, Friedrich-Loeffler-Institute, 17493 Greifswald-Insel Riems, Germany. [4]Division of Microbiology and Animal Hygiene, Department of Animal Sciences, Faculty of Agriculture Sciences, Georg-August-University, 37077 Goettingen, Germany. [5]Institute of Microbiology & Virology, Brandenburg Medical School Fontane, 01968 Senftenberg, Germany. [6]Institute of Aquaculture, University of Stirling, FK9 4LA Stirling, Scotland, UK.

References

1. Sharawi SS, Abd El-Rahim IH. The utility of polymerase chain reaction for diagnosis of lumpy skin disease in cattle and water buffaloes in Egypt. Rev Sci Tech. 2011;30:821–30.
2. El-Tholoth M, El-Kenawy AA. G-Protein-Coupled Chemokine Receptor Gene in Lumpy Skin Disease Virus Isolates from Cattle and Water Buffalo (Bubalus bubalis) in Egypt. Transbound Emerg Dis. 2016;63(6):e288-e295.
3. Tuppurainen ES, Venter EH, Coetzer JA. The detection of lumpy skin disease virus in samples of experimentally infected cattle using different diagnostic techniques. Onderstepoort J Vet Res. 2005;72:153–64.
4. Davies FG. Lumpy skin disease of cattle: A growing problem in Africa and the Near East. World Animal Review. 1991;68:37–42.
5. Weiss KE. Lumpy skin disease. Monogr Virol. 1968;3:111–31.
6. Buller RM, Arif BM, Black DN, Dumbell KR, Esposito JJ, Lefkowitz EJ, McFadden G, Moss B, Mercer AA, Moyer RW, et al. Family Poxviridae. In: Fauquet CM, Mayo MA, Maniloff J, Desselberger U, Ball LA, editors. Virus Taxonomy: Classification and Nomenclature of Viruses. San Diego: Elsevier Academic Press; 2005. p. 117–33.
7. Diallo A, Viljoen GJ. Genus Capripoxvirus. Basel, Switzerland: Birkhauser; 2007.
8. Weiss KE. Lumpy Skin Disease Virus. In: Cytomegaloviruses Rinderpest Virus Lumpy Skin Disease Virus. Berlin Heidelberg: Springer; 1968. p. 111–31.
9. Morris JPA. Pseudo-urticaria. Northern Rhodesia. Dept Anim Health Ann Rpt. 1930:12.
10. Salib FA, Osman AH. Incidence of lumpy skin disease among Egyptian cattle in Giza Governorate, Egypt. Veterinary World. 2011;4:162–7.
11. Ali AA, Esmat M, Attia H, Selim A, Abdel-Hamid YM. Clinical and pathological studies on lumpy skin disease in Egypt. Vet Rec. 1990;127:549–50.
12. Chihota CM, Rennie LF, Kitching RP, Mellor PS. Mechanical transmission of lumpy skin disease virus by Aedes aegypti (Diptera: Culicidae). Epidemiology & Infection. 2001;126:317–21.
13. Bowden TR, Babiuk SL, Parkyn GR, Copps JS, Boyle DB. Capripoxvirus tissue tropism and shedding: A quantitative study in experimentally infected sheep and goats. Virology. 2008;371:380–93.
14. OIE. Lumpy Skin Disease. In: OIE Terrestrial Manual, vol. Chapter 2.4.14. 2010. p. 1–12.
15. Armson B, Fowler VL, Tuppurainen ES, Howson EL, Madi M, Sallu R, Kasanga CJ, Pearson C, Wood J, Martin P, et al. Detection of Capripoxvirus DNA Using a Field-Ready Nucleic Acid Extraction and Real-Time PCR Platform. Transbound Emerg Dis. 2015.
16. Lamien CE, Lelenta M, Goger W, Silber R, Tuppurainen E, Matijevic M, Luckins AG, Diallo A. Real time PCR method for simultaneous detection, quantitation and differentiation of capripoxviruses. J Virol Methods. 2011;171:134–40.
17. Menasherow S, Rubinstein-Giuni M, Kovtunenko A, Eyngor Y, Fridgut O, Rotenberg D, Khinich Y, Stram Y. Development of an assay to differentiate between virulent and vaccine strains of lumpy skin disease virus (LSDV). J Virol Methods. 2014;199:95–101.
18. Balinsky CA, Delhon G, Smoliga G, Prarat M, French RA, Geary SJ, Rock DL, Rodriguez LL. Rapid preclinical detection of sheeppox virus by a real-time PCR assay. J Clin Microbiol. 2008;46:438–42.
19. Piepenburg O, Williams CH, Stemple DL, Armes NA. DNA detection using recombination proteins. PLoS Biol. 2006;4, e204. http://journals.plos.org/plosbiology/article?id=10.1371/journal.pbio.0040204.
20. Abd El Wahed A, Patel P, Heidenreich D, Hufert FT, Weidmann M. Reverse transcription recombinase polymerase amplification assay for the detection of middle East respiratory syndrome coronavirus. PLoS Curr. 2013;5. http://currents.plos.org/outbreaks/article/reverse-transcription-recombinase-polymeraseamplification-assay-for-the-detection-of-middle-east-respiratory-syndrome-coronavirus/.
21. Abd El Wahed A, Weidmann M, Hufert FT. Diagnostics-in-a-Suitcase: Development of a portable and rapid assay for the detection of the emerging avian influenza A (H7N9) virus. J Clin Virol. 2015;69:16–21.
22. Faye O, Faye O, Soropogui B, Patel P, El Wahed AA, Loucoubar C, Fall G, Kiory D, Magassouba N, Keita S, et al. Development and deployment of a rapid recombinase polymerase amplification Ebola virus detection assay in Guinea in 2015. Euro Surveill. 2015;20. http://www.eurosurveillance.org/ViewArticle.aspx?ArticleId=21289.
23. Tulman ER, Afonso CL, Lu Z, Zsak L, Sur JH, Sandybaev NT, Kerembekova UZ, Zaitsev VL, Kutish GF, Rock DL. The genomes of sheeppox and goatpox viruses. J Virol. 2002;76:6054–61.
24. Tulman ER, Afonso CL, Lu Z, Zsak L, Kutish GF, Rock DL. Genome of lumpy skin disease virus. J Virol. 2001;75:7122–30.
25. Abd El Wahed A, El-Deeb A, El-Tholoth M, Abd El Kader H, Ahmed A, Hassan S, Hoffmann B, Haas B, Shalaby MA, Hufert FT, Weidmann M. A portable reverse transcription recombinase polymerase amplification assay for rapid detection of foot-and-mouth disease virus. PLoS One. 2013;8:e71642.
26. Boyle DS, Lehman DA, Lillis L, Peterson D, Singhal M, Armes N, Parker M, Piepenburg O, Overbaugh J. Rapid Detection of HIV-1 Proviral DNA for Early Infant Diagnosis Using Recombinase Polymerase Amplification. MBio. 2013;4.
27. Amer HM, Abd El Wahed A, Shalaby MA, Almajhdi FN, Hufert FT, Weidmann M. A new approach for diagnosis of bovine coronavirus using a reverse transcription recombinase polymerase amplification assay. J Virol Methods. 2013;193:337–40.
28. Whiley DM, Sloots TP. Sequence variation can affect the performance of minor groove binder TaqMan probes in viral diagnostic assays. J Clin Virol. 2006;35:81–3.
29. Cheng Z, Yue J, Li Y, Xu L, Wang K, Zhou B, Chen J, Li J, Jiang N. Development and application of TaqMan-MGB real-time quantitative PCR assay for detection of goat pox virus. Sheng Wu Gong Cheng Xue Bao. 2009;25:464–72.
30. Haegeman A, Zro K, Vandenbussche F, Demeestere L, Van Campe W, Ennaji MM, De Clercq K. Development and validation of three Capripoxvirus real-time PCRs for parallel testing. J Virol Methods. 2013;193:446–51.
31. Tian H, Wu J, Chen Y, Zhang K, Shang Y, Liu X. Development of a SYBR green real-time PCR method for rapid detection of sheep pox virus. Virol J. 2012;9:291.
32. Venkatesan G, Balamurugan V, Bhanuprakash V. TaqMan based real-time duplex PCR for simultaneous detection and quantitation of capripox and orf virus genomes in clinical samples. J Virol Methods. 2014;201:44–50.
33. Zro K, Azelmat S, Bendouro Y, Kuhn JH, El Fahime E, Ennaji MM. PCR-based assay to detect sheeppox virus in ocular, nasal, and rectal swabs from infected Moroccan sheep. J Virol Methods. 2014;204:38–43.
34. Markoulatos P, Mangana-Vougiouka O, Koptopoulos G, Nomikou K, Papadopoulos O. Detection of sheep poxvirus in skin biopsy samples by a multiplex polymerase chain reaction. J Virol Methods. 2000;84:161–7.
35. OIE. Sheep pox and goat pox. In: OIE Terrestrial Manual 2010. 2010. Chapter 2.7.14.
36. Das A, Babiuk S, McIntosh MT. Development of a loop-mediated isothermal amplification assay for rapid detection of capripoxviruses. J Clin Microbiol. 2012;50:1613–20.
37. Venkatesan G, Balamurugan V, Bhanuprakash V, Singh RK, Pandey AB. Loop-mediated isothermal amplification assay for rapid and sensitive detection of

sheep pox and goat pox viruses in clinical samples. Mol Cell Probes. 2016; 30(3):174-7.

38. Zhao Z, Fan B, Wu G, Yan X, Li Y, Zhou X, Yue H, Dai X, Zhu H, Tian B, et al. Development of loop-mediated isothermal amplification assay for specific and rapid detection of differential goat pox virus and sheep pox virus. BMC Microbiol. 2014;14:10.
39. Notomi T, Okayama H, Masubuchi H, Yonekawa T, Watanabe K, Amino N, Hase T. Loop-mediated isothermal amplification of DNA. Nucleic Acids Res. 2000;28, E63.
40. Gari G, Abie G, Gizaw D, Wubete A, Kidane M, Asgedom H, Bayissa B, Ayelet G, Oura CA, Roger F, Tuppurainen ES. Evaluation of the safety, immunogenicity and efficacy of three capripoxvirus vaccine strains against lumpy skin disease virus. Vaccine. 2015;33:3256–61.
41. Liebermann H, Schulze P, Liebermann H. Euterpocken in Deutschland. Archiv für Experimentelle Veterinärmedi. 1967;21:1419–33.
42. Schmidt D. Experimentelle Beiträge zur Kenntnis der Dermatitis pustulosa des Schafes.1. Versuche zur Reinigung des Virus der Dermatitis pustulosa und zur Abtrennung des komplementbindenden Antigens von den Elementarkörpern. Archiv für Experimentelle Veterinärmedi. 1967;21:175–80.
43. Liebermann H, Urbaneck D. Isolierung und Identifizierung von Stomatitis-papulosa Virus mit Hilfe der Zellkultur. Archiv für Experimentelle Veterinärmedi. 1966;20:1268–75.
44. Hoffmann B, Wiesner H, Maltzan J, Mustefa R, Eschbaumer M, Arif FA, Beer M. Fatalities in wild goats in Kurdistan associated with Peste des Petits Ruminants virus. Transbound Emerg Dis. 2012;59:173–6.
45. Hoffmann B, Eschbaumer M, Beer M. Real-time quantitative reverse transcription-PCR assays specifically detecting bluetongue virus serotypes 1, 6, and 8. J Clin Microbiol. 2009;47:2992–4.

14

Application of a new real-time polymerase chain reaction assay for surveillance studies of lymphocystis disease virus in farmed gilthead seabream

Estefania J. Valverde[1], Irene Cano[2], Alejandro Labella[1], Juan J. Borrego[1] and Dolores Castro[1*]

Abstract

Background: Lymphocystis disease (LCD) is the main viral infection reported to affect cultured gilthead seabream (*Sparus aurata*) in Europe. The existence of subclinical Lymphocystis disease virus (LCDV) infection in this fish species has been recognised by using polymerase chain reaction (PCR)-based methods. Nevertheless, these methods do not provide quantitative results that can be useful in epidemiological and pathological studies. Moreover, carrier fish have been involved in viral transmission, therefore the use of specific and sensitive diagnostic methods to detect LCDV will be relevant for LCD prevention.

Results: We have developed a real-time PCR (qPCR) assay to detect and quantify LCDV. The assay was evaluated for viral diagnosis in surveillance studies in gilthead seabream farms, and also to identify viral reservoirs in a hatchery. The prevalence of LCDV infection in the asymptomatic gilthead seabream populations tested varied from 30 to 100 %, including data from one farm without previous records of LCD. Estimated viral load in caudal fin of subclinically infected fish was two to five orders of magnitude lower than in diseased fish. The qPCR assay allowed the detection of carrier fish in broodstock from a farm with a history of clinical LCD in juvenile fish. In addition, the quantitative detection of LCDV was achieved in all samples collected in the hatchery, including fertilized eggs, larvae and fingerlings, and also rotifer cultures and artemia metanauplii and cysts used for larval rearing.

Conclusions: The qPCR assay developed in this study has proved to be a rapid, sensitive, and reliable method for LCDV diagnosis, which could be valuable to identify LCDV reservoirs or to study viral replication in gilthead seabream.

Keywords: Lymphocystis disease virus, Virus surveillance, Farmed gilthead seabream, Real-time PCR

Background

Lymphocystis disease (LCD) affects a wide variety of wild and cultured fish species with an extensive geographical distribution [1]. In Southern Atlantic and Mediterranean aquaculture, this disease is the main viral infection reported to affect cultured gilthead seabream (*Sparus aurata*) [2–4]. The typical sign of lymphocystis disease is the presence of small pearl-like nodules on the skin and fins of affected fish, that may occur singly or more generally grouped in raspberry-like clusters of tumorous appearance [5, 6]. Although this disease is rarely fatal, fish showing these symptoms appear unsightly and cannot be commercialized, causing important economic losses [7]. Moreover, in fish farms, LCD outbreaks may favour secondary bacterial infections, cannibalism and/or parasitic infestations, factors that may increase mortality rates [4, 8–10].

The etiological agent of LCD is the Lymphocystis disease virus (LCDV), a member of the genus *Lymphocystivirus*, family *Iridoviridae*. On the basis of the major capsid protein (MCP) gene sequence, nine genotypes of *Lymphocystivirus* have been proposed [11–15]. All

* Correspondence: dcastro@uma.es
[1]Departamento de Microbiología, Universidad de Málaga, 29071 Málaga, Spain
Full list of author information is available at the end of the article

LCDV isolates from gilthead seabream and Senegalese sole (*Solea senegalensis*) sequenced so far are included in genotype VII [10, 14, 16].

The only adequate measure for LCD prevention in the aquaculture systems is the use of general prophylactic practices, such as good husbandry practices, reduced stocking density and the virological control of fish to be introduced in the farm facilities in order to detect carrier fish [1]. These animals may pose a risk for the introduction of LCDV in fish farms, as direct contact between fish specimens is considered the main route of LCDV spreading [5]. More recently, asymptomatic carrier breeders have also been involved in LCDV transmission to fish larvae [17]. The detection of subclinical viral infections in carrier fish requires the use of sensitive diagnostic methods [18]. In this context, polymerase chain reaction (PCR)-based methods have proved to be adequate for LCDV detection in apparently healthy fish [10, 16, 19–21]. The PCR-hybridization assay developed by Cano et al. [19] not only allowed the detection of LCDV in carrier gilthead seabream, but also in rotifer and artemia used as live food for larval stages, which makes it a valuable tool for the detection of other potential LCDV foci in fish farms [17, 22]. Nevertheless, this assay is relatively time-consuming, not readily applied to screening large sample numbers, and does not provide quantitative results, that can be useful in epidemiological and pathological studies of LCDV.

Real-time PCR (qPCR) has been used for the detection and quantification of numerous viral fish pathogens, including LCDV in yellow perch (*Perca flavescens*) [15], and has been proved to be useful to overcome the disadvantages of conventional PCR above mentioned [23–25]. Recently, a qPCR assay has been developed and applied for the detection and quantification of LCDV in a low number of samples of diseased and recovered gilthead seabream. Nevertheless, the use of the assay for LCDV monitoring in different stages of the fish production cycle was not investigated [26].

The objective of this study was to establish the applicability of a new qPCR assay for LCDV diagnosis in surveillance studies. In addition, this assay has been evaluated using samples from a gilthead seabream hatchery, in order to demonstrate its utility to detect several sources of LCDV in the fish farm.

Methods

Ethics statement

Fish farms owners accepted to participate in the study, and specialized personnel in each farm facility carried out the sampling procedures described below. Fish used in this study have been treated in compliance with the Spanish legislation (Law 32/2007, and RD 53/2013).

Sample collection and DNA extraction

Juvenile gilthead seabream specimens were sampled at four aquaculture farms. In two of these farms (farms A and B), a total of 11 diseased and 25 asymptomatic (i.e., without signs of lymphocystis disease) fish were collected during an outbreak of LCD, whereas in the other two (farms C and D), only asymptomatic fish were observed, and 24 of them were collected. Juvenile fish were euthanized by anaesthetic overdose (MS-222) (Sigma-Aldrich, St. Louis, MO, USA) before sampling. Samples of caudal fin (approximately 1 cm^2 in size) were aseptically cut off, frozen immediately at -20 °C in dry ice and sent to the lab. In addition, 9 gilthead seabream samples were collected at the hatchery in another farm suffering LCD outbreaks over several years (farm E). Samples consisted of fertilized eggs (one sample of 100 mg), larvae (4 pools of 10–15 animals), and fingerlings (up to 2 g of weight) (4 pools of 5–10 animals). No LCD clinical signs were observed in any of the sampled fingerlings. Larvae and fingerlings were also euthanized by anaesthetic overdose. One sample of each rotifers (100 mg), commercial artemia cysts (100 mg), decapsulated artemia cysts (100 mg) and artemia metanauplii (100 mg) used as live food for larvae were also collected. These samples were washed with sterile seawater, gently dried and fresh frozen for shipment to the lab. In this farm, 50 broodstock were also analysed. These animals neither showed symptoms of LCD nor had LCD history, as stated by the farm records. For sampling purposes, these specimens were anaesthetized with MS-222 in seawater at a final concentration of 30 mg/ml. For each specimen, samples of caudal fin and blood were obtained. Blood samples were collected from the branchial arches using S-Monovette 4.5 ml LH (Sarstedt, Nümbrecht, Germany), chilled to 4 °C and sent to the lab for analysis within 24 h, whereas samples of caudal fin were obtained and stored as described above.

Samples were homogenized in Leibovitz's L-15 medium (Gibco, Life Technologies, Carlsbad, CA, USA) (10 % w/v) as described previously [27], except samples of eggs, rotifers and artemia, which were ground in liquid nitrogen. Total DNA was extracted from 200 µl of tissue homogenates or 50 mg of tissue powder using the QIAamp DNA Minikit (Qiagen, Valencia, CA, USA) according to the manufacturer's instructions. Finally, DNA was extracted from 200 µl of heparinised blood using the ReliaPrep Blood gDNA Miniprep System (Promega, Madison, WI, USA). In all cases, DNA was eluted in a final volume of 100 µl and stored at -20 °C until use as template for PCR-hybridization and qPCR. Prior to PCR assays, purified DNA was quantified spectrophotometrically using a NanoDrop 1000 spectrophotometer (Thermo Scientific, West Palm Beach, FL, USA), and DNA was diluted to achieve a final concentration of 20 ng/µl.

PCR-hybridization

LCDV genome was detected using the PCR-hybridization assay described by Cano et al. [19]. Briefly, a 270-bp fragment of the MCP gene of LCDV was amplified by PCR. PCR products were denatured and blotted onto a Hybond-N nylon membrane (GE Healthcare, Waukesha, WI, USA), and hybridization was carried out using an LCDV-specific DIG-labelled probe and the chemiluminescent substrate CSPD (Roche Applied Science, Mannhein, Germany).

Cloning a fragment of MCP gene

Lymphocystis disease virus isolate SA9 was used as source of LCDV DNA [14]. A fragment of the viral MCP gene was amplified by PCR using the primers LCDVs-F and LCDVs-R described by Kitamura et al. [12]. PCR was performed in a 50-µl reaction volume containing 10 µl of 5X Colorless GoTaq Flexi Buffer (Promega), 3 mM $MgCl_2$ (Promega), 5 µl of 0.2 mM dNTP (Roche), 1.25 U of GoTaq DNA polymerase (Promega), and 2 µl of each primer at 15 pmol/µl. DNA was amplified by the use of one denaturation step at 95 °C for 5 min, followed by 35 cycles of denaturation (95 °C for 1 min), annealing (50 °C for 30 s), and extension (72 °C for 1 min), and a final extension step at 72 °C for 10 min. PCR products were run in 2 % agarose gels, purified using the High-Pure PCR Product Purification kit (Roche), and cloned into the pCR4-TOPO vector (TOPO TA cloning kit) (Invitrogen, Life Technologies, Carlsbad, CA, USA) for subsequent transformation in *Escherichia coli* (One Shot competent cells, Invitrogen) following manufacturer's instructions. Recombinant plasmid DNA was purified from *E. coli* cells with a commercial kit (High Pure Plasmid Isolation kit, Roche), and insert size was verified by PCR and sequencing, using the M13 primers provided in the cloning kit. The cloned MCP gene fragment was 609 bp in length, corresponding with nucleotide positions 99 to 707 of the LCDV SA9 MCP gene (GenBank accession no. GU320728).

Real-time PCR assay

Primers for qPCR (RT-LCDV-F: 5′-ACGTTTCTCGAGG CGGAGAT-3′, and RT-LCDV-R: 5′-CGGACGTTTGCTT GACCAA -3′) were designed to target the MCP gene of LCDV genotype VII, using Primer Express Software v3.0 (Applied Biosystems, Life Technologies, Carlsbad, CA, USA). This primer set generates a 150-bp amplicon within the 609-bp cloned fragment of MCP gene (nucleotide positions 173 to 322 of the LCDV SA9 MCP gene).

Real-time PCR reactions were carried out in 96-well plates (Applied Biosystems), in a final volume of 50 µl containing 25 µl of 2x Power SYBR Green PCR Master Mix (Applied Biosystems), 3 µl of each primer at 15 pmol/µl, and 10 µl of DNA. PCR amplifications were performed in a 7500 Real-Time PCR System (Applied Biosystems). The thermal profile was: 50 °C for 2 min; 95 °C for 10 min, and 40 cycles at 95 °C for 15 s and 60 °C for 1 min. Finally, dissociation curve analysis was carried out automatically in order to allow detection of non-specific amplification products.

Standard curve for LCDV quantification

To quantify the amount of viral DNA in different samples, a standard curve was generated using the recombinant plasmid described above. The concentration of the purified plasmid was determined by spectrophotometry as described above, and the plasmid stock was diluted to serve as template for qPCR (10-fold serial dilutions ranging from 10^6 to 10^2 copies, and then two-fold dilutions from 50 to 25 copies, and from 16 copies to 1 copy).

The sensitivity of the qPCR assay was also determined in terms of infective viral particles. LCDV SA9 stock was titrated in SAF-1 cells, using the 50 % cell culture infectious dose ($TCID_{50}$) endpoint dilution assay as described previously [27]. An aliquot of 1 ml of the viral stock with a titre adjusted to 1 x 10^6 $TCID_{50}$/ml was subjected to a 10-fold serial dilution in Leibovitz's L-15 medium. The DNA of each dilution was extracted as previously specified, and used for qPCR. The amount of infective virus analysed per reaction was 1 x 10^5 to 1 x 10^0 $TCID_{50}$.

Milli-Q water and DNA from one LCDV-negative gilthead seabream sample [19] were included within each qPCR run as no-template and negative controls, respectively. In each 96-well, plasmid dilutions for the standard curve were run along with the samples and controls, using three technical replicates. The number of copies of LCDV DNA in each well was calculated from its cycle threshold (C_t) value by interpolation in the standard curve (C_t *versus* log copy number), using the SDS Software v1.3 (Applied Biosystem). The amplification efficiency (E) was calculated from standard curves using the formula $E = (10^{-1/S} - 1) \times 100$ (S being the slope of the linear fit). Viral loads in samples were calculated as the mean of the three replicates, and expressed as viral DNA copies per milligram of tissue (per µl in blood samples).

Assay repeatability and reproducibility

To evaluate the precision of the qPCR, the intra- and inter-assay variability was determined using the recombinant plasmid. To assess intra-assay variation, four plasmid DNA dilution series (from 10^5 to 2 copies per reaction) were prepared and tested simultaneously in the same plate. Four separate PCR runs were carried out to assess inter-assay variation, using also seven dilutions of plasmid DNA. The mean, standard deviation (SD) and coefficient of variation (CV) were calculated independently for each DNA dilution.

Results

Evaluation of the real-time PCR assay

Specificity of the qPCR was determined by analysis of the dissociation curves generated in each experiment. Standard and positive samples gave a single PCR product with a melting temperature of 77.7 ± 0.5 °C, which correspond with that deduced from the sequence of the expected fragment. The size of amplicons was monitored by agarose gel electrophoresis, and bands were observed at the expected size (150 bp).

The linear dynamic range, efficiency and precision of the qPCR assay were evaluated using a recombinant plasmid containing a 609-bp fragment of the LCDV MCP gene. Standard curves generated from four independent assays demonstrated a linear relationship between the amount of plasmid DNA and C_t values over a wide range of concentration, from 10^6 copies ($C_t = 16.25 \pm 0.48$) to 2 copies ($C_t = 34.09 \pm 1.14$) per reaction (Fig. 1a). The regression analysis yielded a correlation coefficient (r) ≥ 0.994 and an amplification efficiency of 101.89 ± 5.11 %. The mean intra-assay variation was 1.38 ± 0.87 % when analysing four replicates of plasmid dilutions, whilst the mean inter-assay variation among four experiments was 2.63 ± 0.48 % (Table 1). These CV values were considered acceptable to validate the repeatability and reproducibility of the assay.

A linear relationship between the infective titre of a viral suspension and C_t values was also observed for viral amounts ranging from 1 x 10^4 to 1 x 10^0 $TCID_{50}$ per reaction ($r = 0.999$) (Fig. 1b), with 1 x 10^0 $TCID_{50}$ yielding a mean viral DNA copy number of 1.2 x 10^2.

Surveillance study of LCDV in gilthead seabream farms

In the present study, individual gilthead seabreams were collected from four farms with different background

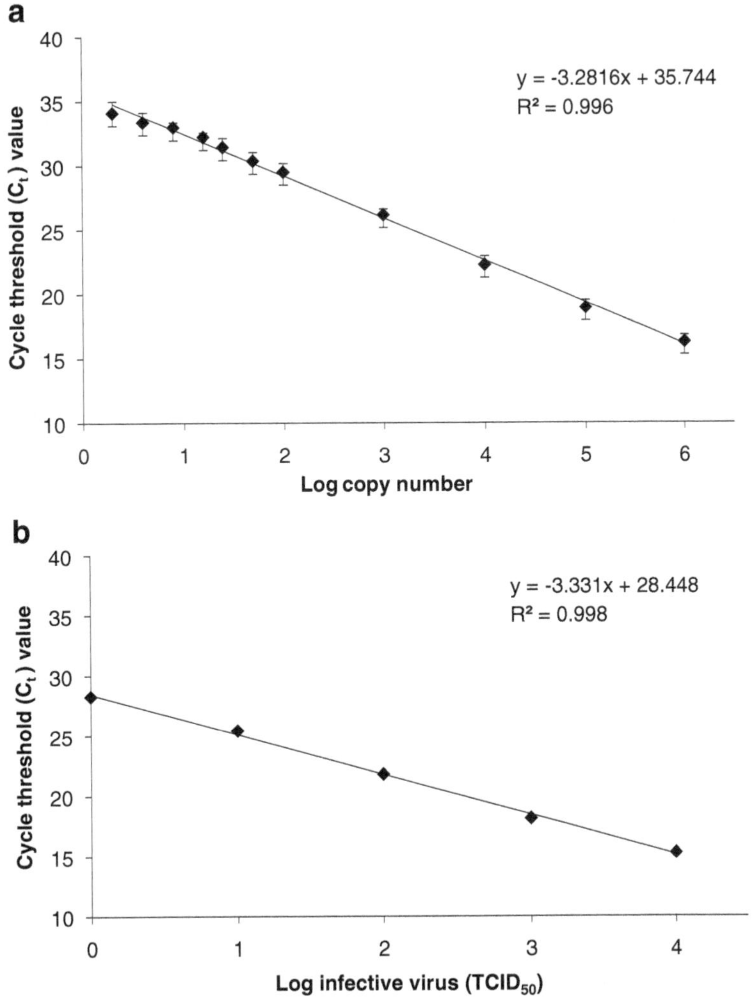

Fig. 1 Dynamic range and sensitivity of the real-time PCR assay for LCDV detection. **a** Standard curve obtained using dilutions of plasmid DNA ranging from 10^6 to 2 copies per reaction. Linear regression was performed on mean data from four separate runs. The logarithm to base 10 (log) of the plasmid copy number *versus* the cycle threshold (C_t) value is represented. **b** Standard curve showing a linear relationship between the log of the amount of infective virus (expressed in $TCID_{50}$) per reaction and their corresponding C_t values

Table 1 Intra- and inter-assay variability of the real-time PCR

	Intra-assay variation[a]		Inter-assay variation[b]	
Copies/reaction	Cycle threshold (C_t)[c]	CV (%)	Cycle threshold (C_t)[c]	CV (%)
1 x 10^5	19.92 ± 0.16	0.78	18.92 ± 0.54	2.83
1 x 10^4	23.34 ± 0.17	0.73	22.27 ± 0.60	2.69
1 x 10^3	26.87 ± 0.18	0.66	26.14 ± 0.46	1.75
1 x 10^2	30.22 ± 0.27	0.89	29.49 ± 0.71	2.39
1.6 x 10^1	32.15 ± 0.47	1.45	32.22 ± 0.87	2.72
4 x 10^0	34.15 ± 0.80	2.34	33.37 ± 0.89	2.68
2 x 10^0	35.23 ± 0.99	2.80	34.09 ± 1.14	3.35
Overall CV[c] (%)		1.38 ± 0.87		2.63 ± 0.48

[a] Intra-assay variation was determined on four replicates of recombinant plasmid dilutions analysed in the same PCR run
[b] Inter-assay variation was calculated on values obtained in four separate PCR runs
[c] Mean ± standard deviation (SD)
CV coefficient of variation

regarding to LCD. Farm C had no records of LCD, either before or after this study, whereas farm D suffered LCD outbreaks in last years. In farms A and B an outbreak of LCD was going on at the time of sampling, affecting several tanks. In these latter farms, fish from two different cycles of production were sampled, one suffering and other unaffected by LCD.

A total of 60 juvenile fish, both asymptomatic and diseased, were analysed by the qPCR assay developed in this study. LCDV was detected in all farms, 30 to 100 % of fish being identified as LCDV-infected (Table 2). In parallel, asymptomatic fish were also analysed by PCR-hybridization, corroborating in all cases their infection status. In asymptomatic fish, viral loads in caudal fin ranged between 1 copy and 3.3 x 10^2 copies of viral DNA per mg of tissue, whereas in animals with signs of the disease, viral loads were between 2.9 x 10^4 and 6.6 x 10^5 copies of viral DNA/mg.

Samples were also collected at the hatchery in another farm with previous LCD records (farm E). Rotifer and artemia metanauplius cultures, and artemia cysts were positive for LCDV. Viral loads estimated for these samples were about 10^2 copies of viral DNA per mg (Table 3). In addition, one sample of decapsulated artemia cysts was analysed, and found to be LCDV-positive (1.2 x 10^1 copies of viral DNA/mg). LCDV was also detected by qPCR in non-disinfected gilthead seabream fertilized eggs, in animals collected at different tanks in the larval rearing unit (1- to 26-d-old larvae), and in fingerlings collected in the weaning area. Viral loads in these gilthead seabream samples ranged from 1.3 x 10^0 to 2.2 x 10^1 copies of viral DNA/mg. All the samples collected at this hatchery were also found to be LCDV-positive by PCR-hybridization.

Finally, broodstock from farm E were analysed using the qPCR assay (Table 4). LCDV was detected in 22 out of the 50 caudal fin samples analysed, with estimated viral loads ranging from 8.7 to 61 copies of viral DNA/mg. When blood samples were considered, only 9 of the fish were identified as LCDV-positive (1.3 ± 1.37 copies of viral DNA/μl).

Table 2 LCDV detection and estimated viral load determined by real-time PCR in caudal fin from diseased and asymptomatic gilthead seabream juveniles

			Viral load[d]	
Fish population[a]	LCD signs[b]	LCDV detection[c]	Load range	Mean ± SD
A	-	73.3 (15)	1–15	(4 ± 3.99) x 10^0
A	+	100 (6)	1.2 x 10^5–6.6 x 10^5	(3.53 ± 2.77) x 10^5
B	-	30.0 (10)	1–330	(1.1 ± 1.89) x 10^2
B	+	100 (5)	2.9 x 10^4–6.9 x 10^4	(5 ± 1.75) x 10^4
C	-	87.5 (16)	1.7–54	(1.6 ± 1.56) x 10^1
D	-	100 (8)	12–140	(5.3 ± 5.88) x 10^1

[a] A, B, C and D are four gilthead seabream farms located in the Mediterranean area. Only farm C had no previous reports of lymphocystis disease (LCD)
[b] Typical lymphocystis disease signs: +, presence; -, absence
[c] Percentage of LCDV-positive fish (total number of fish analysed)
[d] Copies of viral DNA per mg of tissue
SD standard deviation

Table 3 Estimated viral load determined by real-time PCR in samples from a gilthead seabream hatchery

Sample[a]	Viral load[b]
Rotifer culture	1.5×10^2
Artemia cysts	1.9×10^2
Decapsulated artemia cysts	1.2×10^1
Artemia metanauplii	1.5×10^2
Fertilized eggs	4.1×10^0
Larvae (1-d-old)	3.4×10^0
Larvae (6-d-old)	2.5×10^0
Larvae (8-d-old)	3.6×10^0
Larvae (26-d-old)	5.1×10^0
Fingerlings (0.3 g)	1.1×10^1
Fingerlings (0.9 g)	1.3×10^0
Fingerlings (1.6 g)	2.2×10^1
Fingerlings (2 g)	9.7×10^0

[a] Samples consisted of pooled animals
[b] Copies of viral DNA per mg of tissue

Discussion

LCD outbreaks are frequently observed in the Mediterranean gilthead seabream aquaculture. Although it is usually described as a self-limiting disease, there are several reports on mortalities up to 45 % in juvenile fish, which may be related to secondary bacterial infections or with particularly large growth of lymphocysts, which severely impaired fish breathing or feeding [4, 10, 28]. As no effective treatments or commercially available vaccines currently exist, LCD prevention in hatcheries must rely on the selection of LCDV-free broodstock, the use of effective decontamination methods to prevent viral transmission from asymptomatic broodstock to larvae, and the supply of virus - freelive food [17, 22, 29]. During the growing period, the selection of non-infected fish is also advisable, as LCDV-positive juveniles may become symptomatic under stress conditions such us transport to on-growing facilities. Moreover, little information is available on a number of epidemiological questions concerning LCDV infections, as the number of virus particles required to induce the disease, the number of genome copies present in asymptomatic and diseased fish, and the kinetics of viral replication.

Previous studies have demonstrated the applicability of a PCR-based method to detect LCDV in asymptomatic gilthead seabream carriers, independently of its size, as well as in rotifer and artemia cultures [17, 19, 22]. Nevertheless, this method is relatively time-consuming, as an additional step of blot-hybridization of the PCR products is required to detect LCDV-positive samples. Furthermore, this assay is not quantitative and applicable for routine diagnosis.

In the present study a qPCR assay has been developed and applied to detect and quantify LCDV in different samples. The assay was specific for LCDV, as demonstrated by analysis of the melting curves generated from each sample. Its analytical sensitivity, determined as the smallest copy number of the plasmid standard reliably detected, was 2 copies of DNA per reaction. The qPCR assay also showed a wide linear dynamic range, extending to 6 $\log_{10}$ concentrations of plasmid DNA, and infective titres from 10^4 to 1 $TCID_{50}$. In addition, the precision of the assay was supported by the high correlation coefficients obtained for the standard curves, and the intra- and inter-assay variation of C_t values.

Using the protocol as described, the qPCR assay allows the detection of the virus at levels as low as 1 copy of viral DNA per mg of fish tissue. This high sensitivity, combined with its wide dynamic range, makes the qPCR assay suitable to detect low viral loads in subclinical LCDV infections, and, at the same time, to quantify variable viral loads in the course of infection. In addition, it could be useful in searching for potential LCDV reservoirs.

The application of the qPCR assay to LCDV surveillance in fish farms has shown that monitoring the infection in individual fish, both diseased and subclinically infected, is possible by sampling caudal fin as reported previously [16, 19]. The prevalence of LCDV infection in the asymptomatic gilthead seabream populations analysed varied from 30 to 100 %, even in one farm with no previous LCD records. In these fish, estimated viral load in caudal fin was two to five orders of magnitude lower than in diseased fish. Thus viral load seems to correlate with disease manifestation. However, if the low viral loads detected in subclinical infections represent a status associated with viral replication remains to be determined. In addition, the qPCR assay developed could be a valuable tool to study the correlation between viral multiplication and the onset of symptoms in experimental LCDV infections.

Palmer et al. [15] developed a real-time PCR method using fluorogenic primers, specific for LCDV genotype IX sequences, which proved to be reliable in the

Table 4 LCDV detection and estimated viral load determined by real-time PCR in caudal fin and blood from asymptomatic gilthead seabream breeders

Samples	LCDV detection[a]	Viral load[b]	
		Load range	Mean ± SD
Caudal fin	44 (50)	8.7–61	$(2.7 \pm 1.40) \times 10^1$
Blood	18 (50)	0.2–4.4	$(1.3 \pm 1.37) \times 10^0$

[a] Percentage of LCDV-positive fish (total number of fish analysed)
[b] Copies of viral DNA per mg of tissue (caudal fin samples) or per µl (blood samples)
SD standard deviation

detection of subclinically infected yellow perch, although its sensitivity was 5 x 10^2 copies of DNA per mgL^{-1}. LCDV quantification by qPCR has also been carried out in a reduced number of samples from diseased and recovered gilthead seabream [26]. The analytical sensitivity of the former assay was 5.2 copies of DNA per reaction that is more than twice the value reported in the present study. Furthermore, although the authors reported some quantitative data, viral loads were not expressed in terms of viral DNA copies per amount of tissue, which prevents further comparisons [15, 26].

Carrier fish were also identified in the broodstock from a farm with LCD records by analysing caudal fin samples by qPCR. The assay was applied in parallel to blood samples, and although LCDV could be detected, estimated viral load, and also clinical sensitivity, was lower than that obtained in caudal fin analysis. In this farm, the q-PCR assay allowed the quantitative detection of LCDV in all samples collected in the hatchery, including fertilized eggs, larvae and fingerlings, and also rotifer cultures and artemia metanauplii and cysts used for larval rearing. In these samples, as well as in caudal fin samples from asymptomatic juvenile fish, the qPCR assay showed the same clinical sensitivity than the PCR-hybridization protocol described by Cano et al. [19], but is completed in 130 min, including melting curve generation, which considerably reduces the time required for LCDV diagnosis. In addition, the results of this study support the existence of multiple reservoirs of LCDV in the farm facilities, as previously suggested by Cano et al. [17, 22], and the importance of proper application of effective disinfection treatments, as those recommended by the FAO [30], to avoid viral transmission through fish eggs or live food.

Conclusions

The qPCR assay developed in this study is a sensitive, specific and reliable method for detection and quantification of LCDV in gilthead seabream. The method is rapid and appropriate for LCDV surveys for which the detection of subclinical LCDV infections in carrier fish is essential. The assay could also be valuable to identify LCDV reservoirs or to study viral replication in fish.

Competing interests

The authors declare that they have no competing interests.

Authors' contributions

IC designed the qPCR assay, obtained the recombinant plasmid, and contributed to draft the manuscript. EJV evaluated the repeatability and reproducibility of the assay, performed most of the experimental work, and analyzed data. AL assisted with experimental work and data analysis, and contributed to the writing process. DC conceived of the study, participate in its coordination and draft the manuscript. JJB provided essential intellectual contribution to this work, and provided critical revisions to the manuscript content. All authors read and approved the final manuscript.

Acknowledgements

We thank Ms L Cruzado and R Crespillo (Universidad de Málaga) for technical assistance.

Funding

This study has been supported by a project from the Spanish Government (Ministerio de Ciencia e Innovación), co-funded by the FEDER, granted to D Castro (AGL2010-17880), and a project from Junta de Andalucía (P12-RNM-2261) granted to JJ Borrego. EJ Valverde was supported by a fellowship from the Spanish Government (Ref. BES-2011-043607).

Author details

[1]Departamento de Microbiología, Universidad de Málaga, 29071 Málaga, Spain. [2]CEFAS Weymouth Laboratory, Weymouth, Dorset DT4 8UB, UK.

References

1. Anders K. Lymphocystis disease of fishes. In: Ahne W, Kurstak D, editors. Viruses of lower vertebrates. Berlin: Springer; 1989. p. 141–60.
2. Menezes J, Ramos MA, Pereira TG. Lymphocystis disease: an outbreak in *Sparus aurata* from Ria Formosa, south coast of Portugal. Aquaculture. 1987; 67:222–5.
3. Borrego JJ, Castro D, Balebona MC, Garcia-Rosado E, Lopez-Cortes L. Patologías que afectan al cultivo de la dorada (*Sparus aurata*, L.) en la Comunidad Autónoma andaluza. Sevilla: Consejería de Agricultura y Pesca, Junta de Andalucía; 2001.
4. Colorni A, Padrós F. Diseases and health management. In: Pavlidis M, Mylonas C, editors. Sparidae: biology and aquaculture of gilthead sea bream and other species. Oxford: Wiley-Blackwell; 2011. p. 321–57.
5. Wolf K. Fish viruses and fish viral diseases. Ithaca: Cornell University Press; 1988.
6. Smail DA, Munro ALS. The virology of teleosts. In: Roberts RJ, editor. Fish pathology. 3rd ed. Edinburgh: W.B. Saunders; 2001. p. 169–253.
7. Masoero L, Ercolini C, Caggiano M, Rossa A. Osservazioni preliminari sulla linfocisti in una maricoltura intensive italiana. Riv Ital Piscicul Ittiopatol. 1986; 21:70–4.
8. Basurco A, Marcotegui MA, Rueda A, Tidana A, Castellanos A, Tarazona JV, et al. First report of lymphocystis disease in *Sparus aurata* (Linnaeus) in Spain. Bull Eur Ass Fish Pathol. 1990;10:71–3.
9. Moate RM, Harris JE, McMahon S. Lymphocystis infections in cultured gilt-head sea bream (*Sparus aurata*) in the Aegean sea. Bull Eur Ass Fish Pathol. 1992;12:134–6.
10. Haddad-Boubaker S, Bouzgarou N, Fakhfakh E, Khayech M, Mohamed SB, Megdich A, Chéhida NB. Detection and genetic characterization of lymphocystis disease virus (LCDV) isolated during disease outbreaks in cultured gilt-head sea bream *Sparus aurata* in Tunisia. Fish Pathol. 2013;48:101–4.
11. Kitamura SI, Jung SJ, Kim WS, Nishizawa T, Yoshimizu M, Oh MJ. A new genotype of lymphocystivirus, LCDV-RF, from lymphocystis diseased rockfish. Arch Virol. 2006;151:607–15.
12. Kitamura SI, Jung SJ, Oh MJ. Differentiation of Lymphocystis disease virus genotype by multiplex PCR. J Microbiol. 2006;44:248–53.
13. Hossain M, Song JY, Kitamura SI, Jung SJ, Oh MJ. Phylogenetic analysis of lymphocystis disease virus from tropical ornamental fish species based on a major capsid protein gene. J Fish Dis. 2008;31:473–9.
14. Cano I, Valverde EJ, Lopez-Jimena B, Alonso MC, Garcia-Rosado E, Sarasquete C, et al. A new genotype of *Lymphocystivirus* isolated from cultured gilthead seabream, *Sparus aurata* L., and Senegalese sole, *Solea senegalensis* (Kaup). J Fish Dis. 2010;33:695–700.
15. Palmer LJ, Hogan NS, van den Heuvel MR. Phylogenetic analysis and molecular methods for the detection of lymphocystis disease virus from the yellow perch, *Perca flavescens* (Mitchell). J Fish Dis. 2012;35:661–70.
16. Kvitt H, Heinisch G, Diamant A. Detection and phylogeny of *Lymphocystivirus* in sea bream *Sparus aurata* based on the DNA polymerase gene and major capsid protein sequences. Aquaculture. 2008;275:58–63.

17. Cano I, Valverde EJ, Garcia-Rosado E, Alonso MC, Lopez-Jimena B, Ortiz-Delgado JB, et al. Transmission of lymphocystis disease virus to cultured gilthead seabream, *Sparus aurata* L., larvae. J Fish Dis. 2013;36:569–76.
18. Sanz F, Coll J. Techniques for diagnosing viral diseases of salmonid fish. Dis Aquat Org. 1992;13:211–33.
19. Cano I, Ferro P, Alonso MC, Bergmann SM, Römer-Oberdörfer A, Garcia-Rosado E, et al. Development of molecular techniques for detection of lymphocystis disease virus in different marine fish species. J App Microbiol. 2007;102:32–40.
20. Zan J, Sun X, Zhang Z, Qu L, Zhang J. Application of quantitative PCR method in detection of lymphocystis disease virus China (LCDV-cn) in Japanese flounder *(Paralichthys olivaceus)*. Chin J Oceanol Limnol. 2007;25:418–22.
21. Hossain M, Kim SR, Kitamura SI, Kim DW, Jung SJ, Nishizawa T, et al. Lymphocystis disease virus persists in the epidermal tissues of olive flounder, *Paralichthys olivaceus* (Temminch & Schlegel), at low temperatures. J Fish Dis. 2009;32:699–703.
22. Cano I, Lopez-Jimena B, Garcia-Rosado E, Ortiz-Delgado JB, Alonso MC, Borrego JJ, et al. Detection and persistence of Lymphocystis disease virus (LCDV) in *Artemia* sp. Aquaculture. 2009;291:230–6.
23. Pallister J, Gould A, Harrison D, Hyatt A, Jancovich J, Heine H. Development of real-time PCR assays for the detection and differentiation of Australian and European ranaviruses. J Fish Dis. 2007;30:427–38.
24. Pepin JF, Riou A, Renault T. Rapid and sensitive detection of ostreid herpesvirus 1 in oyster samples by real-time PCR. J Virol Methods. 2008;149:269–76.
25. Cutrín JJ, Olveira JG, Bandín I, Dopazo CP. Validation of a real time RT-PCR applied to cell culture for diagnosis of any known genotype of viral haemorrhagic septicaemia virus. J Virol Methods. 2009;162:155–62.
26. Ciulli S, Pinheiro AC, Volpe E, Moscato M, Jung TS, Galeotti M, et al. Development and application of a real-time PCR assay for the detection and quantitation of lymphocystis disease virus. J Virol Methods. 2015;213:164–73.
27. Alonso MC, Cano I, Garcia-Rosado E, Castro D, Lamas J, Barja JL, Borrego JJ. Isolation of lymphocystis disease virus from sole, *Solea senegalensis* Kaup, and blackspot sea bream, *Pagellus bogaraveo* (Brünnich). J Fish Dis. 2005;28:221–8.
28. Dezfuli BS, Lui A, Giari L, Castaldelli G, Mulero V, Noga EJ. Infiltration and activation of acidophilic granulocytes in skin lesions of gilthead seabream, *Sparus aurata*, naturally infected with lymphocystis disease virus. Dev Comp Immunol. 2012;36:174–82.
29. Yoshimizu M. Control strategy for viral diseases of salmonid fish, flounders and shrimp at hatchery and seed production facility in Japan. Fish Pathol. 2009;44:9–13.
30. Moretti A, Fernandez-Criado MP, Cittolin G, Guidastri R. Manual on hatchery production of seabass and gilthead seabream, vol. 1. Rome: Food and Agriculture Organization of the United Nations (FAO); 1999.

15

The whole genomic analysis of orf virus strain HN3/12 isolated from Henan province, central China

Huiqin Chen[1†], Wei Li[1†], Zhenzhan Kuang[1], Daxiang Chen[1], Xiaoqing Liao[1], Ming Li[1], Shuhong Luo[1,2*] and Wenbo Hao[1,3*]

Abstract

Background: The Orf virus (ORFV) is the causative agent of orf, a globally-occurring, acute, pustular, contagious disease affecting sheep, goats and humans with a worldwide distribution. Currently, the genomic analysis of four ORFV strains from the Fujian province in southern China and a NA1/11 strain isolated from the Jilin province in northeast China have been reported. However, little is known about the genomic information of ORFV strains from central China.

Results: From a recent outbreak in a sheep herd in the Henan province of central China, a novel ORFV strain (HN3/12) was isolated and cultured in ovine fetal turbinate (OFTu) cells. The strain was identified as HN3/12 and verified by PCR based on the DNA sequences of *011* and *059* genes. The whole genomic sequence of this isolate was determined by Next Generation Sequencing technology. To determine the genetic characteristics of the HN3/12 strain, phylogenetic analysis of the 011 and 059 genes and amino acid sequence alignment of the HN3/12 strain were performed and compared with reference parapoxvirus strains.

Conclusions: The HN3/12 genome is 136,643 bp in length, contains 63.67% G + C and encodes 132 putative genes. Phylogenetic analysis of the 011 and 059 nucleotide sequences showed that this viral strain was similar to the NA1/11 isolate. The homology analysis indicates that HN3/12 has 93% to 98% identity with published ORFV strains at amino acid level. When open reading frames (ORFs) were aligned among the HN3/12 and four Fujian ORFV strains, most of them have identities greater than 90% and only a few less than 60%. The availability of the whole genomic sequence of HN3/12 aids in our understanding of, and provides new insights into, the genetic diversity of ORFV.

Keywords: Parapoxvirus, ORFV, HN3/12, Phylogenetic analysis, Genomic sequencing

Background

Orf, also known as contagious ecthyma, contagious pustular dermatitis, or scabby mouth, is an acute disease that infects mainly sheep and goats [1–3]. The disease has a worldwide distribution and is characterized by typically self-resolving progress from erythema, via vesicle formation, to pustules and then to scabs [3–6]. It is a zoonotic disease, occasionally causing occupational infections in humans who are in close contact with infected animals [5]. In humans, the common invasion sites of ORFV are the keratinocytes and epithelial cells of the hands and fingers [5, 7]. Although considered a mild disease, orf usually lasts for 3–4 weeks and resolves within 1–2 months. However, mortality rates of up to 93% have been reported in lambs [1, 6, 8, 9]. High mortality rates are generally due to secondary infections or extremely debilitating conditions. Reinfection is commonly observed in sheep [10].

Orf infection has occurred endemically in many countries over the past several years [11]. Since the 1950s, outbreaks of orf have occurred in sheep and goats in more than 20 provinces of China, including the Jilin [6, 9], Hubei [12], Xinjiang and Shaanxi [13], Shandong [14], and

* Correspondence: sluo815@gmail.com; haowa@126.com
†Equal contributors
[1]Institute of Antibody Engineering, School of Laboratory Medicine and Biotechnology, Southern Medical University, Guangzhou 510515, People's Republic of China
Full list of author information is available at the end of the article

Fujian provinces [15, 16]. Although vaccination has been implemented in some regions, morbidity and economic losses remain significant. Attenuated orf virus vaccines can relieve the symptoms of the infection but they are unable to completely prevent the occurrence of orf [17]. Additionally, vaccination is not a common practice in most herds.

The Orf virus (ORFV), the causative agent of orf, is a prototype of the genus Parapoxvirus (PPV), belonging to the family *Poxviridae*, sub-family *Chordopoxvirinae*. The Parapoxvirus genus includes the bovine popular stomatitis virus (BPSV), pseudocowpox virus (PCPV) and parapoxvirus of red deer in New Zealand (PVNZ) [12, 18, 19]. Parapoxviruses can be distinguished from other members of poxvirus genera by their ovoid-shaped virions with relatively small size (about 260 nm in length and 160 nm in width) and the crisscross-pattern tubule-like structure on the particle surface [17].

In spite of the worldwide distribution of ORFV, little information regarding the molecular epidemiology of orf and relatively few molecular characterizations of ORFV strains is available. To date, several complete genomic sequences of ORFV strains isolated from affected sheep or goats have been reported [11, 15, 20–22]. In recent studies, two conserved genes *ORFV011 (B2L)* and *ORFV059 (F1 L)* have been widely used as molecular targets for the phylogenetic analysis of ORFV isolates [6, 23]. Currently, in China, the genomic analysis of four strains (OV-GO, OV-YX, OV-NP and OV-SJ1) from the Fujian province in Southern China [15] and a NA1/11 strain isolated from the Jilin province in Northeast China [22] have been reported. Four Fujian ORFV strain analyses showed gene deletion possibly leads to attenuation of ORFVs, and 47 of the 132 genes can be easily distinguished as originating from sheep or goats. The phylogenetic analysis revealed that the NA1/11 strain was closely related to the Xinjiang and Gansu strains. The nMDS analysis, based on NA1/11 and parapoxvirus reference strains, revealed that geographic locations and animal hosts are likely major factors causing genetic differences among ORFV strains. However, little is known about the genomic information for ORFV viruses from other provinces of China.

Here, we report about an outbreak of orf infection in sheep on a farm located in Wuyang country, Henan province, in the central region of China. The isolated ORFV strain was verified by PCR of the full-length *ORFV011* and *059* genes. Sequence alignment and phylogenetic analysis of *ORFV011*and *059* genes between this strain and other reported stains were carried out. A novel orf virus strain, ORFV-WY-HN (HN3/12), was then successfully isolated and its genomic sequence was determined. The present study provides basic data regarding the new ORFV strain isolated from the north-central region of China, including genomic and phylogenetic analyses.

Results

Clinical gross pathological changes

Orf, which is endemic in China, has not been effectively controlled due to the lack of an implemented vaccination program. In the sheep herd of Wuyang county, skin lesions displaying clinical symptoms characteristic of orf, such as papules, pustules, and scabs, were recorded in 11 lambs and six ewes. Four lambs and two ewes showed ulcerated or proliferative lesions in the epidermis of the lips, nostrils and nipples when examined (Fig. 1a). For all lambs and ewes, the characteristics of weight loss, anorexia, and proliferative papillomatous nodules ranging from 3 to 5 cm in diameter had appeared. All 17 infected sheep recovered about 30 days after the first clinical signs appeared. The morbidity of the outbreak was 4.25% (17 out of 400) and mortality was 0. No farm staff members were infected from the disease in this outbreak.

Isolation and culture of virus

All homogenates from the skin lesions were inoculated in OFTu cells. When about 80% cytopathic effect (CPE) was observed, the inoculated cells were passaged three times. Cells with CPE and the medium were harvested and frozen. Healthy OFTu cells were cultured with 1× MEM, as mentioned previously, and inoculated with a filtered virus suspension. Rounding, pyknosis, detachment and eventual degeneration of the OFTu cells infected with virus were observed at 6–8 days in the fourth blind passage (P4) period, corresponding with CPE. The CPE of OFTu cells progressed slowly, leading to grape-like clusters and cell detachment from the monolayer (Fig. 1b). The cells with specific CPE were confirmed by PCR. The isolated virus from the single plaque caused by a single virus was amplified, purified, titrated and preserved at −80 °C. This ORFV strain was successfully isolated and cultured in OFTu cells, and was named ORFV/Henan-C3/2012 (HN3/12).

PCR amplification

To verify whether or not the ORFV had been isolated, two sets of primers for *ORFV011* (1137 bp) and *ORFV059* (1017 bp) were designed. Two conserved genes were amplified from genomic DNA extracted from inoculated cell cultures or purified viral particles. Viral DNA from NA1/11 strain was used as a positive control. The three samples produced distinct positive bands with sizes corresponding to *B2L* (1137 bp) and *F1 L* (1017 bp) (Fig. 2a). PCR products were purified and cloned into a pMD-19 T vector, sequenced in both orientations, and the nucleotide

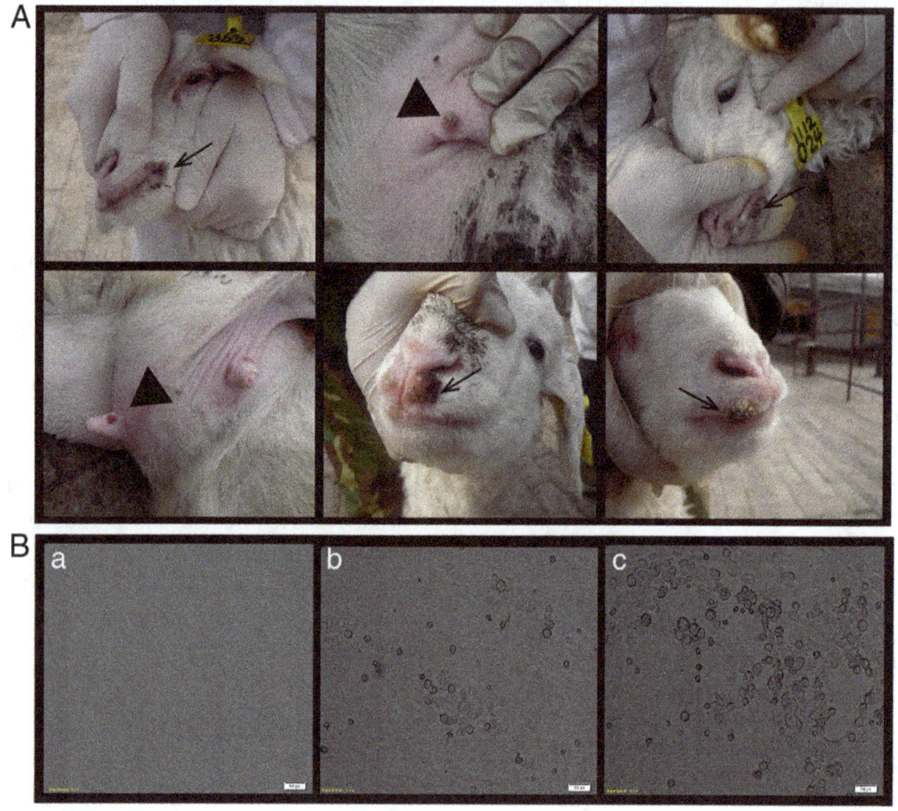

Fig. 1 Typical clinical signs of orf virus infection in sheep and OFTu cells. **a** Skin lesions of 6 infected sheep. Typical proliferative lesions on the skin of nostrils (*arrows*), nipple and mouth (*Triangular arrowheads*). **b** Cytopathic effect (CPE) of ovine fetal turbinate (OFTu) cells infected by orf virus strain HN3/12. **a** Uninfected OFTu cells **b** ORFV-HN-WY in OFTu at six days p.i. **c** ORFV-HN-WY in OFTu at eight days p.i. Scale bars = 100 um

sequence data showed that they were ORFV sequences. *ORFV011* and *059* nucleotide sequences of each sample were identical, indicating that the pathogen of the epidemic disease is the same as on the sheep farm. The *HN3/12–011* and *059* sequences were edited, aligned, and uploaded to GenBank with the following accession numbers: KC569750 (*ORFV011*) and KC569751 (*ORFV059*).

Phylogenetic analysis of ORFV011 and ORFV059 genes

To determine the genetic relation of the HN3/12 isolate to other ORFV strains, the corresponding nucleotide sequences of *ORFV011* and *ORFV059* genes from different strains were obtained from GenBank, aligned and analyzed using the neighbor-joining method by MEGA 5.2. Bootstrap analysis of *HN3/12-ORFV011* showed that these ORFV strains cluster together into two large branches based on the geographical position. In these ORFV strains, most of the strains from the Fujian province of southern China cluster together, while the Henan strain was closer to the isolates from northern China, such as Henan, Shaanxi, Ningxia, Jilin, Xinjiang and Gansu provinces. The HN3/12 strain is 99% identical with these northern Chinese ORFV strains for nucleotide sequences and 99%–100% for deduced amino acid sequences (Table 1). Among these ORFV strains, the Henan orf virus (HN3/12) is closest to ORFV-NA1/11 isolated from the Jilin province (Fig. 2b). Phylogenetic analysis of *ORFV059* showed that all ORFV strains cluster into two branches. HN3/12 was close to NA1/11, similar to *ORFV011*. However, these two strains cluster into the first branch, in which most ORFVs are from the Fujian province (Fig. 2c).

Analysis of genomic sequences of HN3/12

Genomic sequences of ORFV-HN3/12 were assembled into a contiguous sequence of 136,643 bp containing132 genes, with 63.7% G + C content. The left-most nucleotide was arbitrarily designated base 1. Aligned with published reference ORFV strains (OV-GO, OV-YX, OV-NP, OV-SJ1, OV-NZ2, OV-SA00, OV-IA82 and OV-NA1/11) for whole genome sequences, the HN3/12 strain showed the highest homogeneity with NA1/11, having 99% nucleotide identity and 98% amino acid identity. The identities of the HN3/12 strain with other ORFV strains were 97%–98% at the nucleotide level and 93%–97% at the tandem deduced amino acid level

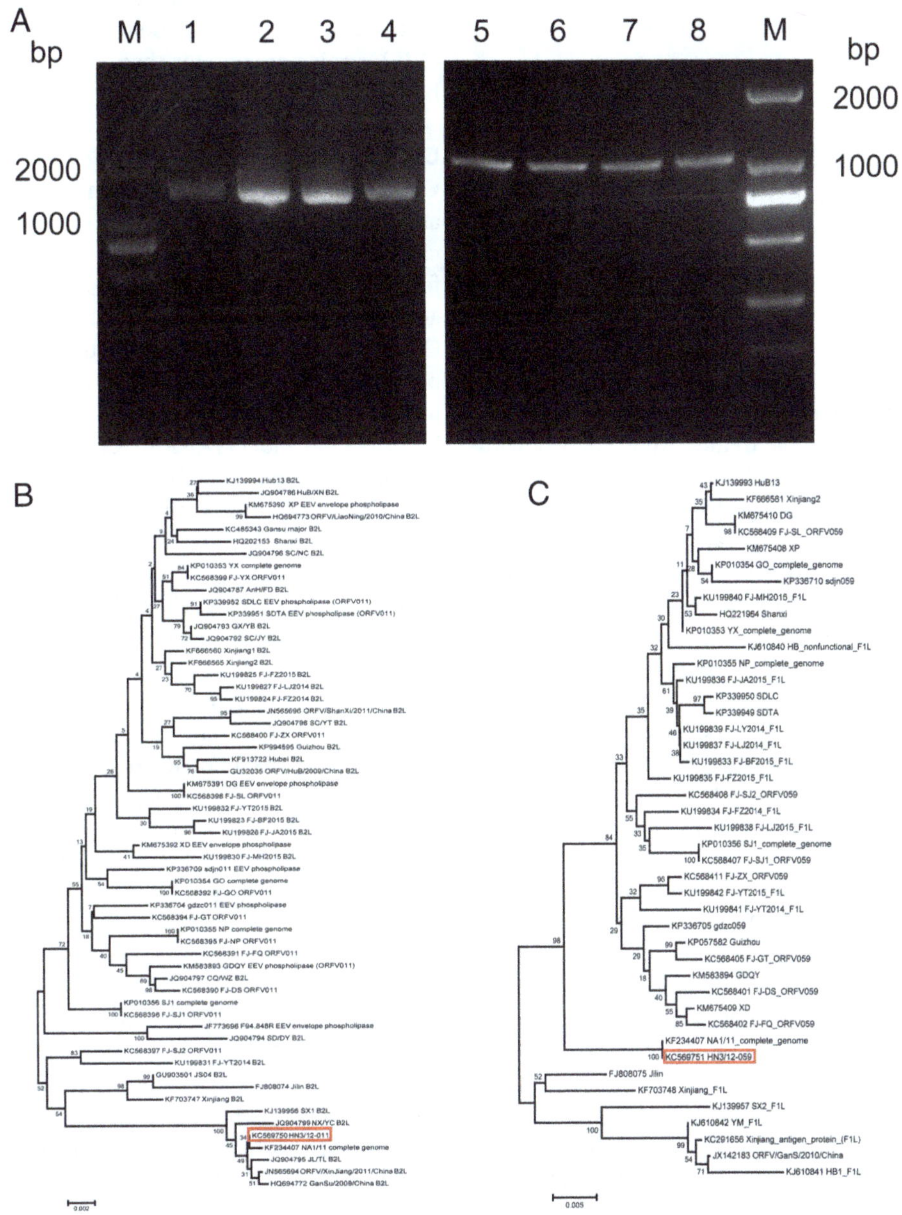

Fig. 2 PCR amplification and phylogenetic analyses of ORFV011 (B2L) and ORFV059 (F1 L) of the HN3/12 strain. **a** Amplification of major envelope genes (ORFV 011 and ORFV 059) by PCR. ORFV011 (lane 1, 2, 4) and ORFV059 (lane 5, 6, 8) were amplified from genomic DNA isolated from HN3/12. Lane 3 and 7: DNA extracted from NA1/11 strain as a positive control. Lane M: 2 kb DNA ladder. Phylogenetic analysis of different ORFV strains around the world, based on nucleotide sequences of ORFV011 (**b**) and ORFV059 (**c**). The phylogenetic trees were constructed by the neighbor-joining algorithm using MEGA version 5.2 software. One thousand bootstrap replicates were subjected to nucleotide sequence distance (cut-off value of 50% from 1000 bootstrap replicates). All bootstrap values are displayed above branches. The *scale bar* indicates the branch length. *Red frame*: HN3/12 in this study

(Table 2). Like the other ORFV isolates, the ORFV-HN3/12 genome contains a large central coding region bounded by two identical inverted terminal repeat (ITR) regions. ITRs of ORFV-HN3/12 contain 2794 bp and are the shortest in length, excepting OV-NP strain (2426 bp) (Table 2).

Phylogenetic analyses based on the complete genomic sequences of 13 PPV strains revealed that five ORFV strains originating in goats and five stains of sheep origination formed two separate branches with 100% bootstrap support. The ORFV strain from the Henan region showed a close relationship with NA1/11. Among strains originating in sheep, HN3/12 was closer to IA82 than to NZ2 or to D1701. Our analysis also showed that ten ORFVs were more closely related to PCPV than to BPSV (Fig. 3).

Table 1 The identity of nucleotide and amino acid sequences between the HN3/11 strain and other ORFV strains

Strain and its Geninfo identifier (gi)		ORFV011	
		Nucleotide	Amino acid
KJ1339956	SX1	99	100
KF234407	NA1/11	99	100
JQ904799	NY/YC	99	99
JQ904795	JL/TL	99	99
JN565694	Xinjiang/2011	99	100
HQ694772	Gansu/2009	99	100

Amino acid sequence alignment in five ORFVs

ORFV-HN3/12 open reading frames were aligned with those of the OV-GO, OV-YX, OV-NP and OV-SJ1 strains under the revision suggested by Chi et al. [15]. Pairwise protein alignments revealed that the HN3/12 strain shared 110 genes, 10 genes, 7 genes and 5 genes with greater than or equal to 90%, 80–89%, 60–79% and <60% amino acid identity, respectively, with OV-GO. Compared with OV-YX, HN3/12 shared 114 genes, 11 genes, 6 genes and one gene with greater than or equal to 90%, 80–89%, 60–79% and <60% the identity of amino acid sequences. With the OV-SJ1 strain, the Henan strain shared 112genes, 11 genes, 4 genes and two genes. HN3/12 shared 111 genes, 7 genes, 2 genes and four genes with OV-NP (Table 3). Multiple amino acid sequence alignments were performed based on four amino acid sequences (001, 005, 116 and 120) from ORFV strains. The open reading frame identities of the pairwise amino acid sequence alignment were <80%. The results of multiple alignments revealed that the homology of ORF001 (72.00%) was higher than ORF005 (61.34%) (Fig. 4), when HN3/12 was compared with four strains from Fujian province. In a comparison of HN3/12 with OV-GO, OV-YX and OV-SJ1 strains, the identity value of ORF120 (71.34%) was greater than ORF116 (55.06%) (Fig. 5). Additionally, the identities of ORF001 and 005 amino acid sequences among the four Fujian ORFV strains are greater than HN3/12. ORF116 and 120 have a similar pattern.

Discussion

Orf, caused by ORFV, is a zoonotic disease that mainly affects sheep and goats globally, and has been listed as a class I animal disease in China [13]. However, little information about the epidemiology and distribution characteristics of this virus is available. Currently, only nine ORFV strains have been isolated and relatively completely sequenced: NZ2 in New Zealand, IA82 and SA00 in America, D1701 in Germany, NA1/11, OV-GO, OV-YX, OV-NP and OV-SJ1 in China [20–22, 24, 25]. No genomic information about ORFV virus has been reported from central China. Therefore, ORFV needs to be explored further in order to effectively prevent and control this disease.

In this study, we successfully isolated and identified a novel orf virus strain named HN3/12 from infected sheep in a village in Wuyang, in the Henan province of central China. The entire genomic sequence of ORFV-HN3/12 is about 136.6-kbp in length, with 63.67% G + C content, and contains 2.79-kbp inverted terminal repeats (ITRs). The features are in agreement with other previously reported ORFV strains, such as OV-GO, OV-YX, OV-NP, OV-SJ1, OV-NZ2, OV-SA00, OV-IA82, OV-NA1/11, and other PPVs. The length of the ITR in HN3/12 strain is the second shortest among these ORFV strains.

Most published phylogenetic analyses and molecular epidemiology of orf virus have been investigated based on the highly conserved genes of *ORFV011 (B2L)*, *ORFV059 (F1 L)* and/or *ORFV020 (VIR)* [23, 26–28]. The sequences of *ORFV011* and *ORFV059*, which were regarded as epidemiologically relevant sequences, are usually used for phylogenetic analysis of orf virus [16, 19, 29]. *ORFV020 (VIR)* as a marker,

Table 2 Summary of complete genomic sequence data of 10 ORFV strains

Isolate	Species of origin	Country of origin	No. predicted genes	Genome size(bp)	ITR size (bp)	Genome G + C (%)	Genbank accession. no.	% ID (nt)	% ID (aa)	References
HN3/12	Sheep	China (HN)	132	136,643	2794	63.7	KY053526	100	100	In this study
NA1/11	Sheep	China (JL)	132	137,080	3020	63.6	KF234407	99	98	Li et al.,2014 [22]
GO	Goat	China (FJ)	132	139,886	3964	63.6	KP010354	97	95	Chi et al.,2015 [15]
YX	Goat	China (FJ)	132	138,231	3446	63.8	KP010353	97	95	Chi et al.,2015 [15]
SJ1	Goat	China (FJ)	129	139,112	4153	63.6	KP010356	97	96	Chi et al.,2015 [15]
NP	Goat	China (FJ)	124	132,111	2426	63.8	KP010355	98	94	Chi et al.,2015 [15]
SA00	Goat	USA	132	139,962	3936	63.4	AY386264	98	93	Delhon et al.,2004 [20]
IA82	Sheep	USA	132	137,241	3092	64.3	AY386263	98	96	Delhon et al.,2004 [20]
NZ2	Sheep	New Zealand	132	137,820	3389	64.3	DQ184476	98	97	Mercer et al.,2006 [21]
D1701	Sheep	Germany	288	134,038			HM133903	97	94	McGuire et al.,2012 [24]

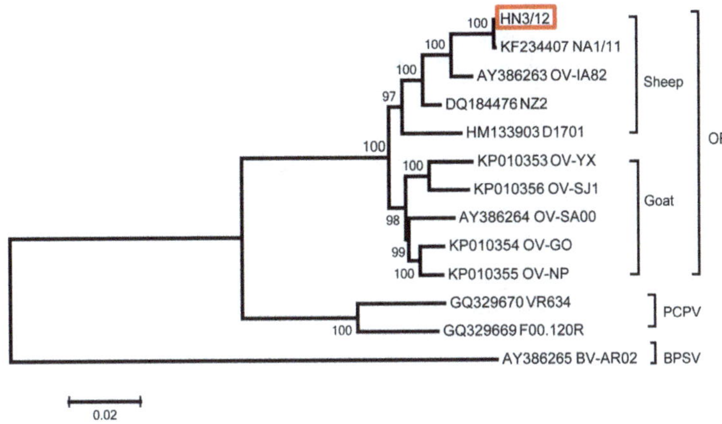

Fig. 3 Phylogenetic comparison of PPVs. Genomic nucleotide sequences, including terminal repetitions, were aligned using Clustal W.Phylogenetic trees were generated using the maximum-likelihood algorithm by MEGA 5.2 software. *Numbers* at the branching points indicate the bootstrap support calculated for 1000 replicates (cut-off value is 50%)

and is also employed in molecular epidemiological studies of ORFV [30, 31].

Phylogenetic analysis of the conserved regions (*011 and 059* genes) indicated that ORFV-HN3/12 is closely related to ORFV-NA1/11, a sequenced orf virus strain isolated from the Jilin province, in the northeast of China [22]. Phylogenetic analysis of the *ORFV011* gene showed that the HN3/12 isolate clusters together with ORFV strains from northern China. However, the strain is closest to the ORFVs coming from the Fujian province, according to the analysis of *ORFV059* gene. This suggests that phylogenetic analysis based on single gene may have some bias.

The results of the phylogenetic analysis based on the genomic sequences of 13 PPV strains revealed that HN3/12 has a closer relationship with NA1/11 than to the others, and this is consistent with the phylogenetic analyses of the *011* and *059* genes. The two virus strains originated in sheep and were isolated from the north of China (NA1/11 from Jilin province and HN3/12 from Henan province), suggesting that they may stem from the same origin. This implies that the strain can be utilized for designing a vaccine to reduce outbreaks of orf in sheep herds at these areas.

Furthermore, 132 amino acid sequences of HN3/12 were compared with that of the four Fujian strains. The results of pairwise sequence alignment showed that the identity of most ORFs are more than 90%, based on protein sequence analysis, and some ORFs are less than 80% (Table 3 and Additional file 1: Table S1). Among the ORFs with low identity, four ORFs (001, 005, 116 and 120) from five ORFV strains were analyzed further based on multiple amino acid sequence alignment. The homology of ORF001 and 120 is greater than the homology of 005 and 116 . Moreover, based on ORF001 and ORF005 sequence alignment analysis, the four Fujian strains share higher identity with each other, while HN3/12 shares a lower identity with the Fujian strains (Fig. 4). The identities of ORF116 and 120 in the Fujian strains, except for OV-NP (there is a deletion of ORF114–120 in OV-NP), are higher than with the HN3/12 strain (Fig. 5). This may be attributed to their having the same origin and fewer mutations between them. In these ORFs with low identity, *ORFV109* and *110* genes encode type II EEV glycoproteins, which are expressed in inter- and extra-cellular enveloped virions [21]. ORFV132 protein is a VEGF-like protein and plays a crucial role in the

Table 3 ORFs of HN3/12compared with the corresponding ORFV strains GO, YX, SJ1, NP

HN3/12	% Id (aa)							
	> = 90		80–90		60–79		<=60	
	Numbers	ORFs	Numbers	ORFs	Numbers	ORFs	Numbers	ORFs
GO	110	002,007,009…	10	012,013,061,080,104,113, 115,118,119,121	7	001,005,059,102,112, 120,134	5	103,109,110,116,132
YX	114	007,008,010…	11	002,012,061,080,110,112,113, 115,118,119,121	6	001,005,109,120,132,134	1	116
SJ1	112	023,053,055…	11	001,012,013,024,061,080,102, 109,113,121,134	4	005,103,120,112	2	116,132
NP	111	023,026,087…	7	012,061,080,104,109,121	2	001,102	4	002,005,103,132

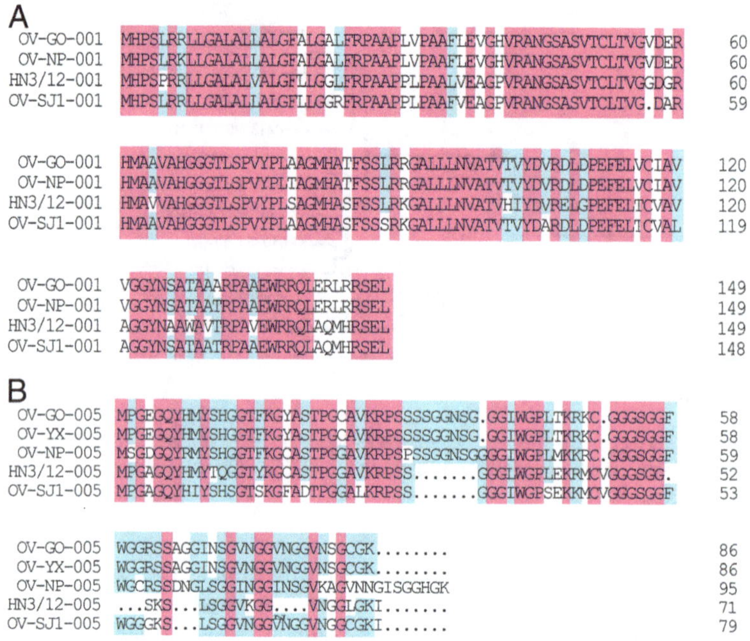

Fig. 4 Amino acid sequence alignment of ORF001 and ORF005 coded by five ORFVs. Multiple alignment was performed by Clustal Omega (available at http://www.ebi.ac.uk/Tools/msa/clustalo/) and DNAMAN software. Five ORFV strain accession numbers are shown in Table 2. The *pink box* indicates 100% ID of amino acid sequence among five ORFV strains. The *cyan box* indicates >50% ID of amino acid sequence among five ORFV strains

development of lesions induced by ORFV [32] (Additional file 1: Table S1). However, the functions of some proteins, such as ORFV001, 005, 116, 120, are still unknown, and require further exploration.

Conclusions

In summary, the isolated HN3/12 virus is a novel ORFV strain based on clinical manifestations, PCR amplification of *ORFV011*and *059*, and genome sequences. New genomic information of this ORFV strain from Wuyang country, in central China's Henan province, was obtained, which provides basic knowledge about ORFV to allow taking reasonable precautions and to control the disease. This may assist other researchers to explore the molecular epidemiology and the diversity of genomic sequences of ORFV. Future studies will reveal more relevant knowledge about ORFV and isolate more strains from different regions in China or worldwide, for a deeper, more comprehensive understanding of ORFV biology and epidemiology.

Methods

Sheep herds and tissue collection

The case described presently originated on a farm keeping about 400 sheep located in a village in Wuyang, Henan province, in the north-central region of China(113.6 E, 33.43 N), in January, 2012. Eleven lambs, aged one to six months, and six ewes presented with typical skin lesions on the muzzle, lips, and teats, possibly due to an Orf virus infection. The afflicted animals were cured within 5 weeks and suffered no deaths. Skin tissue samples with gross pathologic changes and scabs were collected, using a pair of sterilized tweezers, from four lambs and two ewes and stored at −80 °C for virus isolation and further analyses. Sera from the corresponding animals were collected from the jugular vein and preserved at −80 °C for further testing. All animal procedures were reviewed and approved by the Institutional Animal Care and Use Committee at South China Agricultural University (the certification number: CNAS BL0011).

Isolation and culture of Orf virus

The isolation of the virus was performed according to previous methods with some modifications [33, 34]. Briefly, tissue samples were mechanically homogenized with a disposable pestle (Sangon Biotech, Shanghai, China) in 1 × MEM medium (Hyclone, Logan, UT, USA) supplemented with gentamicin (50 μg/ml), penicillin (100 U/ml), and streptomycin (100 μg/ml), followed by centrifugation at 3000×g for 10 min. Clarified supernatant was passed through 0.45 μm filters and inoculated onto OFTu cells. The cells were incubated at 37 °C in 5% CO_2. Cells were observed daily with an inverted microscope for monitoring the progression of virus-induced CPE. Infected cells were passaged thrice after CPE appeared. When 60%–80% CPE was observed, cells and medium were harvested and stored at −80 °C for further experiments. The virus was isolated from the

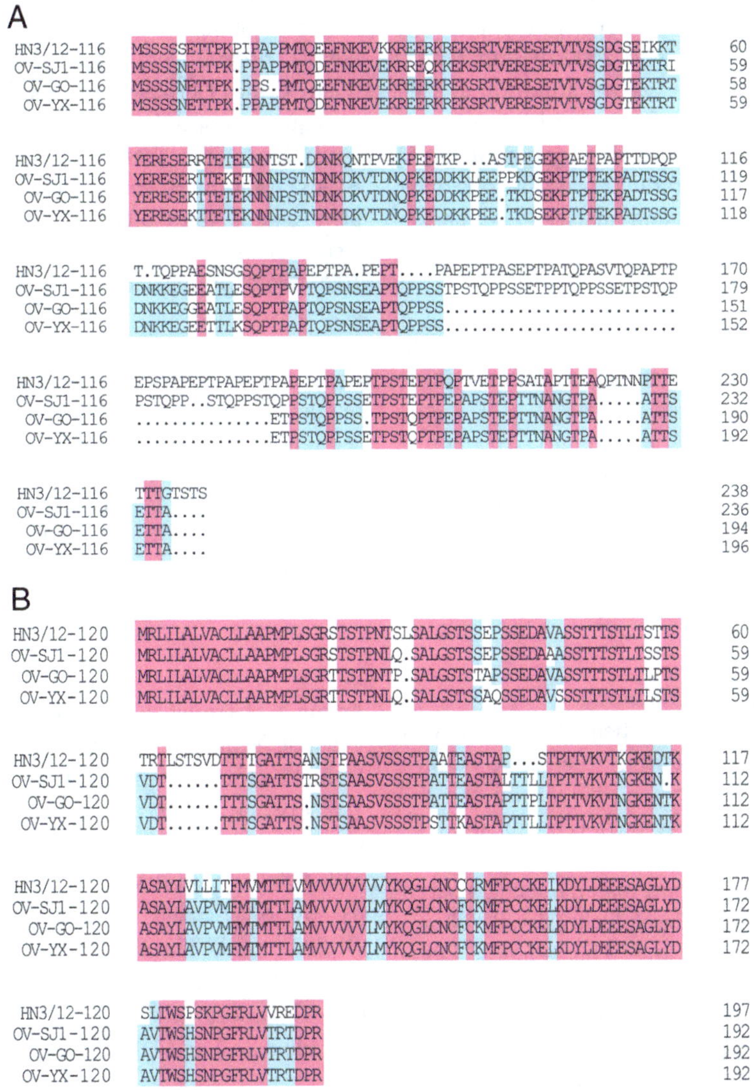

Fig. 5 Amino acid sequence alignment of ORF116 and ORF120 coded by four ORFVs. Multiple alignment was performed by Clustal Omega (available at http://www.ebi.ac.uk/Tools/msa/clustalo/) and DNAMAN software. Four ORFV strain accession numbers are shown in Table 2. The *pink box* indicates 100% ID of amino acid sequence among five ORFV strains. The *cyan box* indicates >50% ID of amino acid sequence among five ORFV strains

OFTu cell culture medium and a single clone of the viral strain was isolated by a plaque assay, performed according to previous reports [6, 9]. Briefly, OFTu cells were infected with serial dilutions of virus from 10^{-1} to 10^{-6} for 1 h at 37 °C in a 5% CO_2 incubator. 3 ml MEM containing 5% FBS and 0.5% low melting point agarose (Sea KemW GTGW, Lonza, Rockland, ME, USA) was added after removing the old medium. Plaques caused by a single virus were visualized and picked at 4 or 5 dpi. Each isolate was acquired with a minimum of 2 or 3 plaques.

Polymerase chain reaction (PCR) and gene sequencing

Total DNA was extracted directly from tissue suspensions (200ul) of the lip lesions or purified virion materials using a QIAamp DNA blood kit (QIAGEN, Duesseldorf, Germany), according to the manufacturer's instructions. PCR of the *ORFV011* and *ORFV059* genes was performed. Two sets of primers were designed based on the OV-NZ2 genomic sequence to amplify these two highly conserved genes [20]. Primer sets were as follows: NZ2-ORFV011Fw: 5′- ACACCTTTCCCCAGAACCCCA-3′; NZ2-ORFV011Rv:5′- GTCCGAGCTCCAGTTGCTGA CTT-3′; NZ2-ORFV059Fw: 5′- ACGTCATCACATGC GGGTCAGAG-3′; NZ2ORFV059Rv:5′- CTTCCTGTT CCTGGCGGGCAT-3′. PCR reactions were carried out in 50 μl reaction volumes, which contained 10 μl of 5 × PCR buffer (10 mMTris–HCl and 50 mMKCl), 2 μl of DNA template, 200 μMof each dNTP, 0.4 μM of each primer, 25 μM $MgCl_2$ and 0.5 μl of Taq polymerase (Takara, Dalian, China). PCR reactions were performed in a thermocycler (GeneAmp PCR 2400, Perkin Elmer, Shelton, CT, USA) for 32 cycles of denaturation at 95 ° C for 1 min, annealing at 56 °C for 30s and extension at 72 °C for 1 min, followed by a final extension at 72 °C for 10 min. The amplified products were resolved by 1% agarose gel electrophoresis and analyzed with an IS-1000 Digital Imaging System (Alpha Innotech Corp. San Leandro, CA, USA).

The PCR products were individually purified using a MiniElute gel extraction kit (QIAGEN, Duesseldorf, Germany), according to manufacturer's procedures. Purified gene fragments were cloned into pMD-19 T vector (Takara, Dalian, China) and transformed into *E.coli* Top10 competent cells. The existence of the insert was determined by restriction endonuclease (EcoRI and BamHI) digestion and agarose gel electrophoresis. Two or three positive clones for each gene were sent to BGI-Shenzhen for sequencing.

Genomic DNA extraction and sequencing

Infected cells were harvested when 80% CPE was observed by scraping the bottom of the tissue culture flasks. The mature virions were purified from the infected cells by sucrose gradient ultra-centrifugation as previously described [9, 16]. Viral genomic DNA was extracted from tissue purified virion material using a Virus DNA purification Kit (Roche, Basel, Switzerland), following the manufacturer's instructions. This genomic DNA preparation was sequenced using the Paired-End method on a high-throughput Illumina system [35, 36]. Briefly, viral genomic DNA was interrupted randomly by sonication to produce a series DNA fragments with sizes less than or equal to 800 bp. The DNA fragments were then repaired and adapters ligated to both ends. Sequence data were assembled with the Phrap and CAP3 software programs. Gaps were closed by primer walking and verified by sequencing of PCR products.

Genomic DNA composition, structure, repeats, and restriction enzyme patterns were analyzed using the Genetics Computer Group (GCG) version 10 software package. Open reading frames (ORFs) longer than 30 codons were evaluated for coding potential and ORFs greater than 60 codons were subjected to homology searches with BLAST in the NCBI database (https://blast.ncbi.nlm.nih.gov/Blast.cgi). In addition, the Hexamer (ftp.sanger.ac.uk/pub/rd) and Glimmer programs were used to evaluate coding potential. Based on these criteria, 132 ORFV putative genes were annotated and orthologous ORFs were similarly numbered. The genome sequence was submitted to GenBank with the Accession Number: HN3/12: KY053526.

Sequences alignment and phylogenetic analysis

The nucleotide and deduced amino acid sequences of the HN3/12 isolate were aligned with Sequencer version 3.0 (Gene Codes Corp., Ann Arbor, MI, USA) and compared to sequences of the corresponding genes of those of PPVs available in the GenBank database using the online BLAST tool (https://blast.ncbi.nlm.nih.gov/Blast.cgi). Two phylogenetic trees of*ORFV011* and *059* gene sequences were constructed by the neighbor-joining method, with 1000 bootstrap replicates, using MEGA version 5.2. Phylogenetic comparisons were done based on the whole genomic nucleotide sequences, including terminal repetition, of PPV strains with MEGA 5.2 software using the maximum-likelihood method. The 13 PPVs genomic sequences were deposited into GenBank with the following Accession Numbers: HN3/12: KY053526, OV-YX: KP010353; OV-GO: KP010354; OV-NP: KP010355; OV-SJ1: KP010356; IA82: AY386263; SA00: AY386264; NZ2: DQ184476and F00.120R: GQ329669; VR634: GQ329670; BV-AR02: AY386265.

Amino acid sequence alignment of ORFVs

Pairwise sequence alignments of 132 ORFs from the HN3/12 strain with eight ORFV strains (OV-GO, OV-YX, OV-NP, OV-SJ1, NA1/11, IA82, NZ2 and SA00) were performed using EMBOSS Needle in the EMBL-EBI database (available at http://www.ebi.ac.uk/Tools/psa/emboss_needle/). Multiple amino acid alignment for ORF001, ORF005, ORF116 and ORF120 from the Fujian ORFV strains and the Henan strain were performed by Clustal Omega (available at http://www.ebi.ac.uk/Tools/msa/clustalo/) and DNAMAN software.

Abbreviations

BLAST: Basic Local Alignment Search Tool; bp: Base pair; BPSV: Bovine popular stomatitis virus; CPE: Cytopathic effect; ITR: Inverted terminal repeat; NGS: Next Generation Sequencing; OFTu: Ovine fetal turbinate; ORF: Open reading frame; ORFV: Orf virus; PCPV: Pseudocowpox virus; PCR: Polymerase chain reaction; PPV: Parapoxvirus; PVNZ: Parapoxvirus of red deer in New Zealand; SPPV: Squirrelparapoxvirus

Funding

This study was supported by grants from the National Natural Science Foundation of China (NSFC) (No. 31170147&31672536). The funding bodies had no role in study design, data collection or analysis, decision to publish or preparation of the manuscript.

Authors' contributions

HC and WL performed the experiments. WL, XL and ML isolated the virus from the clinical tissues. HC, ZK and DC prepared the gene sequence data. HC, WL, WH and SL analyzed the data and wrote the draft. All authors have read and approved the final draft.

Consent for publication
Not applicable

Competing interests
The authors declare that they have no competing interests.

Author details
[1]Institute of Antibody Engineering, School of Laboratory Medicine and Biotechnology, Southern Medical University, Guangzhou 510515, People's Republic of China. [2]Department of Laboratory Medicine, School of Stomatology and Medicine, Foshan University, 5 Hebin Road, Foshan, Guangdong Province 528000, People's Republic of China. [3]Guangdong Provincial Key Laboratory of Tropical Disease Research, School of Public Health, Southern Medical University, Guangzhou 510515, People's Republic of China.

References

1. Haig DM, Mercer AA. Ovine diseases. Orf. Vet Res. 1998;29(3–4):311–26.
2. Hosamani M, Scagliarini A, Bhanuprakash V, et al. Orf: an update on current research and future perspectives. Expert Rev Anti-Infect Ther. 2009;7(7):879–93.
3. Gelaye E, Achenbach JE, Jenberie S, et al. Molecular characterization of orf virus from sheep and goats in Ethiopia, 2008-2013. Virol J. 2016;13:34.
4. McElroy MC, Bassett HF. The development of oral lesions in lambs naturally infected with orf virus. Vet J. 2007;174(3):663–4.
5. Al-Salam S, Nowotny N, Sohail MR, et al. Ecthyma contagiosum (orf)–report of a human case from the United Arab Emirates and review of the literature. J Cutan Pathol. 2008;35(6):603–7.
6. Zhao K, Song D, He W, et al. Identification and phylogenetic analysis of an Orf virus isolated from an outbreak in sheep in the Jilin province of China. Vet Microbiol. 2010;142(3–4):408–15.
7. Thurman RJ, Fitch RW. Contagious Ecthyma. N Engl J Med. 2015;372(8):E12.
8. Yirrell DL, Reid HW, Norval M, et al. Immune response of lambs to experimental infection with Orf virus. Vet Immunol Immunopathol. 1989;22(4):321–32.
9. Li W, Ning Z, Hao W, et al. Isolation and phylogenetic analysis of orf virus from the sheep herd outbreak in northeast China. BMC Vet Res. 2012;8:229.
10. Haig DM, McInnes CJ. Immunity and counter-immunity during infection with the parapoxvirus orf virus. Virus Res. 2002;88(1–2):3–16.
11. Bora DP, Barman NN, Das SK, et al. Identification and phylogenetic analysis of orf viruses isolated from outbreaks in goats of Assam, a northeastern state of India. Virus Genes. 2012;45(1):98–104.
12. Zhang K, Shang Y, Jin Y, et al. Diagnosis and phylogenetic analysis of Orf virus from goats in China: a case report. Virol J. 2010;7:78.
13. Li H, Zhu X, Zheng Y, et al. Phylogenetic analysis of two Chinese orf virus isolates based on sequences of B2L and VIR genes. Arch Virol. 2013;158(7):1477–85.
14. Zhang K, Xiao Y, Yu M, et al. Phylogenetic analysis of three orf virus strains isolated from different districts in Shandong Province, East China. J Vet Med Sci. 2016;77(12):1639–45.
15. Chi X, Zeng X, Li W, et al. Genome analysis of orf virus isolates from goats in the Fujian Province of southern China. Front Microbiol. 2015;6:1135.
16. Chi X, Zeng X, Hao W, et al. Heterogeneity among orf virus isolates from goats in Fujian Province, Southern China. PLoS One. 2013;8(10):e66958.
17. Bora MDP, Bhanuprakash V, Venkatesan G, et al. Effect of Stabilization and Reconstitution on the Stability of a Novel Strain of Live Attenuated Orf Vaccine (ORFV MUK59/05). Asian J Anim Vet Adv. 2015;10(8):365–75.
18. Inoshima Y, Morooka A, Sentsui H. Detection and diagnosis of parapoxvirus by the polymerase chain reaction. J Virol Methods. 2000;84(2):201–8.
19. Hosamani M, Bhanuprakash V, Scagliarini A, et al. Comparative sequence analysis of major envelope protein gene (B2L) of Indian orf viruses isolated from sheep and goats. Vet Microbiol. 2006;116(4):317–24.
20. Delhon G, Tulman ER, Afonso CL, et al. Genomes of the parapoxviruses ORF virus and bovine papular stomatitis virus. J Virol. 2004;78(1):168–77.
21. Mercer AA, Ueda N, Friederichs SM, et al. Comparative analysis of genome sequences of three isolates of Orf virus reveals unexpected sequence variation. Virus Res. 2006;116(1–2):146–58.
22. Li W, Hao W, Peng Y, et al. Comparative genomic sequence analysis of Chinese orf virus strain NA1/11 with other parapoxviruses. Arch Virol. 2014;160(1):253–66.
23. Li H, Ning Z, Hao W, et al. Identification and characterization of monoclonal antibodies against the ORFV059 protein encoded by Orf virus. Virus Genes. 2012;44(3):429–40.
24. McGuire MJ, Johnston SA, Sykes KF. Novel immune-modulator identified by a rapid, functional screen of the parapoxvirus ovis (Orf virus) genome. Proteome Sci. 2012;10(1):4.
25. Friederichs S, Krebs S, Blum H, et al. Comparative and retrospective molecular analysis of Parapoxvirus (PPV) isolates. Virus Res. 2014;181:11–21.
26. Billinis C, Mavrogianni VS, Spyrou V, et al. Phylogenetic analysis of strains of Orf virus isolated from two outbreaks of the disease in sheep in Greece. Virol J. 2012;9:24.
27. Kottaridi C, Nomikou K, Teodori L, et al. Phylogenetic correlation of Greek and Italian orf virus isolates based on VIR gene. Vet Microbiol. 2006;116(4):310–6.
28. Yang H, Meng Q, Qiao J, et al. Detection of genetic variations in Orf virus isolates epidemic in Xinjiang China. J Basic Microbiol. 2014;54(11):1273–8.
29. Hautaniemi M, Ueda N, Tuimala J, et al. The genome of pseudocowpoxvirus: comparison of a reindeer isolate and a reference strain. J Gen Virol. 2010;91(Pt 6):1560–76.
30. Chan KW, Yang CH, Lin JW, et al. Phylogenetic analysis of parapoxviruses and the C-terminal heterogeneity of viral ATPase proteins. Gene. 2009;432(1–2):44–53.
31. Oem JK, Chung JY, Kim YJ, et al. Isolation and characterization of orf viruses from Korean black goats. J Vet Sci. 2013;14(2):227–30.
32. Wise LM, Stacker SA. Vascular endothelial growth factor (VEGF)-like protein from orf virus NZ2 binds to VEGFR2 and neuropilin-1. Proc Natl Acad Sci U S A. 1999;96(6):3071–6.
33. Guo J, Zhang Z, Edwards JF, et al. Characterization of a North American orf virus isolated from a goat with persistent, proliferative dermatitis. Virus Res. 2003;93(2):169–79.
34. Lin FY, Tseng YY, Chan KW, et al. Suppression of influenza virus infection by the orf virus isolated in Taiwan. J Vet Med Sci. 2015;77(9):1055–62.
35. Parkinson NJ, Maslau S, Ferneyhough B, et al. Preparation of high-quality next-generation sequencing libraries from picogram quantities of target DNA. Genome Res. 2012;22(1):125–33.
36. Li R, Zhu H, Ruan J, et al. De novo assembly of human genomes with massively parallel short read sequencing. Genome Res. 2010;20(2):265–72.

16

Diversity of susceptible hosts in canine distemper virus infection

Marlen Martinez-Gutierrez and Julian Ruiz-Saenz*

Abstract

Background: Canine distemper virus (CDV) is the etiological agent of one of the most infectious diseases of domestic dogs, also known as a highly prevalent viral infectious disease of carnivores and posing a conservation threat to endangered species around the world. To get a better panorama of CDV infection in different Orders, a retrospective and documental systematic review of the role of CDV in different non-dog hosts was conducted. The bibliographical data were collected from MedLine/PubMed and Scopus databases. Data related to Order, Family, Genus and Species of the infected animals, the presence or absence of clinical signs, mortality, serological, molecular or antigenic confirmation of CDV infection, geographic location, were collected and summarized.

Results: Two hundred seventeen scientific articles were considered eligible which includes reports of serological evaluation, and antigenic or genomic confirmation of CDV infection in non-dog hosts. CDV infects naturally and experimentally different members of the Orders Carnivora (in 12 Families), Rodentia (four Families), Primates (two Families), Artiodactyla (three Families) and Proboscidea (one Family). The Order Carnivora (excluding domestic dogs) accounts for the vast majority (87.5 %) of the records. Clinical disease associated with CDV infection was reported in 51.8 % of the records and serological evidence of CDV infection in apparently healthy animals was found in 49.5 % of the records. High mortality rate was showed in some of the recorded infections in Orders different to Carnivora. In non-dog hosts, CDV has been reported all continents with the exception of Australasia and in 43 different countries.

Conclusions: The results of this systematic review demonstrate that CDV is able to infect a very wide range of host species from many different Orders and emphasizes the potential threat of infection for endangered wild species as well as raising concerns about potential zoonotic threats following the cessation of large-scale measles vaccination campaigns in the human population.

Keywords: Endangered species, Morbillivirus, Re-emerging virus, Species barrier, Zoonosis

Background

Canine distemper virus (CDV) is the etiological agent of one the most infectious diseases of domestic dogs (*Canis familiaris*). It was first isolated by Carré in 1905 [1] and still remains one of the main problems for veterinarians and owners due to the high morbidity and mortality rates [2]. CDV belongs to the *Paramyxoviridae* family, genus Morbillivirus, that includes viruses with epidemiological relevance for human and animal populations such as measles virus, phocine distemper virus, peste des petits ruminants virus, and the eradicated rinderpest virus [3].

CDV is also known as a highly prevalent viral infectious disease of carnivores, posing a conservation threat to endangered species around the world [4–6]. Even recently, it was proposed to rename the virus "Carnivore Distemper Virus" due to its constant threat for different carnivorous species and to commonly documented outbreaks in non-dog carnivores [7].

In domestic dogs, the major route of CDV transmission is through aerosols from respiratory exudates containing the virus, although other body excretions and secretions (e.g., urine) can be infectious. CDV is highly contagious,

* Correspondence: julianruizsaenz@gmail.com; julian.ruizs@campusucc.edu.co
Grupo de Investigación en Ciencias Animales GRICA, Universidad Cooperativa de Colombia, Calle 30A # 33-51, Bucaramanga, Colombia

and viral shedding may follow infection for 60–90 days [3]. However, the question of how wild animals are exposed to CDV remains to be fully addressed and the role of domestic dogs and wild carnivores in the maintenance and transmission of CDV is still not fully understood [8, 9]. It has been shown that CDV can circulate in wildlife even when levels of infection are extremely low and asynchronous to infections found in domestic dogs, supporting the hypothesis that CDV infection is likely to persist in other wildlife species within complex reservoir systems [10].

CDV has also been found in naturally infected non-canine hosts [11] and recent dramatic outbreaks in breeding colonies of rhesus macaques (*Macaca mulatta*) and cynomolgus macaques (*Macaca fascicularis*), has drawn attention of a possible zoonosis in the post-measles eradication times [12].

In an attempt to consolidate the full list of hosts for CDV, a systematic literature review and data assembly was performed to identify relevant studies published in databases of all possible non-dog hosts for CDV (reported infections in species that are not domestic dogs). The search includes published papers reporting serological evaluations, clinical cases, antigenic/genomic confirmation and experimental infections of CDV in non-dog hosts. The aim was to obtain the most comprehensive information available to determine the range of host species susceptible to natural or experimental infection with CDV.

Methods

Data collection

This is a retrospective and documental study conducted with printed and Epub ahead of print of available online articles published from May 1964 to September, 2014, following the recommendations made by the Preferred Reporting Items for Systematic Reviews and Meta-Analyses (PRISMA) group and the new PRISMA-P2015 guidelines [13, 14]. Given that these recommendations were originally developed to evaluate healthcare interventions, components of this statement have been customized to fit the scope of the current systematic review as has been done by others [15]. The bibliographic data were collected from the databases of the National Library of Medicine on the web MedLine/PubMed® (http://www.ncbi.nlm.nih.gov/Pubmed) and Scopus® database from Elsevier (http://www.scopus.com/). An Excel® database was constructed with the references of the selected papers, country of report, common animal name and animal species reported infected by CDV. The Family and Order of the CDV infected animals were included according to the Handbook of the Mammals of the World, 2009 [16]. Notes, letters, editorials, news and meeting abstracts were excluded. The data set supporting the results of this article is included as Additional file 1: Table S1 in the web site of the journal.

All reports of serological evaluation, antigenic or genomic confirmation of CDV infection in non-dog hosts were included. Active infections were recorded in cases were the presence of virus, genome or antigen were confirmed (by virus isolation, rt-PCR and/or immunohistochemistry); otherwise, prior infections were recorded based on the presence of antibodies to CDV measured by the virus neutralization test or ELISA test. Only confirmed cases were included; by this, papers reporting clinical signs only were not included unless they also had some antigenic confirmation or histopathology report of findings compatible with CDV infection.

Search Strategy

For each search in the PubMed and SCOPUS databases, a sentence consisting of different parts joined together by the so-called Boolean operators, i.e., AND, OR, and NOT was used in the search field. The search strategy was not limited by study design or language and no limits to specific years were used. Manual detection was used to exclude publication types, such as notes, letters, editorials, news and meeting abstracts. The words "Canine Distemper Virus" were selected as "MeSH Terms". As an example of the main search the following text was used: "distemper virus, canine"[MeSH Terms] OR ("distemper"[All Fields] AND "virus"[All Fields] AND "canine"[All Fields]) OR "canine distemper virus"[All Fields] OR ("canine"[All Fields] AND "distemper"[All Fields] AND "virus"[All Fields]. The data was double-checked for all articles included in the qualitative synthesis.

The selection of studies for inclusion was made using a two-step approach. During the first step, researchers selected articles from the search results based on titles and abstracts, excluding those deemed irrelevant to the topic (all those that include dogs as hosts and papers reporting serological evaluation of wildlife CDV vaccination). Disagreements were resolved through mutual consent. The bibliographies of the articles reviewed were scanned for additional older highly relevant literature that could not be indexed in the selected databases. Studies relevant to the research questions were assessed in the second step using the full text, including those studies for which inclusion was uncertain on the basis of title or abstract screen. All articles retained after the first step went through a full-text review performed independently by the two reviewers.

Statistical analysis

Descriptive statistics were used in all cases to evaluate the results (e.g. the frequency in count and percentage); to measure the trend in publication of CDV infections in different orders throughout the years we used the linear regression (R^2) as a measure of linear association with a *p*-value of less than 0.05. Statistical analyses were performed using GraphPad Prism® 6 for Windows®.

Results

The PRISMA flow chart depicting the process for the systematic literature search and selection of the studies is shown in Fig. 1. Relevant records were assembled from May 1964 to September 2014. Due to the impossibility to eliminate the word "Canine" from the search strategy, the initial search yielded 5679 records (3979 from Scopus® and 1700 from MedLine/Pubmed®).

After the two step screening, 217 papers were deemed eligible that included reports of serological evaluation, antigenic or genomic confirmation of CDV infection in non-dog hosts. Also, the presence or absence of clinical signs were recorded. It is important to note that a single paper can include different records of CDV infected animal Species and/or Orders. A total of 272 different records of infected animals was found (See Additional file 1: Table S1).

As mentioned above, papers including serological and/or immunological evaluation of CDV vaccines in wildlife were excluded. As seen in Table 1, the Order *Carnivora* was the main host reported (87.5 % of the records) and within it, the *Canidae* family was the most commonly reported. Natural infection in twelve of the sixteen families within this Order has been reported [16]. It is important to note that CDV infection among members of the *Felidae* family has become the second most common infection reported in the papers evaluated, even with more reports than among members of the *Mustelidae* and the *Procyonidae* families (Table 1). Although other Orders account for only 12.5 % (36 records) of the infections, it is important to indicate that there are important and endangered species within those Orders, such as Primates, Artiodactyla and Proboscidea.

Interestingly, it was found that only 52 % of the records reported clinical disease by CDV. Table 1 show Family by Family the percentage of clinical sings reported on different papers. In these clinical cases, the death of the animals was the most common outcome and CDV was confirmed by immunohistochemical staining of tissues or by rt-PCR. On the other hand, serological reports of CDV infection in healthy animals accounts for almost all the other half of the papers with no clinical signs associated.

Serological evaluation in members of different Orders infected with CDV

Different serological studies have been performed to evaluate natural CDV infections in non-dog hosts. The most common test used was the virus neutralization test (75.4 %), followed by the Enzyme linked immunosorbent assay (13.8 %), the indirect immunofluorescent assay (7.7 %), the direct neutralizing peroxidase-linked antibody assay (1.5 %) and the dot immunobinding assays (1.5 %).

Most studies (129 records) provided evidence of CDV infection through serological studies that demonstrated seropositivity and that the reported seroprevalence ranged widely across host species within different Orders. Independently of the technique used, the median seroprevalence of all studies/populations on which CDV seropositivity was detected in Carnivora Order was 34,9 %, followed by the Artiodactyla Order with 41.7 % seropositivity and 1.3 % in

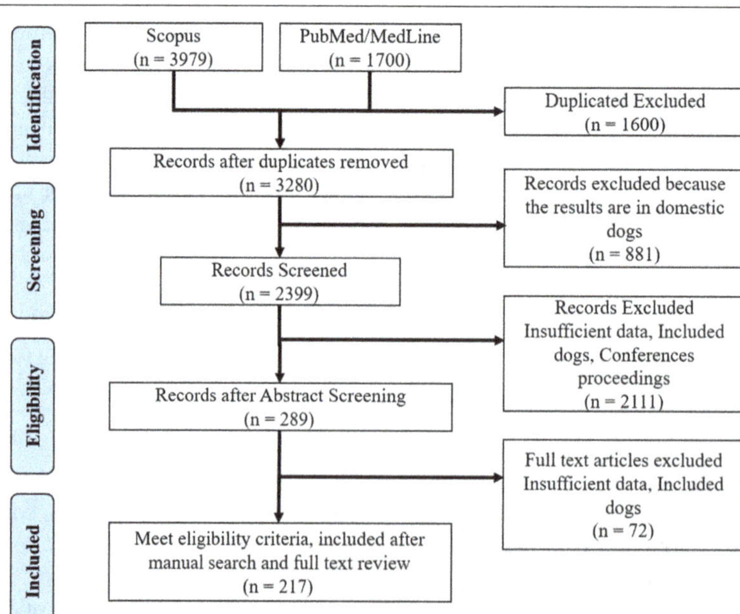

Fig. 1 Summary of study search and inclusion (PRISMA flow diagram)

Table 1 Orders, Families and Species that CDV can infect naturally and/or experimentally

Order	Family	Number of records (% of total)	Number of studies reporting clinical signs in infected animals (%)	Species
Carnivora	*Canidae*	82 (30.0)	27/82 (32.9)	*Canis adustus, Canis aureus, Canis latrans, Canis lupus, Canis lupus baileyi, Canis lupus dingo, Canis lupus signatus, Canis mesomelas, Cerdocyon thous, Chrysocyon brachyurus, Lycalopex culpaeus, Lycalopex griseus, Lycalopex gymnocercus, Lycalopex vetulus, Lycaon pictus, Nyctereutes procyonoides, Nyctereutes procyonoides viverrinus, Urocyon littoralis catalinae, Vulpes chama, Vulpes lagopus, Vulpes macrotis mutica, Vulpes velox, Vulpes vulpes, Vulpes zerda*
	Felidae	49 (17.9)	24/49 (48.9)	*Acinonyx jubatus, Felis lynx, Felis silvestris, Felis silvestris catus, Leopardus geoffroyi, Leopardus pardalis, Lynx Canadensis, Lynx lynx, Lynx pardinus, Lynx rufus, Panthera leo, Panthera leo persica, Panthera onca, Panthera pardus, Panthera pardus japonensis, Panthera tigris, Panthera tigris altaica, Panthera tigris tigris, Panthera uncial, Puma concolor*
	Mustelidae	43 (15.7)	23/43 (67.4)	*Enhydra lutris kenyoni, Galictis vittata, Galictis cuja, Gulo gulo, Lontra Canadensis, Martes foina, Martes martes, Martes melampus, Martes pennanti, Meles meles, Melogale moschata subauantiaca, Mustela erminea, Mustela itatsi sibirica, Mustela lutreola, Mustela nigripes, Mustela nivalis, Mustela putorius, Mustela putorius furo, Mustela vison, Neovison vison, Taxidea taxus*
	Procyonidae	18 (6.5)	9/18 (50.0)	*Nasua nasua, Potos flavus, Procyon lotor, Procyon pygmaeus*
	Ursidae	13 (4.7)	2/13 (15.3)	*Ailuropoda melanoleuca, Ursus americanus, Ursus americanus floridanus, Ursus arctos, Ursus arctos horribilis, Ursus arctos marsicanus, Ursus maritimus, Ursus thibetanus*
	Phocidae	12 (4.4)	8/12 (66.6)	*Halichoerus grypus, Hydrurga leptonyx, Lobodon carcinophagus, Phoca caspica, Phoca sibirica, Phoca vitulina, Pusa caspica*
	Viverridae	9 (3.2)	9/9 (100)	*Arctictis binturong, Gennetta gennetta, Paguma larvata, Paradoxurus hermaphroditus, Viverricula indica*
	Hyaenidae	6 (2.2)	2/6 (33.3)	*Crocuta crocuta, Hyaena hyaena*
	Ailuridae	3 (1.1)	2/3 (66.6)	*Ailurus fulgens*
	Mephitidae	2 (0.7)	2/2 (100)	*Mephitis mephitis*
	Odobenidae	1 (0.4)	0/1 (0)	*Odobenus rosmarus*
	Otariidae	1 (0.4)	1/1 (100)	*Zalophus californianus*
Rodentia	*Muridae*	10 (3.6)	10/10 (100)	*Mus musculus*[a]
	Cricetidae	7 (2.5)	7/7 (100)	*Mesocricetus auratus*[a]
	Sciuridae	1 (0.4)	1/1 (100)	*Marmota caudata*
	Caviidae	1 (0.4)	1/1 (100)	*Cavia porcellus*[a]
Primates	*Cercopithecidae*	7 (2.5)	7/7 (100)	*Macaca fascicularis, Macaca fuscata, Macaca mulatta*
	Cebidae	1 (0.4)	1/1 (100)	*Saimiri sciureus*[a]
Artiodactyla	*Suidae*	2 (0.7)	0/2 (0)	*Sus scrofa domestica*[a], *Sus scrofa*
	Tayassuidae	2 (0.7)	0/2 (0)	*Tayassu tajacu*
	Cervidae	1 (0.4)	0/1 (0)	*Cervus nippon*
Proboscidea	*Elephantidae*	1 (0.4)	0/1 (0)	*Elaphas maximus*
		272 (100)	141/272 (51.8)	

[a]Experimental infections reported

the Proboscidea Order. Within the Carnivora Order, the *Mustelidae* family, has the highest serological seropositivity with 41.1 %, followed by the *Hyaenidae* with 36.7 %, the *Canidae* family with 35.6 %, the *Phocidae* with 34.8 %, the *Felidae* family with 34,1 %, the *Procyonidae* family with 30.7 %, and the *Ursidae* families with 20.3 %. Table 2 summarizes the minimum and maximum prevalence values reported for different Families and Orders on each study. The full list of prevalence reported for each study can be found in Additional file 1: Table S1.

Table 2 Evidence of CDV infection through serological studies. The reported seroprevalence ranged widely across host species within different Orders

Order	Family	[a]Median Seropositivity %	Min % (Sp reported)	Max % (Sp reported)
Carnivora	*Canidae*	35.6	2.0 *Lycalopex culpaeus*	100 *Otocyon megalotis*
	Felidae	34.1	3.0 *Puma concolor*	100 *Panthera uncia*
	Mustelidae	41.1	5.0 *Mustela vison*	100 *Martes melampus*
	Procyonidae	30.7	4.0 *Procyon pygmaeus*	52.0 *Procyon lotor*
	Ursidae	20.3	3.0 *Ursus americanus*	100 *Ursus maritimus*
	Hyaenidae	36.7	5.0 *Crocuta crocuta*	47.0 *Crocuta crocuta*
	Phocidae	34.8	24.0 *Phoca vitulina*	47.5 *Pusa caspica*
	Mephitidae	65.5	-	-
	Ailuridae	100	-	-
	Odobenidae	14	-	-
Artiodactyla	*Suidae*	27	-	-
	Tayassuidae	58	-	-
	Cervidae	40	-	-
Proboscidea	*Elephantidae*	1.3	-	-

[a]Median value of all studies/populations in which CDV seropositivity had been detected in members of the same family. Sp: Specie reported

Worldwide distribution of CDV in non-dog hosts

CDV in non-dog hosts has been reported in almost all continents with the exception of Australasia and in 43 countries. Most reports of CDV came from the United States (24.3 %), followed by Japan, Canada and Germany (11.8, 5.5 and 5.1 % respectively). Table 3 presents the full list of countries in which CDV has been reported in non-dog hosts. It is interesting to note that CDV in non-dog hosts was reported in the same continents in which at least one CDV lineage has been identified (Fig. 2).

CDV is not a new disease in non-dog hosts

CDV has been reported as a pathogen of dogs for more than one century; however, early records of CDV as an

Table 3 Full list of countries in which CDV has been reported in non-dog hosts

Countries	Number of reports
USA	66
Japan	32
Canada	15
Germany	14
Kenya	10
Brazil – China – France	9
Italy – Russia – Spain – Switzerland – United Kingdom – Tanzania	8
Namibia	5
Austria – Norway – Portugal – Thailand	4
Taiwan – South Korea	3
Antarctica – Argentina – Azerbaijan – Bolivia – Chile –Israel – Poland – Zambia - Zimbabwe	2
Botswana – Denmark – Ethiopia – Finland – Guatemala - Greece – India – Luxembourg – Mexico - South Africa – Sudan – Sweden – Uganda	1

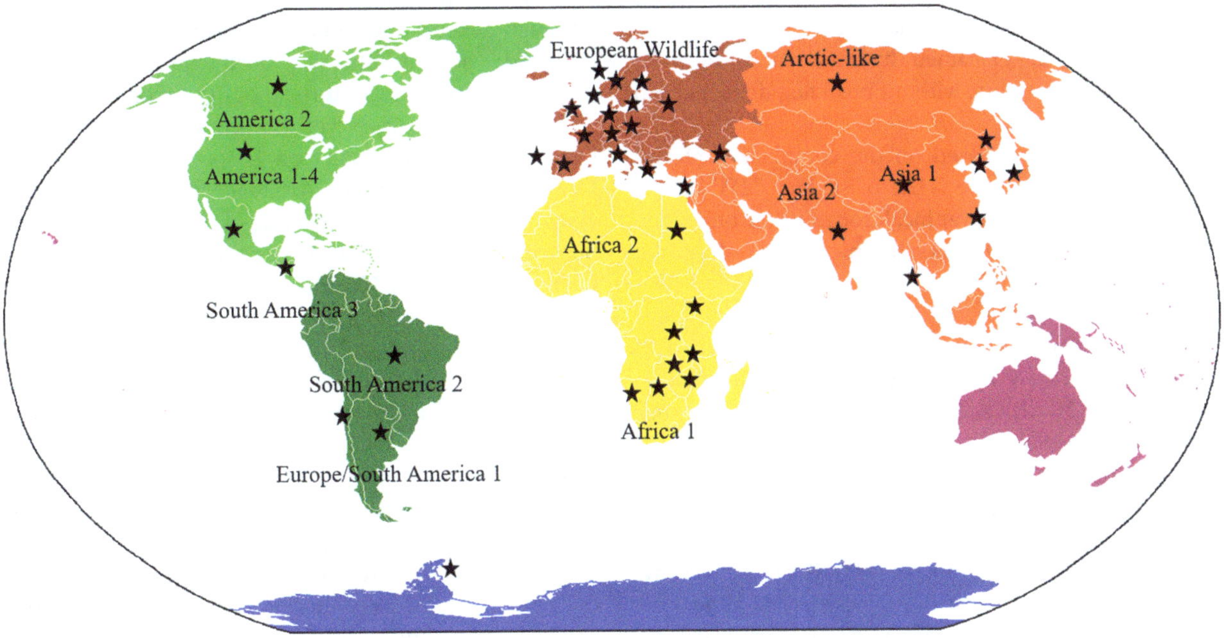

Fig. 2 Areas of the world where CDV has been reported in non-dog species. Different CDV lineages are highlighted. Stars denote punctual countries. Map was created using DIVA-GIS software. See text for references

infectious disease for non-dog species was not reported until 1937 during an outbreak among silver jackals (*Vulpes chama*) in a zoo of Johannesburg [17] and then in the Americas: the first case of CDV in the American badger (*Taxidea taxus)* occurred in Colorado in 1942 [18]. The first inter-Order report of CDV occurred in the early 60's with the development of the hamster model of infection; however due to the non-natural intracerebral inoculation route, this cannot be considered a natural infection. The first report of CDV in clinically healthy wildlife was found during serological evaluation of wolves of Northern Canada, published in 1974; however this report includes samples taken between 1960 and 1964 [19]. Naturally occurring CDV in captive non-human primates (Order Primates) were reported in a Japanese monkey (*Macaca fuscata*) in the late 80´s; however the review shows that experimental infection of macaques could be traced to 1977 [20]. In felids, in 1994, approximately one-third of the lion population in the Serengeti National Park died or disappeared during the best known outbreak of CDV [21]; however, naturally occurring CDV infection in felids was first reported in USA in samples from captive animals infected between 1991 and 1992. It is important to highlight that retrospective tissue evaluations confirmed the presence of CDV antigen in samples from lions and tigers since 1972 in clinical samples belonging to zoos from Switzerland [22].

Taking into account that within the last years, it was claimed that CDV has become an emerging disease for wild animals, we wanted to evaluate if there was a trend in publications of CDV infections in different orders throughout the years. Our results shows that although an exponential tendency is observed (data not shown) we did not find a statistical association between the year of publication and the number of papers reporting CDV infection in different non-dog hosts through the years ($R^2 = 0,6113$; $p > 0,05$). However, it is important to highlight that the lack of statistical association does not reduce the real threat of CDV for wildlife.

Discussion

CDV is a highly contagious virus that has been tagged as the cause of diseases of strong economic, conservation and public health concern. Although different reviews have been written on CDV infection in wildlife Carnivores [23, 24], this is the first systematic review that goes beyond and investigates the role of CDV in different Orders. Our results show that CDV should be evaluated as a possible cause of disease and extinction risk in different species even outside of the Carnivora Order; as has been proposed for the Tasmanian tiger (*Thylacinus cynocephalus,* Order: Dasyuromorphia, *Family Thylacinidae*) [4, 25, 26].

Importantly though, key role of CDV in Tasmanian tiger extinction could not be confirmed on this systematic review; on the contrary, it was shown that evidence is weak for critical reasons: Evidence for disease is anecdotal and was recorded long after the likely time of the epidemics [25], there is no evidence for CDV infection in any Order belonging to the Infraclass *Marsupialia,* instead evidence showed that there are only reports of CDV in canids in the Australasia continent [27] and finally, recent reports using mathematical modelling has shown that thylacine's extinction could be explained by interactions between known historical stressors, without involving diseases such as CDV [28].

Phylogenetic studies based on the complete sequence of the hemagglutinin gene (HA) of several CDV strains isolated in distinct geographical locations around the world have revealed a phylogeographic pattern of genetic diversity. According to this pattern, there are fourteen distinct lineages known as America 1 (that includes almost all commercially available vaccines), America 2, America 3, America 4, Arctic-like, Rockborn-like, Asia 1, Asia 2, Africa 1, Africa 2, European Wildlife, Europe/South America 1, South America 2 and South America 3 [29–34], although recently, a new criterion establishes that strains with <2 % divergence at the HA protein level within a single clade should be classified as subgenotypes [35]. According to the present systematic review, CDV in non-dog hosts has been reported in almost all continents and in 43 countries (Fig. 2); there were no recent reports of CDV infection in Australian non-dog hosts, although CDV is a well known dog pathogen in this continent [27] and it has been reported anecdotally that caused several epidemics in dingoes (*Canis lupus dingo*) in central Australia in the 60s and 70s [36]

It is important to highlight that most of CDV infections reported in this systematic review belong to CDV infections in captive wild animals. It is clear that conditions of captivity and the presence of different mammalian species in and around zoos increase the risk of CDV transmission among many animal species [37, 38]. However, the presence of CDV cases in non-dog hosts could be completely unrelated to the status of CDV in free-ranging wildlife in the same country.

Table 2 demonstrates serological evidence for CDV infection in a wide range of families and orders. Seropositivity was expressed as a median value of all studies within a given Family, however the aim of this review was to show the role of species susceptibility to CDV, independently of the serological technique used or whether the animals were free or captive; that is why these results cannot be taken as a reference of worldwide of CDV prevalence in a determined species and region.

Amino acid variations in the CDV HA protein that bind cellular SLAM (signaling lymphocyte activation molecule) are thought to be important in species specificity. In fact, two mutations have been reported in residues 530 (G/E to R/D/N) and 549 (Y to H) that are involved in the interspecies transmission from domestic dogs to non-dog hosts [4]. Although a recent analysis has suggested a bias with respect to the 530 substitutions [39], two recent papers performing molecular phylogeography of CDV has independently shown, that residues 530 and 549 of the CDV HA have been subject to positive selection [32] and that although genetic flow among domestic and wildlife hosts occurred, the domestic dog host appears as the most probable virus reservoir throughout the evolution [40].

Genbank contains as yet too few CDV sequences isolated from naturally infected hosts belonging to other Orders (such as Primates, Artiodactyla or Proboscidea) to allow evaluating the possible role of these amino acid residues in the ability of CDV to infect members of new Orders and Species. To date, analysis of these residues in pathogenic CDV strains from captive and wild felids has demonstrated no correlation between these amino acid residues and pathogenicity in these felids, and additional factors may be more important than the HA protein in determining the infectivity and pathogenicity of CDV strains in various hosts [7]. We believe that a similar evaluation must be performed for CDV, at the genomic and amino acid sequence levels, isolated from different wild species and from different Orders trying to rule out the role of those mutations in interspecies transmission and in virus pathogenesis in new hosts [41, 42]. Although some efforts have been made in this direction [39], we believe that these studies must include larger datasets not only with sequences belonging to the order Carnivora, but also sequences from other orders that have been shown can become infected.

There have been few reports of CDV in domestic cats (*Felis silvestris catus*). Serological evidences (ranging from 4.5 to 23 % prevalence) [43, 44] have shown that some domestic felines can be exposed to CDV and develop antibodies. In vivo, it was demonstrated years ago that CDV can infect domestic cats [45]; in vitro, it has been shown that feline cell lines can be efficiently infected with CDV [46] either expressing canine [47] or feline SLAM [48]. However, there is as yet no report of distemper disease in domestic cats, maybe due to a natural resistance to the disease by controlling viral replication at initial stages of the disease and only suffering a subclinical disease with a slight increase in temperature as have been experimentally reported [45].

Here we show that only 49 % of the reported records of CDV infections in the *Felidae* family presents clinical sign of the disease (Table 1); moreover, the median serological seropositivity for the *Felidae* Family was 34.1 % (ranging from 3 to 100 %). This serological confirmation of CDV in healthy animals means that some animals can acquire the infection, maybe suffer a subclinical and/or asymptomatic disease and remain seropositive for years.

Different outbreaks of CDV has been recorded in the Order Primates [49, 50], the same Order as *Homo sapiens sapiens*. As shown in Table 1, in Primates, all studies reporting evidence of CDV infection also reported clinical signs, independently of the Species involved. In all studies, the reasons for the epidemic remain unclear and the source of the infection is unknown, because there were no dogs or other animals in the farms. One possible source of infection is contact between the monkeys in the farm and local wild monkeys or the spillover of the virus from a stray animal carrying CDV that became adapted to the new host [50, 51].

Such outbreaks in non-human primates have highlighted the hypothesis of a possible zoonosis in the post-measles eradication era. Until now, due to the fact that SLAM and nectin-4 receptors present high homology in their amino acid sequences between monkeys and humans [49], different studies have shown that CDV could potentially become capable of using human cell receptors [52] indicating that CDV infection could be a potential future threat for humans [53], since it appears that so far, zoonotic CDV potential has been controlled by measles vaccination in humans [12].

Antigenic and/or genetic confirmation of CDV outbreaks in wildlife it is an important tool to evaluate the role of CDV as a threat for non-dog host populations, and it is an optimal approach to confirm interspecies viral transmission among wildlife and dogs that could be driven by the urban ecosystem [54]. Although our results show that 51.8 % of studies report clinical signs in such infected animals (Table 1), the mortality rate could be high for some species, as has been reported in some natural and/or experimentally infections [11, 55]. For example, in some families of the Carnivora Order (such as the *Viverridae*, *Mephitidae* and *Otariidae*), the most common outcome of CDV infection reported in the database was the death of infected animals [56–59]. However, these reports were based on case studies each involving a single individual, and to determine the impact of CDV in these important families, population-level studies would be needed [56–59].

This indicates a high risk of extinction for endangered populations as has been stated for the Amur tigers (*Panthera tigris altaica*) [6, 8] and for the Giant pandas (*Ailuropoda melanoleuca*) [38]; in these populations, recent outbreaks of CDV have become an important cofactor in reducing free-ranging wildlife animals and even in a few breeding centers, demonstrating the need to implement mitigation strategies such as vaccination or antivirals to reduce the heavy impact of this infection on those populations [7, 38, 53]

It is important to highlight that periodic serological and molecular evaluations, and an active search for possible wildlife reservoirs of CDV could help prevent outbreaks of diseases in other susceptible wildlife [60], and that domestic dogs, mesocarnivores or peridomestic wild animals (not only carnivores) should be taken into account as possible sources of CDV infections in wildlife [7, 38, 61]. The wide variety of possible hosts for CDV that we were able to find, agrees with recent papers showing that domestic dogs are not the only potential reservoir of CDV. As has been shown in the case of CDV infection in lions in the Serengeti ecosystem, the virus can circulate in lions even when levels of infection are extremely low and asynchronous to infections found in domestic dogs [10], supporting the hypothesis that CDV infection is likely to persist involving the wider domestic dog population beyond the Serengeti ecosystem and other wildlife species.

The highly common presence of CDV seropositive healthy animals (Table 2) is an indication of viral circulation, infection and recovery of animals belonging to different Orders. We believe that those species may act as wildlife reservoirs and that in some cases, some interconnected populations may function as a "metareservoir" consisting of multiple interconnected populations acting as one single revervoir in nature, on which CDV might be maintained through interaction of multiple subpopulations, each experiencing intermittent but non-simultaneous CDV epizootics [62, 63].

The finding of evidence of CDV infection in naturally infected Orders (Tables 1 and 2) such as Artiodactyla (Family Tayassuidae) [64], Rodentia (Family Sciuridae) [65] and Proboscidea (Family Elephantidae) [66] suggests that further serological and molecular CDV evaluation is warranted to investigate patterns of infection, disease risk and sources of infection in both free-ranging and captive populations. For example, the presence of CDV antibodies in Asian elephants (*Elephas maximus*) in Thailand was not associated with the presence of domestic dogs nor with clinical signs of disease [66], although there is currently no evidence that the Asian elephant is a competent host for virus replication or that CDV may cause disease in this endangered species [67].

Serological data have potential value for estimating pathogen force of infection and transmission rates, and have been used in dynamic disease models [68], as demonstrated by studies of the dynamics of cross-species transmission between domestic dogs and lions in the Serengeti ecosystem [10]. A decrease in seroprevalence could also signal a loss of herd immunity which may have value in assessing risks of potential outbreaks and/or need for implementation of preventive measures [10, 69].

Although the Ferret (*Mustela putorius furo*) has served as the most important animal model to study CDV pathogenesis and transmission [70], there have been many CDV models of infection. For instance as can be seen in Table 1, in all orders on which experimental CDV infection have been performed, natural infection has been shown in at least one other Family of the same Order. Hence, although experimental infection is carried out by an unnatural route, these studies demonstrate the potential for CDV to infect members of the Order. For example, experimental infections have been demonstrated in domestic suids (*Sus scrofa domestica*) with serological evidence for endemic infection in wild populations, as has been reported for the collared peccary (*Tayassu tajacu*) [64] Similarly, experimental infections have been demonstrated in several species of the Order Rodentia, and molecular detection of CDV with clinical signs of disease recorded in captive marmot populations (*Marmota caudate*) [65].

Finally, it is well known that jumps in species barriers is how a pathogen can find novel hosts; it requires a complex process of invasion of and adaptation to a new niche [71]. The new host may present challenges at the level of virus entry into cells, virus replication or transmission from the host to finally cause diseases, outbreaks and pandemics [72]. CDV is not just able to infect multiples species; indeed, the present analysis shows that CDV can infect five different Orders. As far as is known, only a few critically emerging and re-emerging viruses such as the Equid herpesvirus 9 causing fatal encephalitis [73], the West Nile Virus [74] or the Influenza A virus [75] have been reported to infect five or more different Orders.

Although no statistical association was found between the number of articles reporting CDV infection in non-dog host and year of publication, CDV is now being reported more frequently in wild animal populations [8, 10]. However, it cannot be ruled out that this increasing tendency could be biased by the increasing number of international journals indexed in the last years in those databases and the increasing number of papers published in this research area [76, 77].

Strengths and limitations of this review

The major strengths of this systematic review are the characteristics of the selected studies and the wide time window examined. Furthermore, this systematic review allowed us to propose a hypothesis that will be useful to implement future epidemiological research trying to understand the role of mesocarnivores and peridomestic wild animals in the CDV transmission cycle and the role of point mutations in the CDV HA protein in cross species CDV infection.

All of the selected studies were relevant to CDV in non-dog hosts; however, despite of the strength of the search, due to the impossibility to discard the word "canine" from the search keywords, there are some relevant information that could be dismissed because the main focus of the abstract and the title of the paper concerned dogs. Other important limitations were the role of serological techniques used in the different papers reviewed; over the years, authors have used different serological techniques to assess the presence of anti-CDV antibodies in different animal species. Therefore it was not possible to consolidate data related to specific antibody titers, sensitivity or specificity of the techniques used in the papers evaluated.

It is important to note that although the virus neutralization test was shown to be the standard assay used to detect CDV-specific antibodies in serum of different species (75.4 % of records), it requires a large volume of serum, special facilities (biosafety level-2) and a high level of technical skill for the correct manipulation of live virus and cells. Currently, the ELISA test has become a very useful technique to detect anti-CDV antibodies; besides, it does not use live CDV, it requires only a small amount of sample, the procedure to detect antibodies against CDV is simple in many animal species and in many different part of the world that do not have special biosafety laboratories. Also, the ELISA test has shown high specificity and sensitivity in comparison to the virus neutralization test by using anti-dog IgG or IgM antibody as a secondary antibody [78] or by using protein A/G as a secondary antibody to detect the CDV antibody in various mammalian species [79].

Furthermore, the exclusion of studies of CDV vaccine evaluations in wildlife is another limitation of this review; however the aim of the systematic review was focused only on non-vaccinated animals in order to highlight the role of CDV as an important virus for different Species/ Orders. Future reviews are being prepared to clarify the role and efficiency of CDV vaccination in wild, captive and free ranging animals.

Finally, database selection could be introducing some bias in the selection of the studies [80]; however, such bias is accepted due to the importance and worldwide relevance of the selected databases.

Conclusion

The present data support the hypothesis that CDV presents a high potential as emerging virus for wild species as for domestic animals. Also CDV is a worldwide threat for a wider range of host species than is generally recognized and that there is a chance for a possible adaptation of CDV to humans after cessation of measles vaccination as has been suggested by others [12]. The present data also highlights the possible role of CDV as a potential disease threat to a wide range of endangered wild free-ranging and captive species.

Abbreviations

CDV: canine distemper virus; ELISA: enzyme-linked immuno sorbent assay; HA: hemagglutinin gene; PRISMA: preferred reporting items for systematic reviews and meta-analyses; rt-PCR: reverse transcription polymerase chain reaction; SLAM: signaling lymphocyte activation molecule.

Competing interests

The authors declare that they have no competing interests.

Authors' contributions

JRS conceived the study; MMG and JRS were involved in all other aspects of the study: data collection, data analysis, drafting and editing the paper. Both authors read and approved the final manuscript.

Acknowledgement

The authors thank Anne-Lise Haenni for revision of the English and critical reading of the manuscript. This work was financially supported by the Departamento Administrativo de Ciencia, Tecnología e Innovación – COLCIENCIAS Grant No. 123171249669, and partially by CONADI - Universidad Cooperativa de Colombia.

References

1. Carré H. Sur la maladie des jeunes chiens. C R Acad Sci. 1905;140(689–690): 1489–91.
2. Patel JR, Heldens JG, Bakonyi T, Rusvai M. Important mammalian veterinary viral immunodiseases and their control. Vaccine. 2012;30(10):1767–81.
3. Barret T. Rinder pest and distemper viruses. In: Mahy BVRM, editor. Desk encyclopedia of animal and bacterial virology. Elsevier: San Diego; 2010. p. 221–31.
4. McCarthy AJ, Shaw MA, Goodman SJ. Pathogen evolution and disease emergence in carnivores. Proc Biol Sci Royal Soc. 2007;274(1629):3165–74.
5. Martella V, Bianchi A, Bertoletti I, Pedrotti L, Gugiatti A, Catella A, Cordioli P, Lucente MS, Elia G, Buonavoglia C. Canine distemper epizootic among red foxes, Italy, 2009. Emerg Infect Dis. 2010;16(12):2007.
6. Gilbert M, Miquelle DG, Goodrich JM, Reeve R, Cleaveland S, Matthews L, Joly DO. Estimating the potential impact of canine distemper virus on the Amur tiger population (Panthera tigris altaica) in Russia. PLoS One. 2014; 9(10):e110811.
7. Terio KA, Craft ME. Canine distemper virus (CDV) in another big cat: should CDV be renamed carnivore distemper virus? mBio. 2013;4(5):e00702–00713.
8. Seimon TA, Miquelle DG, Chang TY, Newton AL, Korotkova I, Ivanchuk G, Lyubchenko E, Tupikov A, Slabe E, McAloose D.Canine distemper virus: an emerging disease in wild endangered Amur tigers (Panthera tigris altaica). mBio 2013, 4(4).MBio. pii: e00410-13.
9. Müller A, Silva E, Santos N, Thompson G. Domestic dog origin of canine distemper virus in free-ranging wolves in Portugal as revealed by hemagglutinin gene characterization. J Wildl Dis. 2011;47(3):725–9.
10. Viana M, Cleaveland S, Matthiopoulos J, Halliday J, Packer C, Craft ME, Hampson K, Czupryna A, Dobson AP, Dubovi EJ, et al. Dynamics of a morbillivirus at the domestic-wildlife interface: Canine distemper virus in domestic dogs and lions. Proc Natl Acad Sci U S A. 2015;112(5):1464–9.
11. Kapil S, Yeary TJ. Canine distemper spillover in domestic dogs from urban wildlife. Vet Clin North Am Small Anim Pract. 2011;41(6):1069–86.
12. de Vries RD, Ludlow M, Verburgh RJ, van Amerongen G, Yuksel S, Nguyen DT, McQuaid S, Osterhaus AD, Duprex WP, de Swart RL. Measles vaccination of nonhuman primates provides partial protection against infection with canine distemper virus. J Virol. 2014;88(8):4423–33.
13. Moher D, Liberati A, Tetzlaff J, Altman DG, Group P. Preferred reporting items for systematic reviews and meta-analyses: the PRISMA statement. BMJ. 2009;339:b2535.
14. Moher D, Shamseer L, Clarke M, Ghersi D, Liberati A, Petticrew M, Shekelle P, Stewart LA, Group P-P. Preferred reporting items for systematic review and meta-analysis protocols (PRISMA-P) 2015 statement. Syst Rev. 2015;4(1):1.
15. Jacka B, Lamoury F, Simmonds P, Dore GJ, Grebely J, Applegate T. Sequencing of the Hepatitis C Virus: A Systematic Review. PLoS One. 2013;8(6):e67073.
16. Wilson DE, Mittermeier RA. Handbook of the Mammals of the World, vol. Volume 1: Carnivora.; 2009.
17. Armstrong WH, Anthony CH. An epizootic of canine distemper in a zoological park. Cornell Vet. 1942;32(4):286–8.
18. Armstrong WH. Canine distemper in the American badger. Cornell Vet. 1942;32(4):447.
19. Choquette LP, Kuyt E. Serological indication of canine distemper and of infectious canine hepatitis in wolves (Canis lupus L.) in northern Canada. J Wildl Dis. 1974;10(4):321–4.
20. Yamanouchi K, Yoshikawa Y, Sato TA, Katow S, Kobune F, Kobune K, Uchida N, Shishido A. Encephalomyelitis induced by canine distemper virus in non-human primates. Jpn J Med Sci Biols. 1977;30(5):241–57.
21. Roelke-Parker ME, Munson L, Packer C, Kock R, Cleaveland S, Carpenter M, O'Brien SJ, Pospischil A, Hofmann-Lehmann R, Lutz H, et al. A canine distemper virus epidemic in Serengeti lions (Panthera leo). Nature. 1996;379(6564):441–5.
22. Myers DL, Zurbriggen A, Lutz H, Pospischil A. Distemper: not a new disease in lions and tigers. Clin Diagn Lab Immunol. 1997;4(2):180–4.
23. Deem SL, Spelman LH, Yates RA, Montali RJ. Canine distemper in terrestrial carnivores: a review. J Zoo Wildl Med. 2000;31(4):441–51.
24. Harder TC, Osterhaus AD. Canine distemper virus–a morbillivirus in search of new hosts?. Trends Microbiol. 1997;5(3):120–124.
25. Guiler ER. The former distribution and decline of the thylacine. Aust J Sci. 1961;23(7):207–10.
26. Paddle R. The last Tasmanian tiger: the history and extinction of the thylacine. Cambridge: Cambridge University Press; 2002.
27. Norris JM, Krockenberger MB, Baird AA, Knudsen G. Canine distemper: re-emergence of an old enemy. Aust Vet J. 2006;84(10):362–3.
28. Prowse TA, Johnson CN, Lacy RC, Bradshaw CJ, Pollak JP, Watts MJ, Brook BW. No need for disease: testing extinction hypotheses for the thylacine using multi-species metamodels. J Anim Ecol. 2013;82(2):355–64.
29. Espinal MA, Diaz FJ, Ruiz-Saenz J. Phylogenetic evidence of a new canine distemper virus lineage among domestic dogs in Colombia, South America. Vet Microbiol. 2014;172(1-2):168–76.
30. Panzera Y, Calderón MG, Sarute N, Guasco S, Cardeillac A, Bonilla B, Hernández M, Francia L, Bedó G, La Torre J. Evidence of two co-circulating genetic lineages of canine distemper virus in South America. Virus Res. 2012;163(1):401–4.
31. Woma TY, van Vuuren M, Bosman A-M, Quan M, Oosthuizen M. Phylogenetic analysis of the haemagglutinin gene of current wild-type canine distemper viruses from South Africa: lineage Africa. Vet Microbiol. 2010;143(2):126–32.
32. Ke GM, Ho CH, Chiang MJ, Sanno-Duanda B, Chung CS, Lin MY, Shi YY, Yang MH, Tyan YC, Liao PC, et al. Phylodynamic analysis of the canine distemper virus hemagglutinin gene. BMC Vet Res. 2015;11:164.
33. Riley MC, Wilkes RP. Sequencing of emerging canine distemper virus strain reveals new distinct genetic lineage in the United States associated with disease in wildlife and domestic canine populations. Virol J. 2015;12:219.
34. Wilkes RP, Sanchez E, Riley MC, Kennedy MA. Real-time reverse transcription polymerase chain reaction method for detection of Canine distemper virus modified live vaccine shedding for differentiation from infection with wild-type strains. J Vet Diagn Investig. 2014;26(1):27–34.
35. Budaszewski R, Pinto LD, Weber MN, Caldart ET, Alves CDBT, Martella V, Ikuta N, Lunge VR, Canal CW. Genotyping of canine distemper virus strains circulating in Brazil from 2008 to 2012. Virus Res. 2014;180:76–83.
36. Corbett L. The Dingo in Australia and Asia. 2nd ed. Adelaide: JB Books; 2001.
37. Nagao Y, Nishio Y, Shiomoda H, Tamaru S, Shimojima M, Goto M, Une Y, Sato A, Ikebe Y, Maeda K. An outbreak of canine distemper virus in tigers (Panthera tigris): possible transmission from wild animals to zoo animals. J Vet Med Sci. 2012;74(6):699–705.
38. Hvistendahl M. Endangered species. Captive pandas succumb to killer virus. Science. 2015;347(6223):700–1.
39. Nikolin VM, Wibbelt G, Michler FU, Wolf P, East ML. Susceptibility of carnivore hosts to strains of canine distemper virus from distinct genetic lineages. Vet Microbiol. 2012;156(1-2):45–53.
40. Panzera Y, Sarute N, Iraola G, Hernandez M, Perez R. Molecular phylogeography of canine distemper virus: Geographic origin and global spreading. Mol Phylogenet Evol. 2015;92:147–54.
41. Kameo Y, Nagao Y, Nishio Y, Shimoda H, Nakano H, Suzuki K, Une Y, Sato H, Shimojima M, Maeda K. Epizootic canine distemper virus infection among wild mammals. Vet Microbiol. 2012;154(3):222–9.
42. Zhao J, Zhang H, Bai X, Martella V, Hu B, Sun Y, Zhu C, Zhang L, Liu H, Xu S. Emergence of canine distemper virus strains with two amino acid substitutions in the haemagglutinin protein, detected from vaccinated carnivores in North-Eastern China in 2012–2013. Vet J. 2014;200(1):191–4.
43. Millan J, Candela MG, Palomares F, Cubero MJ, Rodriguez A, Barral M, de la Fuente J, Almeria S, Leon-Vizcaino L. Disease threats to the endangered Iberian lynx (Lynx pardinus). Vet J. 2009;182(1):114–24.
44. Lickey AL, Kennedy M, Patton S, Ramsay EC. Serologic survey of domestic felids in the Peten region of Guatemala. J Zoo Wildl Med. 2005;36(1):121–3.
45. Gaskin J. Canine distemper virus in domesticated cats and pigs. Adv Enzymol Relat Areas Mol Biol. 1974;40:803.
46. Fujita K, Miura R, Yoneda M, Shimizu F, Sato H, Muto Y, Endo Y, Tsukiyama-Kohara K, Kai C. Host range and receptor utilization of

canine distemper virus analyzed by recombinant viruses: Involvement of heparin-like molecule in CDV infection. Virology. 2007;359(2):324–35.
47. Nakano H, Kameo Y, Andoh K, Ohno Y, Mochizuki M, Maeda K. Establishment of canine and feline cells expressing canine signaling lymphocyte activation molecule for canine distemper virus study. Vet Microbiol. 2009;133(1-2):179–83.
48. Hara Y, Suzuki J, Noguchi K, Terada Y, Shimoda H, Mizuno T, Maeda K. Function of feline signaling lymphocyte activation molecule as a receptor of canine distemper virus. J Vet Med Sci. 2013;75(8):1085–9.
49. Sakai K, Nagata N, Ami Y, Seki F, Suzaki Y, Iwata-Yoshikawa N, Suzuki T, Fukushi S, Mizutani T, Yoshikawa T. Lethal canine distemper virus outbreak in cynomolgus monkeys in Japan in 2008. J Virol. 2013;87(2):1105–14.
50. Sun Z, Li A, Ye H, Shi Y, Hu Z, Zeng L. Natural infection with canine distemper virus in hand-feeding Rhesus monkeys in China. Vet Microbiol. 2010;141(3):374–8.
51. Qiu W, Zheng Y, Zhang S, Fan Q, Liu H, Zhang F, Wang W, Liao G, Hu R. Canine distemper outbreak in rhesus monkeys, China. Emerg Infect Dis. 2011;17(8):1541–3.
52. Sakai K, Yoshikawa T, Seki F, Fukushi S, Tahara M, Nagata N, Ami Y, Mizutani T, Kurane I, Yamaguchi R. Canine distemper virus associated with a lethal outbreak in monkeys can readily adapt to use human receptors. J Virol. 2013;87(12):7170–5.
53. de Vries RD, Duprex WP, de Swart RL. Morbillivirus Infections: An Introduction. Viruses. 2015;7(2):699–706.
54. Rentería-Solís Z, Förster C, Aue A, Wittstatt U, Wibbelt G, König M. Canine distemper outbreak in raccoons suggests pathogen interspecies transmission amongst alien and native carnivores in urban areas from Germany. Vet Microbiol. 2014;174(1):50–9.
55. Zhao J, Shi N, Sun Y, Martella V, Nikolin V, Zhu C, Zhang H, Hu B, Bai X, Yan X. Pathogenesis of canine distemper virus in experimentally infected raccoon dogs, foxes, and minks. Antivir Res. 2015;122:1–11.
56. Barrett T, Wohlsein P, Bidewell CA, Rowell SF. Canine distemper virus in a Californian sea lion (Zalophus californianus). Vet Rec. 2004;154(11):334–6.
57. Dyer NW, Schamber GJ. Pneumocystosis associated with canine distemper virus infection in a mink. Can Vet J. 1999;40(8):577–8.
58. Lopez-Pena M, Vazquez S, Aleman N, Lopez-Beceiro A, Munoz F, Pereira JL, Nieto JM. Canine distemper in a genet (Gennetta gennetta), associated with endogenous lipid pneumonia. J Comp Pathol. 2001;124(2-3):207–11.
59. Hur K, Bae JS, Choi JH, Kim JH, Kwon SW, Lee KW, Lee KW, Kim DY. Canine distemper virus infection in binturongs (Arctictis binturong). J Comp Pathol. 1999;121(3):295–9.
60. Trebbien R, Chriel M, Struve T, Hjulsager CK, Larsen G, Larsen LE. Wildlife reservoirs of canine distemper virus resulted in a major outbreak in Danish farmed mink (Neovison vison). PLoS One. 2014;9(1):e85598.
61. Cleaveland S, Appel MG, Chalmers WS, Chillingworth C, Kaare M, Dye C. Serological and demographic evidence for domestic dogs as a source of canine distemper virus infection for Serengeti wildlife. Vet Microbiol. 2000; 72(3-4):217–27.
62. Prager K, Mazet JA, Dubovi EJ, Frank LG, Munson L, Wagner AP, Woodroffe R. Rabies virus and canine distemper virus in wild and domestic carnivores in Northern Kenya: are domestic dogs the reservoir? EcoHealth. 2012;9(4):483–98.
63. Begon M, Bowers RG, Kadianakis N, Hodgkinson DE. Disease and community structure: the importance of host self-regulation in a host-host-pathogen model. Am Naturalist. 1992;139(6):1131–1150.
64. Noon TH, Heffelfinger JR, Olding RJ, Wesche SL, Reggiardo C. Serologic survey for antibodies to canine distemper virus in collared peccary (Tayassu tajacu) populations in Arizona. J Wildl Dis. 2003;39(1):221–3.
65. Origgi FC, Sattler U, Pilo P, Waldvogel AS. Fatal combined infection with canine distemper virus and orthopoxvirus in a group of Asian marmots (Marmota caudata). Vet Pathol. 2013;50(5):914–20.
66. Oni O, Wajjwalku W, Boodde O, Chumsing W. Canine distemper virus antibodies in the Asian elephant (Elaphas maximus). Vet Rec. 2006;159(13):420–1.
67. Elephas maximus. The IUCN Red List of Threatened Species. Version 2014.3. [www.iucnredlist.org]
68. Gilbert AT, Fooks AR, Hayman DT, Horton DL, Müller T, Plowright R, Peel AJ, Bowen R, Wood JL, Mills J. Deciphering serology to understand the ecology of infectious diseases in wildlife. EcoHealth. 2013;10(3):298–313.
69. Di Sabatino D, Savini G, Lorusso A. Canine distemper and endangered wildlife: Is it time for mandatory vaccination of dogs? Vaccine. 2015;33(48):6519.
70. Ludlow M, Rennick LJ, Nambulli S, de Swart RL, Duprex WP. Using the ferret model to study morbillivirus entry, spread, transmission and cross-species infection. Curr Opinion Virol. 2014;4:15–23.
71. Ruiz-Saenz J, Villamil-Jimenez LC. Emerging diseases and species barrier: the risk of equine herpesvirus 9. Revista de salud publica. 2008;10(5):840–7.
72. Ohshima K, Akaishi S, Kajiyama H, Koga R, Gibbs AJ. Evolutionary trajectory of turnip mosaic virus populations adapting to a new host. J Gen Virol. 2010;91(Pt 3):788–801.
73. Greenwood AD, Tsangaras K, Ho SY, Szentiks CA, Nikolin VM, Ma G, Damiani A, East ML, Lawrenz A, Hofer H, et al. A potentially fatal mix of herpes in zoos. Curr Biol. 2012;22(18):1727–31.
74. Martin-Acebes MA, Saiz JC. West Nile virus: A re-emerging pathogen revisited. World J Virol. 2012;1(2):51–70.
75. Parrish CR, Murcia PR, Holmes EC. Influenza virus reservoirs and intermediate hosts: dogs, horses, and new possibilities for influenza virus exposure of humans. J Virol. 2015;89(6):2990–4.
76. Sayers EW, Barrett T, Benson DA, Bolton E, Bryant SH, Canese K, Chetvernin V, Church DM, Dicuccio M, Federhen S, et al. Database resources of the National Center for Biotechnology Information. Nucleic Acids Res. 2012; 40(Database issue):D13–25.
77. Coordinators NR. Database resources of the National Center for Biotechnology Information. Nucleic Acids Res. 2015;43(Database issue):D6–D17.
78. Waner T, Mazar S, Keren-Kornblatt E. Application of a dot enzyme-linked immunosorbent assay for evaluation of the immune status to canine parvovirus and distemper virus in adult dogs before revaccination. J Vet Diagn Invest. 2006;18(3):267–70.
79. Suzuki J, Nishio Y, Kameo Y, Terada Y, Kuwata R, Shimoda H, Suzuki K, Maeda K. Canine distemper virus infection among wildlife before and after the epidemic. J Vet Med Sci. 2015;77(11):1457–63.
80. Young JM, Solomon MJ. How to critically appraise an article. Nat Clin Pract Gastroenterol Hepatol. 2009;6(2):82–91.

17

Laboratory investigation into the role of largemouth bass virus (Ranavirus, Iridoviridae) in smallmouth bass mortality events in Pennsylvania rivers

Traimat Boonthai[1], Thomas P. Loch[1], Coja J. Yamashita[2], Geoffrey D. Smith[3], Andrew D. Winters[1,6], Matti Kiupel[1,4], Travis O. Brenden[5] and Mohamed Faisal[1,4,5*]

Abstract

Background: Mortality episodes have affected young-of-year smallmouth bass (*Micropterus dolomieu*) in several river systems in Pennsylvania since 2005. A series of laboratory experiments were performed to determine the potential role of largemouth bass virus (*Ranavirus*, Iridoviridae) in causing these events.

Results: Juvenile smallmouth bass experimentally infected with the largemouth bass virus exhibited internal and external clinical signs and mortality consistent with those observed during die-offs. Microscopically, infected fish developed multifocal necrosis in the mesenteric fat, liver, spleen and kidneys. Fish challenged by immersion also developed severe ulcerative dermatitis and necrotizing myositis and rarely panuveitis and keratitis. Largemouth bass virus-challenged smallmouth bass experienced greater mortality at 28 °C than at 23 or 11 °C. Co-infection with *Flavobacterium columnare* at 28 °C resulted in significant increase in mortality of smallmouth bass previously infected with largemouth bass virus. *Aeromonas salmonicida* seems to be very pathogenic to fish at water temperatures < 23 °C. While co-infection of smallmouth bass by both *A. salmonicida* and largemouth bass virus can be devastating to juvenile smallmouth bass, the optimal temperatures of each pathogen are 7–10 °C apart, making their synergistic effects highly unlikely under field conditions.

Conclusions: The sum of our data generated in this study suggests that largemouth bass virus can be the causative agent of young-of-year smallmouth bass mortality episodes observed at relatively high water temperature.

Keywords: Largemouth bass virus, Smallmouth bass, *Flavobacterium columnare, Aeromonas salmonicida*, Susquehanna River basin, Dermal lesions

Background

Since 2005, mortality episodes of young of the year (YOY) smallmouth bass (*Micropterus dolomieu*; SMB) have been consistently reported from a number of river systems in Pennsylvania, including the Susquehanna, Juniata, and Allegheny Rivers. These mortality events have been more persistent and severe in the Susquehanna and Juniata River systems, occurring annually to varying degrees, than in the Allegheny and other drainages. These SMB die-offs have created considerable concerns among the sport-fishing industry, as well as in state and federal agencies, as decreases in relative abundance of YOY and adult SMB and shifts in size structure have concurrently been noticed [1]. Affected SMB exhibited exophthalmia, dermal lesions (e.g., fin erosions and rounded, shallow ulcers), and organomegaly. The prevalence of moribund fish varied both spatially and temporally and was most prevalent during years with high water temperatures [1]. Several fish-pathogenic bacteria and parasites were reported from fish collected during the course of mortality episode

* Correspondence: faisal@cvm.msu.edu
[1]Department of Pathobiology and Diagnostic Investigation, College of Veterinary Medicine, Michigan State University, 1129 Farm Lane, Room 174, East Lansing, MI 48824, USA
[4]Comparative Medicine and Integrative Biology Program, College of Veterinary Medicine, Michigan State University, East Lansing, MI 48824, USA
Full list of author information is available at the end of the article

examinations, such as *Aeromonas* spp., *Shewanella putrefaciens, Flavobacterium columnare, Pseudomonas aeruginosa*, myxozoa (e.g., *Myxobolus inornatus*) and trematodes [1–4]. Largemouth bass virus (LMBV, genus *Ranavirus*, Family Iridoviridae) has also been isolated from both apparently healthy and moribund SMB during fish-kill episodes in several river watersheds in Pennsylvania (4, https://www.fws.gov/wildfishsurvey/) and the Chesapeake Bay watershed [5]. The contributions of each of these pathogens (single or combined) in causing these recurrent SMB kills have not been thoroughly investigated under controlled laboratory conditions.

Most of the existing knowledge on LMBV is derived from surveys and experiments performed on largemouth bass (*Micropterus salmoides*; LMB), although this virus has been isolated from other centrarchid species. Typically, LMBV-infected LMB exhibit lethargy, external and internal hemorrhages, and organomegaly [6, 7]. However, Deng et al. [8] described an outbreak in LMB in China that was associated with the formation of widespread ulcerative lesions. The causative agent was a ranavirus named largemouth bass ulcerative syndrome virus (LBUSV) by Deng et al. [8]. Upon phylogenetic analysis of LBUSV major capsid protein gene (MCP), it proved to be a ranavirus sharing 100% similarity to the Doctor Fish Virus (DFV) and 98% similarity to LMBV. Most recently, another ranavirus, named LMBV-like, was detected in farmed barcoo grunter (*Scrotum barcoo*) in Thailand during outbreaks that were associated with ulcerative lesions [9]. The MCP gene of Thai ranavirus shared 100% similarity to the Chinese LBUSV, clustered in the same clade with high bootstrap support, and shared 99.3–99.5% similarity to LMBV and DFV.

This study was designed to investigate the role LMBV may play in causing the recurrent YOY SMB mortality episodes. First, we screened five LMBV isolates that were associated with YOY SMB mortality episodes for their pathogenicity to SMB using IP and immersion infection methods. Second, we described gross clinical signs and histopathological alterations of LMBV-experimentally infected fish. Last, we determined the role that two other fish-pathogenic bacteria may play in exacerbating LMBV infection. The series of experiments described herein unravel some of the potential mechanisms leading to the YOY SMB mortality episodes noticed in several watersheds in Pennsylvania.

Methods

Fish

All protocols described in this study involving the use of live fish were approved by the Michigan State University (MSU) Institutional Animal Care and Use Committee (IACUC AUF # 08/15–129-00). Health-certified YOY SMB (fork length: 9.7 ± SD 2.1 cm; weight: 11.2 ± SD 6.3 g) were obtained from Zetts Fish Farm and Hatchery (Drifting, PA), and the New Jersey Department of Environmental Protection Division of Fish and Wildlife. Upon arrival at the MSU-Research Containment Facility, fish were allowed to acclimate to laboratory conditions in 720-L rectangular fiberglass tanks at a water temperature of 22 ± 1 °C for 4 weeks. Fish were fed commercial pellets (Classic Fry – 1.5 mm, Skretting Co., Tooele, UT) and tanks were cleaned daily. A subsample of 10 SMB was screened for the presence of LMBV and other viruses in their visceral organs using the fathead minnow (FHM) cell line as detailed below.

Cell lines and LMBV propagation

FHM cell line was grown and maintained in 150 cm^2 tissue culture flasks (Corning, Inc., Corning, NY) at 25 °C using growth formulation of Hanks' balanced salts minimum essential medium (Invitrogen, Carlsbad, CA) supplemented with 10% fetal bovine serum (GemCell, West Sacramento, CA), 2.0 mM L-glutamine (Invitrogen), penicillin (100 U/ml)/streptomycin (100 μg/ml; Gibco, Grand Island, NY) and amphotericin B (2.5 μg/ml; BioWhittaker, Walkersville, MD).

In this study, we used five LMBV isolates that were isolated from YOY SMB during mortality episodes in the Susquehanna and Allegheny (the principal tributary of the Ohio River) river systems that were designated 13–295 Susquehanna and 15–232 Susquehanna (both isolated from SMB from the lower Susquehanna River sub-basin), 13–286 Juniata and 14–204 Pine Creek (a creek in the West Susquehanna River sub-basin), and 12–342 Allegheny (Fig. 1). These LMBV isolates were originally isolated by the U.S. Fish and Wildlife Northeast Fishery Center, Lamar, PA and Pennsylvania State Animal Health Diagnostic Laboratory, State College, PA and were made available for this study by the Pennsylvania Fish and Boat Commission. Virus stocks were produced using FHM cells grown in 150 cm^2 tissue culture flasks and incubated at 28 °C. To determine the virus concentration, a median tissue culture infectious dose ($TCID_{50}$) was determined using FHM cells and calculations of virus titers were done as described by Reed and Muench [10]. The virus stocks were aliquoted in cryogenic vials (Corning, Inc.) and stored at − 80 °C until used.

Experimental infection of SMB by Pennsylvania LMBV isolates

Two studies were performed. The first experiment was to determine if the five LMBV isolates could induce clinical signs and histopathological changes in juvenile SMB. Twenty groups of fish (n = 5/tank/dose) were housed in 70-L static circular tanks equipped with air-driven sponge filters (Hydro–Sponge III Filter, Aquarium Technologies, Decatur, GA). Water temperature was elevated by 2 °C/day

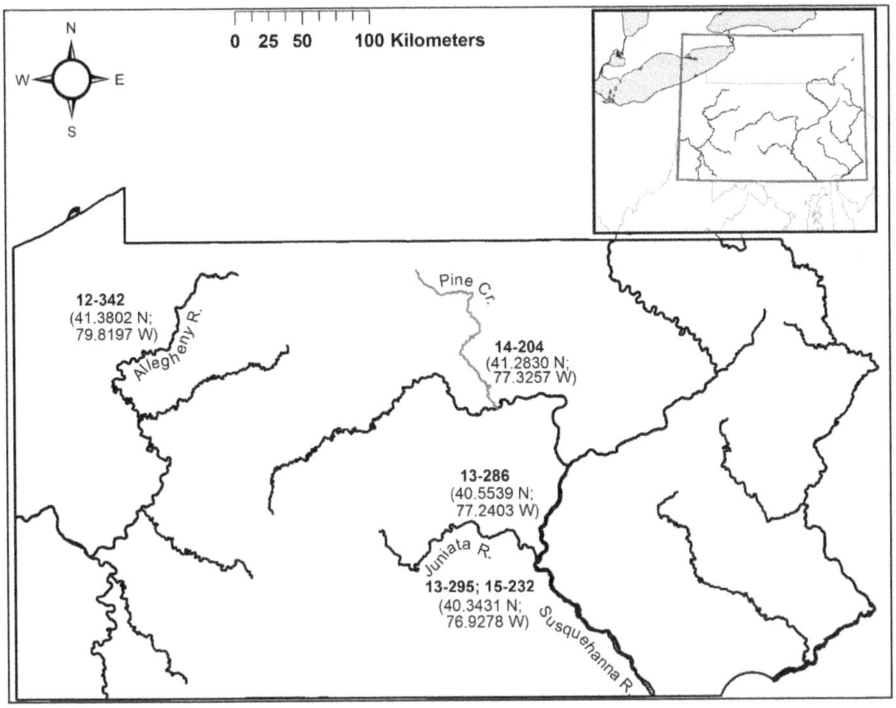

Fig. 1 Geographic origin of the five largemouth bass virus (LMBV) strains used in this study. The designation of the LMBV isolate recovered from moribund fish are indicated in bold, and the latitude and longitude of the smallmouth bass (SMB; *Micropterus dolomieu*) mortality episodes are listed in parentheses

to reach 28 °C ± 1 °C, which is reported to be the optimum temperature for LMBV experimental infection [11], using submersible 150-W heaters (Aqueon®-Pro 150, Central Aquatics™, Franklin, WI). Prior to injection, fish were anesthetized with sodium bicarbonate-buffered tricaine methanesulfonate (100 mg/L; MS-222, Western Chemical, Ferndale, WA). Fish were IP injected with 50 µl of tissue culture medium (TCM) containing LMBV at one of four concentrations: 10^1, 10^3, 10^5 and 10^7 $TCID_{50}$/fish. The negative control consisted of fish ($n = 5$) that were sham-injected with 50 µl of LMBV-free TCM. Fish were monitored daily for 30 days, whereby disease signs, cumulative mortality and behavior were recorded daily.

Based on LMBV intraperitoneal (IP) experimental infection results, the 13–286 Juniata and 13–295 Susquehanna LMBV isolates were selected for SMB waterborne challenge. Immersion exposures ($n = 10$ fish/tank/dose) were performed in aerated water at six final concentrations (10^1, 10^2, 10^3, 10^4, 10^6 and 10^7 $TCID_{50}$/ml) for each of the two LMBV isolates for 1 h and then placed back into their respective tanks. An additional group of fish (n = 10/tank) was subjected to same procedure except that they were immersed in water containing a LMBV-free TCM and were considered negative controls. Fish were kept at 28 ± 1 °C in circular 70-L tanks and clinical signs and mortality were recorded daily. Results of the waterborne experimental infection facilitated estimating a dose of LMBV that would allow the survival of some infected fish after a waterborne encounter with the virus.

Sample collection for LMBV-re-isolation and histopathology

Moribund fish were euthanized with an overdose (250 mg/L) of MS-222. At the end of the observation period for each experiment, all surviving fish were euthanized. Freshly dead and moribund fish, as well as fish that were euthanized at the end of the observation period, were necropsied. Portions of kidneys, spleen, and liver were collected in 1.5-ml centrifuge tubes and kept frozen at − 80 °C until processed for LMBV re-isolation and confirmation.

To examine tissue pathological consequences associated with LMBV infection in SMB, portions of external and internal lesions of each of LMBV-infected fish (moribund and recently dead from IP and water challenge experiments) were collected and fixed in 10% buffered formalin. Fixed samples were then dehydrated in a graded series of alcohol, embedded in paraffin, sectioned and stained with hematoxylin and eosin [12]. Stained tissues were visually examined under a light microscope (Olympus, Model BX41TF, Kyoto, Japan) and photographs were taken using image software (Olympus DP25-BSW, version 2.2) connected to a camera (Olympus DP25).

Molecular characterization of LMBV

Viral DNA from cell culture was purified using a DNeasy® Blood & Tissue Kit (Qiagen, Hilden, Germany) according to the manufacturer's instructions. The full-length major capsid protein gene sequences were PCR amplified using the forward 5′- ATG TCT TCT GTT ACG GGT TCT GGC-3′ and reverse 5′- TTA CAG GAT GGG GAA ACC CAT GG-3′ primer pairs and sequenced. Each PCR reaction contained 12.5 μl of GoTaq Green Master Mix (Promega, Madison, WI), 0.8 μM of each primer, 70 ng of DNA template and DNAase-free water to produce a final volume of 25 μl. Amplification was performed in a GeneAmp® PCR System 9700 thermocycler (AB Applied BioSystems, Foster City, CA) using a single denaturation step at 94 °C for 5 min, followed by 30 cycles of 94 °C for 30 s, 55.0 °C for 30 s and 72 °C for 1.5 min, with an additional elongation at 72 °C for 7 min. The expected amplicon (1392 bp) was visualized in 1.5% (*w*/*v*) agarose gel electrophoresis containing SYBR safe DNA gel stain (Invitrogen, Carlsbad, CA) for 30 min at 100 V under UV transillumination (UVP, Model TFM-26, Upland, CA). The resulting sequences were submitted for basic local alignment search tool analysis (BLAST) [13] against the nr database for sequence similarity searches. The resulting sequences (1392 bp) were deposited in GenBank (Accession #: KY825779-KY825781).

Effect of temperature on SMB susceptibility to LMBV

The effect of temperature on SMB susceptibility to LMBV was evaluated using the 13–286 Juniata LMBV isolate. Water temperature was adjusted to one of three temperatures: 11 ± 1, 23 ± 1 and 28 ± 1 °C (two tanks/temperature). Fish (n = 10/tank/treatment) were randomly chosen for each tank and allowed to acclimate for 7 days. Fish for each of the temperatures were infected with LMBV at a concentration of $10^{2.6}$ $TCID_{50}$/ml in 10-L glass aquaria by immersion for 60 min. Fish in temperature-matched control (three tanks) were immersed in 10-L of diluted sterile TCM. Experimental fish were observed for morbidity and mortality for 30 days and samples were collected as described above.

Role of concurrent infection with *F. columnare* or *Aeromonas salmonicida* on SMB LMBV mortality

Flavobacterium columnare strain 10FC isolated in the authors' laboratory in 2014 and *Aeromonas salmonicida* subspecies *salmonicida* strain 3.205 isolated from SMB during a mass mortality event in 2011 at the southern fork of the Shenandoah River, Millville, WV and provided by Dr. Rocco Cipriano (the US Geologic Survey National Fish Health Center, Leetown, WV) were used in experimental co-infection with LMBV to determine the combined infection effects on fish. All infections were performed via the waterborne immersion route.

For co-infection trials of the 13–286 Juniata LMBV strain and *F. columnare,* 12 tanks (8 SMB/tank), divided into four treatments (3 replicates per treatment), were used. Fish in the first treatment were exposed to neither virus nor bacterium and diluent vehicle was added to their tanks (10-ml TCM/tank added at day 1 and 10-ml phosphate buffered saline [PBS])/tank added at day 10) and were considered a double negative control group. Fish in the second treatment were immersed in suspension of 13–286 Juniata LMBV strain at a concentration of $10^{2.6}$ $TCID_{50}$/ml for 1 h on day 1, and on day 10, 10-ml PBS/tank was added into the water. This treatment was considered the LMBV positive group. In the third treatment, fish were held in water with TCM for 10 days before exposing fish to *F. columnare* at a final concentration of 1.75×10^8 CFU/ml in glass tanks at day 10. The fourth treatment received both LMBV at day 1 and *F. columnare* at day 10 at the same concentrations and conditions described above. Morbidity and mortality of SMB were monitored for 30 days.

The co-infection study with *A. salmonicida* followed the same design, except that following LMBV infection, the water temperature was dropped from 28 to 20 °C over three days, since the optimal temperature for *A. salmonicida* infection ranges from 15 to 20 °C [14]. The bacterial dose used for infection was 1.35×10^8 CFU/ml collected during the logarithmic phase of in vitro growth.

For re-isolation of *F. columnare* 10FC and *A. salmonicida* 3.205 in co-infection trials, kidney tissues and external lesions were collected from dead, moribund and surviving fish that were euthanized using inoculating loops and streaked onto Hsu-Shotts medium supplemented with neomycin sulphate (4 mg/L) for *F. columnare* [15] and Trypticase Soy Agar for *A. salmonicida* [16]. All plates were incubated at 22 °C for up to 72 h. Individual representative colonies were subcultured and confirmed by molecular analyses (below).

Virus and bacteria re-isolation and confirmation

LMBV re-isolation was performed using FHM cells following USFWS and AFS-FHS [16] protocol. Tissue pools (kidney, spleen and liver) were diluted 1:20 (*w*/*v*) in Eagle's minimum essential medium (Gibco) supplemented with 0.3% tryptose phosphate broth (BD Biosciences, Sparks, NY), penicillin (100 U/ml), streptomycin (100 μg/ml), and amphotericin B (2.5 μg/ml) and then homogenized using a hand-held pestle and tissue grinder (Fisherbrand®, Fisher Scientific, Pittsburgh, PA) in a 1.5-ml centrifuge tube. Samples were clarified by centrifugation at 5000 rpm (2711×*g*) for 30 min. Supernatants were inoculated (25 μl) in triplicate wells of 96-well microplates containing s monolayer of FHM cells. Infected plates were incubated at 28 °C and observed for the formation of cytopathic effect (CPE; i.e., cell lysis with wide areas of monolayer detachment). After

7 days post-incubation, cultures with no evidence of CPE were blind passaged by inoculating fresh FHM cells with cell culture supernatant and observed for an additional 7 days. Samples that exhibited the formation of CPE at any time during incubation were considered presumptively positive for LMBV. Confirmatory identification of the virus from cell culture supernatant was made by polymerase chain reaction (PCR) as described below.

To confirm that the virus isolated from experimentally infected fish was LMBV, total DNA was extracted from CPE-positive cell culture using a DNeasy® Blood & Tissue Kit following the manufacturer's protocol and then stored at − 20 °C. For samples that exhibited no signs of CPE at the end of the second passage, DNA extraction was performed directly from collected tissues using the same extraction kit. Extracted DNA was quantified using a Qubit fluorometer (Invitrogen, Eugene, OR). Primer pairs used to confirm LMBV were LMBV288F: 5'-GCG GCC AAC CAG TTT AAC GCA A -3′ and LMBV353R: 5′- AGG ACC CTA GCT CCT GCT TGA T -3′ targeting a portion of LMBV major capsid protein [17]. Each PCR reaction contained 12.5 μl of GoTaq Green Master Mix (Promega, Madison, WI), 0.8 μM of each primer, 70 ng of DNA template and DNAase-free water to produce a final volume of 25 μl. Amplification was performed in a GeneAmp® PCR System 9700 thermocycler (AB Applied BioSystems) using a single denaturation step at 94 °C for 5 min, followed by 30 cycles of 94 °C for 30 s, 56.5 °C for 30 s and 72 °C for 35 s, with an additional elongation at 72 °C for 7 min. The expected amplicon (248 bp) was visualized in 1.5% (*w*/*v*) agarose gel electrophoresis containing SYBR safe DNA gel stain (Invitrogen) for 30 min at 100 V under UV transillumination (UVP, Model TFM-26, Upland, CA).

DNA was extracted from re-isolated bacteria using a DNeasy® Blood & Tissue Kit according to the manufacturer's protocol. Bacterial DNA was quantified as previously described. PCR amplification of *F. columnare* was conducted using the primers FCISRFL (5′ -TGC GGC TGG ATC ACC TCC TTT CTA GAG ACA - 3′) and FCISRR1 (5′ -TAA TYR CTA AAG ATG TTC TTT CTA CTT GTT TG − 3′; detailed in Faisal et al. [18]). To confirm *A. salmonicida*, amplified PCR product was produced using MIY1 (5′- AGC CTC CAC GCG CTC ACA GC- 3′) and MIY2 (5′- AAG AGG CCC CAT AGT GTG GG -3′) primers (detailed in [19]).

Statistical analysis

For examining the effect of temperature on SMB susceptibility to LMBV, differences in Kaplan-Meier survival estimates between LMBV and control treatments were tested with log-rank tests at each experimental temperature. Additionally, differences in overall cumulative mortality between LMBV and control treatments at each experimental temperature were tested using Fisher's exact test for proportions.

For the co-infection experiments, we initially tested for differences in Kaplan-Meier survival estimates among the replicate tanks within each treatment with log-rank tests. If statistically significant differences among the replicates were not detected, we combined the replicate tank results for each treatment and tested for an overall difference in Kaplan-Meier survival estimates among the treatments with a log-rank test. If the overall test was statistically significant, we then conducted pairwise log-rank tests between the infection treatments. Bonferroni corrections were applied to protect the error-rate of the pairwise tests. Differences in overall cumulative mortality among the treatments were tested using a mixed-effects logistic regression model with treatment as a fixed effect and tank as a random effect. Pairwise differences in infection treatments were then tested if there were overall statistically differences among the treatments. As with the pairwise log-rank tests, Bonferroni corrections were applied to protect the error-rate of the pairwise tests. Kaplan-Meier survival curves and log-rank tests were conducted in R [20] using the survive [21] and survminer [22] libraries. Fisher's exact tests and mixed-effect logistic regression models were conducted in SAS Version 9.4 (SAS Institute Inc., Cary, NC) using PROC FREQ and PROC GLIMMIX, respectively [23].

Results

Exposure of SMB to LMBV

Exposure of SMB to LMBV by IP resulted in morbidity and mortality in all LMBV infected groups with variable rates, the 13–295 Susquehanna LMBV and the 13–286 Juniata isolates being the most pathogenic to SMB. Mortality in SMB in the groups that received LMBV at a concentration 10^3–10^7 $TCID_{50}$/fish started at the 2nd day post-infection (pi) and reached a cumulative mortality of 100% within 14 days pi, except the fish exposed to 12–342 Allegheny and 14–204 Pine Creek strains. In the groups challenged with 10^1 $TCID_{50}$/fish, mortality was observed only in 13–295 Susquehanna and 13–286 Juniata infections, reaching a cumulative mortality of 60 and 40%, respectively.

Moribund SMB were lethargic and some displayed gill pallor, abdominal distension, hemorrhages on ventral area, and hemorrhagic protruded vents (Fig. 2a). In some fish, intestinal prolapse, and petechial to diffuse hemorrhages on opercula, isthmus, mandible and maxilla were observed. Visceral organs appeared edematous with hemorrhages of various sizes on visceral fat (Fig. 2b) and heart ventricles (Fig. 2b). Intestines appeared inflamed and contained clear mucus content, while livers were mottled and enlarged with hemorrhages of various sizes (Fig. 2b). Splenomegaly, petechial to ecchymotic hemorrhage within the swim bladder, and diffuse hemorrhage within the

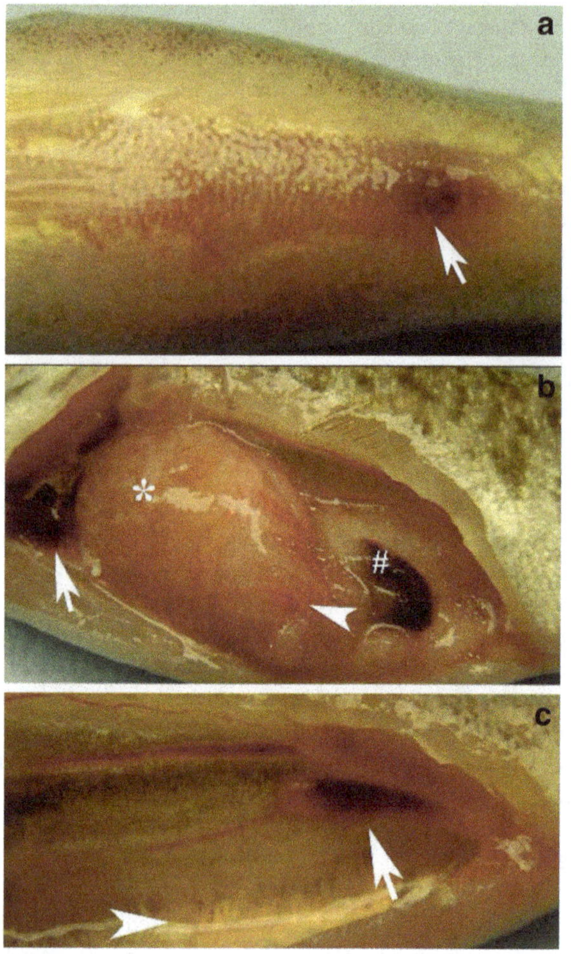

Fig. 2 Clinical signs in largemouth bass virus (LMBV)-IP injected smallmouth bass (SMB; *Micropterus dolomieu*). **a** abdominal distension along with subdermal hemorrhage on ventral area and vent (arrow) of 13–295 Susquehanna-injected SMB; **b** swelling and hemorrhage on heart ventricle (arrow) concomitant with hemorrhage of visceral fat (arrowhead), mottled, friable, edematous and enlarged livers (*) and enlargement with darkening and edema of spleen (#) of SMB exposed to 13–286 Juniata; and **c** severe ascites (arrowhead) and ecchymotic hemorrhage in gonads of 12–342 Allegheny challenged SMB

gonads (Fig. 2c) were observed. Kidneys were enlarged with hemorrhages within the tissues. LMBV was isolated from all dead and surviving SMB and its identity confirmed by conventional PCR. Mock-infected fish showed no clinical signs and no virus was detected in their tissues.

Based on the observations made during the IP infection screening study, the 13–295 Susquehanna and 13–286 Juniata isolates were selected for infecting SMB by immersion. The two LMBV isolates induced mortalities in all challenged SMB at all doses examined, except for dose of 10^1 $TCID_{50}$/ml (Fig. 3). Cumulative mortality of 13–295 Susquehanna-infected SMB in the groups that received the low virus doses (10^2, 10^3 and 10^4 $TCID_{50}$/ml) reached 40–50% within 9 and 12 days pi, while mortality in SMB in the high dose groups (10^6 and 10^7 $TCID_{50}$/ml) began at 2 days pi and continued until 20 days pi, reaching a cumulative mortality of 100% (Fig. 3). Mortality of Juniata-challenged SMB was comparatively more severe than that of the Susquehanna isolate. In the low dose groups (10^2, 10^3 and 10^4 $TCID_{50}$/ml), mortality started between 8 and 12 d pi and peaked to 50–60% by the 21st day pi. In SMB exposed to the high doses (10^6 and 10^7 $TCID_{50}$/ml), mortality started as early as 2nd day pi and continued up to 20 days pi to reach a cumulative value of 100% (Fig. 3).

Gross clinical signs in LMBV-infected SMB by immersion were, to a great extent, similar to those observed in IP-infected fish. In addition, there were some lesions in the two immersion groups that were not observed in the IP infected SMB groups. For examples, ~ 25% of SMB exhibited signs of emaciation, disjointed mandibles (Fig. 4a), uni- or bilateral exophthalmia associated with ecchymotic hemorrhages and corneal opacity (Fig. 4b) that can lead to a rupture of the eye, loss of the vitreous, and subsequent collapse (Fig. 4c) in some survivors. Unique to the immersion group was the presence of external ulcers that began as discoloration of the skin (Fig. 5a) that expanded in size (Fig. 5b) and eventually was accomplanied by hemorrhage and scale loss (Fig. 5c, d). These lesions then progressed to ulcers (0.5-3 cm in diameter) with white centers and hemorrhagic well circumscribed edges that eventually penetrated into the underlying muscular layer (Fig. 5d-f). Moreover, some infected SMB exhibited eroded and ulcerated fins. Internal organs showed lesions that were similar to those observed with the IP infected group; namely, ascites, hemorrhagic visceral fat, enlarged hemorrhagic heart ventricles (Fig. 4d); hemorrhagic, enlarged liver (Fig. 4d), and darkened, friable and enlarged spleens. Hemorrhages within the gonads, and enlarged, hemorrhagic kidneys were also observed (Fig. 4e).

Virus re-isolation and histopathology

LMBV was isolated from all moribund and surviving fish from all dose groups (except the lowest dose group) of all isolates and confirmed by PCR. Neither gross clinical signs were observed, nor was LMBV isolated or detected by PCR from mock-challenged SMB.

In fish challenged with LMBV by IP or by immersion, multifocal hepatic necrosis, multifocal splenic necrosis, multifocal necrotizing steatitis, and to a lesser extent, necrotizing nephritis were the most dominant lesions observed (Fig. 6). Early lesions in the liver included foci of coagulative necrosis characterized by loss of nuclear detail and hypereosinophilia of affected hepatocytes. Lesions expanded quickly involving large portions of the hepatic parenchyma with hepatocytes in affected areas undergoing degeneration and necrosis as evidenced by

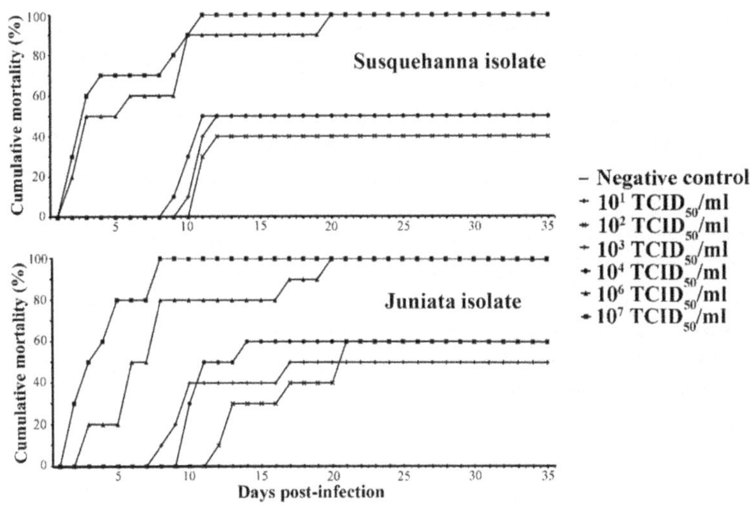

Fig. 3 Cumulative mortality of largemouth bass virus (LMBV) in smallmouth bass (*Micropterus dolomieu*). Fish were experimentally infected with two LMBV strains by immersion

cytoplasmic vacuolation, nuclear pyknosis and ultimately, accumulation of cellular debris admixed with infiltrating heterophils (Fig. 6a, b). Lesions in the spleen were similar, starting as focal areas of necrosis and lymphocytolysis characterized by foci of karyorhectic debris (Fig. 6c) that quickly expanded to confluent areas of coagulative necrosis (Fig. 6d). Necrotizing steatitis, especially affecting the mesenteric fat, was a consistent lesion in all fish regardless of the route of inoculation and presented as focal areas of necrosis as evidenced by nuclear pyknosis and accumulation of karyorhectic debris surrounded by infiltrating heterophils (Fig. 6e). Necrotic adipocytes commonly underwent saponification and were surrounded by large numbers of macrophages. Focal areas of fibrinoid necrosis were observed in the kidneys of some fish and in those animals renal tubules were focally lost and replaced by accumulation of fibrin admixed with cellular debris and macrophages (Fig. 6f). In one fish challenged with the IP route, necrotizing myocarditis was observed. Only fish in the immersion group developed severe skin lesions characterized by severe epithelial necrosis that lead to focally extensive ulcerative dermatitis (Fig. 7a). The affected epithelium was characterized by cytoplasmic swelling and vacuolation of epithelial cells, nuclear pyknosis and ultimately cellular necrosis (Fig. 7b). Severe inflammation extended into the underlying muscle causing massive myofiber necrosis (Fig. 7c). Necrotic myofibers were surrounded by extensive infiltrates of heterophils admixed with macrophages. The necrotizing dermatitis and myositis locally progressed to severe heterophilic and granulomatous inflammation associated with secondary colonization by bacteria and fungal hyphae (Fig. 7d). Exophthalmia observed in SMB challenged via the immersion route and the affected eye had a severe necrotizing panuveitis and keratinitis. There were marked necrosis and heterophilic and histiocytic inflammation expanding the uveal tract including the iris, the ciliary body, and the choroid (Fig. 7e) and causing secondary vitritis (Fig. 7f). The uveal tract also contains multifocal hemorrhage and fibrin, and inflammatory infiltrates fill the ciliary cleft, obscure the trabecular meshwork and extend into the limbus and sclera. Inflammatory cells also dissect underneath Descemet's membrane, commonly extended into the cornea causing perforating ulcers and severe conjunctivitis and infiltrate the episclera. All chambers of the eye contain fibrin and hemorrhage admixed with large numbers of heterophils and fewer macrophages.

Phylogeny of LMBV isolated from SMB mortality episodes

BLAST analysis showed that the sequences from SMB-LMBV are identical to the sequence from LMB-LMBV (FR682503). BLAST analysis also showed that SMB-LMBV sequences shared 99.07% (1379/1392 bp) sequence identity with the two LMBUSV sequences from fish in China and Thailand that were associated with ulcerative lesions (GU256635 and KU507315).

Effect of temperature on LMBV pathogenicity

SMB in the negative control group exhibited no clinical signs or mortality and were free of LMBV regardless of temperature. No mortality or clinical signs were observed in LMBV-infected SMB at a water temperature of 11 °C. At a water temperature of 23 °C, one fish died on day 13 pi, resulting in a cumulative mortality of 10% and a mean survival time (using 30 days as the upper limit for calculations) of 28.3 days (SE = 1.6 days). Log-rank and Fisher's exact tests indicated that differences in Kaplan-Meier survival curves and cumulative mortality

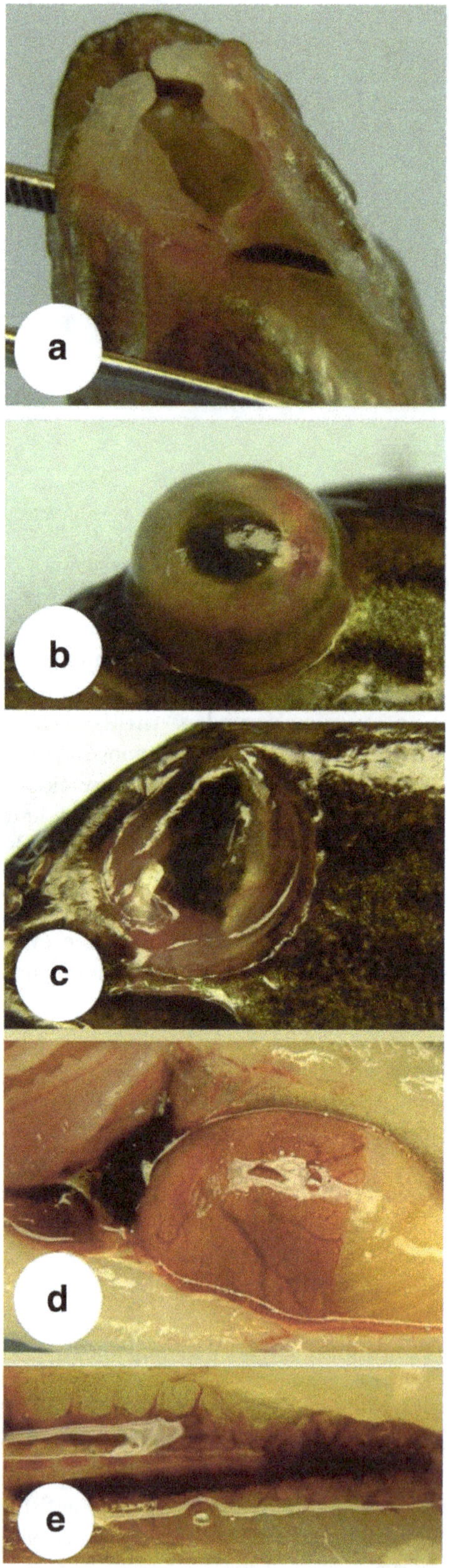

Fig. 4 Clinical signs observed in smallmouth bass (*Micropterus dolomieu*) infected with largemouth bass virus (LMBV) by immersion. **a** broken mandible at the middle with ulceration and hemorrhage in a fish infected with the 13–295 Susquehanna River LMBV isolate; **b** unilateral exophthalmia with the protruding eye ball concurrent with ulceration, intraocular hemorrhage and corneal opacity in a fish infected with the 13–286 Juniata River LMBV isolate, and **c** ruptured eye showing loss of vitreous, lenticular damage and periocular hemorrhage commonly seen in an smallmouth bass that survived infection with the 13–286 Juniata River LMBV isolate. **d** gill pallor, hemorrhagic heart ventricle, severe ascites, ecchymotic hemorrhage with enlargement and edema on liver of 13–286 Juniata LMBV-infected fish; and **e** edematous, friable and ecchymotic hemorrhage observed in kidneys of 13–295 Susquehanna LMBV-infected fish

between the LMBV and control treatments were not statistically significant at this temperature (log-rank test: Chi-square = 1.0, *P*-value = 0.317; Fisher exact test: *P*-value = 0.5). When SMB were immersed in LMBV-tainted water at a concentration of $10^{2.79}$ TCID50/ml and kept at 28 °C, 50% of the fish died with a mean survival time of 22.2 days (SE = 2.6 days) (Fig. 8). Log-rank and Fisher's exact test indicated that differences in Kaplan-Meier survival curves and cumulative mortality between the LMBV and control treatments were statistically significant at this temperature (log-rank test: Chi-square = 6.5, *P*-value = 0.012; Fisher exact test: *P*-value = 0.032).

Gross pathological changes of dead and moribund SMB maintained at 23 and 28 °C were similar to those observed in infected SMB via the immersion route. LMBV was re-isolated and confirmed from tissue samples from all dead and surviving SMB in the LMBV treatment group that were maintained at 23 and 28 °C. However, LMBV was not isolated or detected in tissues by PCR in any of the surviving fish from the LMBV treatment group that were maintained at 11 °C.

Effect of co-infection by *F. Columnare* on LMBV-infected SMB

There was an overall significant difference in cumulative mortality between the treatments ($F_{3,8}$ = 12.03; *P*-value = 0.002). Cumulative mortality for the control treatment was 0.0%. For the LMBV treatment, cumulative mortality was 54.1% (SE = 5.2%). For the *F. columnare* treatment, cumulative mortality was 29.2 (SE = 4.7%). For the co-infection treatment, cumulative mortality was 75.0% (SE = 4.5%) (Fig. 9a). Pairwise comparisons indicated that cumulative mortality in the LMBV and co-infection treatments were significantly greater than in the *F. columnare* treatment (*F. columnare* vs LMBV: – 3.41, df = 8, *P*-value = 0.028; *F. columnare* vs co-infection: – 5.99, df = 8, *P*-value = 0.001); however, the pairwise comparison between the LMBV and co-infection treatments were not significantly different (LMBV vs co-infection: – 2.93, df = 8, *P*-value = 0.057).

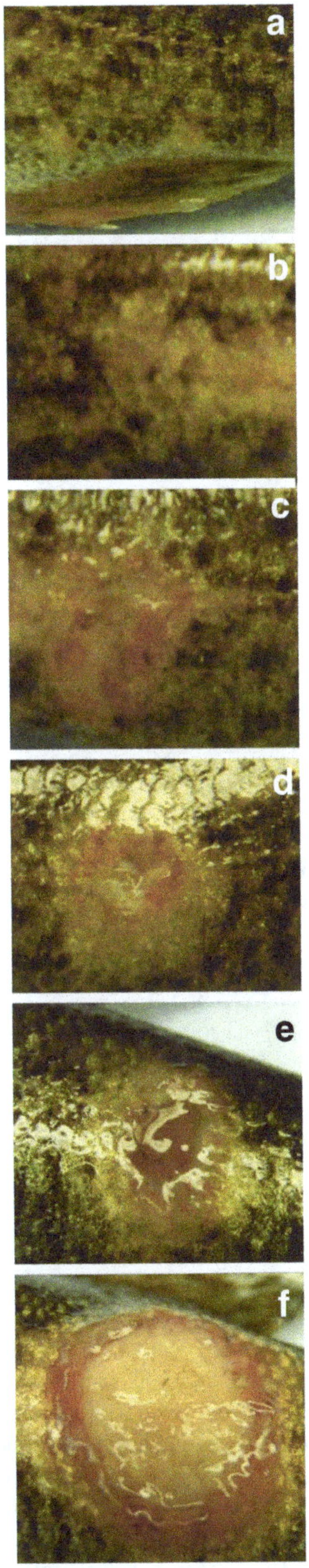

Fig. 5 Progression of dermal lesions in largemouth bass virus-challenged smallmouth bass (*Micropterus dolomieu*). **a** Faint skin discoloration on the trunk. **b** Further progressed skin discoloration. **c** Skin discoloration accompanied by hemorrhage and early stage of scale loss. **d** Skin discoloration surrounding a shallow dermal ulcer with hemorrhagic margins and central scale loss. **e** Deeper ulcer penetrating into the underlying muscular layer with surrounding skin discoloration. **f** Severe ulceration with well-circumscribed, raised, and hemorrhagic edges

There were no significant differences in Kaplan-Meir survival curves among the replicates for any of the treatments based on log-rank tests. However, there was a significant difference in Kaplan-Meier survival curves among the treatments (log-rank test: Chi-square = 31.8, P-value< 0.001). For SMB infected with LMBV, mean survival time (using 30 days as the upper limit for calculations) was 21.7 days (SE = 1.7 days). For SMB infected with *F. columnare*, mean survival time was 25.2 days (SE = 1.6 days). When LMBV-infected SMB were subsequently infected with *F. columnare*, mean survival time was 17.5 days (SE = 0.7 days). Pairwise comparisons of Kaplan-Meir survival curves by log-rank tests indicated that survival curve differences between the *F. columnare* and co-infection treatments were significantly different (P-value = 0.005). Pairwise comparisons between the *F. columnare* and LMBV treatments (P-value = 0.314) and the LMBV and co-infection treatments (P-value = 0.279) were not significantly different.

No gross pathology or clinical signs were observed in the mock-infected SMB. LMBV was recovered from the tissues of kidneys, spleen and liver of all survivors in the LMBV and co-infection treatments. No *F. columnare* was recovered from any SMB that survived the bacterial infection. *F. columnare* and LMBV were re-isolated from the moribund and dead SMB co-infection treatments group and their identities were confirmed by PCR. External and internal clinical signs of dead/moribund and surviving LMBV-infected SMB were consistent with those described above. Immersion of *F. columnare* alone resulted in skin discoloration, subdermal hemorrhage, abdominal distension, and fin erosion and ulceration. Internally, organs appeared edematous with hemorrhage within kidneys, hepatomegaly, and splenomegaly.

Effect of co-infection by *A. salmonicida* on LMBV-infected SMB

There was an overall significant difference in cumulative mortality between the treatments ($F_{3,8} = 12.03$; P-value = 0.002). Cumulative mortality for the control treatment was 0.0%. For the LMBV treatment, cumulative mortality was 16.7% (SE = 4.4%). For the *A. salmonicida* treatment, cumulative mortality was 95.8 (SE = 2.4%). For the

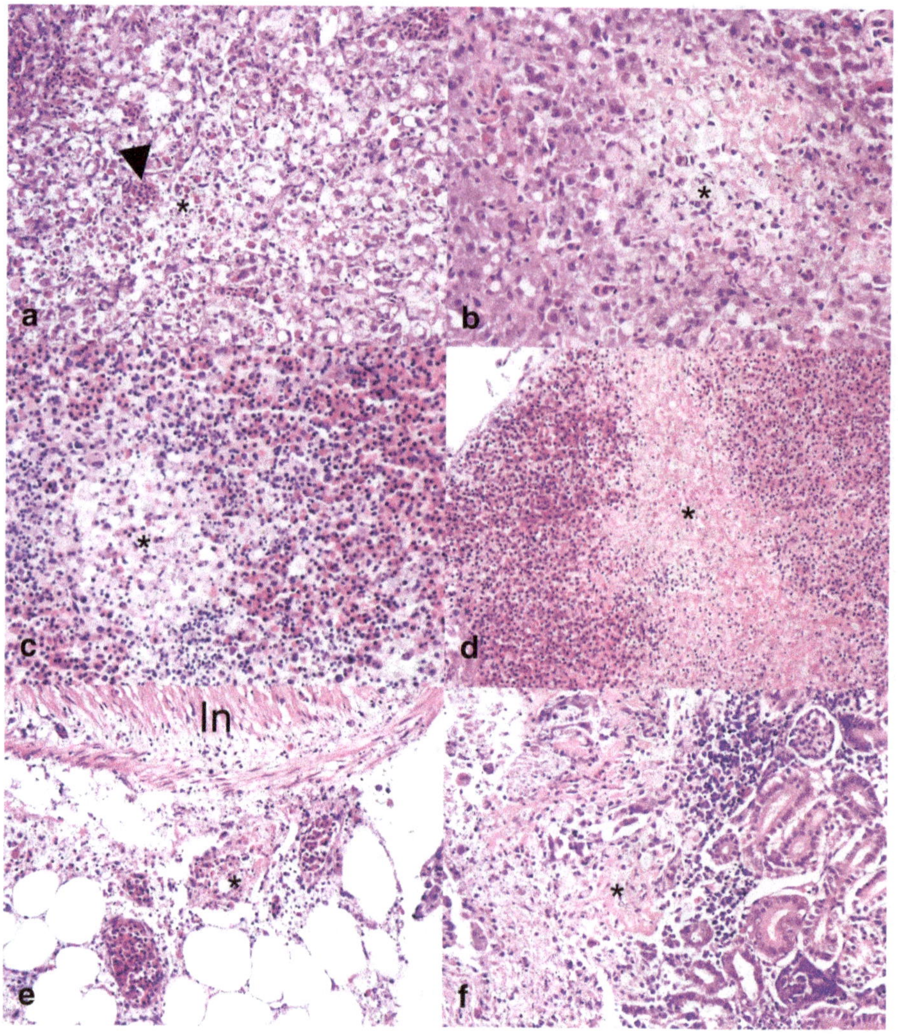

Fig. 6 Histopathological lesions in smallmouth bass (*Micropterus dolomieu*) infected with the largemouth bass virus. **a** Focally extensive hepatocellular degeneration and necrosis (asterisk) with secondary infiltration of heterophils (arrowhead). **b** Liver with focal area of coagulative necrosis (asterisk) characterized by loss of nuclear detail and hypereosinophilia of affected hepatocytes surrounded by cellular debris and few infiltrating heterophils. **c** Focal splenic necrosis (asterisk) with lymphocytolysis and karyorhectic debris. **d** Spleen with confluent area of coagulative necrosis (asterisk). **e** Mesenteric fat with focally extensive necrotizing steatis (asterisk) adjacent to the intestinal wall. **f** Kidney with focal area of fibrinoid necrosis (asterisk) with loss renal tubules and replacement by accumulating fibrin admixed with cellular debris and macrophages. Fish in **a**, **c**, and **e** were infected by intraperitoneal injection, while fish in **b**, **d**, and **f** were infected by immersion

co-infection treatment, cumulative mortality was 100.0% (Fig. 9b). Pairwise comparisons indicated that cumulative mortality in the LMBV treatment was significantly lower than in the *A. salmonicida* treatment (*A. salmonicida* vs LMBV: $t = -7.06$, df = 8, *P*-value = 0.003). Pairwise comparisons of the *A. salmonicida* and LMBV treatments with the co-infection treatment were not estimable presumably because of the lack of variability in cumulative mortality results for the co-infection treatment replicates. Even though this prevents us from attaching statistical significance, we believe there is clear biological significance between the co-infection treatment cumulative mortality of 100% and the LMBV treatment cumulative mortality of 16.7%.

There were no significant differences in Kaplan-Meir survival curves among the replicates for any of the treatments based on log-rank tests. There was a significant difference in Kaplan-Meier survival curves among the treatments (log-rank test: Chi-square = 89.6, *P*-value< 0.001). For SMB infected with LMBV, mean survival time (using 30 days as the upper limit for calculations) was 27.3 days (SE = 1.4 days). For SMB infected with *A. salmonicida*, mean survival time was 13.8 days (SE = 0.7 days). When LMBV-infected SMB were subsequently infected with *A. salmonicida*, mean survival time was 14.8 days (SE = 0.8 days). Pairwise comparisons of Kaplan-Meir survival curves by log-rank tests indicated that survival curve differences between the *A. salmonicida* and LMBV

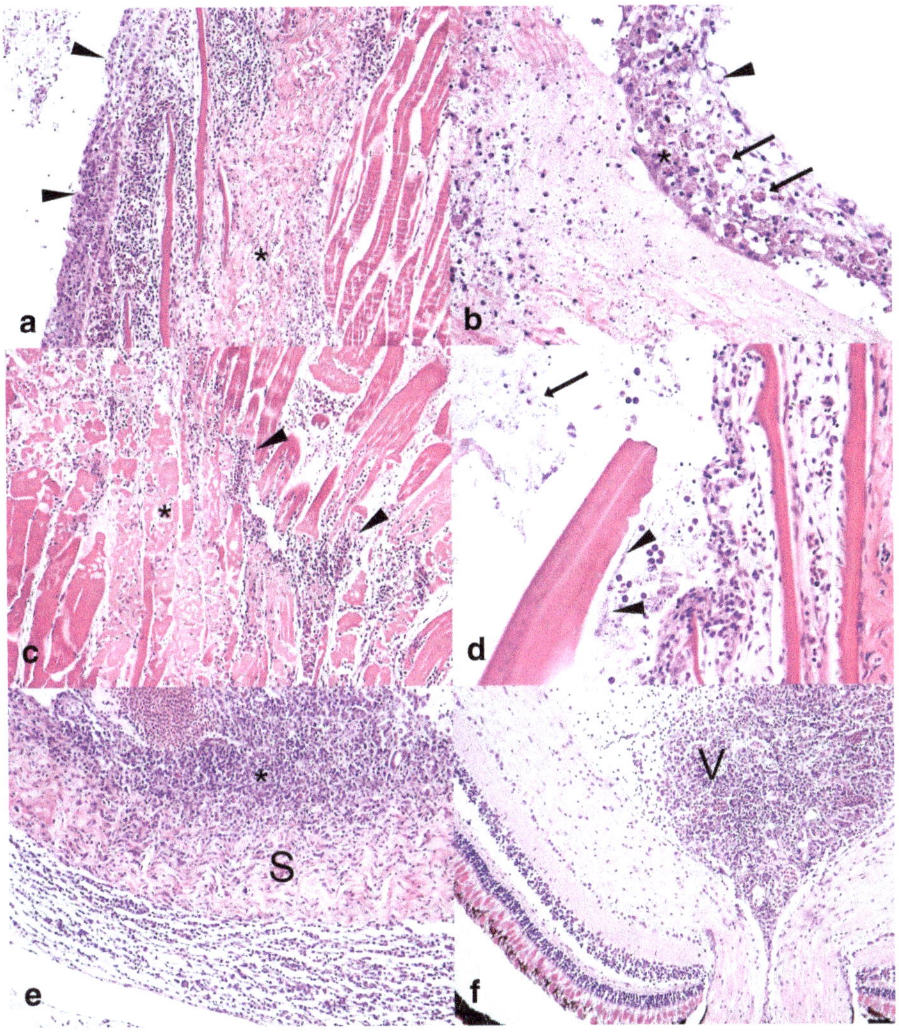

Fig. 7 Histopathological lesions in smallmouth bass (*Micropterus dolomieu*) infected with largemouth bass virus. **a** Extensive ulcerative dermatitis (arrowheads) with severe epithelial necrosis (asterisk). **b** Higher magnification of the affected epithelium with cytoplasmic swelling and vacuolation of epithelial cells (arrowhead), nuclear pyknosis (asterisk) and infiltration of heterophils (arrows). **c** Severe necrotizing myositis with necrotic myofibers (asterisk) being surrounded by extensive infiltrates of heterophils admixed with macrophages (arrowheads). **d** Ulcerative dermatitis was commonly associated with secondary colonization by bacteria (arrowheads) and fungal hyphae (arrow). **e** Severe necrotizing panuveitis with heterophilic and histiocytic inflammation expanding the choroid (asterisk) and extending into the sclera (S) and infiltrating the episclera. **f** Severe heterophilic vitritis with the vitreous chambers (V) containing large numbers of heterophils and fewer macrophages admixed with fibrin and hemorrhage

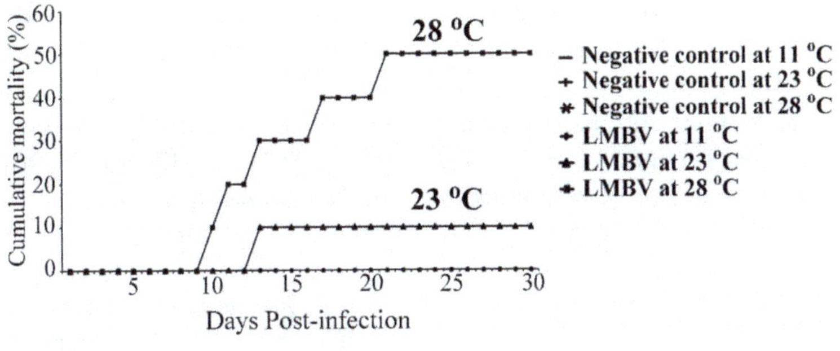

Fig. 8 Effects of water temperature on smallmouth bass mortality. Effects of water temperature on mortality in smallmouth bass (*Micropterus dolomieu*) challenged with largemouth bass virus

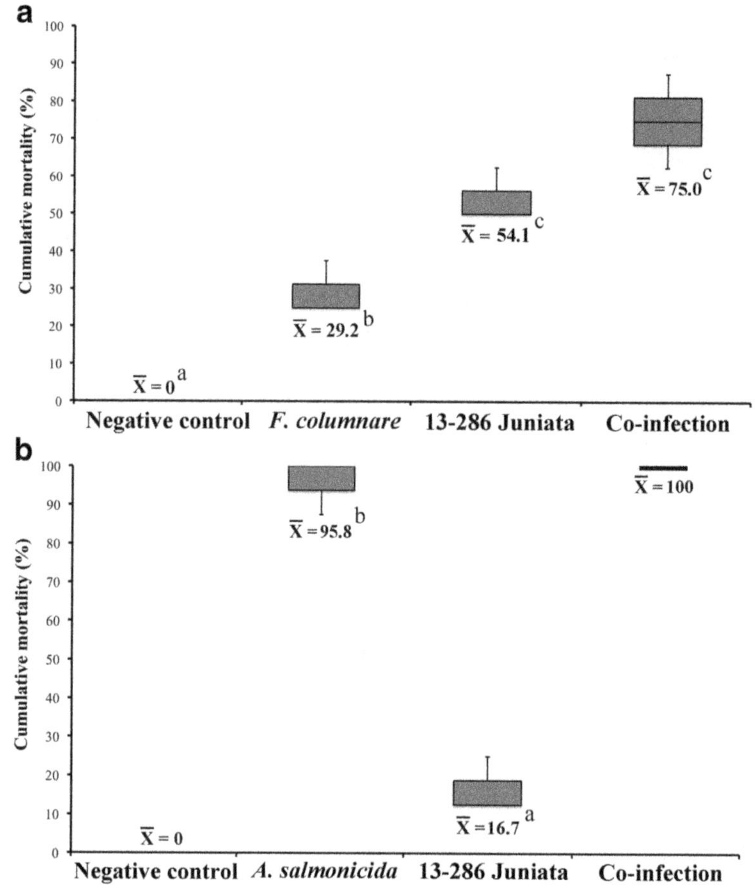

Fig. 9 Effects of co-infecting largemouth bass virus (LMBV)-infected smallmouth bass (*Micropterus dolomieu*) with bacteria: **a** *Flavobacterium columnare*. Both experimental infections were performed at a water temperature of 28 °C. **b** *Aeromonas salmonicida*. Experimental infection with LMBV took place at a water temperature of 28 °C, while that of *A. salmonicida* was performed when the water temperature dropped to 20 °C. Data are displayed as box plots of cumulative mortality (%) displaying the median and upper/lower quartiles; whiskers indicate the maximum and minimum values in each group. Different superscript letters indicate significant difference ($P < 0.05$)

treatments were significantly different (P-value< 0.001). Differences between the LMBV and co-infections treatments were also significantly different (P-value< 0.001). There were not significant differences in the survival curves between the *A. salmonicida* and co-infection treatments (P-value = 1.000).

Gross signs in SMB exposed to *A. salmonicida* only were more severe when compared to *F. columnare* infections (e.g. dermal hemorrhage, ulceration and necrosis on skin, petechial hemorrhage and hyperplasia of gill filaments, hemorrhage on base of all fins along with severe fin erosion and abdominal distension). Internally, ascites, hemorrhage of liver, splenic enlargement and darkening, and distended gastro intestine containing yellowish mucoid content were observed. Kidneys appeared edematous and hemorrhagic.

Discussion

The findings of this study demonstrate that LMBV infection, regardless of the method of exposure, is lethal to YOY SMB. Pairwise sequence analysis based on full-length major capsid protein gene nucleotide sequences demonstrated that the SMB-LMBV isolates were all LMBV strains identical to those isolated from LMB and different from LMBV isolates from fish in China and Thailand that were associated with ulcerative lesions. This finding reveals the ability of LMBV to cause dermal lesions, a pathology not previously reported for this virus.

The disease in the IP-infected SMB group ran an acute course with most mortalities happening within one week pi, which coincides well with disease progression described for LMBV in LMB [6]. Infection by immersion seems to have a prolonged time-to-death as most of the fish died within 2 weeks pi, reaching up to 100% mortality in SMB exposed to 10^6 and 10^7 $TCID_{50}$/ml. In contrast, exposure of LMB to $10^{6.5}$ $TCID_{50}$/ml LMBV by immersion only caused 17% mortality within the same observation period [6]. The fact that LMBV could be re-isolated from apparently healthy SMB that survived experimental infection for up to 5 weeks raises concerns that fish that survives LMBV infection can spread the virus to other geographical locations for perhaps prolonged time periods.

Similar to LMB, water temperature plays an important role in LMBV pathogenicity for SMB under controlled experimental conditions. Raising the water temperature above 23 °C was necessary for successful experimental infection of SMB with LMBV. Grant et al. [11] reported that an optimal temperature of 25 to 30 °C was necessary for LMBV to cause mortality in LMB, which agrees with our observations in SMB. Similar observations have been made during in vitro studies where LMBV was found to replicate in FHM and BF-2 cell lines at optimal incubation temperatures between 25 and 30 °C [11, 24]. This coincides well with the water temperatures recorded during the YOY SMB mortality episodes that fluctuated between 22 and 34 °C. High water temperatures are often associated with other stressors including low dissolved oxygen concentrations. These factors favor LMBV replication and can compromise host defense mechanisms.

In both SMB groups exposed to LMBV by either IP injection or by immersion, multifocal necrotizing steatitis/peritonitis, hepatitis and splenitis were the dominant lesions observed. Necrotizing steatitis/peritonitis as well as necrosis in the liver and spleen have been reported as consistent findings in juvenile LMB experimentally inoculated with LMBV via IP injection [7]. Steatitis/peritonitis and liver necrosis were also reported in another study of juvenile LMBV inoculated with 3 genetically different LMBV isolates [25]. However, it seems that LMBV can also induce local changes at the initial site(s) of contact with the host. For example, small, inflamed, necrotic lesions developed in the skin and muscle at the site of LMBV injection in LMB [6, 7, 26], but not at other skin locations. In contrast, in our study SMB infected by immersion developed multiple ulcerative skin and ocular lesions that were not seen in IP infected SMB. It is apparent that LMBV has tropism to cell types of different origins and that the route of infection can cause different pathology. Skin lesions independent of local injection sites, as observed in SMB infected by immersion, have never been reported in the case of LMB in the USA or Europe, but have been reported in Asia [8, 9]. It is noteworthy, however, that the two Asian strains are phylogenetically distinct when compared with the LMBV isolates of this study. A similar disease course has been described for other ranaviruses (e.g., ranavirus 3) in several amphibian species, where lesions ranged from ulcerative dermatitis to wide spread necrosis in parenchymal organs [27].

Based on the gross and microscopical lesions, it is possible that the dermal lesions observed in SMB in affected rivers are initiated primarily by LMBV and that affected areas became colonized by opportunistic bacteria and fungi; both of which are abundant in the aquatic environment. It is also possible that the rapidly developing LMBV-induced necrotic changes in hematopoietic tissue may have compromised the host defense mechanisms leading to secondary infections. The wide tissue distribution of LMBV in the infected SMB and variation of lesions based on route of infection are highly suggestive that different routes of infection are effective for transmitting disease. These factors combined can lead to explosive propagation of a deadly virus among a naïve susceptible population, and can lead to die offs of the magnitude reported in the affected rivers.

One alternative explanation is that bacteria known to cause lethal disease outbreaks and associated with dermal lesions at warmer water temperatures, such as *F. columnare* or motile *Aeromonas* spp. [28], might be the primary cause of YOY SMB mortality without the involvement of LMBV. While this hypothesis is plausible, no bacterium has consistently been isolated from affected SMB. On the contrary, our study demonstrated that *F. columnare* is more likely a contributor to overall SMB mortality in natural disease outbreaks. In our study, SMB infected with *F. columnare* alone developed skin lesions and mortalities at a much lower magnitude compared to LMBV-infected SMB, despite large numbers of bacteria having been added to the water at environmentally unrealistic levels (~ 10^8 cfu/ml). Instead, co-infection of LMBV-infected SMB with *F. columnare* significantly elevated mortalities. This finding further supports the hypothesis that SMB are either immunocompromised through infection with LMBV or with a damaged skin barrier due to viral infection, and can therefore easily contract secondary bacterial infections.

At the same water temperature at which LMBV and *F. columnare* were able to infect SMB causing dermal lesions, *A. salmonicida*, when added to the water at a concentration of 10^8 cfu/ml, was unable to cause mortalities or lesions in SMB (data not shown). It is therefore unlikely that *A. salmonicida* plays a causative role in SMB mortalities during the summer months. In contrast to LMBV, *A. salmonicida* was highly pathogenic to SMB at a lower temperature, 20 °C, at which LMBV pathogenicity was substantially diminished. Our findings clearly demonstrate that *A. salmonicida* alone can cause high mortality associated with dermal lesions albeit at much lower water temperature.

Conclusions

Co-infection of LMBV with *F. columnare* or *A. salmonicida* may have important implications for YOY SMB mortality across a wide temperature range. During warmer summer months, LMBV alone or in combination with *F. columnare* can cause YOY SMB mortality at the magnitude noticed in the multiple river systems. As discussed earlier, *F. columnare* alone cannot be the primary cause of mortality since, even at extremely high concentrations in experimental settings, it does not cause mortality levels as high as reported for the Susquehanna and Potomac River basins. In addition, since *F. columnare* has a wide host range, other fish species should have been affected as well. In contrast, LMBV has a much narrower host range and primarily infects centrarchids [6, 7, 27]. While at lower water temperatures, certain bacterial pathogens such as *A. salmonicida* could become a major contributor to mortality episodes, though their host range is also wide and such episodes of high mortality should have involved other fish species as well. The observed YOY SMB fish kills in PA occur at warmer temperatures and as a result most likely are not the result of an *A. salmonicida*, however the results of this study show that the pathogen could play a role in SMB fish kills in other river systems or under different conditions.

The sum of the data generated in this study, including LMBV ability to cause, without co-infection, high mortality rates associated with dermal lesions under laboratory conditions that are visually similar to the skin lesions observed in YOY SMB during the mortality episodes, and its relatively high optimal temperature which coincides with those prevailing at the affected rivers during the peak of mortality episodes, strongly suggest that this iridovirus is the most likely primary cause of this large-scale mortality afflicting SMB, a local recreationally and economically important fish. While chemicals and other adverse environmental factors could be indirectly involved (e.g., immune suppressor), their role in the mortality episodes remains unclear.

Abbreviations

BLAST: Basic local alignment search tool; CPE: Cytopathic effect; DFV: Doctor fish virus; FHM: Fathead minnow cell line; IACUC: Institutional Animal Care and Use Committee; IP: Intraperitoneal; LBUSV: Largemouth bass ulcerative syndrome virus; LD_{50}: Median lethal dose; LMB: Largemouth bass; LMBV: Largemouth bass virus; MCP: Major capsid protein gene; MSU: Michigan State University; PBS: Phosphate buffered saline; SMB: Smallmouth bass; $TCID_{50}$: Tissue culture infectious dose; TCM: Tissue culture medium; YOY: Young of the year

Acknowledgements

We thank Michelle Gunn Van Deuren for her indispensable help throughout the study, the New Jersey Department of Environmental Protection Division of Fish and Wildlife for providing some of the fish used and the US Fish and Wildlife Service for providing viral isolates. We acknowledge the NOAA National Sea Grant College Program for providing the funding for this research.

Funding

This study was generously supported by the Pennsylvania Sea Grant College Program through the NOAA National Sea Grant College Program (grant no. 5031-COP-NOAA-0063), through the Pennsylvania Fish and Boat Commission (grant no. 4100070848).

Authors' contributions

TB performed all experimental infections, sampling, and processing of the data and interpretation of results; TPL and MF assisted with experimental design, infections, histopathology, microbiological analyses, and manuscript edits; CJY and GDS were involved in the conception and design of the study, acquisition of fish, interpretation of data, and editing of manuscript; ADW performed all genetic analyses; MK prepared and interpreted the histopathology; TOB performed statistical analyses. All authors were involved in drafting the manuscript or revising it critically for important intellectual content, and have given final approval of the version to be submitted for publication. Each author agrees to be accountable for all aspects of the work in ensuring that questions related to the accuracy or integrity of any part of the work are appropriately investigated and resolved.

Consent for publication

Not applicable

Competing interests

The authors declare that they have no competing interests.

Author details

[1]Department of Pathobiology and Diagnostic Investigation, College of Veterinary Medicine, Michigan State University, 1129 Farm Lane, Room 174, East Lansing, MI 48824, USA. [2]Division of Fish Production Services, Pennsylvania Fish and Boat Commission, State College, PA 16801, USA. [3]Division of Fisheries Management, Pennsylvania Fish and Boat Commission, Harrisburg, PA 17106, USA. [4]Comparative Medicine and Integrative Biology Program, College of Veterinary Medicine, Michigan State University, East Lansing, MI 48824, USA. [5]Department of Fisheries and Wildlife, College of Agriculture and Natural Resources, Michigan State University, East Lansing, MI 48824, USA. [6]Present address: Department of Microbiology, Immunology, and Biochemistry, School of Medicine, Wayne State University, Detroit, MI 48201, USA.

References

1. Smith GD, Blazer VS, Walsh HL, Iwanowicz LR, Starliper C, Sperry AJ. The effects of disease-related mortality of young-of-year smallmouth bass on population characteristics in the Susquehanna River Basin, Pennsylvania and the potential implications to conservation of black bass diversity; 2015. p. 319–332. In Tringali, M.D., Long, J.M., Birdsong, T.W., and Allen, M.S. (eds.), Black Bass Diversity: Multidisciplinary Science for Conservation. American Fisheries Society, Symposium 82, Bethesda, Maryland.
2. Chaplin JC, Crawford JK, Brightbill RA. Water-quality monitoring in response to young-of-the-year smallmouth bass (*Micropterus dolomieu*) mortality in the Susquehanna River and major tributaries, Pennsylvania-2008: U.S. Geological survey open-file report 2009–1216; 2009.
3. Walsh HL, Blazer VS, Iwanowicz LR, Smith G. A redescription of *Myxobolus inornatus* from young-of-the-year smallmouth bass (*Micropterus dolomieu*). J Parasitol. 2012;98:1236–42.
4. Starliper C, Blazer V, Iwanowicz L, Walsh H. Microbial isolates in diseased fishes, primarily smallmouth bass (Micropterus dolomieu), within the Chesapeake Bay drainage in 2009-2011. Proceedings of the West Virginia Academy of Science 2013;85(2).
5. Blazer VS, Iwanowicz LR, Starliper CE, Iwanowicz DD, Barbash P, Hedrick JD, et al. Mortality of centrarchid fishes in the Potomac drainage: survey results and overview of potential contributing factors. J. Aquat. Anim. Hlth. 2010;22: 190–218.
6. Plumb JA, Zilberg D. The lethal dose of largemouth bass virus in juvenile largemouth bass and the comparative susceptibility of striped bass. J. Aquat. Anim. Hlth. 1999;11:246–52.
7. Zilberg D, Grizzle JM, Plumb JA. Preliminary description of lesions in juvenile largemouth bass injected with largemouth bass virus. Dis Aquat Org. 2000;39:143–6.
8. Deng G, Li S, Xie J, Bai J, Chen K, Ma D, et al. Characterization of a ranavirus isolated from cultured largemouth bass (*Micropterus salmoides*) in China. Aquaculture. 2011;312:198–204.

9. Kayansamruaj P, Rangsichol A, Dong HT, Rodkhum C, Maita M, Katagiri T, et al. Outbreaks of ulcerative disease associated with ranavirus infection in barcoo grunter, *Scortum barcoo* (McCulloch & Waite). J Fish Dis. 2017;40: 1341-50.
10. Reed LJ, Muench H. A simple method of estimating fifty percent endpoints. Am J Hyg. 1938;27:493–7.
11. Grant EC, Philipp DP, Inendino KR, Goldberg TL. Effects of temperature on the susceptibility of largemouth bass to largemouth bass virus. J Aquat Anim Hlth. 2003;15:215–20.
12. Prophet E, Mills B, Arrington J, Sobin LH. Laboratory methods in histotechnology. Washington, D.C.: Armed Forces Institute of Pathology, American Registry of Pathology; 1992.
13. Altschul S, Gish W, Miller W, Myers E, Lipman D. Basic local alignment search tool. J Mol Biol. 1990;215:403–10.
14. Ishiguro EE, Kay WW, Ainsworth T, Chamberlain JB, Austen RA, Buckley JT, et al. Loss of virulence during culture of *Aeromonas salmonicida* at high temperature. J Bacteriol. 1981;148:333–40.
15. Bullock G, Hsu TC, Shotts E Jr. Columnaris disease of fishes: fish disease leaflet 72. Washington DC: U.S. Fish and Wildlife Service; 1986. p. 1–9.
16. USFWS and AFS-FHS (U.S. Fish and Wildlife Service and American Fisheries Society-Fish Health Section). AFS-FHS. FHS Blue Book: Suggested Procedures for the Detection and Identification of Certain Finfish and Shellfish Pathogens, 2016 ed; 2016. http://afs-fhs.org/bluebook/bluebook-index.php. Accessed 4 Jan 2016.
17. Grizzle JM, Altinok I, Noyes AD. PCR method for detection of largemouth bass virus. Dis Aquat Org. 2003;54:29–33.
18. Faisal M, Diamanka A, Loch TP, LaFrentz BR, Winters AD, Garcia JC, et al. Isolation and characterization of *Flavobacterium columnare* strains infecting fishes inhabiting the Laurentian Great Lakes basin. J Fish Dis. 2017;40:637–48.
19. Loch TL, Faisal M. Isolation of *Aeromonas salmonicida* subspecies *salmonicida* from lake whitefish (*Coregonus clupeaformis*) inhabiting lakes Michigan and Huron. J Great Lakes Res. 2010;36:13–7.
20. R Development Core Team. R: a language and environment for statistical computing. R Foundation for Statistical Computing, Vienna, Austria, 2016. https://www.R-project.org. Accessed 23 Oct 2017.
21. Therneau, T. A package for survival analysis in S. Version 2.38. 2015. https://CRAN.R-project.org/package=survival. Accessed 23 Oct 2017.
22. Kassambara A, Kosinski M. Survminer: drawing survival curves using 'ggplot2' R package version 0.4.0. 2017. http://www.sthda.com/english/rpkgs/survminer. Accessed 23 Oct 2017.
23. SAS Institute Inc. SAS/STAT® 12.3 User's Guide. Cary: SAS Institute Inc; 2013.
24. Piaskoski TO, Plumb JA, Roberts SR. Characterization of the largemouth bass virus in cell culture. J Aquat Anim Hlth. 1999;11:45–51.
25. Goldberg TL, Coleman DA, Grant EC, Inendino KR, Philipp DP. Strain variation in an emerging iridovirus of warm-water fishes. J Virol. 2003;77(16):8812–8.
26. Plumb JA, Grizzle JM, Young HE, Noyes AD, Lamprecht S. An iridovirus isolated from wild largemouth bass. J. Aquat. Anim. Hlth. 1996;8:265–70.
27. Forzán MJ, Jones KM, Ariel E, Whittington RJ, Wood J, Markham RJ, et al. Pathogenesis of frog virus 3 (Ranavirus, *Iridoviridae*) infection in wood frogs (*Rana sylvatica*). Vet Pathol. 2017;54:531–48.
28. Austin B, Austin DA. Bacterial fish pathogens: diseases of farmed and wild fish. Chichester: Praxis Publishing Ltd.; 2007.

18

Molecular detection and genomic characterization of porcine circovirus 3 in pigs from Northeast China

Zhuo Ha[1], Chang-zhan Xie[2,3], Jin-feng Li[5], Shu-bo Wen[2], Ke-long Zhang[6], Fu-long Nan[5], He Zhang[2], Ying-cheng Guo[4], Wei Wang[2,7], Hui-jun Lu[2,7*] and Ning-yi Jin[1,2,7*]

Abstract

Background: First identified in the United States in 2016, porcine circovirus type 3 (PCV3) is a newly emerging porcine circovirus exhibiting a wide range of clinical syndromes, which may be associated with the pathogenicity observed in pigs.

Results: The aim of this study was to identify and characterize the full genome sequence of PCV3 strains circulating in Northeast China. Herein, 105 lung samples isolated from sick pigs in Northeast China during 2018 were analyzed for PCV3. Using PCR, the total PCV3-positive rate was 33.3% (35/105), with rates of 17.8% (8/45), 66.7% (10/15), and 37.8% (17/45) in Heilongjiang, Jilin, and Liaoning province, respectively. Additionally, our findings showed that PCV3-positive samples had a high rate of co-infection with PCV2, PPV6, and PPV7. To study the evolution of the PCV3 in Northeast China, we sequenced the entire genome of 13 strains of PCV3. The results of phylogenetic analyses revealed that PCV3 could be divided into two clades, PCV3a and PCV3b. Interestingly, a G deletion at position 1072 was found in the 1999 nt genome of PCV3-CN2018LN-4 (MH277118). The G deletion terminated replicase protein translation and induced a truncated replicase protein.

Conclusion: These results contribute to the understanding of PCV3 molecular epidemiology and evolution in Northeast China. A new strain of PCV3 with truncated replicase protein was identified.

Keywords: PCV3, Northeast China, Co-infection, Complete genome, Replicase protein

Background

Porcine circovirus is a small non-enveloped virus with a circular, single-stranded DNA genome, belonging to the family *Circoviridae* [1]. Porcine circovirus 1 (PCV1) was initially identified in the 1970s as a contaminating agent in pig kidney cells and was considered nonpathogenic for swine [2, 3]. Porcine circovirus type 2 (PCV2), known as an essential pathogen of porcine circovirus-associated disease (PCVAD) clinically manifests as postweaning multisystemic wasting syndrome (PMWS), porcine dermatitis and nephropathy syndrome (PDNS), and reproductive failure, resulting in huge economic losses for the swine industry [4–6]. Currently, a novel circovirus termed porcine circovirus 3 (PCV3), was identified in the United States by metagenomic sequencing. PCV3 is characterized by PDNS, reproductive failure, as well as cardiac and multisystemic inflammation [7, 8]. Subsequently, other researchers found that PCV3 might be associated with congenital tremors (CT) and porcine respiratory disease complex (PRDC) [9, 10]. In addition, several strains of circovirus were found to be associated with different clinical diseases, such as fox circovirus, dog circovirus and duck circovirus [11–13]. Therefore, these data indicate that PCV3 might be associated with pathogenicity in pigs.

Similar to PCV2, PCV3 has a circular single-stranded DNA genome ranging in size from 1999 to 2001 nucleotides, containing two major open reading frames (ORFs), ORF1 and ORF2, which code for a 296 amino acid (aa) replicase protein (rep) and 214 aa capsid protein (cap),

* Correspondence: huijun_lu@126.com; ningyik@126.com
[2]Institute of Military Veterinary medicine, Academy of Military Medical Sciences, Changchun 130122, China
[1]College of Veterinary Medicine, Northeast Agricultural University, Harbin 150030, China
Full list of author information is available at the end of the article

respectively [7, 8]. PCV3 is widely circulated across the world, including the United States, China, Italy, Brazil, Korea, German, Denmark, and Spain [14–19]. In addition, increasing evidence has shown that PCV3 co-infections with other pathogens might be associated with increased pathogenicity in pigs [8, 20]. Moreover, the study by Li et al. demonstrated that PCV3 could be divided into two clades using the complete coding sequences [21, 22]. However, a greater number of PCV3 sequences are required to verify the division of PCV3 into different clades. In the present study, we investigated the extent of infection and co-infection of PCV3 in Northeast China. Furthermore, 62 complete coding sequences (13 in this study) were used for phylogenetic analysis and dividing PCV3 into different clades. More importantly, a new strain of PCV3 with a 13 aa deletion in the replicase protein was identified.

Results

Characteristics of the PCV3 epidemic in Northeast China

Of the 105 clinical lung samples obtained from sick pigs in Northeast China, the total PCV3-positive rate was 33.3% (35/105), with 17.8% (8/45) positivity in Heilongjiang, 66.7% (10/15) in Jilin, and 37.8% (17/45) in Liaoning. In addition, both the present and previous studies demonstrate that the presence of PCV3 is extensive in China (Fig. 1).

PCV3 co-infection with other pathogens

Among the 35 PCV3-positive samples, co-infection of PCV3 with other pathogens, including CSFV, PRRSV, SIV, PRV, PPV2, PPV6, PPV7, TTSuV1, TTSuV2, and PCV2 was analyzed. As shown in Table 1, PCV3 co-infections with PRRSV, PCV2, TTSuV1, TTSuV2, PPV2, PPV6, and PPV7 were detected in 11.4% (4/35), 45.7% (16/35), 34.3% (12/35), 25.7% (9/35), 25.7% (9/35), 60.0% (21/35), and 74.3% (26/35) of the samples, respectively. In contrast, neither CSFV, SIV, nor PRV were detected in the PCV3-positive samples. These data indicate that a high co-infection rate of PCV3 with PCV2, PPV6, and PPV7 exists, which provide valuable information for further study into the pathology of PCV3 in association with PCV2, PPV6, and PPV7.

Sequence comparison and phylogenetic analysis of PCV3

To analyze the genetic relationship of PCV3 strains collected in Northeast China, 13 complete sequences of

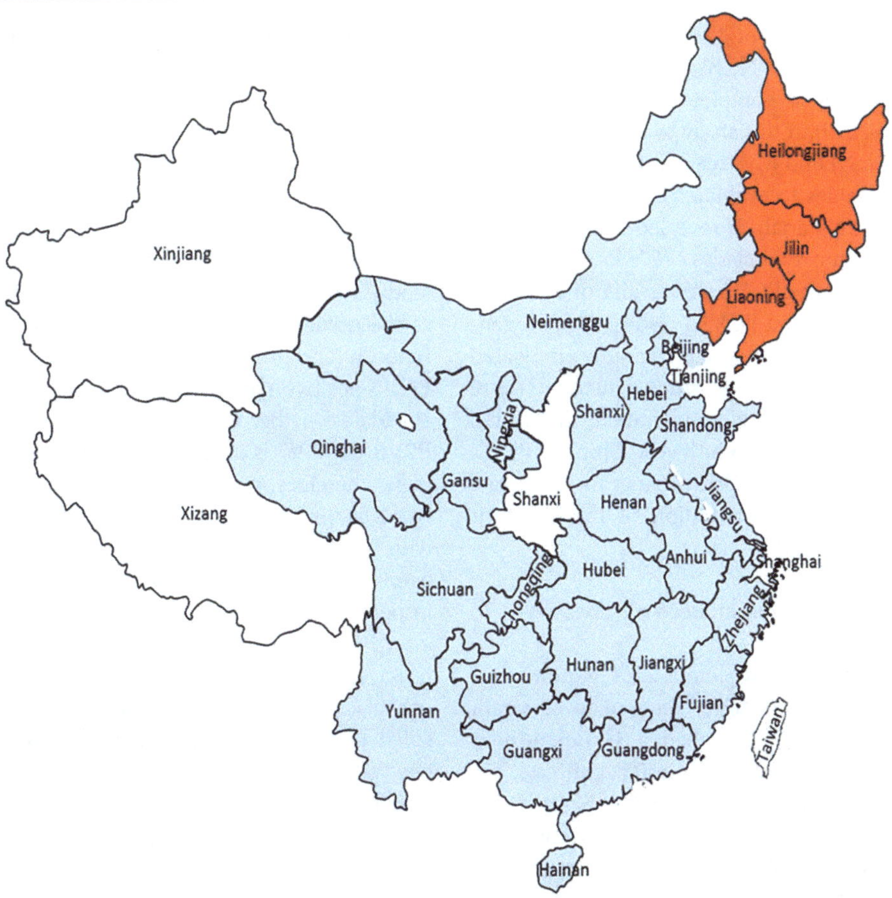

Fig. 1 Geographical distributions of PCV3 in China. Red represents the PCV3-positive provinces in this study. Light blue represents the PCV3-positive provinces in previous reports [14, 20, 26, 27]

Table 1 Detection of PCV3 co-infections with PRRSV, PCV2, TTSuV1, TTSuV2, PPV2, PPV6, PPV7, CSFV, PRV, and SIV in tissue samples isolated from sick pigs during 2018

Geographical origin	Number of samples	PCV3 positive	Co-infection									
			PRRSV	PCV2	TTSuV1	TTSuV2	PPV2	PPV6	PPV7	CSFV	PRV	SIV
Heilongjiang	45	8/45	3/8	3/8	4/8	2/8	2/8	6/8	6/8	0/8	0/8	0/8
Jilin	15	10/15	0/10	6/10	1/10	2/10	3/10	5/10	5/10	0/10	0/10	0/10
Liaoning	45	17/45	1/17	7/17	7/17	5/17	4/17	10/17	15/17	0/17	0/17	0/17
Northeast in China (total)	105	35/105	4/35	16/35	12/35	9/35	9/35	21/35	26/35	0/35	0/35	0/35

the PCV3 genome were amplified and sequenced. The complete genome sequences of the 13 samples infected with PCV3 identified in this study were deposited in GenBank under accession numbers MH277107-MH277119. Their genomes were two sizes: 1999 (MH277118) and 2000 nucleotides in length. The alignment of multiple sequences within these 13 PCV3 samples shared 97.9% to 100% and 98.8% to 99.9% nucleotide similarities at the ORF2 and complete genome sequences, respectively. The samples also shared 97.5% to 100% and 97.6% to 99.8% nucleotide similarities with available PCV3 ORF2 and complete genome sequences from the NCBI GenBank, respectively. The method described by Li et al. for dividing clades of PCV3 was used in this study [21, 22]. A total of 49 complete genome sequences were available in the NCBI database, which were used together with the 13 complete genome sequences (MH277107-MH277119) in this study to divide PCV3 into different clades. The NJ and ML tree was performed to reconstruct the phylogenies to evaluate the PCV3 complete genome sequences. This analysis revealed that the PCV3 strains were divided into two clades, PCV3a and PCV3b (Fig. 2). The majority of the PCV3 strains identified in this study were of the PCV3a and PCV3b clades. A phylogenetic analysis based on the complete genomes indicated that the 13 PCV3 strains in this study clustered more closely around the PCV3 strains identified in United States, South Korea, Italy and Southwest China (Fig. 2). The results revealed that the PCV3 variants in Northeast China exhibited a uniform distribution of the different PCV3 strains across the world.

PCV3 genome with a G deletion induced a truncated replicase protein

Surprisingly, from the 13 complete PCV3 genome sequences in our study, the genome sequences of strain PCV3-CN2018LN-4 (MH277118) had a G deletion at position 1072 compared with the total genome sequences of the PCV3 strains available in the NCBI database (Fig. 3a). The G deletion was found to prematurely terminate Rep protein translation, inducing a truncated Rep protein of 283 aa (Fig. 3b). Thus, the influence of this truncated Rep protein on the pathogenicity of PCV3 requires further study.

Discussion

Since PCV3 was first identified, PCV3 has been associated with PDNS, CT, reproductive failure, as well as cardiac and multi-systemic inflammation in infected pigs [7, 8]. However, whether PCV3 is capable of inducing a broad range of pathological effects similar to PCV2 requires further study. In this study, the co-infection of PCV3 with other pathogens was investigated using samples isolated from sick pigs. Moreover, PRRSV, PCV2, PRV, CSFV, SIV, TTSuV1, TTSuV2, PPV2, PPV6, and PPV7 were detected in the PCV3-positive tissue samples. Although no co-infections with CSFV, SIV, or PRV were detected in the PCV3-positive tissue samples, a high prevalence of PCV2, PPV6, and PPV7 existed in the PCV3-positive pigs. Previous studies have identified PCV3 and TTSuV1 co-infections in PDNS sows from the United States [8]. Moreover, a high co-infection rate of TTSuV1 and TTSuV2 with PCV3 was detected among clinically healthy sows [23], whereas a co-infection of PCV3 with PRRSV existed in pigs exhibiting severe respiratory disease [20]. Furthermore, a single PCV3 infection was found in pigs with reproductive failure [15]. In the present study, a single PCV3 infection was observed in four tissue of the tissue samples. In addition, this is the first study to report a high prevalence of PPV6 and PPV7 co-infection in PCV3-positive pigs. However, further study is required to elucidate whether PCV3 alone or co-infection with PCV2, PPV6, or PPV7 is involved in the pathogenicity exhibited in pigs. Therefore, there is an urgent need to isolate various PCV3 strains in vitro and evaluate the pathogenicity in pigs with PCV3 infections or co-infections with the above pathogens. In the present study, we attempted to isolate PCV3 in porcine kidney (PK-15) and swine testis (ST) cells; however, PCV3 was not found in either of the cells after four passages. In addition, an infectious molecular clone was constructed using PK-15 cells to isolate PCV3 but it also failed (data not shown). Thus, it is important to explore new approaches that can be used for successful PCV3 isolation.

PCV3 is widely circulated across the world, especially in China, where it has been detected almost provinces (Fig. 1). Recent epidemiological survey showed the positive rate of PCV3 infection between 19.1 and 39.4% in some provinces of China [15, 24–26]. In the present

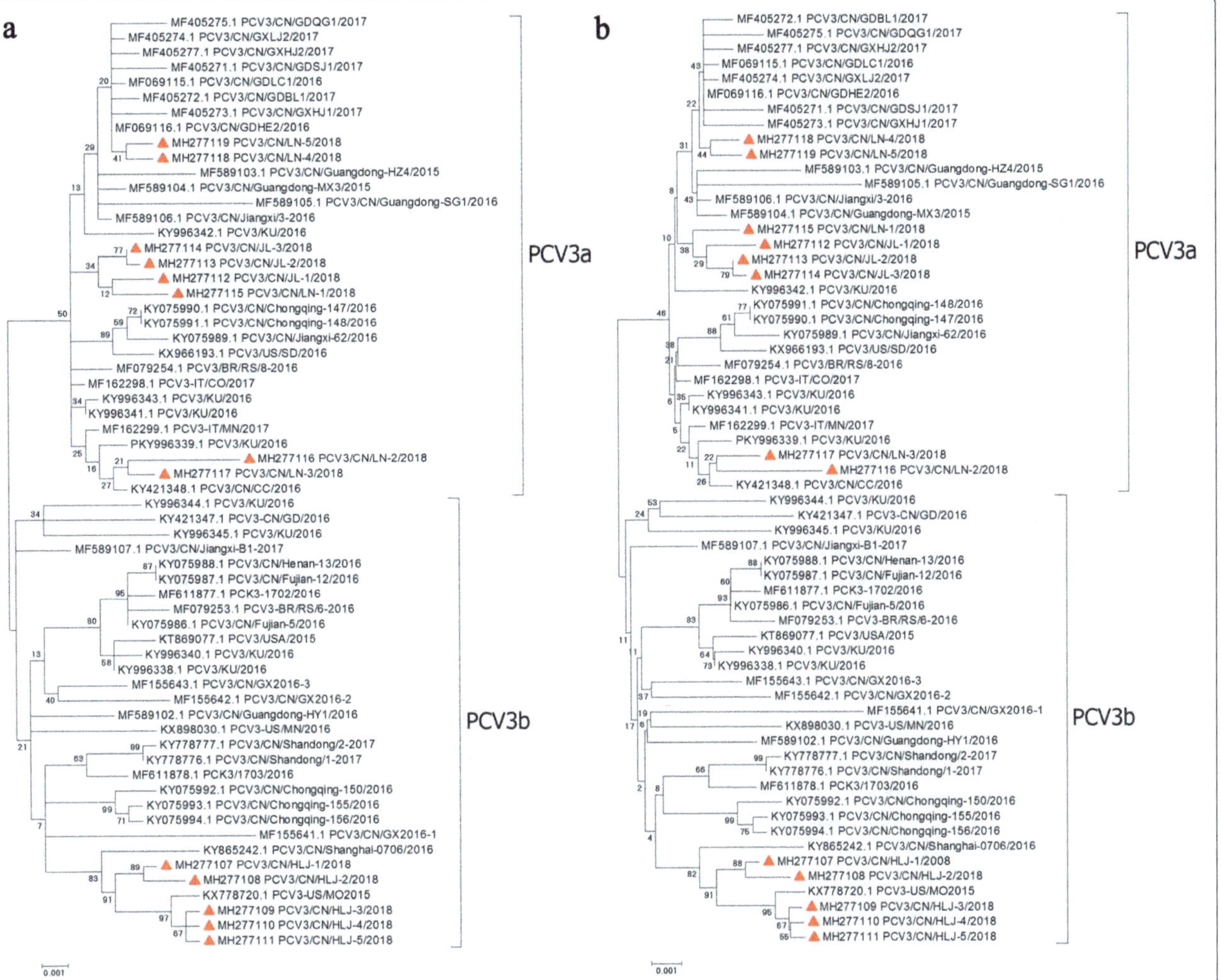

Fig. 2 Phylogenetic analysis of the 13 complete PCV3 genomes isolated in this study, together with 49 complete PCV3 genomes obtained from GenBank. The tree was constructed using MEGA version 6.06 with 1000 bootstraps replicates, p-distance model. PCV3 strains are denoted by its accession number at GenBank, isolation year, and country of origin. The 13 strains in this study are indicated with a red triangle. **a** maximum-likelihood method. **b** neighbor joining method

study, the positive rates of PCV3 were 17.8%, 66.7% and 37.8% in Heilongjiang, Jilin, and Liaoning province, respectively. Limited detection of sample numbers may result in the high prevalence in Jilin and low prevalence in Heilongjiang. However, a greater number of samples are required to verify the positive rate of PCV3 in Northeast China. The phylogenetic analysis of the PCV3 genome sequences revealed that the PCV3 strains in this study are closely related to strains isolated in United States (KX778720), South Korea (KY996339), Italy (MF162299), and Southwest China (KY421348). These results indicate that the PCV3 variants in Northeast China have a uniform distribution with different PCV3 strains across the world. A possible reason for this might be the presence of PCV3 infections within swine herds over long periods of time. Previous studies have found that PCV3 infections in China can be traced back to 1996 [27]. In addition, a common recent ancestor analysis suggests that PCV3 lineages have been circulating among swine herds over the past 50 years [26, 28].

The PCV2 strains were divided into different genotypes based on an analysis of the ORF2 gene sequences, from which a distance genotype was calibrated [29]. Fu et al. divided PCV3 was divided into three clades based on the aa codons in ORF2 (24, 27, 77, 104, and 150 aa) [26]. Fux et al. divided PCV3 into a1, a2, b1, and b2 subtypes based on the aa codons in ORF1 (122 aa), ORF2 (24, 27, 77, and 150 aa), and ORF3 (1, 4, and 27 aa) [30]. Subsequently, Li et al. study showed the phylogenetic analysis of PCV3 did not show clear clusters and consistent in different references based on the sequences of the ORF2 gene. But, by ML, maximum clade credibility (MCC), and NJ methods to reconstruct the phylogenies of PCV3 using complete coding sequences, PCV3 could

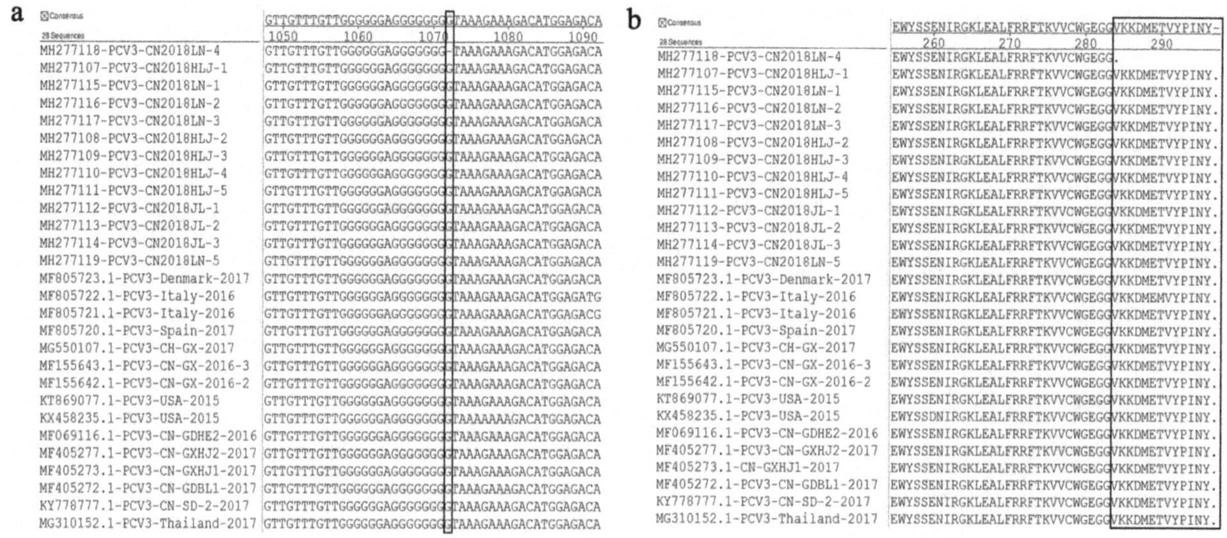

Fig. 3 Multiple alignments of the complete PCV3-CN2018LN-4 genome sequences and amino acids of the Rep protein with the other 27 PCV3 strains. (**a**) Complete PCV3 genome sequences between the sites 1048 and 1092. PCV3-CN2018LN-4 contains a G deletion at position 1072 compared with the other PCV3 strains. The deletion of G is indicated by a block. (**b**) PCV3 Rep protein between amino acid sites 255 and 296. There is a 13-amino acid deletion of PCV3-CN2018LN-4 from the amino acid positions 284 to 296. The deletion of 13 amino acids is indicated with a block

be stably divided into two clades, PCV3a and PCV3b, and further confirmed by principle component analysis (PCA) [21, 22]. Li et al. study provided a comprehensive genotype identification. In the present study, we referred to the methods used by Li et al. to divide the strains of PVC3 into different clades. We used the NJ and ML tree to reconstruct the phylogenies of PCV3 complete genome sequences. Two different trees displayed similar structures in the division of PCV3 into different clades. PCV3 strains could be divided into two clades, PCV3a and PCV3b. Therefore, phylogenetic analysis of complete coding sequences might be considered as PCV3 clade division in the future.

A previously study showed that the PCV3 genome was 1999–2001 nucleotides in length [8, 25, 30]. Moreover, the genome consisted of two inverse ORFs, coding for the Rep (296 aa) and cap (214 aa) proteins, respectively [8]. In this study, the 13 complete PCV3 genomes were 2000 or 1999 nucleotides in length. However, a G deletion at position 1072 of the PCV3-CN2018LN-4 (MH277118) strain was observed, which differs from previous reports. Interestingly, the G deletion at position of 1072 was in the coding region of the Rep protein, as the termination codon, TAA, is situated after the G gene. Thus, the G deletion induced a truncated Rep protein of 283 aa. This finding suggests that two different lengths (296 aa and 283 aa) of the Rep protein exist in PCV3. However, the impact of the truncated Rep protein (283 aa) in PCV3 infections requires further study.

Conclusions

PCV3 could be divided into two clades using complete coding sequences. A new strain PCV3-CN2018LN-4 (MH277118) had a G deletion in the coding region of the Rep protein and induced a truncated Rep protein of 283 aa, this finding suggests that two different lengths (296 aa and 283 aa) of the Rep protein exist in PCV3. There is a high prevalence of PPV6 and PPV7 co-infection in PCV3-positive pigs.

Methods

Tissue samples

In January 2018, a total of 105 lung tissue samples isolated from sick pigs were collected from seven large pig farms in Northeast China, three farms in Heilongjiang, one farm in Jilin, and three farms in Liaoning. All pigs were euthanized by an anesthetic overdose with the pentobarbital (100 mg/kg of body weight) before collecting the samples. Each pig farm consisted of a herd of over 10,000 sows. The age of all sampled pigs ranged from 4 to 16 weeks.

PCV3 detection

Viral DNA was extracted from the tissue samples using a Tissue DNA Kit (OMEGA Bio-Tek, Georgia, USA) according to the manufacturers' instructions and tested for PCV3 using PCR, as described previously [9]. Briefly, the detection of PCV3 by PCR was performed in a 25 μL final volume, consisting of 2 μL DNA, 1 μL of each 10 μM primer, 2 μL (2.5 mmol/L) dNTPs, 5 μL PCR buffer, 0.5 μL DNA polymerase (TransGen Biotech, Beijing, China), and ddH_2O up to 25 μL. The profile of the PCR conditions were as follows: 95 °C for 2 min, 35 cycles of 95 °C for 20 s, 56 °C for 20 s and 72 °C for 20 s, and a final extension at 72 °C for 5 min. The amplified products were analyzed on 1% agarose gels and the positive amplicons were sequenced (Comate Biosciences Co., Jilin, China).

Co-infection detection

For PCV3-positive tissue samples, viral RNA was extracted using a commercial RNA extraction kit (Sangon Biotech, Shanghai, China) in accordance with the instruction manual. PRRSV, SIV, and CSFV were detected using a one-step reverse transcription PCR Kit (TransGen Biotech, Beijing, China); the primers used for detection were the same as that described previously [31–33]. In addition, the DNA from PCV3-positive tissue samples was selected for the detection of PCV2, TTSuV1, TTSuV2, PPV2, PPV6, PPV7, and PRV, using the same primers as those previously described [34–38].

PCV3 genome sequencing and phylogenetic analysis

To obtain a full-length sequence of PCV3 for phylogenetic analysis, three pairs of overlapping PCR primers were utilized for whole genome sequencing as previously described [8]. PCR assays were performed using TransGen Biotech DNA polymerase (TransGen Biotech, Beijing, China). The PCR profile conditions were as follows: 95 °C for 2 min, 35 cycles at 95 °C for 20 s, 50 °C for 20 s, and 72 °C for 40 s, with a final extension at 72 °C for 5 min. The PCR products were purified using a Gel Extraction Kit (Bioer Technology, Hangzhou, China) and cloned into a pEASY-Blunt vector (TransGen Biotech, Beijing, China) for sequencing (Comate Biosciences Co., Jilin, China). A total of 13 complete PCV3 genome sequences were obtained in this study and all of the available complete PCV3 genomes from the NCBI GenBank were used for alignment and phylogenetic analysis. Multiple sequence alignments were performed using Lasergene software with the Clustal W program implemented in DNAStar software. A phylogenetic analysis of the complete PCV3 genome was reconstructed using MEGA 6.06 software with the p-distance-based, maximum-likelihood (ML) method and neighbor joining (NJ) method with 1000 bootstrap replicates.

Abbreviations

A: Alanine; K: Lysine; ORFs: Open reading frames; PCV3: Porcine circovirus type 3; PPV6: Porcine parvovirus 6; PPV7: Porcine parvovirus 7; R: Arginine; aa: amino acid; rep: Replicase protein; V: Valine

Acknowledgements

We would like to thank the native English speaking scientists of Elixigen Company (Huntington Beach, California) for editing our manuscript.

Funding

This work was supported by the following Grants: National Key Research and Development Program of China (grant number 2017YFD0500101 and 2016YFD0500401), National Natural Science Foundation of China (grant number 31272573). The funders did not play any role in the design, conclusions or interpretation of the study.

Authors' contributions

NYJ and HJL designed the experiments. ZH, CZX, SBW and JFL performed the experiments. ZH, KLZ, FLN, HZ analyzed the data and drew the graphs. ZH, YCG and WW wrote the paper. All authors approved the final manuscript.

Consent for publication

Not applicable.

Competing interests

All authors have declared no conflict of interest.

Author details

[1]College of Veterinary Medicine, Northeast Agricultural University, Harbin 150030, China. [2]Institute of Military Veterinary medicine, Academy of Military Medical Sciences, Changchun 130122, China. [3]College of Animal Science and Technology, Jilin Agricultural University, Changchun 130118, China. [4]Jilin Fengman area Animal Prevention and Control Center, Jilin 132013, China. [5]College of Veterinary Medicine, Jilin University, Changchun 130012, China. [6]College of Animal Science and Technology, Guangxi University, Nanning 530004, China. [7]Jiangsu Co-Innovation Center for the Prevention and Control of Important Animal Infectious Disease and Zoonoses, Yangzhou University, Yangzhou 225009, China.

References

1. Rosario K, Breitbart M, Harrach B, Segales J, Delwart E, Biagini P, Varsani A. Revisiting the taxonomy of the family Circoviridae: establishment of the genus Cyclovirus and removal of the genus Gyrovirus. Arch Virol. 2017; 162(5):1447–63.
2. Saha D, Lefebvre DJ, Ducatelle R, Doorsselaere JV, Nauwynck HJ. Outcome of experimental porcine circovirus type 1 infections in mid-gestational porcine foetuses. BMC Vet Res. 2011;7:64.
3. Tischer I, Rasch R, Tochtermann G. Characterization of papovavirus-and picornavirus-like particles in permanent pig kidney cell lines. Zentralbl Bakteriol Orig A. 1974;226(2):153–67.
4. Baekbo P, Kristensen CS, Larsen LE. Porcine circovirus diseases: a review of PMWS. Transbound Emerg Dis. 2012;59 Suppl 1:60–7.
5. Karuppannan AK, Ramesh A, Reddy YK, Ramesh S, Mahaprabhu R, Jaisree S, Roy P, Sridhar R, Pazhanivel N, Sakthivelan SM, et al. Emergence of porcine circovirus 2 associated reproductive failure in southern India. Transbound Emerg Dis. 2016;63(3):314–20.
6. Opriessnig T, Meng XJ, Halbur PG. Porcine circovirus type 2 associated disease: update on current terminology, clinical manifestations, pathogenesis, diagnosis, and intervention strategies. J Vet Diagn Invest. 2007;19(6):591–615.
7. Phan TG, Giannitti F, Rossow S, Marthaler D, Knutson TP, Li L, Deng X, Resende T, Vannucci F, Delwart E. Detection of a novel circovirus PCV3 in pigs with cardiac and multi-systemic inflammation. Virol J. 2016;13(1):184.
8. Palinski R, Pineyro P, Shang P, Yuan F, Guo R, Fang Y, Byers E, Hause BM. A novel porcine circovirus distantly related to known circoviruses is associated with porcine dermatitis and nephropathy syndrome and reproductive failure. J Virol. 2017;91(1).
9. Chen GH, Tang XY, Sun Y, Zhou L, Li D, Bai Y, Mai KJ, Li YY, Wu QW, Ma JY. Development of a SYBR green-based real-time quantitative PCR assay to detect PCV3 in pigs. J Virol Methods. 2018;251:129–32.

10. Kedkovid R, Woonwong Y, Arunorat J, Sirisereewan C, Sangpratum N, Lumyai M, Kesdangsakonwut S, Teankum K, Jittimanee S, Thanawongnuwech R. Porcine circovirus type 3 (PCV3) infection in grower pigs from a Thai farm suffering from porcine respiratory disease complex (PRDC). Vet Microbiol. 2018;215:71–6.
11. Li L, McGraw S, Zhu K, Leutenegger CM, Marks SL, Kubiski S, Gaffney P, Dela Cruz FN, Jr., Wang C, Delwart E et al: Circovirus in tissues of dogs with vasculitis and hemorrhage. Emerg Infect Dis 2013, 19(4):534–541.
12. Bexton S, Wiersma LC, Getu S, van Run PR, Verjans GM, Schipper D, Schapendonk CM, Bodewes R, Oldroyd L, Haagmans BL, et al. Detection of circovirus in foxes with meningoencephalitis, United Kingdom, 2009-2013. Emerg Infect Dis. 2015;21(7):1205–8.
13. Hong YT, Kang M, Jang HK. Pathogenesis of duck circovirus genotype 1 in experimentally infected Pekin ducks. Poult Sci. 2018.
14. Chen GH, Mai KJ, Zhou L, Wu RT, Tang XY, Wu JL, He LL, Lan T, Xie QM, Sun Y, et al. Detection and genome sequencing of porcine circovirus 3 in neonatal pigs with congenital tremors in South China. Transbound Emerg Dis. 2017;64(6):1650–4.
15. Ku X, Chen F, Li P, Wang Y, Yu X, Fan S, Qian P, Wu M, He Q. Identification and genetic characterization of porcine circovirus type 3 in China. Transbound Emerg Dis. 2017;64(3):703–8.
16. Kwon T, Yoo SJ, Park CK, Lyoo YS. Prevalence of novel porcine circovirus 3 in Korean pig populations. Vet Microbiol. 2017;207:178–80.
17. Franzo G, Legnardi M, Hjulsager CK, Klaumann F, Larsen LE, Segales J, Drigo M. Full-genome sequencing of porcine circovirus 3 field strains from Denmark, Italy and Spain demonstrates a high within-Europe genetic heterogeneity. Transbound Emerg Dis. 2018;65(3):602–6.
18. Tochetto C, Lima DA, Varela APM, Loiko MR, Paim WP, Scheffer CM, Herpich JI, Cerva C, Schmitd C, Cibulski SP, et al. Full-genome sequence of porcine circovirus type 3 recovered from serum of sows with stillbirths in Brazil. Transbound Emerg Dis. 2018;65(1):5–9.
19. Shen H, Liu X, Zhang P, Wang L, Liu Y, Zhang L, Liang P, Song C. Genome characterization of a porcine circovirus type 3 in South China. Transbound Emerg Dis. 2018;65(1):264–6.
20. Zhai SL, Zhou X, Zhang H, Hause BM, Lin T, Liu R, Chen QL, Wei WK, Lv DH, Wen XH, et al. Comparative epidemiology of porcine circovirus type 3 in pigs with different clinical presentations. Virol J. 2017;14(1):222.
21. Li G, He W, Zhu H, Bi Y, Wang R, Xing G, Zhang C, Zhou J, Yuen K, Gao G, et al. Origin, genetic diversity, and evolutionary dynamics of novel porcine circovirus 3. Advanced science. 2018. https://doi.org/10.1002/advs.201800275.
22. Li G, Wang H, Wang S, Xing G, Zhang C, Zhang W, Liu J, Zhang J, Su S, Zhou J. Insights into the genetic and host adaptability of emerging porcine circovirus 3. Virulence. 2018. https://doi.org/10.1080/21505594.2018.1492863.
23. Zheng S, Shi J, Wu X, Peng Z, Xin C, Zhang L, Liu Y, Gao M, Xu S, Han H, et al. Presence of torque Teno sus virus 1 and 2 in porcine circovirus 3-positive pigs. Transbound Emerg Dis. 2018;65(2):327–30.
24. Zou Y, Zhang N, Zhang J, Zhang S, Jiang Y, Wang D, Tan Q, Yang Y, Wang N. Molecular detection and sequence analysis of porcine circovirus type 3 in sow sera from farms with prolonged histories of reproductive problems in Hunan, China. Arch Virol. 2018. https://doi.org/10.1007/s00705-018-3914-7.
25. Wen S, Sun W, Li Z, Zhuang X, Zhao G, Xie C, Zheng M, Jing J, Xiao P, Wang M, et al. The detection of porcine circovirus 3 in Guangxi, China. Transbound Emerg Dis. 2018;65(1):27–31.
26. Fu X, Fang B, Ma J, Liu Y, Bu D, Zhou P, Wang H, Jia K, Zhang G. Insights into the epidemic characteristics and evolutionary history of the novel porcine circovirus type 3 in southern China. Transbound Emerg Dis. 2018; 65(2):e296–303.
27. Sun J, Wei L, Lu Z, Mi S, Bao F, Guo H, Tu C, Zhu Y, Gong W. Retrospective study of porcine circovirus 3 infection in China. Transbound Emerg Dis. 2018;65(3):607–13.
28. Saraiva GL, Vidigal PMP, Fietto JLR, Bressan GC, Silva Junior A, de Almeida MR. Evolutionary analysis of porcine circovirus 3 (PCV3) indicates an ancient origin for its current strains and a worldwide dispersion. Virus Genes. 2018.
29. Segales J, Olvera A, Grau-Roma L, Charreyre C, Nauwynck H, Larsen L, Dupont K, McCullough K, Ellis J, Krakowka S, et al. PCV-2 genotype definition and nomenclature. The Veterinary record. 2008;162(26):867–8.
30. Fux R, Sockler C, Link EK, Renken C, Krejci R, Sutter G, Ritzmann M, Eddicks M. Full genome characterization of porcine circovirus type 3 isolates reveals the existence of two distinct groups of virus strains. Virol J. 2018;15(1):25.
31. Nilubol D, Tripipat T, Hoonsuwan T, Tipsombatboon P, Piriyapongsa J. Genetic diversity of the ORF5 gene of porcine reproductive and respiratory syndrome virus (PRRSV) genotypes I and II in Thailand. Arch Virol. 2013; 158(5):943–53.
32. Paton DJ, McGoldrick A, Greiser-Wilke I, Parchariyanon S, Song JY, Liou PP, Stadejek T, Lowings JP, Bjorklund H, Belak S. Genetic typing of classical swine fever virus. Vet Microbiol. 2000;73(2–3):137–57.
33. Richt JA, Lager KM, Clouser DF, Spackman E, Suarez DL, Yoon KJ. Real-time reverse transcription-polymerase chain reaction assays for the detection and differentiation of north American swine influenza viruses. J Vet Diagn Invest. 2004;16(5):367–73.
34. Xiao CT, Gerber PF, Gimenez-Lirola LG, Halbur PG, Opriessnig T. Characterization of porcine parvovirus type 2 (PPV2) which is highly prevalent in the USA. Vet Microbiol. 2013;161(3–4):325–30.
35. Schirtzinger EE, Suddith AW, Hause BM, Hesse RA. First identification of porcine parvovirus 6 in North America by viral metagenomic sequencing of serum from pigs infected with porcine reproductive and respiratory syndrome virus. Virol J. 2015;12:170.
36. Xing X, Zhou H, Tong L, Chen Y, Sun Y, Wang H, Zhang G. First identification of porcine parvovirus 7 in China. Arch Virol. 2018;163(1):209–13.
37. Pogranichnyy RM, Yoon KJ, Harms PA, Swenson SL, Zimmerman JJ, Sorden SD. Characterization of immune response of young pigs to porcine circovirus type 2 infection. Viral Immunol. 2000;13(2):143–53.
38. Kekarainen T, Lopez-Soria S, Segales J. Detection of swine torque Teno virus genogroups 1 and 2 in boar sera and semen. Theriogenology. 2007;68(7): 966–71.

19

Molecular characterization of a porcine teschovirus HuN-1 isolate proliferating in PK-15 cell

Molin Chen[1], Wei Tang[2] and Xiuguo Hua[1*]

Abstract

Background: Porcine teschoviruses (PTVs) are small non-enveloped viruses with single-stranded, positive sense genomic RNA, belonging to the family *Picornaviridae*. Natural infections of teschoviruses are limited to pigs.

Results: In this study, a PTV HuN-1 was found that it could be proliferated in PK-15 cell, and it came from the pig fecal samples from Hunan province, in central China. The complete genome of the HuN-1 was amplified by RT-PCR and sequenced. The complete genome of HuN-1 isolate is 7098 nt, which shares the highest sequence identity (85. 9%) with the PTV 8 strain of Jilin/2003/2 and Fuyu/2009/2. The HuN-1 isolate contains only one ORF (from 320 to 7039 nt) coding a 2240 amino acid polyprotein. Aligned sequences show that more mutations occurred in the structural region than in the nonstructural region. Phylogenetic analysis showed that HuN-1 isolate did not clustered with the hitherto reported strains, according to P1 sequences, forming a subgroup in the PTV cluster.

Conclusion: In this study, complete genome of PTV HuN-1 was cloned and sequenced. Detection and characterization of further PTV strains from different geographic areas are important to understand the worldwide distribution and heterogeneity (serotype) of PTVs and their association with symptomatic infections in pigs.

Keywords: Swine, Teschovirus, Complete genome, PK-15 cell

Background

Porcine teschoviruses (PTVs) are small non-enveloped viruses with single-stranded, positive sense genomic RNA, belonging to the family *Picornaviridae*. Because of the nucleotide acid stability of the PTV, it was considered originally as porcine enteroviruses (PEVs) of cytopathogenic effect (CPE) group I, but has been classified as a separate genus, including former PEVs 1–7 and 11–13. Now, PTVs comprise at least thirteen serotypes identified [1–6]. Currently, PTV infections are diagnosed by RT-PCR [5–8] which replaced virus isolation in cell cultures and differentiation of serotypes by serological assays [9, 10].

Natural infections of teschoviruses are limited to pigs [11]. PTVs are the causative agents of severe and mild neurological disorders known as Teschen/Talfan disease, reproductive failure, pneumonia, and dermal lesions of swine [12–16]. Marked differences in neurovirulence among various strains of each serotype have been reported [17].

The PTV genome is 7.0–7.2 thousand nucleotides in length, and encodes a single polyprotein. The teschoviruses have the same genome organization: 5′-UTR, leader (L) protein, four structural proteins (VP4, VP2, VP3, and VP1), seven non-structural proteins (2A-2C, 3A-3D) and 3′-UTR [3, 18].

In this study, the complete nucleotide sequences and detailed genomic organization of PTV HuN-1 isolate are presented, and an analysis of the complete nucleotide sequences is reported. The existence of diversity and genetic recombination in porcine teschovirus are further confirmed.

Methods

Propagation and isolation of PTVs

Propagation and isolation of PTVs were performed following procedures. Briefly, PK-15 cells in our lab were maintained in Dulbecco's modified Eagle's medium

* Correspondence: hxg@sjtu.edu.cn
[1]Shanghai Key Laboratory of Veterinary Biotechnology, School of Agriculture and Biology, Shanghai Jiao Tong University, Shanghai 200240, China
Full list of author information is available at the end of the article

(DMEM), and 10% (*v*/v) fetal bovine serum. Fecal sample of PTV positive is filtrated by 0.22 μm filter. Cell monolayers (25 cm^2 flasks) were covered with the Filtrate for adsorption of one hour. And then, discuss the filtrate and add fresh media with 2% fetal bovine serum for viral propagation at 37 °C, 5% CO_2. Observing the cytopathic effect (CPE), incubation was ended when 90% of the monolayers were destroyed. Blind passages three time. Then for ten generations. The sample of PTVs was isolated and purified by the plaque three times. After three freeze–thaw cycles, the specimen was clarified prior to storage at − 80 °C until used. Collection of pig fecal samples was performed after obtaining consent from the pig farm. All study protocols were approved by the Institutional animal care and use committee of the Shanghai Jiao Tong University. Experimental animals license Number: SYXK (shanghai) 2013–0052.

RT-PCR detection of PTVs

RNA was extracted from 450 μl of the specimen with TRIzol Reagent (Invitrogen, USA), following the manufacturer's instructions. The isolated RNA was dissolved in 25 μl RNase-free dH_2O. cDNA synthesis was performed using a PrimeScript_RT Reagent Kit (Takara, Dalian, China). Briefly, purified viral RNA 16 μl was mixed with 4 μl of PrimeScript_RT Master Mix to a total volume of 20 μl. The reaction mixture was heated to 42 °C for 5 min, chilled on ice and then incubated for 1.5 h at 37 °C followed by 5 s at 85 °C to inactivate the reverse transcriptase. According to the reference [6], a pairs of primers were synthesized to detect PTVs based on the conserved sequences in 5'-UTR region (primer F: 5'-GTGGCGACAGGGTACAGAAGAC-3'; primer R: 5'-GGCCAGCCGCGACCCTGTCAG-3').

PCR amplification of teschovirus HuN-1 genome

The primers were designed with Primer 5.0 and synthesized by Life Technologies of Shanghai, China. According to the reference genomic sequences of porcine teschoviruses from GenBank, Eight pairs of primers (as Table 1 showed) was designed to amplify the teschovirus HuN-1 isolate genome.

PCR was carried out using 2 μl of cDNA and a master mix containing 5 μl 10x LA PCR buffer, 2 μl of each primer (20 μM), 8 μl dNTP mixture (2.5 mM each), 0.5 μl LA Taq (Takara, Dalian, China), and 30.5 μl of ddH_2O in a total reaction volume of 50 μl. The mixture was denatured at 94 °C for 1 min, followed by 33 cycles of 45 s at 94 °C, 45 s at 50 °C and 2 min at 72 °C, and a final extension at 72 °C for 10 min. There were minor modifications to the cycling conditions depending on the primers and the length of the products.

Nucleotide sequencing and analysis

PCR products were extracted from an agarose gel using an AxyPrepTM DNA Gel Extraction Kit. Purified PCR products were then ligated into a pMD18-T vector (Takara, Dalian, China). For each product, five positive colonies were selected and sequenced. The sequence

Table 1 Primers were designed to amplify the Full-length genome of PTV HuN-1

Primers	Nucleotide Sequences	Position	Length(nt)
P1-F	5'-CTCCCTTTGAATTTGTAA-3'	1–18	382
P1-R	5'-GGCCAGCCGCGACCCTGTCAG-3'	362–382	
P2-F	5'-GGACTGGACTTGTGCTGCC-3'	344–362	1328
P2-R	5'-ATRTCAACRCTRGGTGTTCCTCC-3'	1648–1671	
P3-F	5'-CCCTAGGACAAATTCMTCAGCAA-3'	1522–1544	978
P3-R	5'-CCTGTTTCTGCAGGTTGMAGGGG-3'	2477–2499	
P4-F	5'-GGTCACGGGGATACATCACTA-3'	2316–2336	988
P4-R	5'- AACAGGGAGAAGTTTGTAGCA –3'	3262–3282	
P5-F	5'-ATCTTATTCAAATGAATCTAC-3'	3172–3192	797
P5-R	5'-YTCTGTCTGGRTGCCTGTAATT-3'	3947–3968	
P6-F	5'- CGGCTCAAAACCTGGAGAACT –3'	3839–3859	789
P6-R	5'- TAGGGTATGTTTGCCATGTTTA –3	4606–4627	
P7-F	5'-AAGCCTGACGGGACACTTGAT-3	4493–4513	1457
P7-R	5'-GGTTCAAGAAAGTCTGGTGGC-3	5929–5949	
P8-F	5'- GCCAACATTTGTGTGTGGTGATC -3	5743–5765	1356
P8-R	5'-AACTAAAACTACTCAAGCAACAGGC-3	7074–7098	

Reference strains were used to design the primers are as follows: CH/IMH/03 (DQ355222); JF613 (GU446660); 10BJ02 (JQ975417); HB-2010 (JQ664746); Jilin/2003/2 (JN710381); NC_003985

data were first checked for the quality using software Chromas, and then assembled and aligned by DNAstar software package. Phylogenetic tree based on the P1 sequences was constructed by the maximum-likelihood method and using the best model, TN93 (Tamura-Nei) with 1000 bootstrap replicates in MEGA version 5.1. The bootstrap values are shown at the branch nodes representing the most recent common ancestor of the clade they support (values< 70% not shown).

Results

Detection of the CPE samples was PTV positive. The results showed that the PTVs could persistently proliferating in PK-15 cell. The sample of PTVs was isolated and purified by the plaque three times. Based on the published genomic sequence of PTVs, the whole genome of PTV isolate named HuN-1 was sequenced by using specific primers. The genome sequences of the PTV HuN-1 isolate were 7098 nucleotides in length, and contains one ORF (from 320 to 7039 nt) coding a 2240 amino acid polyprotein. This was preceded by a 319-nt-long 5′-UTR and followed by a 59-nt-long 3′-UTR. The coding regions contain four parts: L region(354 nt) coding L-protein; P1 regions coding structural proteins VP4(222 nt), VP2(840 nt), VP3(726 nt) and VP1(792 nt); P2 regions coding nonstructural proteins 2A(63 nt), 2B(438 nt) and 2C(963 nt); P3 regions coding nonstructural proteins 3A(273 nt), 3B(75 nt), 3C(615 nt) and 3D(1356 nt).The base composition of the full-length genome of HuN-1was found to be 27.97% A, 22.03% G, 28.18% U and 21.82% C. Sequence analysis based on the complete genomic sequences of the isolate in this study and the other known serotype reference strains, the results show that HuN-1 shares the highest nucleotide sequences identity (85.9%) with the PTV 8 strain of Jilin/2003/2(JN710381) and Fuyu/2009/2(KC757344), and as Fig. 1 showed.

To determine genetic relationships of PTV HuN-1 isolate with the reference strains [19], twenty two representative strains were selected to construct the phylogenetic tree (as Fig. 2 showed) on the basis of P1 sequences. The result showed that HuN-1 isolate did not cluster with the hitherto reported strains, forming a subgroup in the PTV cluster.

The genomic sequence of PTV HuN-1 isolate has been deposited in GenBank under accession number: KU297677.

Discussion

PTVs were identified during serious outbreaks of polioencephalomyelitis in Europe in 1929 and 1957 respectively [12, 13]. PTVs were first reported in Inner Mongolia, China, 2003. Subsequently, PTVs were reported in Hebei, Beijing, Shanghai, and Heilongjiang Province [20, 21]. Now, a porcine teschovirus HuN-1 was found that it could be proliferated in PK-15 cell, and it came from the pig fecal samples from China. The present study showed that the isolation of PTV strains from domestic pigs is easily accomplished in PK-15 cell directly from pig stools.

A pair of primers (Table 1, P4-F and P4-R) were designed to amplify PTV fragments of the CPE samples for the high-mutation region VP1. The results showed that the CPE samples' product sequences were identical. No discrepancies of sequence fragments were found in the cultures purified subsequently. Therefore, we proposed

Percent Identity (upper triangle); Divergence (lower triangle)

	1	2	3	4	5	6	7	8	9	10	11	12	13	14	15	16	17		
1		84.1	84.7	84.7	85.3	81.3	81.5	81.5	84.7	83.2	83.4	84.7	86.6	84.1	84.2	86.8	84.0	1	PTV-6 PS 37
2	18.2		81.9	81.9	84.6	81.9	80.8	81.3	81.5	85.1	85.4	82.1	86.6	83.5	81.6	83.9	86.3	2	PTV-7 F 43
3	17.4	21.0		100.0	87.4	81.6	81.6	82.0	85.9	81.2	81.6	85.2	84.1	81.3	84.9	84.4	81.9	3	PTV-8 Fuyu 2009 2
4	17.4	21.0	0.0		87.4	81.6	81.6	82.0	85.9	81.2	81.6	85.2	84.1	81.3	84.9	84.4	81.9	4	PTV-8 Jilin 2003-2,
5	16.6	17.4	14.1	14.1		81.1	81.0	81.0	84.0	83.6	83.9	84.4	86.8	81.6	84.0	85.1	84.1	5	PTV-8 UKG 173 74
6	21.8	21.0	21.4	21.4	22.1		82.9	81.7	82.3	81.1	81.4	81.4	81.0	81.8	81.3	81.3	81.8	6	PTV-9 Vir 2899 84
7	21.5	22.6	21.5	21.5	22.3	19.7		83.8	82.1	83.2	83.4	80.7	80.7	83.3	82.3	80.7	81.2	7	PTV-10 Vir 460 88
8	21.6	21.8	20.9	20.9	22.3	21.3	18.7		81.5	84.9	85.4	81.2	80.4	84.0	81.0	80.9	81.7	8	PTV-11 Dresden
9	17.5	21.7	16.0	16.0	18.4	20.5	20.7	21.6		80.6	80.8	84.3	83.9	80.6	85.7	83.6	81.0	9	PTV HuN-1
10	19.3	16.8	21.9	21.9	18.7	22.1	19.6	17.3	22.8		99.5	81.6	84.3	85.9	81.1	82.6	85.4	10	PTV-1 CH IMH 03
11	19.1	16.5	21.5	21.5	18.4	21.8	19.2	16.6	22.6	0.5		81.8	84.5	86.1	81.3	82.8	85.6	11	PTV-1 Talfan
12	17.4	20.8	16.8	16.8	17.8	21.8	22.8	21.9	18.1	21.4	21.2		86.7	81.2	85.7	83.7	82.0	12	PTV-2 JF613
13	15.0	14.9	18.3	18.3	14.9	22.3	22.7	23.1	18.5	17.9	17.5	15.1		82.8	85.0	86.0	84.9	13	PTV-2 T80
14	18.1	18.9	21.9	21.9	21.5	21.2	19.4	18.4	22.8	16.0	15.8	22.0	19.9		80.8	83.7	84.0	14	PTV-3 O 2b
15	18.1	21.5	17.2	17.2	18.5	21.9	20.5	22.2	16.2	22.1	21.9	16.2	17.2	22.6		84.3	81.6	15	PTV-4 10BJ02
16	14.8	18.5	17.8	17.8	17.0	21.9	22.7	22.5	18.9	20.2	19.8	18.8	15.8	18.6	18.1		83.6	16	PTV-4 PS 36
17	18.2	15.3	21.0	21.0	18.1	21.2	22.0	21.3	22.3	16.5	16.3	20.9	17.0	18.2	21.4	18.8		17	PTV-5 F 26
	1	2	3	4	5	6	7	8	9	10	11	12	13	14	15	16	17		

Fig. 1 Identity of genome sequences of PTV HuN-1 isolate and other serotype reference strains

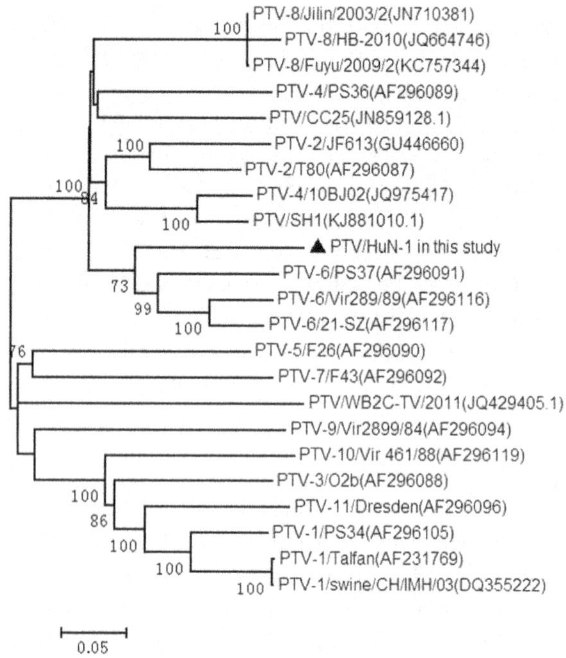

Fig. 2 Phylogenetic analysis of PTV HuN-1 together with those of reference representative strains based on the P1 gene (2580 nt). Filled triangle HuN-1 in this study

that only one teschorvirus isolate was separated from the pig feces' sample. A pig farm may have multiple serotypes of teschorvirus, but only this virus was isolated from the experiment. To my way of thinking the reason may be that HuN-1 is a strong virulent strain, the others are weak strains, and the rapid increase of HuN-1 inhibits the increase of other strains. After many passages, HuN-1 occupies an absolute advantage, so the detected sequence is HuN-1 and no similar sequences were yielded from the isolate.

The genome of the HuN-1 isolate was amplified and sequenced, exclusive of the 5′poly(C) and the 3′poly (A) tract. The single ORF is translated into a polyprotein, which is subsequently processed. Initiation of protein synthesis on the PTV RNA could occur at one of two different AUG codons [22]. In the PTV HuN-1 sequences, there were two initiation codon, the first one at position 320, and the second one at position 416. However, comparison with other PTV sequences indicated that the first of these AUGs was not conserved, even though an extremely high level of sequence identity between different strains of PTV in coding region of leader protein. The basic organization of the product is similar in several picornaviruses. The primary cleavages separate the polyprotein into three or four regions, L, P1, P2, and P3 [3, 18]. The P1 region is precursor to the structural proteins, and P2 and P3 regions split into the nonstructural proteins responsible for replication and proliferation. The leader protein, P2, and P3 is quite conserved among the teschoviruses.

For PTVs, most genomic variations occur in coding region of the structural protein [4]. Based on the molecular comparisons presented in this study, the entire P1 region encoding structural proteins displayed high rates of mutations [18]. The complete P1 nucleotide sequences were used for phylogenetic analysis and serotype typing in this study, the result showed that this virus HuN-1 did not cluster to reported reference strains. So we speculate the HuN-1 might belongs to another new serotype, although there is still insufficient data to support this proposition. Until now, more than thirteen serotypes have been identified [5]. They were popularly mixed distribution in pig farms. In China, PTV2, PTV4, and PTV8 were the main serotypes in epidemic [23].

Conclusions

In this study, complete genome of PTV HuN-1 was cloned and sequenced. The genome sequences of the HuN-1 isolate were 7098 nucleotides in length, and contains one ORF (from 320 to 7039 nt) coding a 2240 amino acid polyprotein. Phylogenetic analysis showed that HuN-1 did not cluster with the hitherto reported strains, forming a subgroup in the PTV cluster. Detection and characterization of further PTV strains from different geographic areas are important to understand the worldwide distribution and heterogeneity of PTVs and their association with symptomatic infections in pigs.

Abbreviations

nt: Nucleotide; ORF: Open reading frame; PK: Porcine Kidney; RT-PCR: Reverse transcription-polymerase chain reaction; UTR: Untranslated Region; VP1: Viral protein 1

Funding

XH was funded by the National Key Research and Development Program of China No.2017YFC1200203 and the National Natural Science Foundation of China (Grant No.31572525).

Authors' contributions

MC designed the method, collected the data, and prepared the manuscript. WT and XH planned the study, contributed to and reviewed the manuscript. All authors read and approved the final manuscript.

Competing interests

The authors declare that they have no competing interests.

Author details
[1]Shanghai Key Laboratory of Veterinary Biotechnology, School of Agriculture and Biology, Shanghai Jiao Tong University, Shanghai 200240, China. [2]Department of Library, Hunan University of Science and Engineering, Yongzhou 425199, People's Republic of China.

References

1. Knowles NJ, Buckley LS, Pereira HG. Classification of porcine enteroviruses by antigenic analysis and cytopathic effects in tissue culture: description of 3 new serotypes. Arch Virol. 1979;62:201–8.
2. Knowles NJ. The association of group III porcine enteroviruses with epithelial tissue. Vet Rec. 1988;122:441–2.
3. Zell R, Dauber M, Krumbholz A, Henke A. Birch- Hirschfeld E, et al. porcine teschoviruses comprises at least eleven distinct serotypes: molecular and evolutionary aspects. J Virol. 2001;75:1620–31.
4. Cano-Gómez C, Palero F, Buitrago MD, et al. Analyzing the genetic diversity of teschoviruses in Spanish pig populations using complete VP1 sequences. Infect Genet Evol. 2011;11:2144–50.
5. Cano-Gómez C, Jiménez-Clavero MA. Complete coding genome sequence of a putative novel Teschovirus serotype 12 strain. Genome Announc. 2016; 4(2):e00107_16.
6. Palmquist JM, Munir S, Taku A, et al. Detection of porcine teschovirus and enterovirus type II by reverse transcription–polymerase chain reaction. J Vet Diagn Investig. 2002;14:476–80.
7. Zell R, Krumbholz A, Henke A, Birch-Hirschfeld E, Stelzner A, et al. Detection of porcine enteroviruses by nRT-PCR: differentiation of CPE groups I-III with specific primer sets. J Virol Methods. 2000;88:205–18.
8. Krumbholz A, Wurm R, Scheck O, Zell R, et al. Detection of frequent porcine teschoviruses and enteroviruses by LightCycler real-time PCR. J Virol Methods. 2003;113:51–63.
9. Knowles NJ, Buckley LS. Differentiation of porcine enterovirus serotypes by complement fixation. Res vet Sci 29: 113–115.Serotypes. Arch. Virol. 1980;62:201–8.
10. Auerbach J, Prager D, Neuhaus S, Loss U, Witte H. Grouping of porcine enteroviruses by indirect immunofluorescence and description of two new serotypes. Zbl Vet Med B. 1994;41:277–82.
11. Boros Á, Nemes C, Pankovics P, Kapusinszky B, Delwart E, Reuter G. Porcine teschovirus in wild boars in Hungary. Arch Virol. 2012;157(8):1573–8.
12. Trefny L. Massive illness of swine in Teschen area. Zvoroleki Obzori. 1930;23: 235_6.
13. Harding JOJ, Done JT, Kershaw GF. A transmissible polio-encephalomyelitis of pigs (Talfan disease). Vet Rec. 1957;69:824–32.
14. Edington N, Christofinis GJ, Betts AO. Pathogenicity of Talfan and Konratice strains of Teschen virus in gnotobiotic pigs. J Comp Pathol. 1972;82:393–9.
15. Long JF, Koestner A, Kasza L. Infectivity of three porcine polioencephalomyelitis viruses for germfree and pathogen-free pigs. Am J Vet Res. 1966;27:274_9.
16. Chiu SC, Shu CH, Chang CC, Chang CY, Huang CC, Pang VF, Wang FI. The role of porcine teschovirus in causing diseases in endemically infected pigs. Vet Microbiol. 2012;161:88–95.
17. Deng MY, Millien M, Jacques-Simon R, Flanagan JK, et al. Diagnosis of porcine teschovirus encephalomyelitis in the Republic of Haiti. J Vet Diagn Investig. 2012;24:671–8.
18. Doherty M, Todd D, McFerran N, Hoey EM. Sequence analysis of a porcine enterovirus serotype 1 isolate: relationships with other picornaviruses. J Gen Virol. 1999;80:1929_41.
19. Kaku Y, Murakami Y, Sarai A, Wang Y, Ohashi S, Sakamoto K. Antigenic properties of porcine teschovirus 1 (PTV-1) Talfan strain and molecular strategy for serotyping of PTVs. Arch Virol. 2007;152:929–40.
20. Qiu Z, Wang Z, Zhang B, Zhang J, Cui S. The prevalence of porcine teschovirus in the pig population in northeast of China. J Virol Methods. 2013;193:209–14.
21. Zhang CF, Cui SJ, Hu S, Zhang Z, Guo Q, Zell R. Isolation and characterization of the first Chinese strain of porcine Teschovirus-8. J Virol Methods. 2010;167:208–13.
22. Kaku Y, Chard LS, Inoue Y, Belsham GJ. Unique characteristics of a picornavirus internal ribosome entry site from the porcine Teschovirus-1 Talfan. J Virol. 2002;76(22):11721–8.
23. Sun H, Gao H, Chen M, Lan D, Hua X, Wang C, Yuan C, Yang Z, Cui L. New serotypes of porcine teschovirus identified in shanghai. China Arch Virol. 2015;160:831–5.

Evolutionary analysis of rabies virus isolates from Guangxi Province of southern China

Xian-Kai Wei[1,2], Xiao-Xia He[2], Yan Pan[1,2], Cheng Liu[2], Hai-Bo Tang[1,2], Yi-Zhi Zhong[2], Xiao-Ning Li[1,2], Jing-Jing Liang[1,2] and Ting Rong Luo[1,2*]

Abstract

Background: Rabies is a severe epidemic in Guangxi province, China, with hundreds of deaths occurring each year. In the past six decades, rabies has emerged three times in Guangxi, and the province has reported the largest number of rabies cases in China. The domestic dog is the principal vector for rabies, and 95% of human cases are associated with transmission from dogs.

Results: To understand the genetic relationship between street rabies virus (RABV) from Guangxi, genetic diversity analysis was performed using RABV isolates collected between 1999 and 2012. The N gene of 42 RABV isolates, and the P and M genes, as well as fragments of the 3′ terminus (L^{1-680}) and the polymerase activity module of the L gene (L^{pam}) of 36 RABV isolates were sequenced. In addition, whole genome sequencing was performed for 5 RABV isolates. There was evidence of topological discrepancy in the phylogenetic trees based on different genes of the RABV isolates. Amino acid variation of the deduced N protein exhibited different patterns to those obtained from the P and M proteins reported here, and the previously reported G protein (Tang H. et al., PLoS Negl Trop Dis, 8(10): e3114, 2014), and L^{1-680} and L^{pam}. These RABV isolates were divided into three main branches against fixed strains.

Conclusion: RABV is prevalent in Guangxi province and strains collected over the last two decades belong mainly to three groups (I, II, III). These RABV isolates reveal genetic diversity. Individual RABV genes from Guangxi exhibit different evolutionary characteristics. The results will have benefits for continuing comprehensive rabies surveillance, prevention and control in China.

Keywords: Rabies virus, Genetic diversity, Evolution

Background

The rabies virus (RABV), a member of the Lyssavirus genus, which is found worldwide, causes lethal viral encephalitis in a wide range of host species. Rabies is of specific concern as it is fatal to humans and has a significant impact on public health.

Previous research on the phylogenetic analysis of the RABV N gene has identified differences in RABVs found in bats, compared to those found in terrestrial mammals [1, 2]. A better understanding of the N gene evolutionary trajectory can assist the development of control measures [3, 4]. Evolutionary analysis based on the lyssavirus surface glycoprotein (ectodomain) revealed that point mutations are the most frequent mutation in lyssavirus evolution; additionally, all lyssavirus lineages have similar evolutionary rates [5]. Phylogenetic analyses of N, P, and G gene sequences among bat lyssaviruses from central Asia have demonstrated that quantitative overlap between the currently established genotypes likely occurs at the amino acid level [6, 7]. Phylogenetic analysis based on the full RABV genome, or based on N, P, M, G, and L genes, resulted in phylogenetic trees with similar topologies, indicating that individual lyssavirus genes are likely sufficient to establish phylogenetic relationships [8]. This suggests that rigorous phylogenetic techniques based on full-length genome sequences provide considerable discriminatory power for genotype classification within the lyssaviruses [9]. The current global understanding of RABV phylogeography is that there

* Correspondence: tingrongluo@gxu.edu.cn
[1]State Key Laboratory for Conservation and Utilization of Subtropical Agro-Bioresources, Guangxi University, Nanning 530004, Guangxi, China
[2]Laboratory of Veterinary Microbiology and Animal Infectious Diseases, College of Animal Sciences and Veterinary Medicine, Guangxi University, Nanning 530004, Guangxi, China

are six clades of RABV in non-flying mammals, each with a distinct geographical distribution, likely reflecting major physical barriers to gene flow.

In China, human rabies has re-emerged since 1997. Two distinct clades of RABV isolates found in China were identified by genetic analysis [10, 11]. Investigation of the molecular epidemiology of rabies in southern China has demonstrated that long-distance migration, or trans-provincial movement of dogs (by humans) from high-incidence regions may be one of the causes of the recent human rabies epidemics in southern China [12]. Evolutionary dynamic analysis based on the G gene shows that the RABV currently circulating in China consists of three main groups [13], and that the RABV in China and Southeast Asia share a common ancestor [14]. Phylogenetic analysis based on the 3′ terminus of the N gene shows that RABV isolates from Guangxi province, south China can be divided into four groups [15]. Further studies have demonstrated that isolates from groups I, II, and III are lethal once introduced in mice, whereas isolates of group IV are not fatal to either adult or suckling mice [15].

In this study we sequenced the N, P and M gene as well as L^{1-680} and L^{pam} of the Guangxi isolates. In addition, we performed whole-genome sequencing for 5 of the isolates. The goal of this study was to identify novel genetic features, in several different RABV genes, that may have occurred in the evolutionary process of Guangxi RABV. Due to the fact that live attenuated rabies vaccines have been used in Guangxi in the past, and these vaccines contain RABV strains with the potential for replication and reversion to the pathogenic form, all field isolates were compared against these vaccine strains.

Methods

Isolation of virus

Between 1999 and 2012, 42 RABV isolates were obtained from rabid dogs, cattle, pigs, and asymptomatic dogs that were received from different regions of Guangxi. All samples were provided by the Guangxi Center for Animal Diseases Control and Prevention, with permission from the Veterinary Administration of the Guangxi Provincial Government. Samples were subjected to RT-PCR, and the positive samples were further used for RV isolation by mouse inoculation test [15]. Mice were purchased from the Animal Centre of Guangxi Medical University. To comply with Animal Research as Reporting In Vivo Experiments (ARRIVE) guidelines, all husbandry and experimental procedures were conducted in compliance with the Animal Welfare Act and the Guide for the Care and Use of Laboratory Animals. The mice were euthanized in a container after application of halothane inhalant, with the container closed once the aenesthesized mouse displayed a lack of righting reflex (mouse unable to right itself within 10 s after being placed on its side). Reference sequences of Lyssaviruses sequences used for constructing the phylogenetic tree were sourced from GenBank (Additional file 1: Table S1).

RNA extraction and reverse transcription

Total viral RNA was extracted from original host or mouse brain using Trizol (Invitrogen Biotechnology Co., Ltd, California, America). Following the manufacturer's instructions, cDNA was synthesized using 2.5 μg total RNA, 1 μL (25 pMol/μL) sense primer of each pair, and 100 U MuMLV RTase (Promega Trading Co., Ltd, Wisconsin, America) in a 25 μL reaction volume using standard methods. Each viral gene or fragment was amplified by RT-PCR using ExTaq (Takala Biomedical Technology Co., Ltd, Dalian, China) DNA polymerase.

Cloning and sequencing of viral genes

Primers used for amplification of RABV genes are shown in Additional file 2: Table S2. This table includes gene sequences, nucleotide positions, lengths, and regions.

PCR products were separated on 1% agarose and stained with ethidium bromide, purified and cloned into the pMD18-T cloning vector, and sequenced by Takara Corp. Three clones were analyzed for each amplicon of each virus. Sequence information was aligned and edited using DNAStar software.

Phylogenetic analysis

The coding regions of the N, P, and M genes and the L^{1-680} and L^{pam} regions of the genome of the isolates from Guangxi (accession numbers in Additional file 3: Table S3) were used to construct a phylogenetic tree. Homologous sequences were aligned using the Clustal method of the MegAlign program of DNAStar version 7.1 (DNAS_{TAR} Inc., USA) [16]. A Maximum likelihood (ML) tree for all DNA sequences was constructed using the Kimura 2-parameter model with MEGA5.0 software [17, 18].

Results

Phylogenetic analysis of RABV using the N, P, and M genes and regions L^{1-680} and L^{pam}

A total of 42 RABV isolates were obtained from different locations in Guangxi between 1999 and 2012. The N of 42 RABV isolates, and the P and M genes, as well as fragments of the 3′ terminus (L^{1-680}) and the polymerase activity module of the L gene (L^{pam}) of 36 RABV isolates, and the whole genomes of 5 RABV isolates were sequenced (Additional file 3: Table S3). Maximum likelihood phylogenetic trees were constructed for 113 complete N sequences (including the isolates (from Asia) downloaded from GenBank), 84 complete P sequences, 84 complete M sequences, 83 L^{1-680}, 83 L^{pam}, and 49 whole genome sequences, including a set of laboratory-passaged strains and street RABV strains from other locations (Additional file 1: Table S1).

Constructing phylogenetic trees for each of the N, P, and M genes, L^{1-680}, L^{pam} and the whole genome, revealed different topologies with strong bootstrap values. Isolates from Guangxi could be divided into three groups, designated I, II, and III (Figs. 1, 3, 4, 5, 6 and 7). Group I included isolates from the Guizhou, Hunan, Jiangxi, Fujian and Zhejiang provinces. Group II contained isolates from the Yunnan, Guizhou, Hunan, Anhui, Jiangsu, and Henan provinces. Group III contained isolates from Guangxi and Yunnan, and from the Southeast Asia countries. Of which, the two main groups (I and II) are related to China I (Clade I) and II (Clade II) [19–21], also associated with Asia1 and Asia2 [14]. We compared the N gene of 113 isolates from the world and constructed the phylogenetic tree, indicating that an India isolate and a Sri Lanka isolate are classified as Asia1, the China I and II are classified as Asia2 and Asia3. Compared with the Asia area, the isolates of group I in Guangxi (GX I) belong to the Asia2, including the isolates from Chinese Hunan, Jiangxi, Zhejiang, Fujian provinces, and including some isolates (94280PHI/dog/1994/Philippines/EU086202 and 03006PHI/human/2000/Philippines/EU086203) from the Philippines. The isolates of group II in Guangxi (GX II) belong to the Asia3, including the isolates from Chinese Yunnan, Guizhou, Hunan, Anhui, Jiangsu, Henan provinces and Shanghai. The RABV isolates of GX I and GX II are principally from the epidemic in Guangxi or from some other provinces of China. The isolates of group III in Guangxi (GX III) belong to Asia4. In the past two decades only three isolates were collected from China, GXN119 was isolated from Guangxi in 2000, and N11 was also from Guangxi, Tc06 from Yunnan; the other isolates were reported in the Southeast Asia countries Thailand, Vietnam, Myanmar, Cambodian and Laos, and were classified as Asia4 [15], indicating that GXIII (Asia4) is mainly prevalent in the Southeast Asia countries (Fig. 2), and the group III is associated with SEA3, as designated in a previous study [21].

Furthermore, the relationship between the three branches varied depending on the gene segment employed. The tree generated from the full N gene, the previously reported G gene [22] and L^{pam} had a branching pattern where groups II and I were linked while group III formed a separate branch. For trees generated from the P gene, groups I and II were clustered most closely while group III formed a separate, outlying branch. However, for the M, L^{1-680} and whole genome trees, groups I and III were most closely related, while group II formed a separate, outlying branch (Figs. 1, 3, 4, 5, 6 and 7 and Table 1).

Amino acid variation in RABV isolates

Totally, the nucleotide sequence data from RABV isolates showed that N, M genes and two fragments L^{1-680} and L^{pam} were highly conserved, with the exception that a few nucleotides of the P gene varied. On comparison of deduced amino acid (aa) sequences from N, P, M genes, the fragments of L^{1-680} and L^{pam}, as well as the whole genome of 5 isolates, we found that most of the functional motifs mapped in the different genes of RABV isolates were extremely conserved. Details are described as follows.

N amino acid variations

Based on the deduced amino acid sequences, the specific epitope (358-367aa) of B cells, the principal epitope (404-418aa) of Th and RNA binding site (298-352aa) were highly conserved [23]. A phosphorylation site S389, related to viral transcription and replication, was also highly conserved [24]. Comparison of the entire N protein of all isolates with that of the ERA, commonly used as a reference strain, showed two specific amino acid substitutions at positions 90 and 110 of group I: T90 N and E110D. In group II, the threonine in ERA was replaced by serine (T42S). The single isolate in group III, GXN119, and isolate 8743THA from Thailand showed 3 different substitutions (L128 V, P135A, and T375 M). In addition, all isolates from Guangxi and other provinces of China had variations at 5 locations that were conserved across regions I, II and III: H26Y, C40S, S61 N, V95 L, and G106D (Additional file 4: Table S4).

P amino acid variations

For the P protein, several functional domains – L protein binding region [25] (1-19aa), LC8 binding motif [26] (144-148aa) and N protein binding region [27] (209-216aa) – were highly conserved. Nuclear export signal [28] (49-58aa) had two variations: G54R/H57Q in the three groups and one variation E51D in group II. Th/Tc epitope (191-206aa) had one variation, K192E, in the three groups. It is unclear whether the functions of these domains have been influenced or not by these mutations. A phosphorylation site serine at 63aa that was changed to proline (S63P) removed the phosphorylation function.

There were three specific substitutions (A70T, A130M and V131 T) in group I, five specific substitutions (P134S, N135 T, S140P, R151K and A174V) in group II, and six specific substitutions (G73 V, S162 L, Q167K, K239R, D253E, and D281E) in group III. At residue 130, the A130M substitution was specific to group I, while the A130T substitution was specific to group II. At residue 174, the A174V substitution was specific to group II, while the A174E substitution was specific to group III. Four substitutions (H57Q, S63P, S90G, and A241S) were common to all isolates from Guangxi (Additional file 5: Table S5).

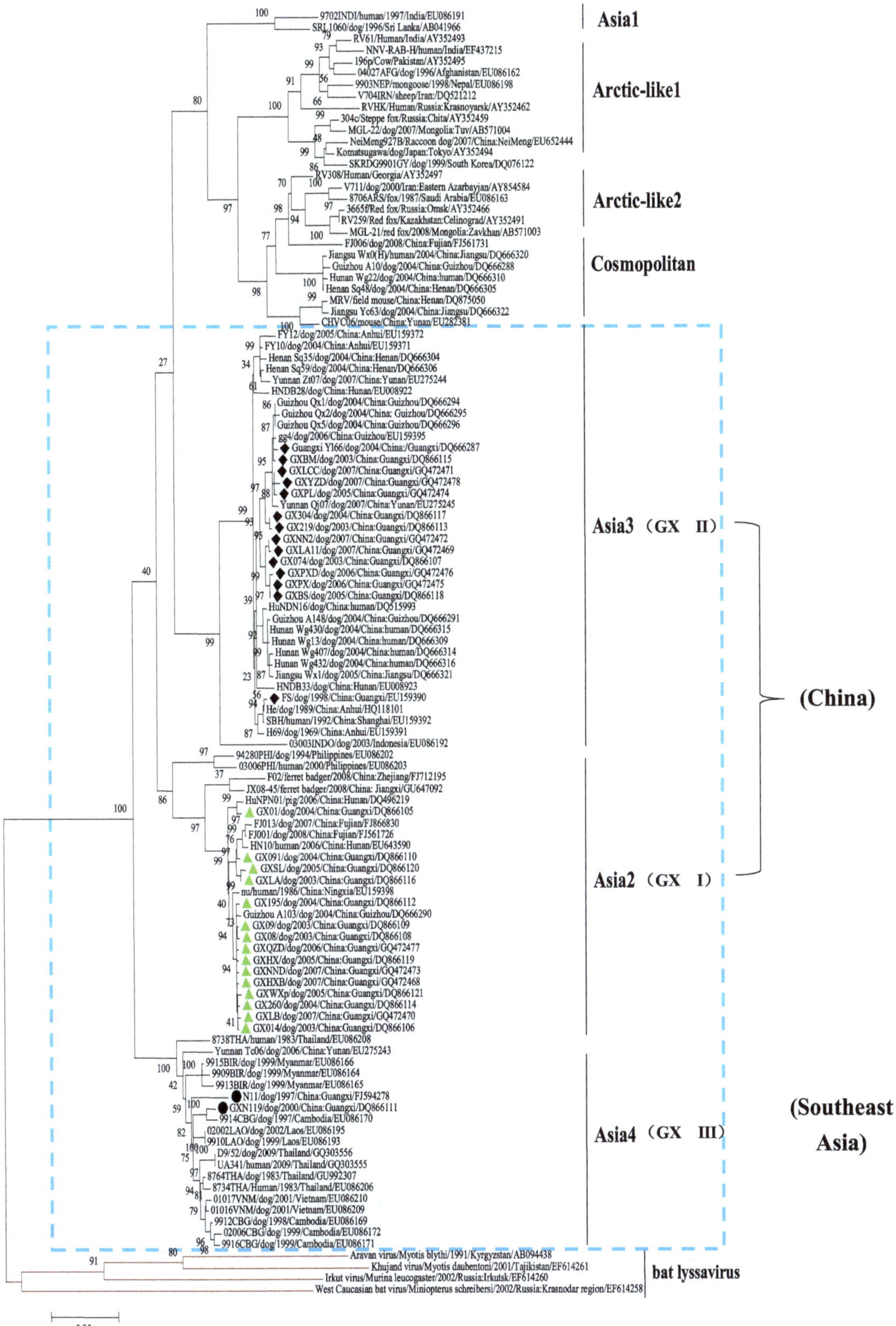

Fig. 1 Phylogenetic tree based on nucleotide sequences of N gene

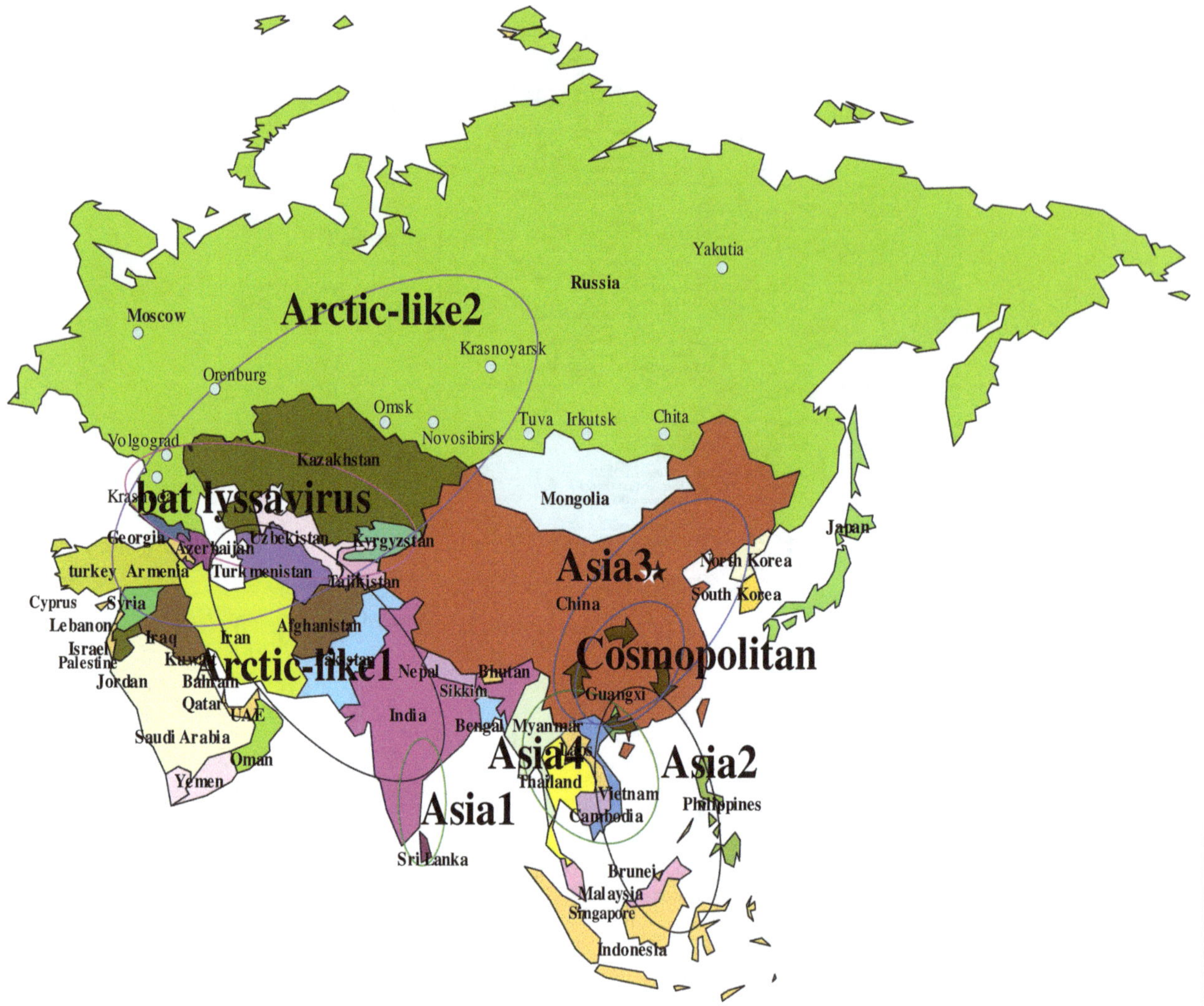

Fig. 2 Distribution of RABV isolates from Asia

Compared with the other genes, P gene also included several sporadic variations in group I and II, resulting in the variation rate of the P gene being higher than the other genes. In group I, four isolates (GXS822010, GXBS13201, GXNNSL and GXLB19) had H57F sporadic variation and three isolates (GXNND, GXLB and GXHX82) had M69 V variation. In group II, there were eight sporadic variations. Of which, five isolates (GXBS89201, GXBA09201, GXLQ2010, GXLB2010 and GXBN2011) had three sporadic variations (H57F, M69G and A70T); four isolates (GXNN2, GXLCC, GXPL, and GXYZD) had four sporadic variations (G61R/K, K62 N, T157I and A170V); four isolates (GX074, GXPX, GXPXD and GXLA11) had one sporadic variation (at N292S); GXHXN isolates had three sporadic variations (H57P, M69G and A70T; Additional file 5: Table S5).

M amino acid variations

For the M protein, there were nine substitutions (L26P, S46G, G58E, K77R, S104A, F120 L, I158S, K160R and P175S) common to the three groups I, II and III, one specific substitution I168V in group I, and four specific substitutions (Q17H, S20F, P21S and V22A) in group II. And a functional motif PxSAP [29] mapped at 21-25aa included P21S and V22A variations; its P21S change indicated that the PxSAP motif was abolished in the group II. Another motif PPxY at 35-38aa, relating to viral budding [29], was highly conserved (Additional file 6: Table S6). In addition, the amino acid Y138 that was highly conserved in virulent or avirulent RABV strains was mapped as a functional residue corresponding to viral replication (data not shown).

L^{1-680} and the L^{pam} amino acid variations

Alignment of the 226 amino acids of the L^{1-680} fragment revealed four substitutions (R115K, I117M, A168S, and

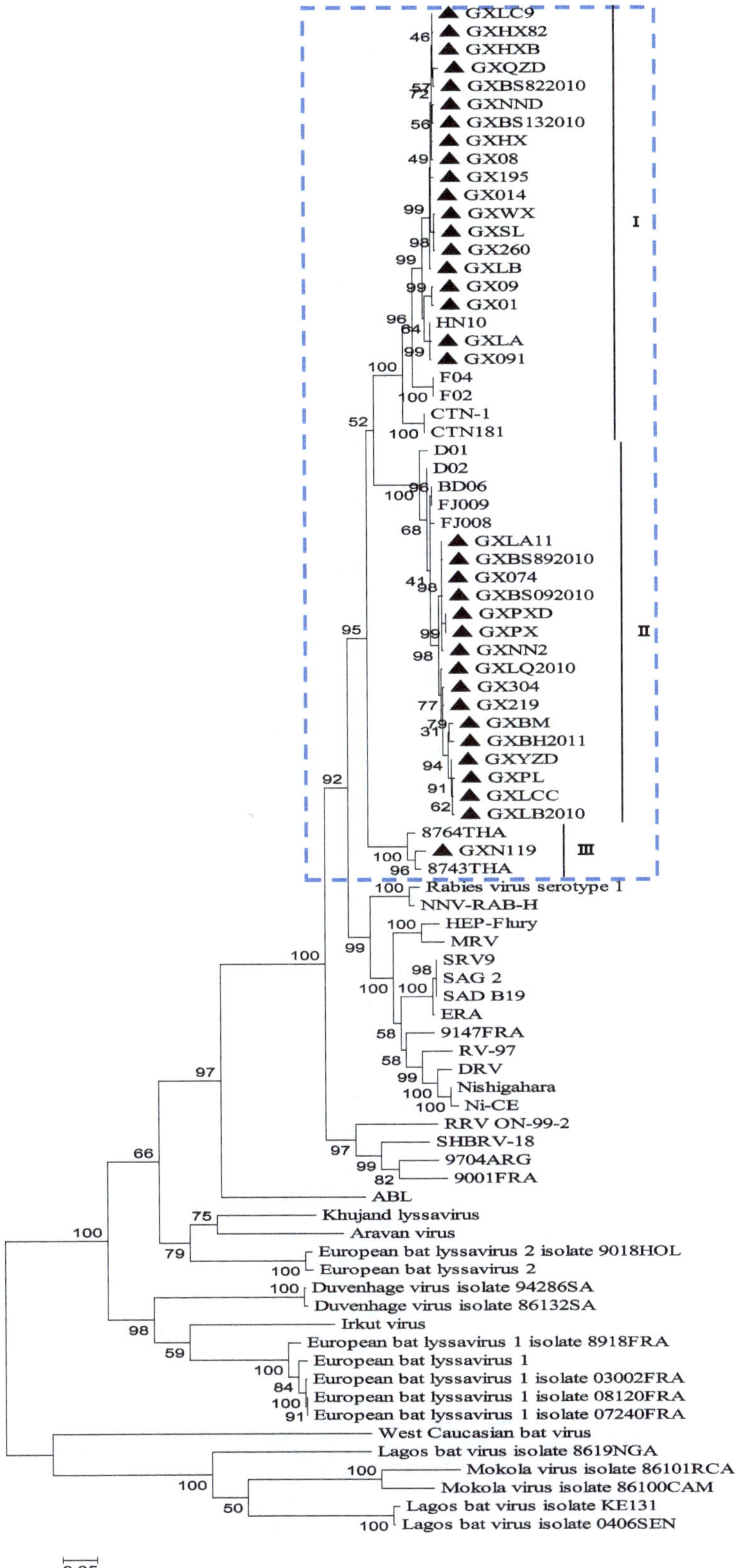

Fig. 3 Phylogenetic tree based on nucleotide sequences of the RABV P gene

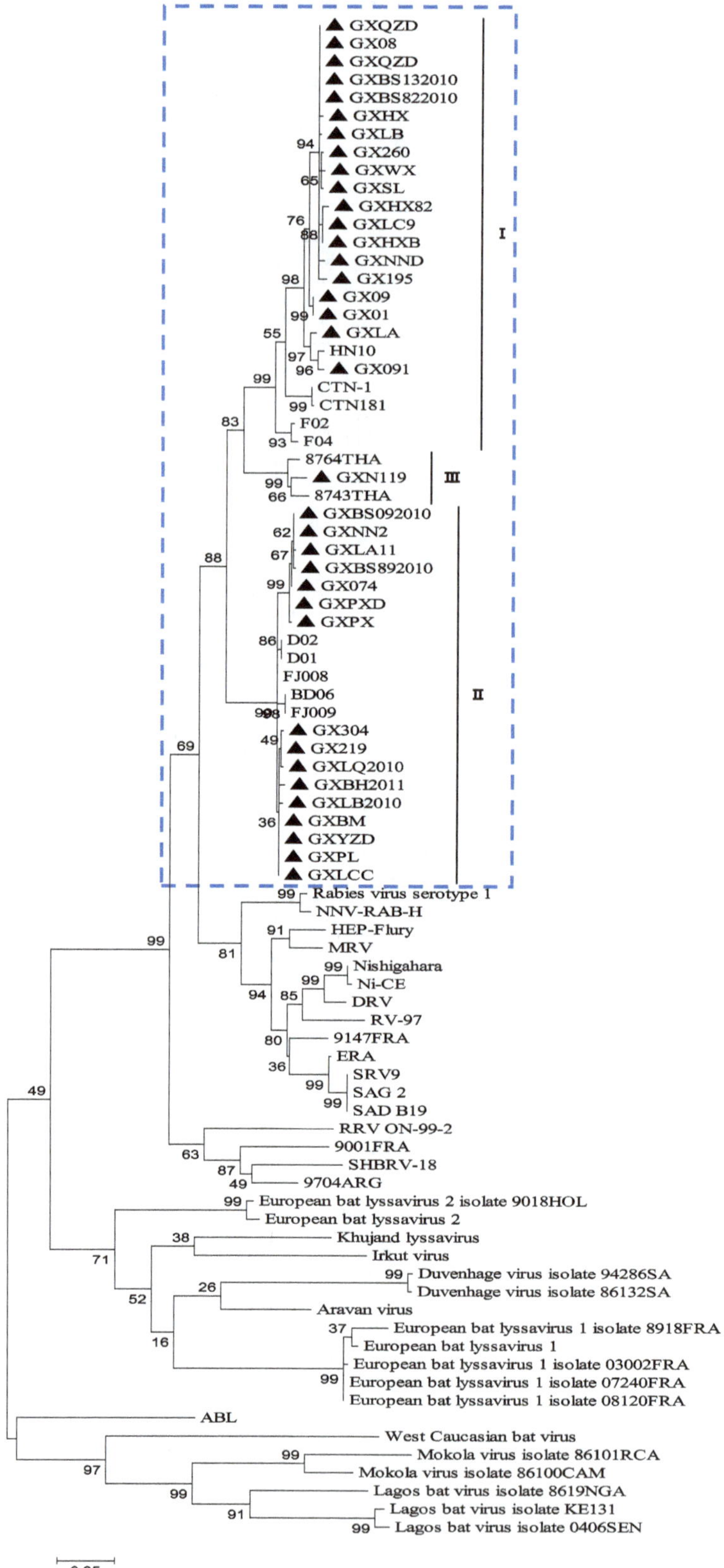

Fig. 4 Phylogenetic tree based on nucleotide sequences of the RABV M gene

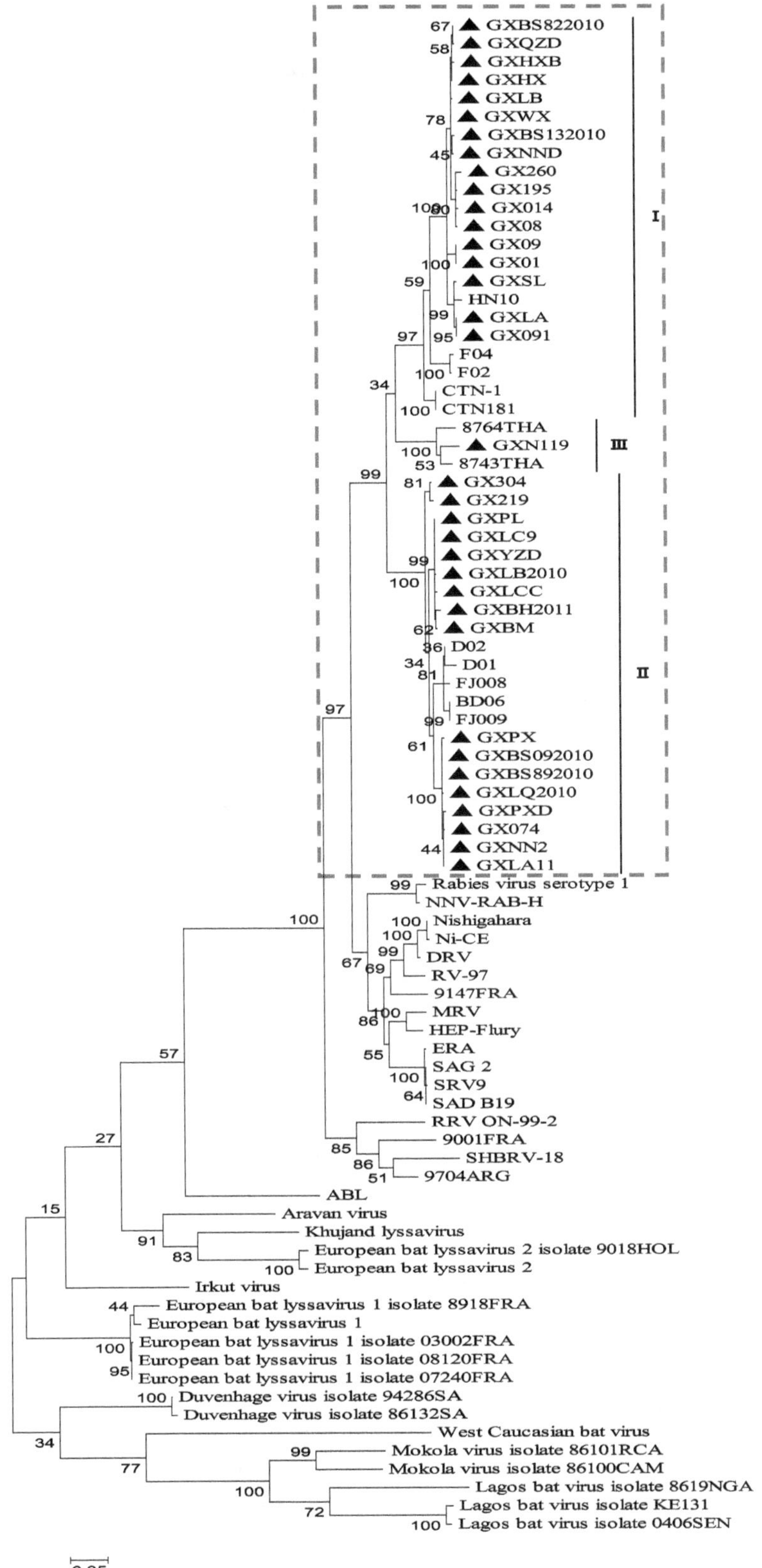

Fig. 5 Phylogenetic tree based on nucleotide sequences of the RABV 3′ terminal in the L gene (L^{1-680})

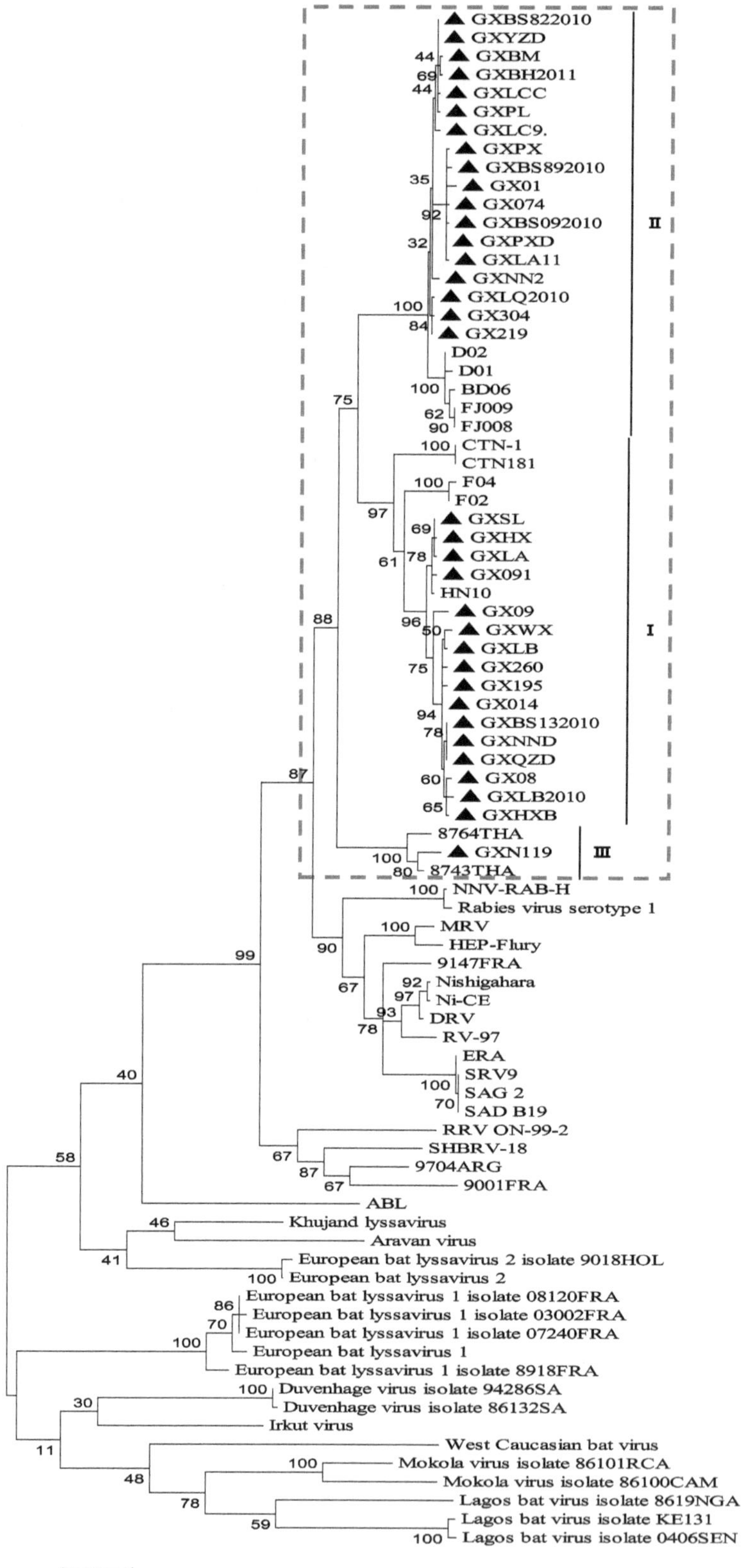

Fig. 6 Phylogenetic tree based on nucleotide sequences of the RABV polymerase activity module in the L gene (L^{pam})

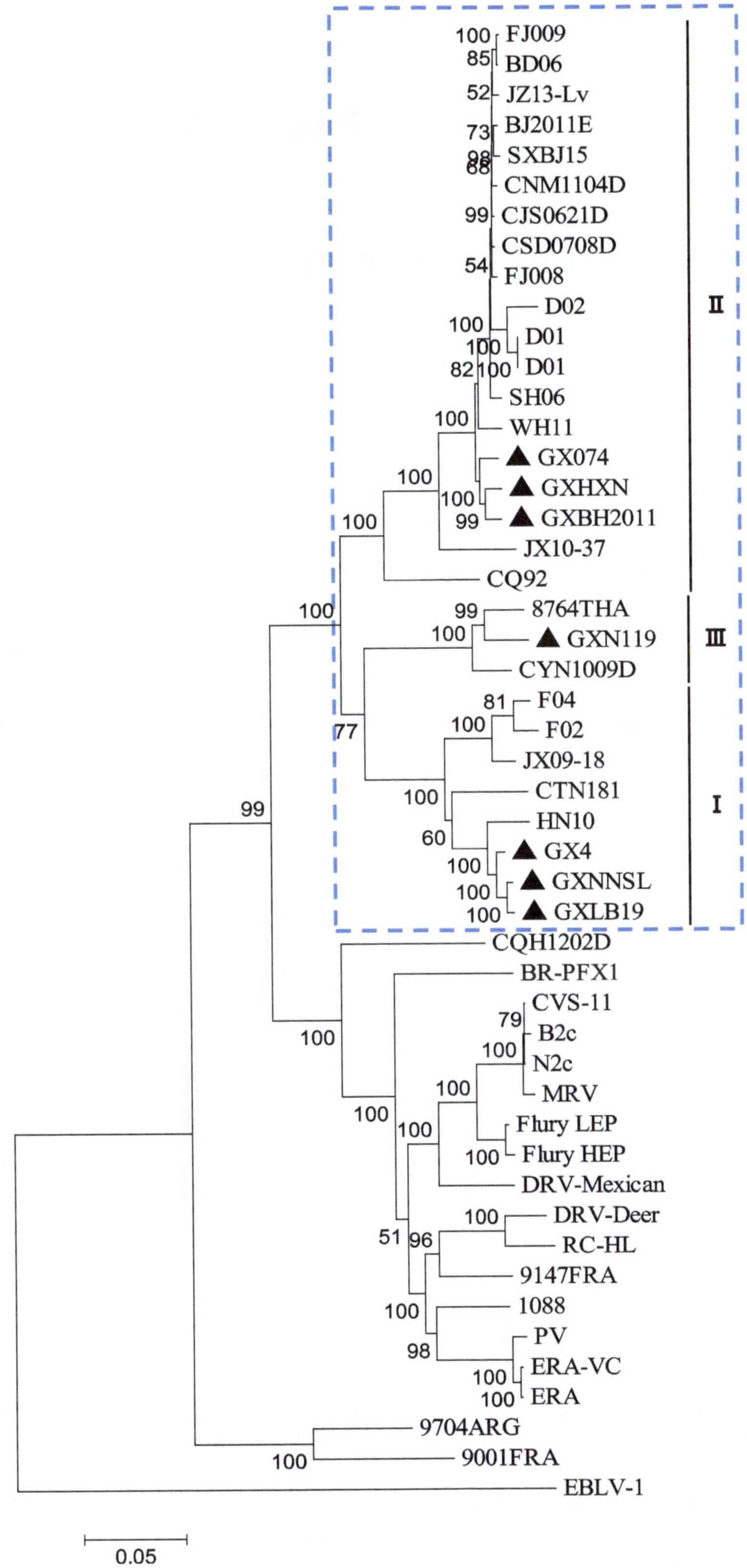

Fig. 7 Phylogenetic tree based on RABV whole genome nucleotide sequences

Table 1 Comparison of genetic patterns based on different genes of rabies virus from Guangxi.

Virus gene	Group pattern		
Virus genome	II	III	I
N	II	I	III
G	II	I	III
L^{pam}	II	I	III
P	I	II	III
M	I	III	II
$L^{1\text{-}680}$	I	III	II

Shading illustrates which groups were most closely related.

I207V) that were specific to group I, one substitution (T64A) that was specific to group II, and five substitutions (L76F, L88 V, T118A, V157I, and D190E) that were specific to group III. The R48K substitution was common to groups I and II, while V83 L was common to groups II and III. Notably seven substitutions (L2I, L17S, D19A, F73Y, R74K, L136C, and N161 K) were common to all three groups (Table 2).

Among the 200 amino acids of the L^{pam} fragment we found one substitution, S162A, specific to group I and another, I51V, specific to group II (Table 2).

These data are summarized in Table 2 and Additional file 4: Table S4, Additional file 5: Table S5, Additional file 6: Table S6, which demonstrate that amino acid variations differ across the three groups and serve as viral genetic markers in each of the proteins of wild RABV isolates from Guangxi.

Whole genome amino acid variation

The sizes of the individual structural genes, functional motifs and important functional sites of the five RABV isolates for which whole genome sequencing was performed were mostly consistent, with few sites differing. Relative to the coding regions, the non-coding regions were more variable. The full genome of five RABV isolates contained 11,921-11,924 nt in length: 11921 nt/GXLB19; 11,922 nt/GXNNSL and GX4 isolate (from Guangxi downloaded from GenBank); and 11,924 nt/GXBH2011, GXN119, GX074. The P-M non-coding regions were 86-87 nt in length, while the 5' UTR regions were 129-131 nt in length (Table 3).

The nAchR-binding region located at 189-214aa of G protein [30] had one common variation E205K in the five isolates. Transcription initiation (AACA) was extremely conserved. In the G-L non-coding region, there are two transcription termination poly:A_7 (TTP) motifs located downstream of the G protein stop codon. According to the whole genome sequences of the five RABV isolates from Guangxi, the 1st TTP motif (70-77 nt) had 3–5 nt changed, while the second TTP motif located 470-477 nt was conserved and observed in all five isolates (Table 4).

Discussion

Rabies is a severe epidemic in Guangxi, China, with hundreds of deaths occurring each year [22], and globally the number of rabies cases in China is second only to India [31]. In the past six decades, rabies has emerged three times in Guangxi, which has the largest number of rabies cases in China. The 1st outbreak of rabies was from 1968 to 1976, with the peak of human rabies cases at 560 in 1972. The 2nd time occurred in 1978, reaching a peak of 879 human rabies cases in 1981, and then gradually decreasing to just 24 cases in 1995. However, in the 3rd time, the number of human rabies cases increased from 50 in 1996, rose steeply to 203 in 2003, and reached a peak of 602 in 2004 [22].

The domestic dog is the principal vector for rabies, and 95% of human cases are associated with transmission from dogs. Our research group began surveillance of the RABV-carriage rate of at least 500 clinically healthy dogs from rural areas of Guangxi from 1999, and isolated RABV from RABV-positive cases. Of these isolates, several from rabid and normal dogs taken at different times showed similar pathogenicity in mice, indicating that the RABV from Guangxi has stable virulence [22]. Nevertheless, following an increase in dog vaccination in rural areas, the RABV-carriage rate in dogs appears to be gradually decreasing (data not shown). Between 2013 and 2016, we did not obtain any positive samples even though at least 500 samples from different areas in Guangxi were tested each year. Therefore, the data shown in this study consists of RABV isolates collected up until 2012. After reviewing a molecular epidemiological study conducted in Guangxi [15], we decided to further examine the genetic properties of these RABV isolates.

Generally, similar phylogenetic trees imply similar evolutionary paths [32–34]. In the phylogenetic analysis of Wu et al., trees constructed with the N, P, M, G, and L

Table 2 Specific amino acid mutations on the 3′ terminal and polymerase activity module of the L gene

Isolate	Group	L^{1-680}																				(L^{pam})								
		2	17	19	48	64	73	74	76	83	88	93	115	117	118	136	157	161	168	190	207	49	51	63	72	108	136	145	157	162
ERA		L	L	D	R	T	F	R	L	V	L	M	R	I	T	L	V	N	A	D	I	A	I	R	A	I	Q	R	V	S
GXLA	I	I	S	A	K		Y	K				T	K	M		C		K	S		V	S		W	M	T	R	S	I	A
GX08		I	S	A	K		Y	K				T	K	M		C		K	S		V	S		W	M	T	R	S	I	A
GX09		I	S	A	K		Y	K				T	K	M		C		K	S		V	S		W	M	T	R	S	I	A
GX014		I	S	A	K		Y	K				T	K	M		C		K	S		V	S		W	M	T	R	S	I	A
GX01		I	S	A	K		Y	K				T	K	M		C		K	S		V									
GX091		I	S	A	K		Y	K				T	K	M		C		K	S		V	S		W	M	T	R	S	I	A
GX195		I	S	A	K		Y	K				T	K	M		C		K	S		V	S		W	M	T	R	S	I	A
GX260		I	S	A	K		Y	K				A	K	M		C		K	S		V	S		W	M	T	R	S	I	A
GXHX		I	S	A	K		Y	K				T	K	M		C		K	S		V	S		W	M	T	R	S	I	A
GXWX		I	S	A	K		Y	K				T	K	M		C		K	S		V	S		W	M	T	R	S	I	A
GXSL		I	S	A	K		Y	K				T	K	M		C		K	S		V	S		W	M	T	R	S	I	A
GXQZD		I	S	A	K		Y	K				A	K	M		C		K	S		V	S		W	M	T	R	S	I	A
GXHXB		I	S	A	K		Y	K				T	K	M		C		K	S		V	S		W	M	T	R	S	I	A
GXNND		I	S	A	K		Y	K				A	K	M		C		K	S		V	S		W	M	T	R	S	I	A
GXLB		I	S	A	K		Y	K				A	K	M		C		K	S		V	S		W	M	T	R	S	I	A
GXBS822010		I	S	A	K		Y	K				T	K	M		C		K	S		V	S		W	M	T	R	S	I	A
GXBS132010		I	S	A	K		Y	K				T	K	M		C		K	S		V	S		W	M	T	R	S	I	A
GXYZD	II	I	S	A	K	A	Y	K		L		T				C		K				S	V	W	M	T	R	S	I	
GXLA11		I	S	A	K	A	Y	K		L		T				C		K				S	V	W	M	T	R	S	I	
GXLCC		I	S	A	K	A	Y	K		L		T				C		K				S	V	W	M	T	R	S	I	
GXNN2		I	S	A	K	A	Y	K		L		T				C		K				S	V	W	M	T	R	S	I	
GXPL		I	S	A	K	A	Y	K		L		T				C		K				S	V	W	M	T	R	S	I	
GXPXD		I	S	A	K	A	Y	K		L		T				C		K				S	V	W	M	T	R	S	I	
GX074		I	S	A	K	A	Y	K		L		T				C		K				S	V	W	M	T	R	S	I	
GX219		I	S	A	K	A	Y	K		L		T				C		K				S	V	W	M	T	R	S	I	
GX304		I	S	A	K	A	Y	K		L		T				C		K				S	V	W	M	T	R	S	I	
GXBM		I	S	A	K	A	Y	K		L		T				C		K				S	V	W	M	T	R	S	I	
GXPX		I	S	A	K	A	Y	K		L		T				C		K				S	V	W	M	T	R	S	I	
GXLB2010		I	S	A	K	A	Y	K		L		T				C		K				S	V	W	M	T	R	S	I	
GXBH2011		I	S	A	K	A	Y	K		L		T				C		K				S	V	W	M	T	R	S	I	

Table 2 Specific amino acid mutations on the 3′ terminal and polymerase activity module of the L gene *(Continued)*

Isolate	Group	L^{1-680}																				(L^{pam})								
		2	17	19	48	64	73	74	76	83	88	93	115	117	118	136	157	161	168	190	207	49	51	63	72	108	136	145	157	162
GXBS092010		I	S	A	K	A	Y	K		L		T				C		K				S	V	W	M	T	R	S	I	
GXBS892010		I	S	A	K	A	Y	K		L		T				C		K				S	V	W	M	T	R	S	I	
GXLQ2010		I	S	A	K	A	Y	K		L		T				C		K				S	V	W	M	T	R	S	I	
GXN119	III	I	S	A			Y	K	F	L	V	T			A	C	I	K	V	E		S		W	M	T	R	S	I	

Table 3 Non-coding regions, coding regions and genome sizes of rabies virus isolates. Numbers represent sizes in base pairs

	GXLB19	GXNNSL	GXBH2011	GXN119	GX074	GX4
3′ UTR	70	70	70	70	70	70
N	1353	1353	1353	1353	1353	1353
N-P	91	91	91	91	91	91
P	894	894	894	894	894	894
P-M	86	86	87	87	87	86
M	609	609	609	609	609	609
M-G	211	211	211	211	211	211
G	1575	1575	1575	1575	1575	1575
G-L	516	516	516	516	516	516
L	6387	6387	6387	6387	6387	6387
5′ UTR	129	130	131	131	131	130
genome	11,921	11,922	11,924	11,924	11,924	11,922

genes were found to have similar topologies [8]. In this study, the phylogenetic trees constructed from the complete N, P, and M genes as well as the L^{1-680} and L^{pam} fragments exhibited different topologies with strong bootstrap values as well as G gene (Table 1) [22], although the Guangxi RABV isolates of three groups were closely related (Figs. 1, 3, 4, 5, 6, and 7). The possible reason might be a difference of variation rate (varied nucleotides/total nucleotides of each gene) in each gene [35, 36]. The comprehensive datasets of the N, P, M, L^{1-680}, and L^{pam} genes, widely distributed across different provinces of China, corroborated the assumption that the Guangxi RABV genes were likely undergoing co-evolution.

It is worth mentioning that although phylogenetic trees of the N, P, and M genes and the L^{1-680} and L^{pam} fragments consistently had three groups, branching of the three viral groups actually revealed four different patterns. The tree generated from the N, G gene and L^{pam} has a branching pattern in which groups II (Asia 3) and I (Asia2) are linked with group III (Asia4) lying on a separate branch; the trees generated from P gene had groups I and II clustered most closely with group III forming an outlying branch; trees generated from the M and L^{1-680} genes and whole genome sequences had groups I and III most closely related, with group II as an outlying branch. This finding indicates that the rate of evolution might vary depending on the RABV gene examined (Table 1).

Based on the phylogenetic analysis and amino acid variation, the RABV isolates from Guangxi were divided into two main groups (I and II) and a minor group (III). However, the phylogenetic trees constructed from the complete N, P and M genes as well as the L^{1-680} and L^{pam} fragments exhibited different topologies with strong bootstrap values as well as G gene. In fact, most of the isolates from the south China including Hunan, Guizhou, Guangdong, Fujian, Jiangsu, Anhui and Henan provinces belong to two main groups, the same as those isolates from Guangxi. Nevertheless, some isolates from Hunan, Guizhou, Jiangsu, Anhui, and Henan provinces are classified into the group Cosmopolitan (Fig. 1).

On the basis of differences identified by the phylogenetic analysis of nucleotide sequences, the downstream significance of these variations at the protein level was explored. Protein alignment revealed several specific amino acid residue mutations in each protein, which coincided with the phylogenetic analysis and grouping of isolates from Guangxi. Construction of phylogenetic trees and comparison of amino acids of each protein revealed an overall picture of significant genetic diversity for the isolates from Guangxi.

Table 4 Functional domain of rabies virus

Virus	nAchR-binding domain (189-214 aa) of G gene	TTP motif of G—L noncoding region	
	205	TTP1	TTP2
ERA	CDIFTNSRGKRASKGSETCGFVDERG	GAAAAAAA	GAAAAAAA
GXLB19	----------------K---------	—GGG—C—T	--------
GXNNSL	----------------K---------	—GGG—C—T	--------
GXBH2011	R--------------GK---------	—GG——C—T	--------
GXHXN	----------------K---------	—GG——C—T	--------
GXN119	----------------K---------	—GGG—C—T	--------

In this study, we present the sequences of the entire N, P, and M genes and the L^{1-680} and L^{pam} fragments of the L gene from 42 RABV isolates from Guangxi. We previously also sequenced the full length G gene for which we performed phylogenetic analysis [22]. The final results revealed that Maximum likelihood (ML) of the N gene sequences generated a tree with a similar overall structure to that obtained with the G gene and L^{pam} sequences [22], while different to that obtained using P, M gene and L^{1-680}. In addition, the deduced amino acid sequences of the N, P, and M proteins and L^{1-680} and L^{pam} for all 42 isolates from Guangxi were aligned and compared to other terrestrial strains. Variations in the N protein demonstrated different patterns to those obtained for the P and M proteins, and for the L^{1-680} and L^{pam} fragments of the L protein, as well as for the G protein [22]. RNA variation in RABV isolates from Guangxi revealed a significant genetic diversity with differences observed from other geographical regions, and there are strong geographical associations among RABV isolates including the three groups in Guangxi.

Although live attenuated oral rabies vaccines could revert to virulent strains and have residual pathogenicity in certain rodents, they have been shown to be safe in foxes, dogs and skunks [37, 38]. Intensive molecular investigation of SAD B19 strain passaged several times in mice has demonstrated their sequence conservation and genetic stability in vivo [39]. However, there is always a risk that vaccine strains could revert to a fully pathogenic form, and thus, all RABV isolates collected from the field should be sequenced and subjected to phylogenetic analysis. We found that the attenuated vaccine ERA strain used across Guangxi was genetically distributed in a different group compared with the Guangxi RABV isolates (Figs. 1, 3, 4, 5, 6 and 7).

Here, we performed a detailed genetic analysis of RABV isolates from Guangxi. These data provide rich genetic information on nucleotide and amino acid variation patterns in RABV proteins and reveal genetic diversity in the RABV epidemic in Guangxi.

Additional files

Additional file 1: Table S1. Reference sequences of Lyssaviruses used in the present study. (DOC 282 kb)

Additional file 2: Table S2. Primers used in this study. (DOC 184 kb)

Additional file 3: Table S3. Origin of rabies virus isolates from Guangxi used in this study. (DOC 288 kb)

Additional file 4: Table S4. Specific amino acids mutations in the nucleoprotein (N) of rabies virus isolates from Guangxi. (DOCX 19 kb)

Additional file 5: Table S5. Specific mutational amino acid on phosphoprotein (P) protein of rabies virus isolates from Guangxi. (DOCX 23 kb)

Additional file 6: Table S6. Specific mutational amino acid on matrix protein of rabies virus isolates from Guangxi. (DOCX 22 kb)

Abbreviations

G: Glycoprotein; L^{1-680}: 3' terminal 1–680 amino aicd in L gene; L^{pam}: Polymerase activity module in L gene; M: Matrix protein; N: Nucleoprotein; P: Phosphoprotein; RABV: Rabies virus

Acknowledgements

The authors wish to thank the study participants for their contribution to the research, as well as current and past investigation and staff.

Funding

The study was supported by the National Natural Science Foundation of China (31570147), and the Fund Program of the Director of the Key Laboratory of the Ministry of Education for Microbial and Plant Genetic Engineering, Guangxi University. The funding body was solely involved in funding and had no role in the design of the study, the collection, analysis, and interpretation of the data, nor in writing the manuscript.

Authors' contributions

XKW collected and analyzed the data, and led the preparation of the manuscript. XXH, YP, HBT, CL, YZZ, XNL, JJL contributed to the project by collecting and analyzing the data. TRL supervised the project and provided substantial contributions to the analysis and interpretation of the data, and the preparation of the manuscript. All authors approved the final manuscript.

Competing interests

All authors declare that they have no competing interests.

References

1. Bourhy H, Kissi B, Tordo N. Taxonomy and evolutionary studies on lyssaviruses with special reference to Africa. Onderstepoort J Vet Res. 1993; 60(4):277–82.
2. Kissi B, Tordo N, Bourhy H. Genetic polymorphism in the rabies virus nucleoprotein gene. Virology. 1995;209(2):526–37.
3. He W, Zhang H, Zhang Y, Wang R, Lu S, Ji Y, Liu C, Yuan P, Su S. Codon usage bias in the N gene of rabies virus. Infect Genet Evol. 2017;54:458–65.
4. Zhang J, Zhang Z, Deng Y, Wu S, Wang W, Yan Y. Incidence of human rabies and characterization of rabies virus nucleoprotein gene in dogs in Fujian Province, Southeast China, 2002-2012. BMC Infect Dis. 2017;17(1):599.
5. Badrane H, Bahloul C, Perrin P, Tordo N. Evidence of two lyssavirus phylogroups with distinct pathogenicity and immunogenicity. J Virol. 2001; 75(7):3268–76.
6. Kuzmin I, Orciari L, Arai Y, Smith J, Hanlon C, Kameoka Y, Rupprecht C. Bat lyssaviruses (Aravan and Khujand) from Central Asia: phylogenetic relationships according to N, P and G gene sequences. Virus Res. 2003; 97(2):65–79.
7. Kuzmin I, Hughes G, Botvinkin A, Orciari L, Rupprecht C. Phylogenetic relationships of Irkut and west Caucasian bat viruses within the lyssavirus genus and suggested quantitative criteria based on the N gene sequence for lyssavirus genotype definition. Virus Res. 2005;111(1):28–43.
8. Wu X, Franka R, Velasco-Villa A, Rupprecht C. Are all lyssavirus genes equal for phylogenetic analyses? Virus Res. 2007;129(2):91–103.
9. Delmas O, Holmes E, Talbi C, Larrous F, Dacheux L, Bouchier C, Bourhy H. Genomic diversity and evolution of the lyssaviruses. PLoS One. 2008; 3(4):e2057.
10. Zhang Y, Xiong C, Zou Y, Wang D, Jiang R, Xiao Q, Hao Z, Zhang L, Yu Y, Fu Z. Molecular characterization of rabies virus isolates in China during 2004. Virus Res. 2006;121(2):179–88.
11. Zhang Y, Xiong C, Lin X, Zhou D, Jiang R, Xiao Q, Xie X, Yu X, Tan Y, Li M, et al. Genetic diversity of Chinese rabies viruses: evidence for the presence of two distinct clades in China. Infect Genet Evol. 2009;9(1):87–96.
12. Tao X, Tang Q, Li H, Mo Z, Zhang H, Wang D, Zhang Q, Song M, Velasco-Villa A, Wu X, et al. Molecular epidemiology of rabies in southern People's Republic of China. Emerging Infect Dis. 2009;15(8):1192–8.
13. Ming P, Yan J, Rayner S, Meng S, Xu G, Tang Q, Wu J, Luo J, Yang X. A history estimate and evolutionary analysis of rabies virus variants in China. J Gen Virol. 2010;91(Pt 3):759–64.

14. Gong W, Jiang Y, Za Y, Zeng Z, Shao M, Fan J, Sun Y, Xiong Z, Yu X, Tu C. Temporal and spatial dynamics of rabies viruses in China and Southeast Asia. Virus Res. 2010;150(1–2):111–8.
15. Liu Q, Xiong Y, Luo T, Wei Y, Nan S, Liu F, Pan Y, Feng L, Zhu W, Liu K, et al. Molecular epidemiology of rabies in Guangxi Province, south of China. J Clin Virol. 2007;39(4):295–303.
16. Thompson J, Gibson T, Higgins D. Multiple sequence alignment using ClustalW and ClustalX. Curr Protoc Bioinformatics. 2002;Chapter 2(Unit 2):3.
17. Tamura K, Dudley J, Nei M, Kumar S. MEGA4: molecular evolutionary genetics analysis (MEGA) software version 4.0. Mol Biol Evol. 2007;24(8): 1596–9.
18. Su S, Wong G, Shi W, Liu J, Lai A, Zhou J, Liu W, Bi Y, Gao G. Epidemiology, genetic recombination, and pathogenesis of coronaviruses. Trends Microbiol. 2016;24(6):490–502.
19. Lang SL, Tao XY, Guo ZY, Tang Q, Li H, Yin CP, Li Y, Liang GD. Molecular characterization of viral G gene in emerging and re-emerging areas of rabies in China, 2007 to 2011. Virol Sin. 2012;27(3):194–203.
20. Tao XY, Tang Q, Rayner S, Guo ZY, Li H, Lang SL, Yin CP, Han N, Fang W, Adams J, et al. Molecular phylodynamic analysis indicates lineage displacement occurred in Chinese rabies epidemics between 1949 to 2010. PLoS Negl Trop Dis. 2013;7(7):e2294.
21. Yu F, Zhang G, Zhong X, Han N, Song Y, Zhao L, Cui M, Rayner S, Fu ZF. Comparison of complete genome sequences of dog rabies viruses isolated from China and Mexico reveals key amino acid changes that may be associated with virus replication and virulence. Arch Virol. 2014; 159(7):1593–601.
22. Tang H, Pan Y, Wei X, Lu Z, Lu W, Yang J, He X, Xie L, Zeng L, Zheng L, et al. Re-emergence of rabies in the Guangxi province of southern China. PLoS Negl Trop Dis. 2014;8(10):e3114.
23. Kouznetzoff A, Buckle M, Tordo N. Identification of a region of the rabies virus N protein involved in direct binding to the viral RNA. The Journal of general virology. 1998;79(Pt 5):1005–13.
24. Dietzschold B, Wunner WH, Wiktor TJ, Lopes AD, Lafon M, Smith CL, Koprowski H. Characterization of an antigenic determinant of the glycoprotein that correlates with pathogenicity of rabies virus. Proc Natl Acad Sci U S A. 1983;80(1):70–4.
25. Chenik M, Schnell M, Conzelmann KK, Blondel D. Mapping the interacting domains between the rabies virus polymerase and phosphoprotein. J Virol. 1998;72(3):1925–30.
26. Lo KW, Naisbitt S, Fan JS, Sheng M, Zhang M. The 8-kDa dynein light chain binds to its targets via a conserved (K/R)XTQT motif. J Biol Chem. 2001; 276(17):14059–66.
27. Jacob Y, Real E, Tordo N. Functional interaction map of lyssavirus phosphoprotein: identification of the minimal transcription domains. J Virol. 2001;75(20):9613–22.
28. Toriumi H, Kawai A. Association of rabies virus nominal phosphoprotein (P) with viral nucleocapsid (NC) is enhanced by phosphorylation of the viral nucleoprotein (N). Microbiol Immunol. 2004;48(5):399–409.
29. Jayakar HR, Murti KG, Whitt MA. Mutations in the PPPY motif of vesicular stomatitis virus matrix protein reduce virus budding by inhibiting a late step in Virion release. J Virol. 2000;74(21):9818–27.
30. Lentz T, Wilson P, Hawrot E, Speicher D. Amino acid sequence similarity between rabies virus glycoprotein and snake venom curaremimetic neurotoxins. Science. 1984;226(4676):847–8.
31. Tan J, Wang R, Ji S, Su S, Zhou J. One health strategies for rabies control in rural areas of China. Lancet Infect Dis. 2017;17(4):365–7.
32. Song M, Tang Q, Wang D, Mo Z, Guo S, Li H, Tao X, Rupprecht C, Feng Z, Liang G. Epidemiological investigations of human rabies in China. BMC Infect Dis. 2009;9:210.
33. Hafner M, Nadler S. Phylogenetic trees support the coevolution of parasites and their hosts. Nature. 1988;332(6161):258–9.
34. Korn E. Coevolution of head, neck, and tail domains of myosin heavy chains. Proc Natl Acad Sci U S A. 2000;97(23):12559–64.
35. Bourhy H, Reynes J, Dunham E, Dacheux L, Larrous F, Huong V, Xu G, Yan J, Miranda M, Holmes E. The origin and phylogeography of dog rabies virus. J Gen Virol. 2008;89(Pt 11):2673–81.
36. Talbi C, Holmes E, de Benedictis P, Faye O, Nakouné E, Gamatié D, Diarra A, Elmamy B, Sow A, Adjogoua E, et al. Evolutionary history and dynamics of dog rabies virus in western and Central Africa. J Gen Virol. 2009;90(Pt 4):783–91.
37. Vos A. Oral vaccination against rabies and the behavioural ecology of the red fox (Vulpes vulpes). J Vet Med B Infect Dis Vet Public Health. 2003; 50(10):477–83.
38. Vos A, Pommerening E, Neubert L, Kachel S, Neubert A. Safety studies of the oral rabies vaccine SAD B19 in striped skunk (Mephitis mephitis). J Wildl Dis. 2002;38(2):428–31.
39. Beckert A, Geue L, Vos A, Neubert A, Freuling C, Müller T. Genetic stability (in vivo) of the attenuated oral rabies virus vaccine SAD B19. Microbiol Immunol. 2009;53(1):16–21.

The prevalence and genetic characteristics of porcine circovirus type 2 and 3 in Korea

Seung-Chai Kim[1], Salik Nazki[1], Sam Kwon[1], Jhung-Hyun Juhng[1], Kyeong-Hwan Mun[1], Do-Young Jeon[1], Chang-Gi Jeong[1], Amina Khatun[1], Seog-Jin Kang[2] and Won-Il Kim[1*]

Abstract

Background: Porcine circovirus-associated diseases (PCVAD), caused by porcine circovirus type 2 (PCV2), threaten the pig industry worldwide. Five genotypes of PCV2 were recently identified: PCV2a, PCV2b, PCV2c, PCV2d and PCV2e. In addition, a novel porcine circovirus from a case of a sow with dermatitis, nephropathy syndrome and reproductive failure has been identified based on metagenomic analysis and classified as porcine circovirus type 3 (PCV3). Therefore, the current study was conducted to determine the prevalence and genetic characteristics of PCV2 and PCV3 in clinical samples.

Results: A total of 471 samples (161 tissue samples of lungs and lymph nodes from 34 farms and 310 serum samples from 47 farms) were tested for PCV2. Among them, 171 samples from 59 farms that had been positive for PCV2 were genotyped. Another 690 samples (296 tissue samples of lungs and lymph nodes from 91 farms, 108 samples of aborted foetuses from 26 farms, and 286 serum samples from 47 farms) were tested for PCV3. Based on PCV2 genotyping results, PCV2d was the most prevalent genotype (107 of 171 samples), and co-infections with combinations of PCV2a, 2b and 2d were identified in 48 samples from 17 farms. A total of 14 samples from 11 farms were also positive for both PCV2 and PCV3. For PCV3, 57 samples (9.8%) from 32 farms (23.2%) were positive. Among the 108 aborted foetuses from 26 farms, only 2 samples were positive for PCV3. Based on sequence comparisons, PCV2d shares 89.6–91.0% and 93.2–94.3% homology with PCV2a and PCV2b, respectively; 98.6–100% homology is shared among PCV2d strains. The PCV3 strains identified in this study share 98.0–99.5% homology.

Conclusions: Our study concludes that PCV2d has become the most predominant genotype in Korea. PCV3 was also identified in clinical samples, though no significant association with clinical symptoms was observed in PCV3-positive cases.

Keywords: PCV2, PCV3, Prevalence, Genotyping, Genetic characteristics

Background

Porcine circovirus (PCV), belonging to the family *Circoviridae* and the genus *Circovirus*, is the smallest virus with a circular, ambisense, single-stranded DNA genome. Two types of PCVs are known to be infectious to pigs: PCV1 and PCV2. PCV1 was first detected in 1974 [1]; non-pathogenic to pigs, PCV1 was found as a contaminant of PK-15 cell culture [2]. Reported as a new syndrome, post-weaning multi-systemic wasting syndrome (PMWS), PCV2 was first identified in 1996 [3, 4]. Unlike PCV1, PCV2 is one of the most important pathogens in the swine industry because of its association with numerous types of syndromes and diseases in pigs under the umbrella of porcine circovirus-associated disease (PCVAD) [5, 6], including reproductive failure [7], porcine respiratory disease complex (PRDC) [8], porcine dermatitis and nephropathy syndrome (PDNS) [9], granulomatous enteritis [10, 11], proliferative and necrotizing pneumonia (PNP) [12], necrotizing lymphadenitis, and possibly exudative epidermitis [13].

The capsid protein of PCV2, which is encoded by ORF2, binds to the host receptor and triggers immune responses [14, 15]. Recombination mainly occurs within ORF1, though it can occur in ORF2 [16]. As the range of nucleotide variation is greater for ORF2 than for ORF1 [17–19], ORF2 genome analysis is mainly used for phylogenetic and epidemiological markers and is considered similar to PCV2 whole-genome analysis [20, 21]. In 2008, the EU consortium on PCVAD set standardized nomenclature guidelines

* Correspondence: kwi0621@jbnu.ac.kr
[1]College of Veterinary Medicine, Chonbuk National University, 79 Gobong-ro, Iksan 54596, Jeonbuk, Republic of Korea
Full list of author information is available at the end of the article

for PCV2 genotypes [22], indicating that the p-distance cut-off value should be greater than 0.035 [23, 24]. With this criterion, 5 genotypes of PCV2 have been identified: PCV2a, PCV2b, PCV2c, PCV2d and PCV2e. Until the early 2000s, PCV2a was the dominant PCV2 genotype worldwide, and it can be subdivided into four clusters (2A to 2D) [20, 21]. In contrast, PCV2b, which can be subdivided into three clusters (1A to 1C), was the dominant strain worldwide after 2000 [20, 21, 25]. PCV2c has only been detected in archived swine serum samples from Denmark [25]. PCV2d was first identified in China in 2009 [26]. After worldwide debate differentiating mPCV2b and PCV2d, PCV2d was finally proposed as an independent genotype that includes the mPCV2b cluster [21, 23, 27, 28]. PCV2d is currently the most dominant genotype [21] and is a source of much concern to the swine industry, which has reported worldwide PCV2 vaccine failure [29–32]. In 2016, PCV2e was identified in the US through diagnostic phylogenetics [33].

Recently, a novel porcine circovirus was identified through metagenomic analysis from a sow in the US suffering from dermatitis, nephropathy syndrome and reproductive failure; this isolate was classified as porcine circovirus type 3 (PCV3) [34]. PCV3 has also been detected in pigs with cardiac and multisystemic inflammation in the US [35]. Furthermore, PCV3 is being reported in China [36, 37] and Korea [38] as a new threat to the swine industry. However, insufficient evidence indicates that PCV3 will be as significant a pathogen as PCV2 because PCV3 was detected without any significant clinical symptoms [39]. As little information exists on overall porcine circovirus infection in Korea, this study was conducted to determine the prevalence and genetic characteristics of PCV2 and PCV3 in Korea.

Methods

Sample information

During a period of 1 year between April 2015 and March 2016, 471 samples (161 tissue samples of lungs and lymph nodes from 34 farms and 310 serum samples from 47 farms) were submitted to Chonbuk National University-Veterinary Diagnostic Center (CBNU-VDC) for PCV2 testing. Among the samples, 30 serum samples from 25 farms and 141 tissue samples from 34 farms were positive for PCV2 and genotyped. In addition, another set of 690 samples (296 tissue samples of lungs and lymph nodes from 91 farms, 108 samples of aborted foetuses from 26 farms, and 286 serum samples from 47 farms) submitted to CBNU-VDC between April 2016 and June 2017 were tested for PCV3.

Nucleic acid extraction and PCR detection of PCV2

Tissue samples were homogenized, mixed with phosphate-buffered saline (PBS; 0.1 M, pH 7.4) and centrifuged at 2500 rpm for 10 min at 4 °C. Viral nucleic acid was immediately extracted from the supernatant using Patho Gene-spin DNA/RNA Extraction Kit (iNtRON Biotechnology Inc., Seongnam, Korea) according to the manufacturer's instructions. Four sets of primers were used. One set of primer was used for detection and ORF2 genome sequencing [40], and three were used for subtype differential PCR [14, 41]. Two microlitres of extracted DNA and 2× F-Star Taq PCR Master Mix (BIOFACT Co., Daejeon, Korea) were mixed with 10 pmol of each subtype-specific primer (Table 1). The PCR conditions were as follows: pre-denaturation at 94 °C for 1 min, 35 cycles of denaturation at 94 °C for 30 s, annealing at 60 °C for 30 s, and extension at 72 °C for 1 min, and a final extension at 72 °C for 10 min.

Table 1 Primers used in this study

Primer name	Nucleotide sequence (5' - 3')	Product size	Purpose	Reference
F-PCV2C	GCT GGC TGA ACT TTT GAA AGT	1767 bp	PCV2 detection and sequencing	L. Li et al., 2016
R-PCV2C	AAA TTT CTG ACA AAC GTT ACA			
PCV2ab 2NF	GGT TGG AAG TAA TCA ATA GTG GA	277 bp	PCV2a-specific	T. Kwon et al., 2017
PCV2a 2NR	GGG GAA CCA ACA AAA TCT C			Hesse et al., 2008
PCV2ab 2NF	GGT TGG AAG TAA TCA ATA GTG GA	277 bp	PCV2b-specific	T. Kwon et al., 2017
PCV2b 2NR	GGG GCT CAA ACC CCC GCT C			Hesse et al., 2008
PCV2d 2NF	GGT TGG AAG TAA TCG ATT GTC CT	343 bp	PCV2d-specific	T. Kwon et al., 2017
PCV2d 2NR	TCA GAA CGC CCT CCT GGA AT			
PCV3-1-F	TTA CTT AGA GAA CGG ACT TGT AAC G	649 bp	PCV3 detection	Ku et al., 2016
PCV3-1-R	AAA TGA GAC ACA GAG CTA TAT TCA G			
PCV3-genome-2-F	TTG CAC TTG TGT ACA ATT ATT GCG	1075 bp	PCV3 sequencing	Ku et al., 2016
PCV3-genome-2-R	ATC TTC AGG ACA CTC GTA GCA CCA C			

Table 2 PCR results for genotyping of PCV2-positive serum and tissue samples

Sample type	PCV2 genotype	Number of samples		Number of farms		PCV3 co-infection (samples/farms)
Serum Samples	2a	1	(1/30, 3.3%)	1	(1/25, 4%)	1 (1/1, 100%) /1 (1/1, 100%)
	2b	1	(1/30, 3.3%)	1	(1/25, 4%)	0
	2d	25	(25/30, 83.3%)	20	(20/25, 80%)	4 (4/25, 16%) /4 (4/20, 20%)
	2b, 2d	3	(3/30, 10%)	3	(3/25, 12%)	1 (1/3, 33.3%) /1 (1/3, 33%)
Tissue Samples	2a	8	(8/141, 5%)	1	(1/34, 2.9%)	0
	2b	5	(5/141, 3.1%)	1	(1/34, 2.9%)	0
	2d	82	(82/141, 51.3%)	17	(17/34, 50%)	6 (6/82, 7.3%) /3 (3/17, 17.6%)
	2a, 2b	1	(1/141, 0.6%)	1	(1/34, 2.9%)	1 (1/1, 100%) /1 (1/1, 100%)
	2a, 2d	20	(20/141, 12.5%)	3	(3/34, 8.8%)	1 (1/20, 5%) /1 (1/3, 33.3%)
	2b, 2d	16	(16/141, 10%)	8	(8/34, 23.5%)	0
	2a, 2b, 2d	9	(9/141, 5.6%)	3	(3/34, 8.8%)	0

PCR detection of PCV3

Samples suspected of harbouring PCV3 had already been tested for porcine reproductive and respiratory syndrome (PRRS) and PCV2, as they are routinely diagnosed pathogens of pigs in the CBNU-VDC. Using 2× F-Star Taq PCR Master Mix (BIOFACT Co., Daejeon, Korea), a pair of primers was used to detect PCV3, and another pair of primers was utilized for ORF2-region genome sequencing, as described in a previous study [36] (Table 1). The following conditions were used for PCR: pre-denaturation at 94 °C for 2 min, 35 cycles of denaturation at 94 °C for 30 s, annealing at 56 °C for 30 s, and extension at 72 °C for 1 min, and a final extension at 72 °C for 10 min.

Phylogenetic analysis

The ORF2 regions of PCV2 and PCV3 were amplified with the sequencing primers listed in Table 1. The PCR products were then sequenced using a commercial sequencing service (BIOFACT Co., Daejeon, Korea), and assembly was completed with SeqMan v5.06 (DNASTAR, Madison, Wisconsin, USA). A total of 32 sequences were submitted to GenBank, 27 of which were PCV2 and 5 PCV3 (Accession numbers MF631803-MF631834). A phylogenetic tree for PCV2 genotypes was inferred by using the maximum-likelihood (ML) method with 1000 replicates for bootstrap values based on the ORF2 scale and utilizing the software MEGA 6.06; Korean strains detected since 2015 and reference strains for each genotype were employed [42]. In the case of PCV3, the same method was used to reconstruct a phylogenetic tree on the ORF2 scale with all PCV3 ORF2 sequences in GenBank.

Results

PCR detection of PCV2 and genotyping

PCV2-positive samples were examined by genotyping PCR (Table 2). Serum samples were positive for PCV2a (1/30, 1 farm), PCV2b (1/30, 1 farm), PCV2d (25/30, 20 farms), and co-infection with PCV2b and 2d (3/30, 3 farms). Tissue samples were positive for PCV2a (8/141, 1 farm), PCV2b (5/141, 1 farm), PCV2d (82/141 17 farms), PCV2a and 2b (1/141, 1 farm), PCV2a and 2d (20/141, 3 farms), PCV2b and 2d (16/141, 8 farms), and PCV2a, 2b and 2d (9/141, 3 farms). In addition, 14 samples from 11 farms were positive for both PCV2 and PCV3 (Table 2). The age-wise distribution of PCV2-positive samples revealed that among five groups, finisher pigs were infected most (24.0%) prevalently, followed by growing pigs (21.1%), weaning pigs (10.5%), suckling pigs (4.1%) and sows and gilts (1.2%) (Fig. 1).

Phylogenetic analysis of PCV2 ORF2

The 27 PCV2 ORF2 sequences identified in the current study were classified into three groups (PCV2a, PCV2b, and PCV2d), with minor mutant groups. All of the PCV2d sequences identified in this study belong to the PCV2d-2 clade (Fig. 2).

The ORF2 length of PCV2a and PCV2b is 702 bp, while that of PCV2d is 705 bp. Korean PCV2a, PCV2b, and PCV2d exhibit 99.4 ± 0.2% (99.1–99.6%), 98.7 ± 0.5% (98.1–99.4%), and 99.5 ± 0.3% (98.6–100%) within-group homology, respectively. In addition, PCV2d shares 90.4 ± 0.2% (89.6–91.0%) and 93.9 ± 0.3% (93.2–94.3%)

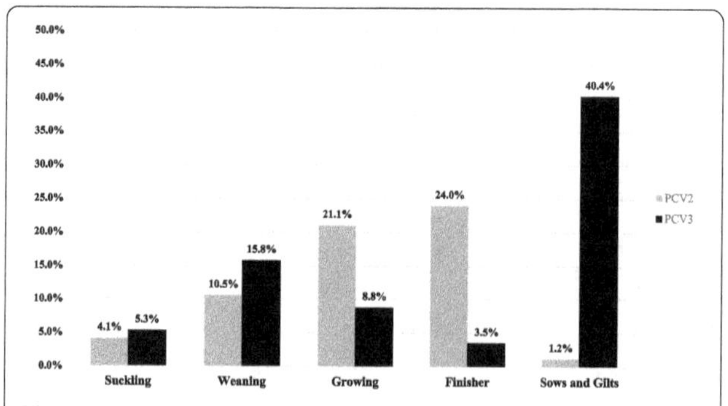

Fig. 1 Distribution of PCV2 and PCV3 infection by age group

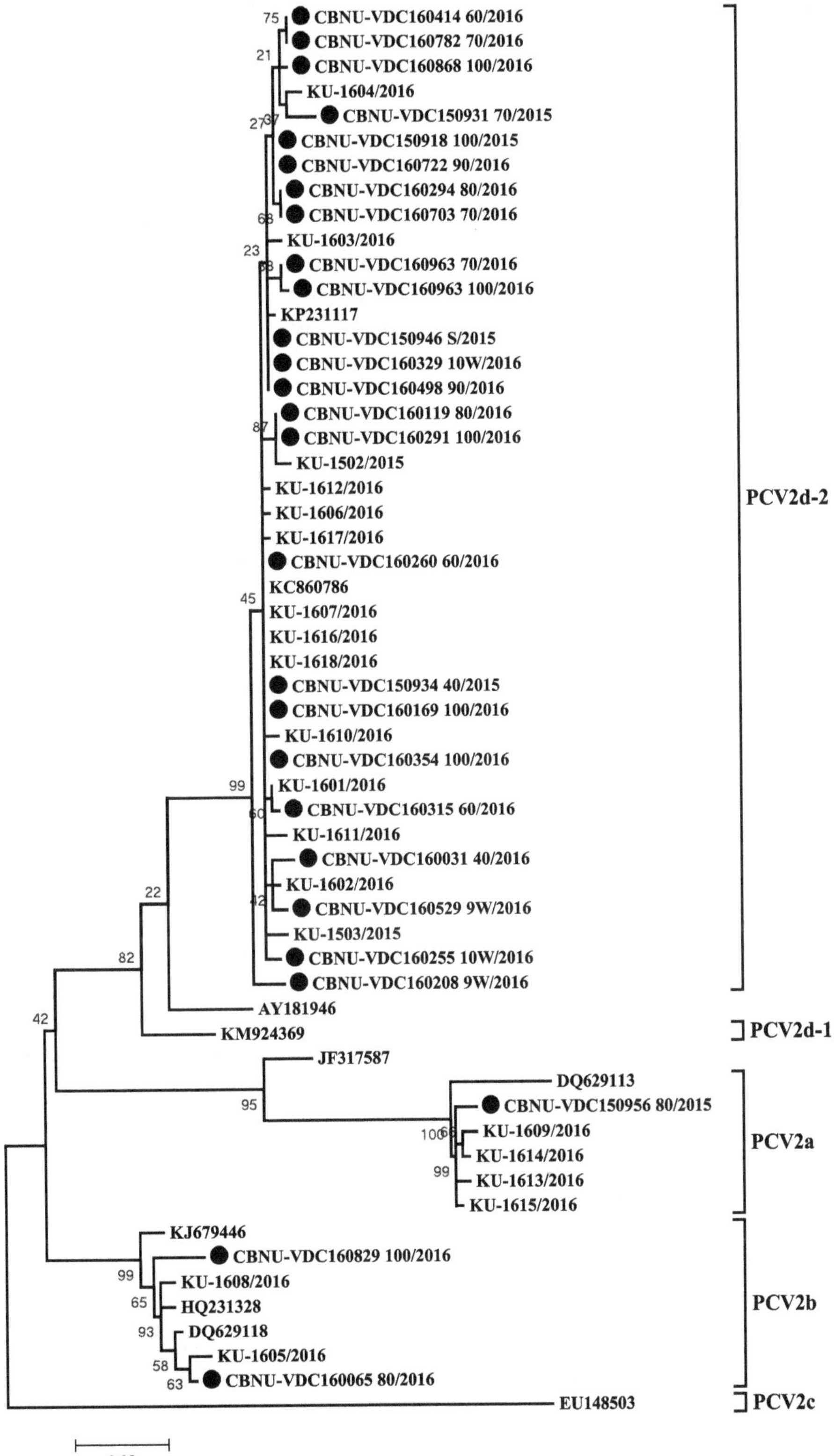

Fig. 2 Phylogenetic trees of PCV2 ORF2 sequences constructed using the maximum-likelihood method based on the generalized time-reversible (GTR) model with G + I in MEGA 6.06. Bootstrap values were calculated with 1000 replicates. Filled circles indicate the PCV2 strains identified in this study

Table 3 Average nucleotide sequence homology within and between PCV2 genotypes

Nucleotide homology within genotypes (%)	Genotype	Nucleotide homology between PCV2 genotypes (%)		
		PCV2a	PCV2b	PCV2d
99.4 ± 0.2 (99.1–99.6)	PCV2a	–	–	–
98.7 ± 0.5 (98.1–99.4)	PCV2b	91.4 ± 0.3 (91.0–92.0)	–	–
99.5 ± 0.3 (98.6–100)	PCV2d	90.4 ± 0.2 (89.6–91.0)	93.9 ± 0.3 (93.2–94.3)	–

Homology was determined by the maximum-likelihood method based on the GTR model with G + I in MEGA 6.06 software. Bootstrap values were calculated with 1000 replicates. The analysis includes Korean ORF2 sequences isolated after 2015

homology with PCV2a and PCV2b, respectively, and PCV2a and PCV2b share 91.4 ± 0.3% homology (91.0–92.0%) (Table 3).

PCR detection of PCV3 and co-infection with PRRS virus (PRRSV) and PCV2

Among 286 serum samples from 47 farms, 37 samples (12.9%) from 20 farms (42.6%) were PCV3 positive. Of 296 tissue samples from 91 farms, 20 samples (6.8%) from 12 farms (6.8%) were positive. The positive rate of PCV3 was higher for serum samples than for tissue samples. Of 108 samples (26 farms) of aborted foetuses, only 2 samples (2 farms) were positive. The age-wise distribution of PCV3-positive samples revealed that among five groups, sows and gilts were infected most (40.4%) prevalently, followed by weaned pigs (15.8%), growing pigs (8.8%), suckling pigs (5.3%) and finisher pigs (3.5%) (Fig. 2). In addition, co-infection with PRRSV or PCV2 was identified in 12 serum and 13 tissue samples and in 4 serum and 7 tissue samples, respectively (Table 4).

Phylogenetic analysis of PCV3 ORF2

The length of all PCV3 ORF2 sequences is 645 bp. Five PCV3 ORF2 sequences identified in this study were compared with those available in GenBank, and 98.7 ± 0.4% (98.0–99.5%) sequence homology is shared among the sequences. However, attempts at full-length sequencing were not successful. By comparing p-distances of all PCV3 ORF2 sequences present in GenBank, 3 clades, designated Clades I, II, and III, are proposed. Clade II can also be sub-grouped as Clade IIa and IIb. The Korean PCV3 strains are grouped into all three major clades (Fig. 3). Average p-distances of 0.0065 ± 0.0035, 0.0079 ± 0.0045, and 0.0050 ± 0.0026 were calculated for PCV3 Clades I, II, and III, respectively, and the p-distances between clades (Clade I/II: 0.0144 ± 0.0027, Clade I/III: 0.0152 ± 0.0027, and Clade II/III: 0.0155 ± 0.0030) were significant. However, four strains could not be classified into any of these three clades due to their long p-distances, suggesting the possibility of new clades or intermediate clades (Table 5).

Discussion

In the current study, PCV2 isolates detected in samples from 50 farms of 60 PCV2-positive farms were identified as PCV2d (Table 2 and Fig. 2), suggesting a major genotype shift from PCV2b to PCV2d on swine farms in Korea [14]. Detection of PCV2d alone was predominant in both serum and tissue samples, but co-detection of PCV2a, PCV2b or PCV2d was more prevalent in tissue samples such as lungs and lymph nodes than in serum samples. Since it is not possible to differentiate between PCV2 detected in tissue samples with current or previous infection and only actively replicating virus can be detected in circulating blood, PCV2 genotyping in serum samples was concluded to appropriately identify the major genotype causing clinical problems on farms at the specific time of the current study.

When the age-wise distribution of PCV2-positive cases was analysed, the highest positive rate was detected in finishers (24.0%), followed by growing pigs (21.1%). PCV2-positive rates were also reported in previous studies to be higher in growing and finisher pigs than in other groups, suggesting the higher susceptibility of growing and finisher pigs to PCV2 infection and maternal antibodies interfering with vaccination [43–45]. In addition, the PCV2-positive rate has increased in suckling and weaned pig populations (Fig. 1). Opriessnig et al. [46] reported that the current PCV2 vaccines, which were developed based on PCV2a, can prevent PCV2d transmission to naive pigs and the vaccinated pigs showed reduced levels of PCV2d viraemia. Because mass vaccination with PCV2a-based inactivated vaccines are applied to 3–4-week-old piglets and sows in Korean farms, it was concluded that the current PCV2 vaccines reduce clinical

Table 4 PCR results for PCV3-positive serum and tissue samples

Sample type	Number of samples	Number of farms	PRRS co-infection (samples/farms)	PCV2 co-infection (samples/farms)
Serum	37 (37/286, 12.9%)	20 (20/47, 42.6%)	12 (12/37, 32.4%)/10 (10/20, 50%)	4 (4/37, 10.8%)/4 (4/20, 20%)
Tissue	20 (20/296, 6.8%)	12 (12/91, 13.2%)	13 (13/20, 65%)/10 (10/12, 83.3%)	7 (7/20, 35%)/6 (6/12, 50%)
Aborted foetus	2 (2/108, 1.9%)	2 (2/26, 7.7%)	–	–

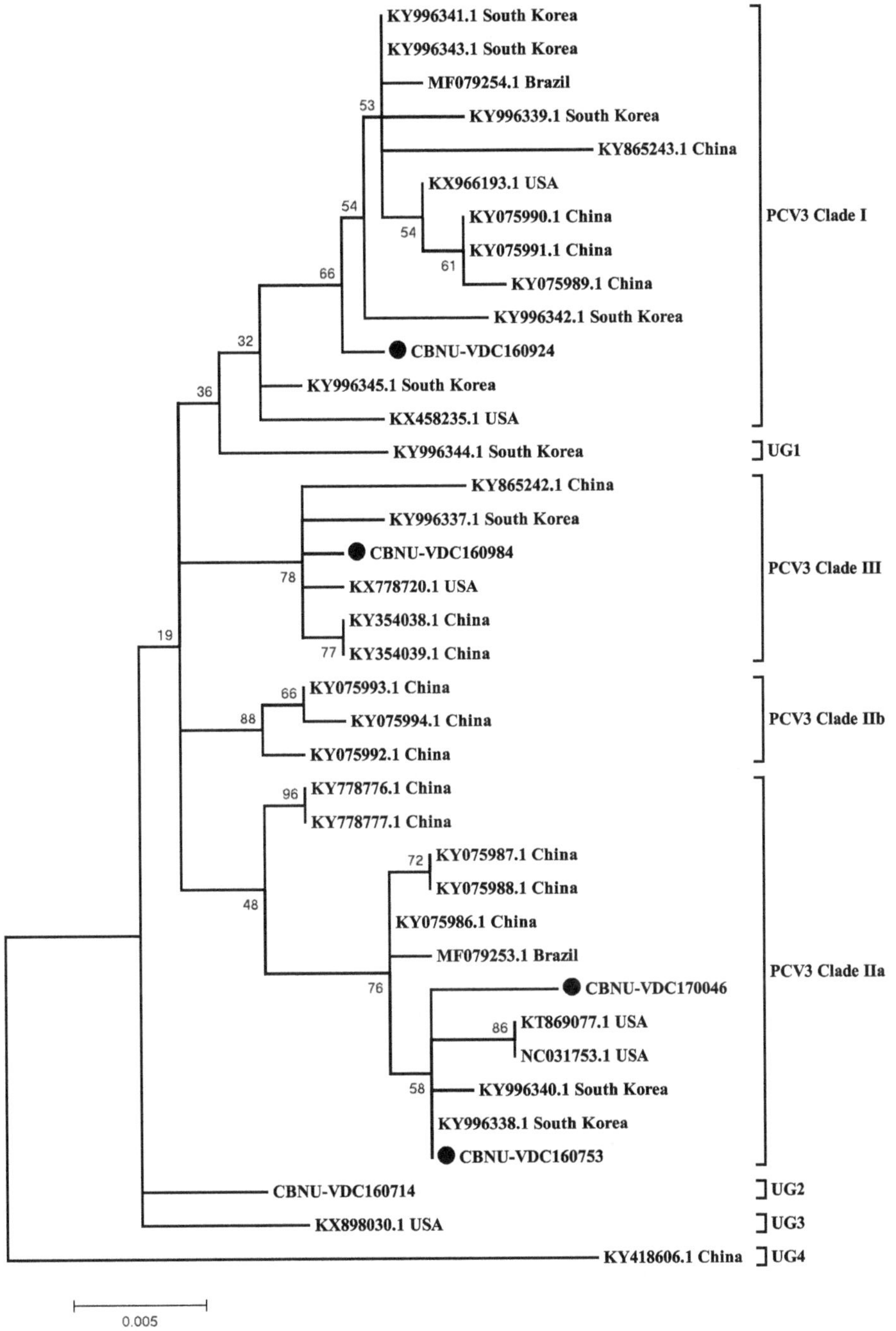

Fig. 3 Phylogenetic trees of PCV3 ORF2 sequences of Korean PCV3 constructed using the maximum-likelihood method based on the GTR model with G + I in MEGA 6.06. Bootstrap values were calculated with 1000 replicates. Filled circles indicate the PCV3 strains identified in this study

symptoms and lesions caused by PCV2d but do not provide sterile immunity against PCV2d infection.

Recently, clinical signs similar to those of PCVAD were reported from PCV2 negative pigs, and a novel porcine circovirus, PCV3, was identified from these cases [34]. Another research group reported a case of cardiac and multi-systemic inflammation due to PCV3 infection [35]. A Chinese research group detected PCV3 in China (34.7% of individual samples and 68.6% at the farm level were positive), suggesting the wide distribution of PCV3 in multiple tissues and the possibility of vertical transmission [36]. Nationwide surveillance for PCV3 has been conducted in Korea, reporting approximately 72.6% of investigated farms to be positive for this infection [38]. In the present study, serum and tissue samples from various farms were tested for PCV3, and 12.9% of serum samples

Table 5 Average *p*-distances within and between PCV3 clades

Average *p*-distance within clades (mean ± SE)	Genotype	Average *p*-distance between PCV3 clades (mean ± SE)						
		Clade I	Clade II	Clade III	UG1	UG2	UG3	UG4
0.0065 ± 0.0035	Clade I	–	–	–	–	–	–	–
0.0079 ± 0.0045	Clade II	0.0144 ± 0.0027	–	–	–	–	–	–
0.0050 ± 0.0026	Clade III	0.0152 ± 0.0027	0.0155 ± 0.0030	–	–	–	–	–
–	UG1	0.0136 ± 0.0025	0.0163 ± 0.0031	0.0150 ± 0.0019	–	–	–	–
–	UG2	0.0132 ± 0.0022	0.0127 ± 0.0020	0.0134 ± 0.0019	0.0140	–	–	–
–	UG3	0.0148 ± 0.0022	0.0143 ± 0.0020	0.0150 ± 0.0019	0.0155	0.0109	–	–
–	UG4	0.0308 ± 0.0024	0.0293 ± 0.0017	0.0328 ± 0.0012	0.0341	0.0295	0.0279	–

The *p*-distance was determined by the neighbour-joining method based on the GTR model with G + I in MEGA 6.06 software. Bootstrap values were calculated with 1000 replicates. The analysis includes ORF2 sequences of 13 PCV3 Clade I, 15 PCV3 Clade II, 6 PCV3 Clade III and 4 ungrouped (UG) sequences (UG1 = KY996344.1, UG2 = CBNU-VDC160714, UG3 = KX898030.1 and UG4 = KY418606.1)

(42.6% at the farm level) and 6.8% of tissue samples (13.2% at the farm level) were positive. Although the overall positive rate was less than that of the previous study by another Korean research group [38], PCV3 is clearly prevalent in the Korean swine industry.

Analysis based on age-wise distribution of PCV3-positive samples revealed the highest prevalence in the group of sows and gilts (40.4%), whereas the suckling pig group showed a relatively low positive rate (5.3%) (Fig. 1). In previous studies, PCV3 has been identified from sows that experienced abortion, and cardiac and multi-systemic inflammation [34–36]. Thus, the age susceptibility and physio-pathologic characteristic of PCV3 might have a close relationship with the high positive rate in the sow and gilt group. Reproductive failures and stillbirth cases have been reported to be caused by PCV3 [34, 36, 39]. In our study, however, PCV3 was detected from only 2 aborted foetuses from 2 farms (of 108 samples from 26 farms). In fact, the association of PCV3 with the clinical condition remains controversial. For example, Franzo G et al. [47] was unable to find statistically significant relevance of PCV3 co-infection with any clinical condition, yet Zhai et al. [48] reported that a higher genome load of PCV3 was detected in cases of severe respiratory disease or diarrhea than in mild cases. Thus, the relationship between PCV3 infection and clinical symptoms should be investigated further.

Genotyping PCV2 has been an important issue because different genotypes of PCV2 have resulted in outbreaks and vaccine failures in the global swine industry. PCV2 genotypes are divided by a *p*-distance cut-off of 0.035 [22]. PCV3 being one of the possible causes of PCVAD outbreak, it is indeed important to set criteria for genotyping of PCV3 and monitoring trends in genotype distribution. In a previous study, PCV3 strains were divided into 2 clades (PCV3a and PCV3b) based on the partial capsid protein gene of 474 bp [36]. In the present study, all PCV3 sequences available in GenBank were analysed based on the ORF2 sequence, and PCV3 was tentatively divided into three clades (Clades I, II and III). To define the *p*-distance cut-off for genotyping PCV3, more PCV3 ORF2 sequences should be identified worldwide.

Conclusion

Our study summarized the recent evolution of PCV2 and PCV3 in Korea. PCV2d is most prevalent in Korea, even though PCV2a-based vaccines are currently used for regular vaccination. In addition, a novel porcine circovirus, PCV3, has recently emerged in Korea. Although no significant association was demonstrated between PCV3 infection and clinical symptoms, continuous surveillance for PCV3 should be performed in future studies.

Abbreviations

CBNU-VDC: Chonbuk National University-Veterinary Diagnostic Center; PCV2: Porcine circovirus type 2; PCV3: Porcine circovirus type 3; PCVAD: Porcine circovirus-associated disease; *p*-distance: Pairwise distance

Acknowledgements

The authors wish to acknowledge the assistance of the lab technicians and undergraduate students from the College of Veterinary Medicine, Veterinary Diagnostic Center, Chonbuk National University.

Funding

The experiments related to the prevalence and genetic characteristics of porcine circovirus type 2 were carried out with the support by grants from the Technology Development Program for Bio-industry (315029-3). In addition, the experiments related to the prevalence and genetic characteristics of porcine circovirus type 3 were and the Cooperative Research Program for Agriculture Science & Technology Development (PJ012612) in Rural Development Administration, Republic of Korea.

Authors' contributions

SCK conducted the experiments and drafted the manuscript. SN participated in the sequence and data analysis and helped in drafting the manuscript. SK, JHJ, KHM and DYJ contributed to the collection and processing of the samples. AK and CGJ contributed to the data analysis. SJK assisted in designing the study and critically revising the manuscript. WIK designed the entire study and prepared the manuscript. All authors read and approved the final manuscript.

Consent for publication
Not applicable.

Competing interests
The authors declare that they have no competing interests.

Author details
[1]College of Veterinary Medicine, Chonbuk National University, 79 Gobong-ro, Iksan 54596, Jeonbuk, Republic of Korea. [2]National Institute of Animal Science, Rural Development Administration, Cheonan 55365, South Korea.

References

1. Tischer I, Rasch R, Tochtermann G. Characterization of papovavirus-and picornavirus-like particles in permanent pig kidney cell lines. Zentralbl Bakteriol Orig A. 1974;226(2):153–67.
2. Tischer I, Mields W, Wolff D, Vagt M, Griem W. Studies on epidemiology and pathogenicity of porcine circovirus. Arch Virol. 1986;91(3–4):271–6.
3. Clark E. Pathology of the post-weaning multisystemic wasting syndrome of pigs. Proc Western Can Assoc Swine Pract. 1996;1996:22–5.
4. Harding JC. Postweaning multisystemic wasting syndrome: epidemiology and clinical presentation. J Swine Health Prod. 1998;6(6):249–54.
5. Opriessnig T, Meng XJ, Halbur PG. Porcine circovirus type 2 associated disease: update on current terminology, clinical manifestations, pathogenesis, diagnosis, and intervention strategies. J Vet Diagn Investig. 2007;19(6):591–615.
6. Grau-Roma L, Fraile L, Segales J. Recent advances in the epidemiology, diagnosis and control of diseases caused by porcine circovirus type 2. Vet J. 2011;187(1):23–32.
7. West KH, Bystrom JM, Wojnarowicz C, Shantz N, Jacobson M, Allan GM, Haines DM, Clark EG, Krakowka S, McNeilly F, et al. Myocarditis and abortion associated with intrauterine infection of sows with porcine circovirus 2. J Vet Diagn Investig. 1999;11(6):530–2.
8. Kim J, Chung HK, Chae C. Association of porcine circovirus 2 with porcine respiratory disease complex. Vet J. 2003;166(3):251–6.
9. Rosell C, Segales J, Ramos-Vara JA, Folch JM, Rodriguez-Arrioja GM, Duran CO, Balasch M, Plana-Duran J, Domingo M. Identification of porcine circovirus in tissues of pigs with porcine dermatitis and nephropathy syndrome. Vet Rec. 2000;146(2):40–3.
10. Kim J, Ha Y, Jung K, Choi C, Chae C. Enteritis associated with porcine circovirus 2 in pigs. Can J Vet Res. 2004;68(3):218–21.
11. Jensen TK, Vigre H, Svensmark B, Bille-Hansen V. Distinction between porcine circovirus type 2 enteritis and porcine proliferative enteropathy caused by Lawsonia intracellularis. J Comp Pathol. 2006;135(4):176–82.
12. Drolet R, Larochelle R, Morin M, Delisle B, Magar R. Detection rates of porcine reproductive and respiratory syndrome virus, porcine circovirus type 2, and swine influenza virus in porcine proliferative and necrotizing pneumonia. Vet Pathol. 2003;40(2):143–8.
13. Chae C. A review of porcine circovirus 2-associated syndromes and diseases. Vet J. 2005;169(3):326–36.
14. Kwon T, Lee DU, Yoo SJ, Je SH, Shin JY, Lyoo YS. Genotypic diversity of porcine circovirus type 2 (PCV2) and genotype shift to PCV2d in Korean pig population. Virus Res. 2017;228:24–9.
15. Nawagitgul P, Morozov I, Bolin SR, Harms PA, Sorden SD, Paul PS. Open reading frame 2 of porcine circovirus type 2 encodes a major capsid protein. J Gen Virol. 2000;81(9):2281–7.
16. Cheung AK. Homologous recombination within the capsid gene of porcine circovirus type 2 subgroup viruses via natural co-infection. Arch Virol. 2009; 154(3):531–4.
17. Fenaux M, Halbur PG, Gill M, Toth TE, Meng X-J. Genetic characterization of type 2 porcine circovirus (PCV-2) from pigs with postweaning multisystemic wasting syndrome in different geographic regions of North America and development of a differential PCR-restriction fragment length polymorphism assay to detect and differentiate between infections with PCV-1 and PCV-2. J Clin Microbiol. 2000;38(7):2494–503.
18. Hamel AL, Lin LL, Sachvie C, Grudeski E, Nayar G. PCR detection and characterization of type-2 porcine circovirus. Can J Vet Res. 2000;64(1):44.
19. Mankertz A, Domingo M, Folch JM, LeCann P, Jestin A, Segalés J, Chmielewicz B, Plana-Durán J, Soike D. Characterisation of PCV-2 isolates from Spain, Germany and France. Virus Res. 2000;66(1):65–77.
20. Olvera A, Cortey M, Segales J. Molecular evolution of porcine circovirus type 2 genomes: phylogeny and clonality. Virology. 2007;357(2):175–85.
21. Xiao C-T, Halbur PG, Opriessnig T. Global molecular genetic analysis of porcine circovirus type 2 (PCV2) sequences confirms the presence of four main PCV2 genotypes and reveals a rapid increase of PCV2d. J Gen Virol. 2015;96(7):1830–41.
22. Segalés J, Olvera A, Grau-Roma L, Charreyre C, Nauwynck H, Larsen L, Dupont K, McCullough K, Ellis J, Krakowka S. PCV-2 genotype definition and nomenclature. Vet Rec. 2008;162(26):867.
23. Chae C: An emerging porcine circovirus type 2b mutant (mPCV2b) originally known as PCV2d. Vet J 2015, 203(1):6.
24. Kumar S, Tamura K, Jakobsen IB, Nei M. MEGA2: molecular evolutionary genetics analysis software. Bioinformatics. 2001;17(12):1244–5.
25. Dupont K, Nielsen E, Baekbo P, Larsen L. Genomic analysis of PCV2 isolates from Danish archives and a current PMWS case–control study supports a shift in genotypes with time. Vet Microbiol. 2008;128(1):56–64.
26. Wang F, Guo X, Ge X, Wang Z, Chen Y, Cha Z, Yang H. Genetic variation analysis of Chinese strains of porcine circovirus type 2. Virus Res. 2009;145(1):151–6.
27. Guo LJ, Lu YH, Wei YW, Huang LP, Liu CM. Porcine circovirus type 2 (PCV2): genetic variation and newly emerging genotypes in China. Virol J. 2010;7(1):273.
28. Guo L, Fu Y, Wang Y, Lu Y, Wei Y, Tang Q, Fan P, Liu J, Zhang L, Zhang F. A porcine circovirus type 2 (PCV2) mutant with 234 amino acids in capsid protein showed more virulence in vivo, compared with classical PCV2a/b strain. PLoS One. 2012;7(7):e41463.
29. Eddicks M, Fux R, Szikora F, Eddicks L, Majzoub-Altweck M, Hermanns W, Sutter G, Palzer A, Banholzer E, Ritzmann M. Detection of a new cluster of porcine circovirus type 2b strains in domestic pigs in Germany. Vet Microbiol. 2015;176(3):337–43.
30. Salgado RL, Vidigal PM, de Souza LF, Onofre TS, Gonzaga NF, Eller MR, Bressan GC, Fietto JL, Almeida MR, Júnior AS. Identification of an emergent porcine circovirus-2 in vaccinated pigs from a Brazilian farm during a postweaning multisystemic wasting syndrome outbreak. Genome Announc. 2014;2(2):e00163–14.
31. Seo HW, Park C, Kang I, Choi K, Jeong J, Park S-J, Chae C. Genetic and antigenic characterization of a newly emerging porcine circovirus type 2b mutant first isolated in cases of vaccine failure in Korea. Arch Virol. 2014; 159(11):3107–11.
32. Xiao C-T, Halbur PG, Opriessnig T. Complete genome sequence of a novel porcine circovirus type 2b variant present in cases of vaccine failures in the United States. J Virol. 2012;86(22):–12469.
33. Davies B, Wang X, Dvorak CM, Marthaler D, Murtaugh MP. Diagnostic phylogenetics reveals a new porcine circovirus 2 cluster. Virus Res. 2016;217:32–7.
34. Palinski R, Piñeyro P, Shang P, Yuan F, Guo R, Fang Y, Byers E, Hause BM. A novel porcine circovirus distantly related to known circoviruses is associated with porcine dermatitis and nephropathy syndrome and reproductive failure. J Virol. 2017;91(1):e01879–16.
35. Phan TG, Giannitti F, Rossow S, Marthaler D, Knutson TP, Li L, Deng X, Resende T, Vannucci F, Delwart E. Detection of a novel circovirus PCV3 in pigs with cardiac and multi-systemic inflammation. Virol J. 2016;13(1):184.
36. Ku X, Chen F, Li P, Wang Y, Yu X, Fan S, Qian P, Wu M, He Q. Identification and genetic characterization of porcine circovirus type 3 in China. Transbound Emerg Dis. 2017;64(3):703–8.
37. Shen H, Liu X, Zhang P, Wang L, Liu Y, Zhang L, Liang P, Song C. Genome characterization of a porcine circovirus type 3 in South China. Transbound Emerg Dis. 2017.
38. Kwon T, Yoo SJ, Park CK, Lyoo YS. Prevalence of novel porcine circovirus 3 in Korean pig populations. Vet Microbiol. 2017;207:178–80.
39. Zheng S, Wu X, Zhang L, Xin C, Liu Y, Shi J, Peng Z, Xu S, Fu F, Yu J. The occurrence of porcine circovirus 3 without clinical infection signs in Shandong Province. Transbound Emerg Dis. 2017;64(5):1337–41.
40. Li L, Yuan W, Guo H, Ma Z, Song Q, Wang X, Li H. Prevalence and genetic variation of porcine circovirus type 2 in Hebei, China from 2004 to 2014. Gene. 2016;586(2):222–7.
41. Hesse R, Kerrigan M, Rowland RR. Evidence for recombination between PCV2a and PCV2b in the field. Virus Res. 2008;132(1):201–7.

42. Tamura K, Stecher G, Peterson D, Filipski A, Kumar S. MEGA6: molecular evolutionary genetics analysis version 6.0. Mol Biol Evol. 2013;30(12):2725–9.
43. Fraile L, Sibila M, Nofrarias M, Lopez-Jimenez R, Huerta E, Llorens A, Lopez-Soria S, Perez D, Segales J. Effect of sow and piglet porcine circovirus type 2 (PCV2) vaccination on piglet mortality, viraemia, antibody titre and production parameters. Vet Microbiol. 2012;161(1–2):229–34.
44. Oliver-Ferrando S, Segales J, Lopez-Soria S, Callen A, Merdy O, Joisel F, Sibila M. Evaluation of natural porcine circovirus type 2 (PCV2) subclinical infection and seroconversion dynamics in piglets vaccinated at different ages. Vet Res. 2016;47(1):121.
45. Shen H-G, Loiacono CM, Halbur PG, Opriessnig T. Age-dependent susceptibility to porcine circovirus type 2 infections is likely associated with declining levels of maternal antibodies. J Swine Health Prod. 2012;20(1):17–24.
46. Opriessnig T, Xiao CT, Halbur PG, Gerber PF, Matzinger SR, Meng XJ. A commercial porcine circovirus (PCV) type 2a-based vaccine reduces PCV2d viremia and shedding and prevents PCV2d transmission to naive pigs under experimental conditions. Vaccine. 2017;35(2):248–54.
47. Franzo G, Legnardi M, Tucciarone CM, Drigo M, Klaumann F, Sohrmann M, SegalEs J. Porcine circovirus type 3: a threat to the pig industry? Vet Rec. 2018;182(3):83.
48. Zhai SL, Zhou X, Zhang H, Hause BM, Lin T, Liu R, Chen QL, Wei WK, Lv DH, Wen XH, et al. Comparative epidemiology of porcine circovirus type 3 in pigs with different clinical presentations. Virol J. 2017;14(1):222.

22

Hypothalamus-pituitary-adrenal axis involves in anti-viral ability through regulation of immune response in piglets infected by highly pathogenic porcine reproductive and respiratory syndrome virus

Jie Tong[1†], Ying Yu[1†], Linlin Zheng[1†], Chong Zhang[1], Yabin Tu[1], Yonggang Liu[1], Jianan Wu[1], Hai Li[1], Shujie Wang[1], Chenggang Jiang[1], En-Min Zhou[2], Gang Wang[1*] and Xuehui Cai[1*]

Abstract

Background: The highly pathogenic porcine reproductive and respiratory syndrome virus (HP-PRRSV) has been responsible for several viral attacks in the Asian porcine industry, since the first outbreak in China in 2006. During the early stages of the HP-PRRSV infection, high levels of proinflammatory cytokines are noted in the host peripheral blood, which are accompanied by severe lesions in the lungs and immune system organs; these are considered as the greatest contributors to the overall disease burden. We hypothesized that the anti-PRRSV response in piglets might be mediated by the hypothalamus-pituitary-adrenal (HPA) axis, which led to a decrease in the psycho-neuroendocrinological manifestation of HP-PRRSV etiology via immune response regulation.

Results: We investigated the regulation of the HPA axis in HP-PRRSV-infected piglets that were treated with 1 mg/kg body weight (b. w.)/day mifepristone (RU486) or 2 mg/kg b.w./day dexamethasone (DEX). Both RU486 and DEX enhanced the disease status of the piglets infected by the HP-PRRSV HuN4 strain, resulting in high mortality and more severe pathological changes in the lungs.

Conclusions: HP-PRRSV infection activates the HPA axis, and artificial regulation of the immune-endocrine system enhances disease severity in HP-PRRSV-infected piglets. Thus, DEX and RU486 should be avoided in the clinical treatment of HP-PRRS.

Keywords: HP-PRRSV, Hypothalamus-pituitary-adrenal axis, Proinflammatory cytokines

Background

Porcine reproductive and respiratory syndrome (PRRS) is caused by PRRS virus (PRRSV) [1]. Since the first outbreak in 2006, HP-PRRS has been the leading cause of serious economic losses in the pig industry in China [2–4]. It is generally believed that PRRSV induces lesions in immune organs in piglets, causing severe disorders of the host immune response [5–8].

Apart from the direct effect of the virus infection, the inefficient immune response may also be caused by an unbalanced neuro-endocrino-immunological (NEI) status after PRRSV infection. In this case, the hypothalamus-pituitary-adrenal (HPA) axis is considered to play a crucial role as it changes the host's susceptibility to some infectious diseases. Under stressful conditions, such as during a robust proinflammatory response in the early stage of

* Correspondence: wanggang@caas.cn; cai139@hvri.ac.cn
†Equal contributors
[1]State Key Laboratory of Veterinary Biotechnology, Harbin Veterinary Research Institute of Chinese Academy of Agriculture Science, Harbin 150001, People's Republic of China
Full list of author information is available at the end of the article

virus infection, the HPA axis may be triggered by high levels of proinflammatory cytokines, particularly IL-1β, IL-6, and TNF-α [9]. It has been found that the plasma levels of these cytokines increased after HP-PRRSV infection [10], which may possibly activate the HPA axis after infection. Following the activation of the whole HPA neuroendocrine-pathway, glucocorticoids (GCs) secreted by the adrenal glands are the final effector molecules that suppress violent inflammations and balance the immune response [11]. The anti-inflammatory effects of GCs are mediated via the glucocorticoid receptor (GR) [9, 12], which is a member of the steroid hormone-receptor family of ligand-dependent transcription factors (NR3C1). Accordingly, pharmacologic GCs such as dexamethasone (DEX) have been used as potential therapeutic options for virus-induced autoimmune disease and inflammations, including the Kilham rat virus (KRV) and severe acute respiratory syndromes (SARS) [13, 14]. However, the administration of excess DEX may impede the secretions of ACTH and cortisol through negative feedback loops of the HPA axis, which may also lead to other problems [15]. Hence, DEX treatment has multiple effects on the immune response in the clinical setting. In some other cases, excess GCs induce the apoptosis of lymphocyte cells, which are responsible for immune suppression during viral infection. Apharmacy GC inhibitor, mifepristone (RU486), has been used for GR blockade, and the treatment is termed as a temporary adrenalectomy. However, reports on the interactions between HP-PRRSV infection and HPA axis regulation are currently rare.

Our previous studies showed that HP-PRRSV infection consistently induced high levels of proinflammatory cytokines in the peripheral blood of infected piglets, which resulted in long-lasting high body temperatures and considerably higher mortality as compared to that induced by classical PRRSV infection. Interestingly, most of the infected piglets displayed severe thymus atrophy and lymphocyte apoptosis from 3 to 10 days after the virus infection [7, 10, 16–18]. These symptoms may develop under NEI deficient conditions, which suggests that some neuroendocrine hormones released by the HPA axis failed to modulate the anti-viral innate immune response during the viral infection [19–21]. Thus, we hypothesized that the HPA axis was affected by the HP-PRRSV infection, which then failed to sustain homeostasis in the infected piglets. In this study, we investigated the functions of the HPA axis in HP-PRRSV-infected piglets by assessing the effects of daily treatment with 1 mg/kg body weight (b.w.) RU486 or 2 mg/kg b. w. DEX. At 10 days post infection, higher mortality and more severe pathological changes in the lungs were observed in pharmacy-treated animals, which indicate that disorders of the HPA axis enhance the disease status of piglets infected by the HP-PRRSV HuN4 strain. Furthermore, significant changes in the proinflammatory cytokine levels in peripheral blood were observed in both DEX- and RU486-treated piglets, which was consistent with our hypothesis of incomplete HPA axis function. These results provide new insights into the NEI pathophysiology associated with HP-PRRSV infection.

Methods

Virus

The HP-PRRSV HuN4 strain (GenBank accession no. EF635006) was used in this study as a viral inoculum after three passages through porcine alveolar macrophages (PAMs, which were isolated using a lung lavage technique from 4 to 6-week-old specific-pathogen-free piglets that were free of PRRSV, PCV_2, CSFV, PPV, PRV, swine influenza virus, and Mycoplasma hyopneumoniae infections as previously described [22]) with a titer of $10^{5.0}$ $TCID_{50}$/mL [23].

Ethics statement

The animal experiment protocols were approved by the Animal Ethics Committee of Harbin Veterinary Research Institute of the Chinese Academy of Agricultural Sciences (CAAS), and the methods were conducted in accordance with the approved animal ethics guidelines. The Animal Ethics Committee approval number was SYXK (Hei) 2,015,042.

Experimental design

20 PRRSV-negative piglets (Landrace× Yorkshire× crossbred, 12 males, weighting 7.5 to 9 kg and aged 28 days) were purchased from a local PRRSV free farm (Xinli farm), randomly divided into four groups (5 piglets/group) and maintained separately in isolated rooms. After 1 week of acclimation, Groups A, B and C were inoculated intranasally (i.n., without anesthesia) with 3 mL of HP-PRRSV HuN4 ($10^{5.5}$ $TCID_{50}$ in 3 mL DMEM medium), and Group D were sham-inoculated with 3 mL of DMEM medium. Group A was injected intramuscularly (i.m.) with DEX (Dexamethasone Sodium Phosphate Injection solution, Sanchine Pharmaceutical Co., China) at 2 mg/kg b. w. daily during the HuN4 infection. Group B was injected with RU486 (mifepristone; Sigma-Aldrich, dissolved in 50% ethanol) intra-peritoneally at 1 mg/kg b. w. within 1 day prior to the viral infection. Blood samples collected at 0 (before inoculation), 3, 5, 7 and 10 days after inoculation (days post-inoculation; DPI) were used for virological analysis. Some piglets died without euthanasia during the experimental intervention, and the other piglets were anesthetized by barbiturate overdose (intravenously), bled and euthanized humanely at 14 DPI.

Clinical observation

Piglets were monitored daily for clinical signs including anorexia, lethargy, fever, and emaciation prior to feeding, including anorexia, lethargy, fever, and emaciation.

Serum cytokine levels

Serum samples were collected at the designated DPI. Cytokine concentrations were measured in duplicate using commercial ELISA kits (Cloud Clone Corp, USA) according to the manufacturer's instructions. The serum concentrations of cytokines (pg/mL) were calculated according to the recombinant standards supplied in the kits.

Quantitative real-time PCR for detection of viral loads

Viral loads in peripheral blood were detected by TaqMan fluorescent quantitative RT-PCR (RT-qPCR) as described previously [10].

Necropsy

The macroscopic lesions in the lungs were recorded at necropsy. Sections of the thymus and lungs were fixed in 10% neutrally-buffered formalin for histological examination using hematoxylin and eosin staining.

Statistical analysis

No formal calculation of sample size was done due to the characteristics of the experiment. It was expected that more than three piglets per group would allow obtaining appropriate results data.

Statistical analysis was performed using GraphPad Prism software (version 5.02 for Windows; GraphPad Software). Comparisons between groups were analyzed using the analysis of variance (ANOVA) test. A *P*-value less than 0.05 was considered to indicate statistical significance.

Results

Disease status of piglets infected by HP-PRRSV was enhanced after treatment with RU486 or DEX

Group A (2 mg/kg b. w. DEX) maintained a high fever (40–42 °C) from 2 DPI (Fig. 1a) and showed symptoms of severe HP-PRRS disease, reaching 100% mortality at 14 DPI (Fig. 1b). Similar results were observed in Group B (RU486 1 mg/kg b. w.), reaching 100% mortality at 7 DPI (Fig. 1b). Group C showed symptoms typical of HP-PRRS infection including high fever and one piglet died as a result of HP-PRRS infection at 9 DPI. During the experiment, Groups A and Group B exhibited more severe disease than Group C, which was infected with HuN4 alone. Group D showed no symptoms during the experiment.

Visual and histological observations

The macroscopic lesions of the lungs were recorded at necropsy. The mortality in Groups A and Group B reached 100%, and severe interstitial pneumonia accompanied by edema and congestion was observed in the lungs of these piglets (Fig. 2a and b). Observation of histopathological changes revealed suppurative pneumonia characterized by severe diffuse interstitial proliferation of small lymphocytes (Fig. 2e and f). The lungs of Group C piglets infected with HuN4 alone showed typical signs of interstitial pneumonia (Fig. 2c and g), while the lungs in Groups D piglets were normal (Fig. 2d and h).

Viremia

Group A piglets were PRRSV-positive at 3 DPI (mean titer, $10^{5.69}$ copies/mL), and peaked at 10 DPI ($10^{8.8}$ copies/mL). Group B piglets were also PRRSV-positive at 3 DPI ($10^{5.13}$copies/mL), and peaked at 6 DPI ($10^{9.86}$ copies/mL). The viral load in sera of Group C was $10^{5.14}$copies/mL at 3 DPI and peaked at 10 DPI ($10^{7.31}$copies/mL) (Table 1).

Dysregulation of the HPA axis altered the proinflammatory levels in the peripheral blood of HP-PRRSV-infected piglets

The concentrations of the proinflammatory cytokines IL-1β, IL-6 and TNF-α were determined for all serum samples (Fig. 3). The concentrations of IL-1β, IL-6 and TNF-α in Group A began to rise at 3 DPI, and peaked at 6 DPI. No significant changes in the serum concentrations of IL-1β, IL-6 and TNF-α were detected in Group B during the experiment. The concentrations of IL-1β, IL-6 and TNF-α in Group C also began to increase at 3 DPI, although the levels were significantly lower than those of Group A at 6 DPI.

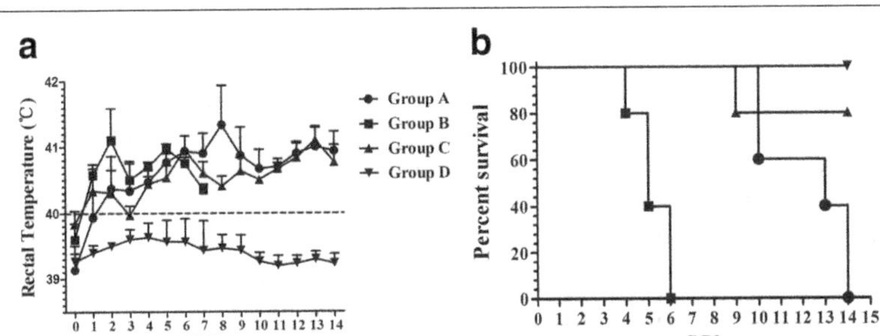

Fig. 1 Rectal temperature and percentage survival in piglets after HuN4 infection. Daily average rectal temperatures in the four groups (**a**), each point represents the mean values (±S.D.) generated from all pigs at each DPI; and percentage survival of piglets from the four groups (**b**)

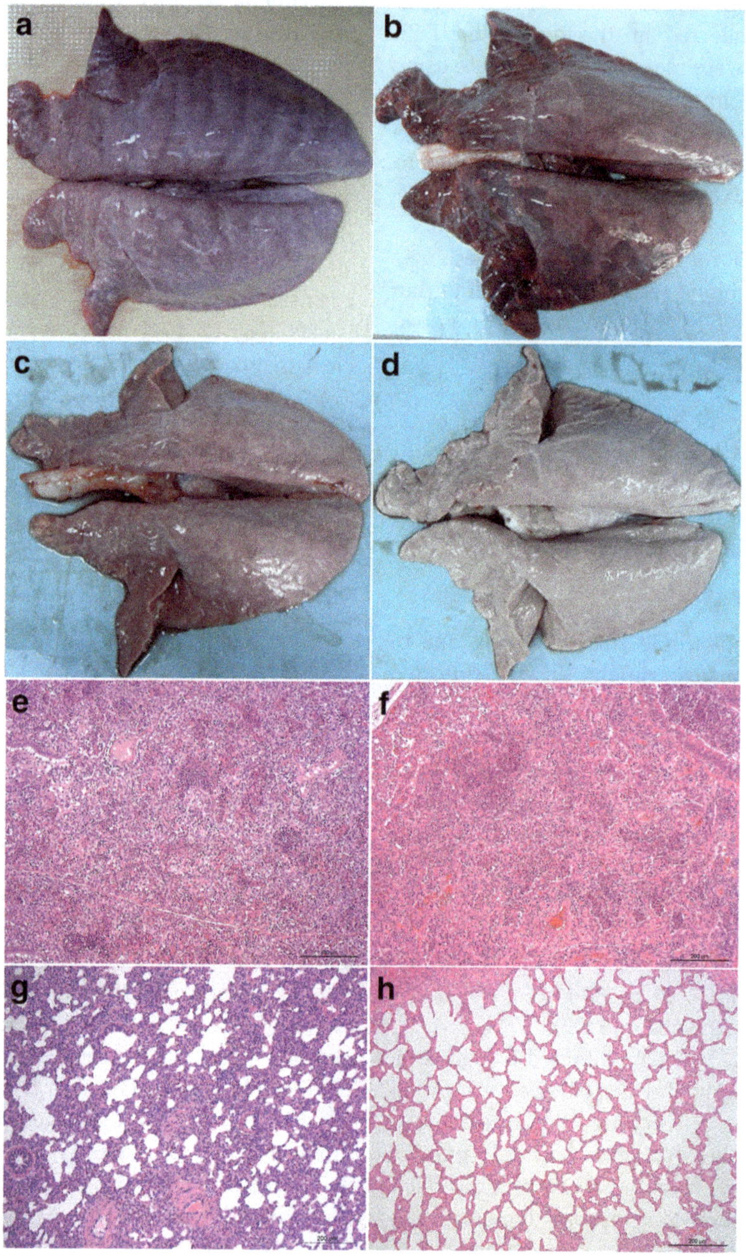

Fig. 2 Representative images showing the gross pathological findings as well as the pathological changes in the lung of piglets from the four groups. Lung of one piglet that died in group A following HP-PRRS infection at 14 DPI (**a** and **e**), in group (**b**) at 6 DPI (**b** and **f**), humanely euthanized from Groups (**c**) (**c** and **g**) and (**d**) (**d** and **h**) at 14 DPI. **e**, **f**, **g** and **h** magnification: 100×

Discussion

Our current animal experiment was based on our previous result that HP-PRRSV infection activated the HPA axis by changing the peripheral blood hormone levels (Additional file 1: Figure S1). The present study showed that both RU486 and DEX enhanced disease in piglets infected with HuN4, with higher mortality and more severe pathological changes in the lungs of infected piglets.

Previous study has shown that low dose of DEX (1.5 mg/kg b.w.) therapy attenuates pulmonary injury and chronic lung disease in premature animals by improving pulmonary compliance [24]. However, after viral infection, for example PCV2, even such low dose of DEX treatment may accelerate the presence of post-weaning multisystemic wasting syndrome [25]. Similar to the case of PCV2, our results showed that daily treatment of DEX also suppresses the cell-mediated immunity of piglets after HP-PRRSV infection (Fig. 3). RU486 are generally characterized as progesterone and glucocorticoid receptor antagonist, and because of this

Table 1 Detection of viremia and amounts of virus at different DPIs

DPI	Group A		Group B		Group C	
	Viremia[a]	PRRSV amount[b]	Viremia	PRRSV amount	Viremia	PRRSV amount
0	0/5	0	0/5	0	5/5	0
3	5/5	$10^{5.69 \pm 0.2}$	5/5	$10^{5.13 \pm 0.2}$	5/5	$10^{5.14 \pm 0.1}$
6	5/5	$10^{7.65 \pm 0.2}$	2/2[d]	$10^{9.86 \pm 0.4}$	5/5	$10^{6.64 \pm 0.4}$
10	3/3[c]	$10^{8.8 \pm 0.3}$	–	–	4/4[e]	$10^{7.31 \pm 0.3}$

[a]Viremia was detected by TaqMan fluorescent quantitative PCR (Liu al., 2010);
[b] Each number represents the average amount of virus (copies/mL) generated from the blood of all PRRSV-positive piglets at each DPI;
[c] Two piglets died from HP-PRRS at 10 DPI;
[d] One piglet died from HP-PRRS at 4 DPI and two piglets died from PRRS at 5 DPI;
[e]One piglet died from HP-PRRS at 9 DPI

activity, high dose (more than 100 mg) treatment of RU486 are commonly used as a contraceptive [26]. RU486 rarely has detrimental effects on the immune response of animals. However in our case, when the piglets were pre-infected by HP-PRRSV, the additionally treatment of RU486 significantly accelerates the development and severity of the disease. As indicated in the survival rates analysis, piglets in Group B died very early after the infection (Fig. 1b). Given the evidence of much higher levels of proinflammatory cytokines in the peripheral blood and sever lung lesions, the lethal outcome may due to the multisystemic wasting syndrome induced by severe inflammations. The uncontrolled inflammations may be related to insufficient HPA regulation that induced by RU486 treatment.

Although some studies have shown that the secretion of proinflammatory cytokines were involved in the activation of the NF-κB pathway after PRRSV infection [27, 28], our results indicated that it may also influenced by HPA axis regulation. The HPA axis is generally activated as the first line of defense against viral infection in humans [29]. GCs secreted by the adrenal glands after HPA axis activation have been found to suppress immune functions through negative feedback control of the immune system [30, 31]. Predisposition to inflammatory or autoimmune disease can cause insufficient GCs responses; however, chronic stress, predisposition to infectious diseases and other sequelae of immunosuppression can induce excessive GCs production [11, 32]. Although many types of immune-mediated diseases lead to the dysregulation of the HPA axis and impropriate GC production, GC analogues, such as DEX, have long been used as effective anti-viral agents in both humans and animals [33].

In the present study, RU486 and DEX were used to regulate the function of the HPA axis in order to improve the health status of piglets during HP-PRRSV infection. Surprisingly, neither RU486 nor DEX improved the health status of virus-infected piglets, but instead, enhanced the disease. After evaluating the proinflammatory cytokine levels in infected piglets, we found that RU486 exerted a negative effect on the host anti-inflammatory response during HP-PRRSV infection by suppressing the physiological concentrations of GCs, which play a vital role in the anti-viral process. In contrast, DEX inhibited the inflammation induced by HP-PRRSV, although the levels of proinflammatory cytokines in the peripheral blood were significantly decreased and long-lasting high fever and lung lesions were also observed in these HuN4-infected piglets. Despite the solvent of RU486 contained 50% ethanol (30 mg/ml), the dose used for each piglet was no more than 0.1 g/kg

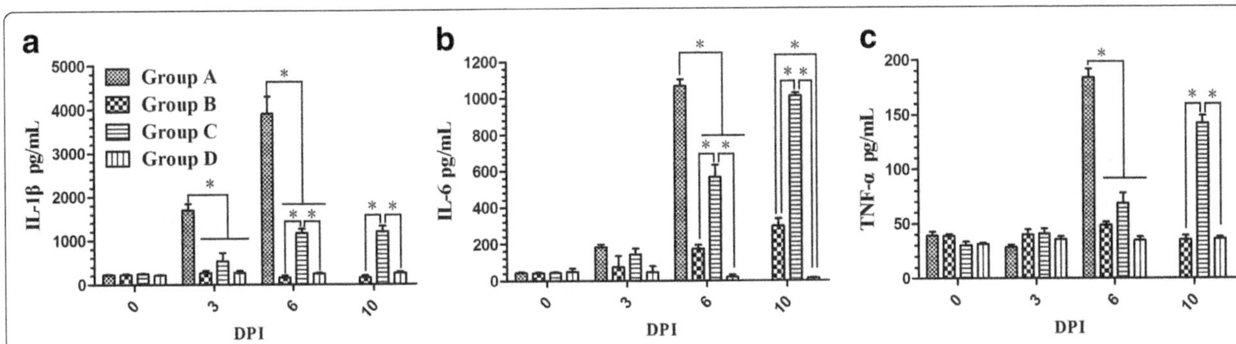

Fig. 3 Levels of proinflammatory cytokines in the peripheral blood of piglets from the four groups. The levels of IL-1β (**a**) IL-6 (**b**) and TNF-α (**c**) were measured using commercial ELISA kits. Each point represents the mean values (±S.D.) generated from all piglets at each DPI. *: Values were significantly different ($P < 0.05$)

b.w., which has been demonstrated to have neither significant effect on the plasma cortisol levels nor anti-viral cell-mediate immune response, as well as no perceptible depression of the central nervous system [22, 25]. Thus, we believe that DEX induces immunosuppression during HP-PRRSV infection, allowing enhanced viral replication and leading to high mortality. These results demonstrate that both RU486 and DEX influence the anti-inflammatory responses in HP-PRRSV -infected piglets, leading to more severe disease.

Conclusions

Our study demonstrates that HP-PRRSV infection activates the HPA axis, while artificial regulation of this immune-endocrine system enhanced the severity of disease in HP-PRRSV-infected piglets. These results indicate that DEX and RU486 should be avoided in the clinical therapy of HP-PRRS.

Abbreviations

b.w.: Body weight; DEX: Dexamethasone; DPI: days post-inoculation; GCs: Glucocorticoids; GR: Glucocorticoid receptor; HPA: Hypothalamus-pituitary-adrenal; HP-PRRSV: Highly pathogenic PRRSV; i.m.: Intramuscularly; PRRS: Porcine reproductive and respiratory syndrome; PRRSV: Porcine reproductive and respiratory syndrome virus; RU486: Mifepristone

Acknowledgements

Not applicable.

Funding

This work was supported by grants from the Heilongjiang Province Natural Science Foundation of China [grant number C2016068] and the National Science Foundation for Young Scholars of China [grant number 31201885] to GW.

Authors' contributions

GW and JT performed the experiment, arranged the data for statistical analysis and drafted the manuscript. YY, LLZ, CZ, YBT were involved in the histopathological analysis. YGL, JNW, HL, SJW and CGJ participated in the detection of viral loads in peripheral blood. GW and XHC designed the study, analyzed the data and revised the manuscript. JT, LLZ and EMZ revised the manuscript. All authors read and approved to the final manuscript.

Consent for publication

Not applicable.

Competing interests

The authors declare that they have no competing interests.

Author details

[1]State Key Laboratory of Veterinary Biotechnology, Harbin Veterinary Research Institute of Chinese Academy of Agriculture Science, Harbin 150001, People's Republic of China. [2]Department of Preventive Veterinary Medicine, College of Veterinary Medicine, Northwest A&F University, Yangling, Shaanxi 712100, People's Republic of China.

References

1. Neumann EJ, Kliebenstein JB, Johnson CD, Mabry JW, Bush EJ, Seitzinger AH, Green AL, Zimmerman JJ. Assessment of the economic impact of porcine reproductive and respiratory syndrome on swine production in the United States. J Am Vet Med Assoc. 2005;227(3):385–92.
2. Li Y, Wang X, Bo K, Tang B, Yang B, Jiang W, Jiang P. Emergence of a highly pathogenic porcine reproductive and respiratory syndrome virus in the mid-eastern region of China. Vet J. 2007;174(3):577–84.
3. Tian K, Yu X, Zhao T, Feng Y, Cao Z, Wang C, Hu Y, Chen X, Hu D, Tian X, et al. Emergence of fatal PRRSV variants: unparalleled outbreaks of atypical PRRS in China and molecular dissection of the unique hallmark. PLoS One. 2007;2(6):e526.
4. Tong GZ, Zhou YJ, Hao XF, Tian ZJ, An TQ, Qiu HJ. Highly pathogenic porcine reproductive and respiratory syndrome, China. Emerg Infect Dis. 2007;13(9):1434–6.
5. Li L, Zhao Q, Ge X, Teng K, Kuang Y, Chen Y, Guo X, Yang H. Chinese highly pathogenic porcine reproductive and respiratory syndrome virus exhibits more extensive tissue tropism for pigs. Virol J. 2012;9:203.
6. Wang G, Song T, Yu Y, Liu Y, Shi W, Wang S, Rong F, Dong J, Liu H, Cai X, et al. Immune responses in piglets infected with highly pathogenic porcine reproductive and respiratory syndrome virus. Vet Immunol Immunopathol. 2011;142(3–4):170–8.
7. Li X, Qiu L, Yang Z, Dang R, Wang X. Emergency vaccination alleviates highly pathogenic porcine reproductive and respiratory syndrome virus infection after contact exposure. BMC Vet Res. 2013;9:26.
8. Diaz I, Darwich L, Pappaterra G, Pujols J, Mateu E. Immune responses of pigs after experimental infection with a European strain of porcine reproductive and respiratory syndrome virus. J Gen Virol. 2005;86(Pt 7):1943–51.
9. DeRijk RH, Petrides J, Deuster P, Gold PW, Sternberg EM. Changes in corticosteroid sensitivity of peripheral blood lymphocytes after strenuous exercise in humans. J Clin Endocrinol Metab. 1996;81(1):228–35.
10. Liu Y, Shi W, Zhou E, Wang S, Hu S, Cai X, Rong F, Wu J, Xu M, Li L. Dynamic changes in inflammatory cytokines in pigs infected with highly pathogenic porcine reproductive and respiratory syndrome virus. Clin Vaccine Immunol. 2010;17(9):1439–45.
11. Sternberg EM. Neuroendocrine regulation of autoimmune/inflammatory disease. J Endocrinol. 2001;169(3):429–35.
12. Rhen T, Cidlowski JA. Antiinflammatory action of glucocorticoids - new mechanisms for old drugs. New Engl J Med. 2005;353(16):1711–23.
13. So LKY, Lau ACW, Yam LYC, Cheung TMT, Poon E, Yung RWH, Yuen KY. Development of a standard treatment protocol for severe acute respiratory syndrome. Lancet. 2003;361(9369):1615–7.
14. Londono P, Komura A, Hara N, Zipris D. Brief dexamethasone treatment during acute infection prevents virus-induced autoimmune diabetes. Clin Immunol. 2010;135(3):401–11.
15. Cole MA, Kim PJ, Kalman BA, Spencer RL. Dexamethasone suppression of corticosteroid secretion: evaluation of the site of action by receptor measures and functional studies. Psychoneuroendocrinology. 2000;25(2):151–67.
16. He Y, Wang G, Liu Y, Shi W, Han Z, Wu J, Jiang C, Wang S, Hu S, Wen H, et al. Characterization of thymus atrophy in piglets infected with highly pathogenic porcine reproductive and respiratory syndrome virus. Vet Microbiol. 2012;160(3–4):455–62.
17. Li Y, Wang G, Liu Y, Tu Y, He Y, Wang Z, Han Z, Li L, Li A, Tao Y, et al. Identification of apoptotic cells in the thymus of piglets infected with highly pathogenic porcine reproductive and respiratory syndrome virus. Virus Res. 2014;189:29–33.
18. Wang G, Yu Y, Tu Y, Tong J, Liu Y, Zhang C, Chang Y, Wang S, Jiang C, Zhou EM, et al. Highly pathogenic porcine reproductive and respiratory syndrome virus infection induced apoptosis and autophagy in Thymi of infected piglets. PLoS One. 2015;10(6):e0128292.
19. Liddicoat DR, Kyparissoudis K, Berzins SP, Cole TJ, Godfrey DI. The glucocorticoid receptor 1A3 promoter correlates with high sensitivity to glucocorticoid-induced apoptosis in human lymphocytes. Immunol Cell Biol. 2014;92(10):825–36.
20. Planey SL, Litwack G. Glucocorticoid-induced apoptosis in lymphocytes. Biochem Biophys Res Commun. 2000;279(2):307–12.

21. Smith LK, Cidlowski JA. Glucocorticoid-induced apoptosis of healthy and malignant lymphocytes. Prog Brain Res. 2010;182:1–30.
22. Wang LT, Hu SP, Liu Q, Li YR, Xu L, Zhang Z, Cai XH, He XJ. Porcine alveolar macrophage polarization is involved in inhibition of porcine reproductive and respiratory syndrome virus (PRRSV) replication. J Vet Med Sci. 2017; 79(11):1906–15.
23. Tian ZJ, An TQ, Zhou YJ, Peng JM, Hu SP, Wei TC, Jiang YF, Xiao Y, Tong GZ. An attenuated live vaccine based on highly pathogenic porcine reproductive and respiratory syndrome virus (HP-PRRSV) protects piglets against HP-PRRS. Vet Microbiol. 2009;138(1–2):34–40.
24. Holopainen R, Laine J, Halkola L, Aho H, Kaapa P. Dexamethasone treatment attenuates pulmonary injury in piglet meconium aspiration. Pediatr Res. 2001;49(2):162–8.
25. Kawashima Y, Tsunemitsu H, Horino R, Katsuda Y, Onodera T, Shoji T, Kubo M, Haritani M, Murakami Y. Effects of dexamethasone on the pathogenesis of porcine circovirus type 2 infection in piglets. J Comp Pathol. 2003;129(4): 294–302.
26. Vallet JL, Christenson RK. Effect of progesterone, mifepristone, and estrogen treatment during early pregnancy on conceptus development and uterine capacity in swine. Biol Reprod. 2004;70(1):92–8.
27. Fang Y, Fang L, Wang Y, Lei Y, Luo R, Wang D, Chen H, Xiao S. Porcine reproductive and respiratory syndrome virus nonstructural protein 2 contributes to NF-kappaB activation. Virol J. 2012;9:83.
28. Luo R, Fang L, Jiang Y, Jin H, Wang Y, Wang D, Chen H, Xiao S. Activation of NF-kappaB by nucleocapsid protein of the porcine reproductive and respiratory syndrome virus. Virus Genes. 2011;42(1):76–81.
29. Fontana A, Weber E, Dayer JM. Synthesis of interleukin 1/endogenous pyrogen in the brain of endotoxin-treated mice: a step in fever induction? J Immunol. 1984;133(4):1696–8.
30. Turnbull AV, Rivier CL. Regulation of the hypothalamic-pituitary-adrenal axis by cytokines: actions and mechanisms of action. Physiol Rev. 1999;79(1):1–71.
31. Webster JI, Tonelli L, Sternberg EM. Neuroendocrine regulation of immunity. Annu Rev Immunol. 2002;20:125–63.
32. Sternberg EM. Neural-immune interactions in health and disease. J Clin Invest. 1997;100(11):2641–7.
33. Cupps TR, Fauci AS. Corticosteroid-mediated immunoregulation in man. Immunol Rev. 1982;65:133–55.

Natural peste des petits ruminants virus infection in Black Bengal goats: virological, pathological and immunohistochemical investigation

Emdadul Haque Chowdhury[1*], Ataur Rahman Bhuiyan[1,2], Mohammad Mushfiqur Rahman[1], Mohammad Sahinur Alam Siddique[2] and Mohammad Rafiqul Islam[1]

Abstract

Background: Peste des Petits Ruminants (PPR), also known as Goat Plague, occurs in goats, sheep and related species. It is caused by a *morbillivirus* in the family *Paramyxoviridae*. In Bangladesh PPR is endemic and it causes serious economic losses. Pathology of PPR has been reported in different goat and sheep breeds from natural and experimental infections. Field results are better indicators of pathogenicity of the circulating virus. The severity of the disease varies with species, breed and immune status of the host. Pathological investigations of natural outbreaks of PPR in Balck Bengal goats are very limited. The current investigation was aimed at describing pathology and antigen localization in natural PPR infections in Black Bengal goats.

Results: A total of 28 outbreaks were investigated clinically and virologically. Average flock morbidity and mortality were 75% and 59%, respectively, with case fatality rate of 74%. Necropsy was conducted on 21 goats from 15 outbreaks. The major gross lesions were congestion of gastrointestinal tract, pneumonia, engorged spleen, and oedematous lymphnodes. Histopathological examination revealed severe enteritis with denudation of intestinal epithelium, severe broncho-interstitial pneumonia with macrophages within lung alveoli and extensive haemorrhages with depletion of lymphoid cells and infiltration of macrophages in the sinuses of spleen. In lymph nodes, the cortical nodules were replaced by wide sinusoids with severe depletion of lymphocytes, infiltration of mononuclear cells and some giant cells in sub-capsular areas and medullary sinuses. PPR virus antigen was found in pneumocytes and alveolar macrophages in lungs. Viral RNA could be detected by RT-PCR in 69 out of 84 nasal swab, 59 out of 84 blood and 21 out of 21 lymph node samples. Sequence analyses revealed closeness of Bangladeshi strains with other recent Asian isolates.

Conclusion: Natural outbreaks of PPR in Black Bengal goats in Bangladesh resulted in 75% and 59% flock morbidity and mortality, respectively, with a case fatality rate of 74%. The striking histo-morphologic diagnosis of PPR was acute pneumonia and severe gastro-enteritis. A detailed experimental pathological study on Black Bengal goats infected with recent isolates is required.

Keywords: PPR, Natural outbreak, Pathology, Antigen detection, Nucleic acid detection

Background

Peste des Petits Ruminants (PPR), also known as Goat Plague and Ovine Rinderpest, occurs in goats, sheep and related species. It is caused by a *morbillivirus* in the family *Paramyxoviridae*. It is closely related to Rinderpest, measles, canine distemper and morbilliviruses of marine mammals and is the most economically important viral disease of small ruminants [1-3]. In the field, PPR virus causes disease in goats and sheep. Goats are usually considered to be more susceptible than sheep, but this is not always the case; cattle and pigs can be infected subclinically by experimental infections [4,5]). The disease is characterized by high fever, discharges from nose, eyes and mouth; profuse diarrhoea; pneumonia; and oral erosion, with high morbidity [6-8]. In susceptible populations, morbidity and mortality rate are 5-90% and 50-80%,

* Correspondence: emdad001@yahoo.com
[1]Department of Pathology, Faculty of Veterinary Science, Bangladesh Agricultural University, Mymensingh, Bangladesh
Full list of author information is available at the end of the article

respectively [9-11]. Post mortem examination reveals frothy exudates in respiratory tract, congestion and partial consolidation of lungs, congested mesenteric and bronchial lymph nodes, severe congestion, haemorrhages and edema in gastro-intestinal tract [6,12-14]. Histologically characteristic lesions are usually seen in digestive and respiratory systems [15]. In intestine histologic findings of natural PPR virus infection include atrophic villi with partial denudation of epithelial lining and intense diffusion of mononuclear cells in the lamina propria and sub-mucosa [16,17]. The lungs show broncho-interstitial pneumonia characterized by proliferation of bronchiolar lining epithelium, intense diffusion of mononuclear cells mainly in lymphoid, macrophages and plasma cells in the pericardial, the interstitial tissue and alveolar lumina [17]. In Bangladesh, the first outbreak of PPR was recorded in 1993 [18]. Since then outbreaks are being reported regularly across the country. In 2010, there were 84,000 veterinary clinic cases, causing an estimated loss of Taka: 1,842 million (US$ 24.6 million) [19], but the actual number of cases may be even more because infected cases from remote rural areas were not brought to the veterinary clinic. Although prevention is the main strategy against viral diseases, supportive treatment may prevent some loss. Knowledge of pathology and pathogenesis may help in formulation of supportive treatment. Pathology of PPR has been reported in different goat and sheep breeds from experimental infections [6,16,17,20]. Pathological data from field cases are very important as they could better characterize the pathogenicity of the circulating virus. The severity of the disease varies with species, immunity and breed of the host [21]. Pathological investigations of natural outbreaks of PPR in Black Bengal goats are very limited [18].The current investigation was aimed at describing the pathology and antigen localization in natural PPR infections in Black Bengal goats.

Results

Clinical findings

This investigation examined 28 outbreaks of PPR in Black Bengal goats from different parts of the country having average 75% (63% to 100%) morbidity, 59% (23% to 100%) mortality and 74% (26% -100%) case fatality (Table 1). Mortality was higher in the young (5–12 month of age) goats (field veterinarian's observation). The veterinarians treated 250 – 300 out of 947 affected goats with antibiotic, antihistamine, astringent and 5% dextrose saline for a week. A few (±30) of the treated goats survived after treatment but 5 goats died after a month due to secondary bacterial infections (field veterinarian's report, data not shown). The goat that died after a month was not included in the mortality calculation. The most frequently observed signs were abrupt rise of body temperature (105-106°F) that lasted for 3 to 5 days. The affected animals were severely depressed, standing apart and had impaired appetite and constipation. Rise of body temperature was accompanied by watery discharges (nasal, ocular and oral), which lasted for 4 to 5 days. Very often ocular discharges were associated with conjunctivitis; nasal discharge became purulent and blocked nostril in advanced stages. Medial canthus revealed some crusts at later stages. Small areas of necrosis were seen on the visible nasal mucous membranes. The erosive and necrotic stomatitis was seen on hyperaemic gums, cheeks, dental pad and on tongue, with frothy salivation in some cases. In some cases circular raised non-bleeding lesions were present on the tongue. Lesions similar to orf developed at mucocutaneous junction of mouth in many animals at later stages of the disease. Abortion was frequent at all stages of pregnancy. Diarrhoea was common with sub-normal body temperature usually 5 to 6 days after the first appearance of clinical signs. The hindquarters of diarrhoeic goats were soiled with liquid greenish feces. Bronchopneumonia, evidenced by coughing, was common at the later stages of PPR. In severe cases, most animals died within a week. A subnormal temperature preceded death in animals when severe diarrhoea continued for a few days.

Necropsy findings

The carcasses were dehydrated and emaciated with sunken eyes, but some goats were in good bodily condition after death at early infection. The lesions of respiratory tract included necrotic areas on the mucosa of nostrils and turbinate and severely congested tracheal mucous membrane with white frothy mucus in lumen (Figure 1). The lungs were dark red or purple with areas firm to touch, mainly in the anterior and cardiac lobes (Figure 2). In the digestive tract, rumens of three goats revealed ecchymotic haemorrhages (Figure 3) and streaks of haemorrhages were also seen in duodenum and the terminal ileum (Figure 4). The lymph nodes, especially from the mesentery were severely oedematous, congested and enlarged (Figure 5). The large intestine was usually more severely affected with congestion around the ileocaecal valve, at the caeco-colic junction, and in the rectum, although not in all the carcasses. Spleen was atrophied in cases that died after a couple of weeks (Figure 6). Erosive vulvo-vaginitis was observed in eight animals.

Histopathological findings

Details of the histopathological findings are listed in Table 2. The most remarkable lesions were found in respiratory, alimentary and lymphatic systems. Goats that died within 48 hours of the onset of clinical signs were mostly haemorrhagic and showed severe exudation in the upper respiratory tract and in the lung parenchyma. The exudates in the lung parenchyma often proceeded to fibrinous organization (Figure 7). In goats that died

Table 1 Morbidity and mortality of goats in different outbreaks of PPR in Bangladesh during May 2008 to June 2010

Outbreaks	Location	Breed	Flock size	Age (m)	No. of goats affected	No. of goats died	Flock Morbidity (%)	Flock Mortality (%)	Case fatality (%)	No. of necropsy
1	Chittagong	BB	16	5-30	11	10	69	63	91	2
2	Narayangong	BB	47	2-36	47	41	100	87	87	nd
3	Rajshahi	BB	22	1-36	22	18	100	82	82	2
4	Dhaka	BB	7	6-24	6	4	86	57	67	1
5	Narayangong	BB	6	6-8	5	4	83	67	80	2
6	Chittagong	BB	8	5-24	5	2	63	25	40	nd
7	Sylhet	BB	6	6-30	6	3	100	50	50	1
8	Dhaka	JP	31	1-36	27	7	87	23	26	nd
9	Dhaka	BB	8	6-8	8	8	100	100	100	1
10	Sylhet	BB	6	6-24	5	4	83	67	80	nd
11	Mymensingh	BB	6	6-24	5	4	83	67	80	1
12	Dhaka	JP	12	5-30	12	9	100	75	75	nd
13	Dhaka	BB	69	1-36	60	58	88	85	97	nd
14	Sathkira	BB	805	1-36	540	425	67	53	79	nd
15	Jessore	JP	7	6-24	6	4	86	57	67	nd
16	Mymensingh	BB	25	8-12	23	19	92	76	83	nd
17	Dhaka	BB	22	1-36	22	16	100	73	73	2
18	Mymensingh	BB	22	3-36	17	11	77	50	65	2
19	Dhaka	BB	15	8-24	12	10	80	67	83	1
20	Dhaka	JP	15	5-24	13	11	87	73	85	nd
21	Jessore	BB	8	4-24	6	4	75	50	67	1
22	Dhaka	JP	12	5-24	11	6	92	50	55	nd
23	Rajshahi	BB	12	5-30	8	6	67	50	75	nd
24	Dhaka	BB	8	5-30	6	4	75	50	67	1
25	Rajshahi	BB	6	8-15	6	6	100	100	100	1
26	Mymensingh	BB	6	6-15	4	3	67	50	75	2
27	Narayangong	BB	7	6-30	6	4	86	57	67	1
28	Jessore	BB	50	1-36	48	41	96	82	85	nd
Total	1264		947	742	74.92	58.71	74.32	21		

BB: Black Bengal Goat, JP: Jamuna Pari, m: month, nd: Not done, only clinical history and nasal swabs and/or blood smeared filter papers were received from the veterinary surgeons for diagnosis.

after 3–5 days, lesions of lungs were more severe, with additional involvement of alimentary tract. The lung parenchyma was infiltrated with large mononuclear cells and clumps of these cells were found in the lung alveoli (Figure 8). In some places, alveoli lost its lining of squamous epithelium, which were partially replaced by cuboidal type epithelial cells. The entire alimentary tract revealed haemorrhagic gastroenteritis with infiltration of mononuclear cells in the lamina propria and loss of laminar epithelia. Clumps of epithelial cells were aggregated in the lumen of the intestine. Liver was severely congested and haemorrhagic. Changes in the lymphatic systems appeared more haemorrhagic in goats that died within 2–3 days. Lymphatic organs were depleted of lymphocytes (Figure 9). These lesions were more severe in goats that survived more than a week. Conspicuous lymphoid depletion was seen in Peyer's patches in 6 cases, in lymph nodes in 7 cases, and in spleen (Figure 10) in 7 cases.

Localization of antigen

Only lung tissue was positive for PPR virus antigen. Specific staining was characterized by a diffuse red granular reaction in the cytoplasm and nucleus, often coalescing with each other. specifically antigen was localized in the cytoplasm and nuclei of alveolar and bronchiolar epithelia, macrophages and syncytia (Figures 11 and 12). Other organs were also analyzed but positive reaction was not detected.

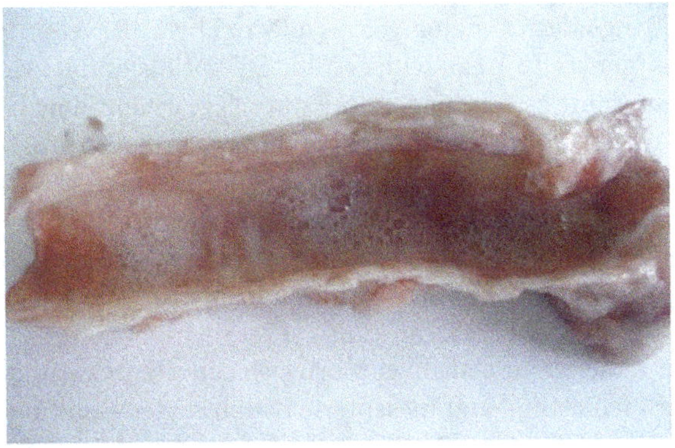

Figure 1 Necropsy finding of trachea of a PPR virus infected goat. Trachea revealed severe congestion in tracheal mucous membrane with frothy exudates in the lumen.

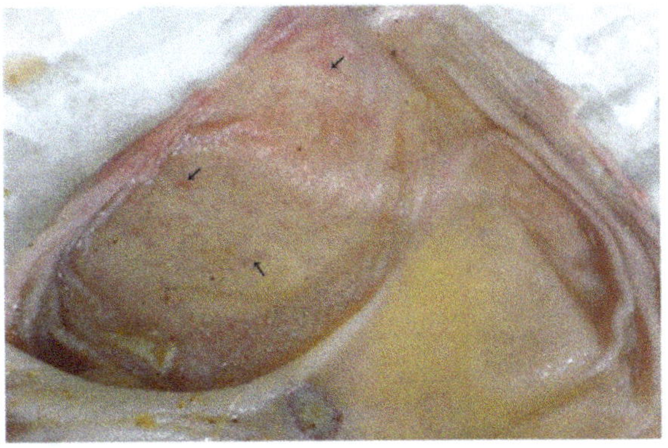

Figure 3 Necropsy finding of rumen of a PPR virus infected goat. Ecchymotic haemorrhages (arrow) were present on the mucosal surface of rumen.

Viral nucleic acid detection in lymph node, blood and nasal swabs

All samples tested from 28 outbreaks yielded PCR products of 448 bp (F gene) and 351 bp (N gene) as stated by Forsyth and Barrett (1995) [22] for PPR virus. Details of the samples are given in Table 3. All of the 21 lymph node homogenates were found positive from 15 outbreaks, where either blood or nasal swabs or both were positive from 13 outbreaks. Viral RNA could be detected in 69 out of 84 nasal swabs and 59 out of 84 blood samples (Table 3). Lymphnode samples were not available from all outbreaks. All the three nasal swab samples from one outbreak were positive but not the blood samples (outbreak no. 20). On the contrary, in another outbreak all the three blood samples were positive but not the nasal swabs (outbreak no. 4). Goats which were positive with nasal swab but not with blood were sampled at the non-febrile stage (diarrhoeic phase) 7 days after the onset of clinical signs. The animal that was positive with blood but negative with nasal swab were found dead at morning within 24 hours of onset of high temperature (107°F).

Sequence analyses

The representative PCR products of F and N genes of one isolate were sequenced from a commercial source and confirmed by comparing with known PPR sequence. The sequences have been submitted to the GenBank [GenBank Accession No. HQ898003 & JF276436]. On phylogenetic analysis the present Bangladeshi strain clustered in Lineage IV and formed a sub-cluster along with recent isolates from Tibet, Tajikistan and India. These isolates have two unique amino acid substitutions (K423Q and E426G) in N protein, which were not evident in other Lineage IV isolates.

Discussion

Peste des petits ruminant virus (PPRV) produced severe pathological lesions in respiratory tract, alimentary tract

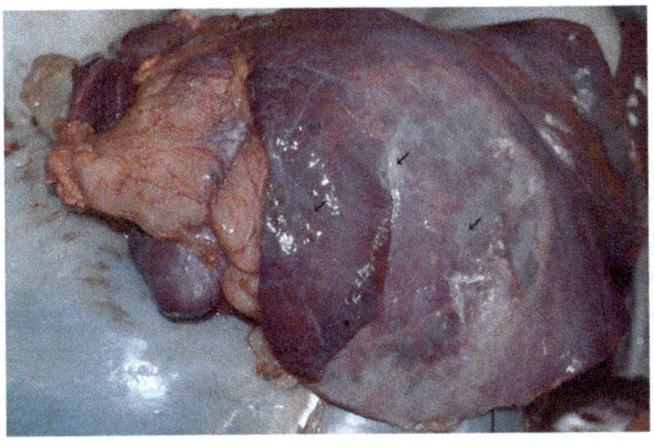

Figure 2 Necropsy finding of lung of a PPR virus infected goat. Lung showed pneumonia with consolidation and accumulation of fibrin (arrow) over the surface of the lung. Lung showed muscular appearance.

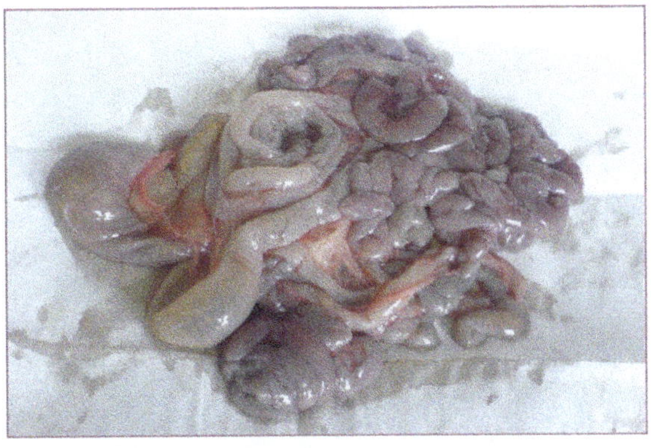

Figure 4 Necropsy finding of intestine of a PPR virus infected goat. Severe enteritis with haemorrhages and congestion was present in small and large intestine. The intestine contained diarrheic faeces and gas.

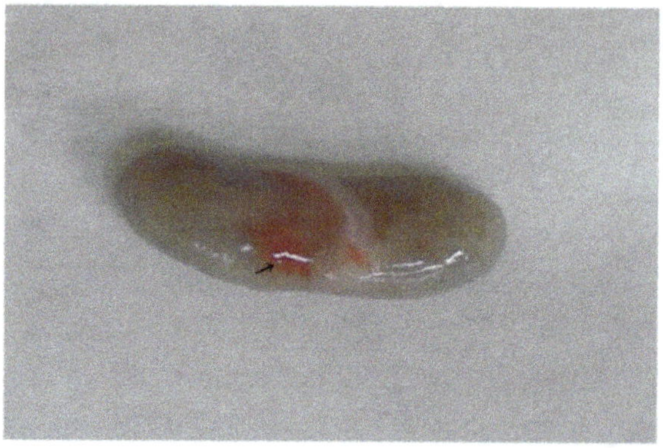

Figure 5 Mesenteric lymph node of a PPR virus infected goat. Lymph node was oedematous, congested (arrow) and enlarged.

and lymphatic system in natural outbreaks in Black Bengal goats. PPR has been one of the most prevalent infectious diseases among goats in Bangladesh and is considered an emerging economically important disease. In the present study, 28 outbreaks in flocks having 1264 goats were investigated. The suspected samples were first screened by RT-PCR for PPR virus. The flock morbidity and mortality in this study were 63 to 100% and 23 – 100%, respectively, whereas few other authors found 5-90% and 50 – 80%, respectively [9-11]. According to field veterinarian's observations, young goats (6–12 months) were more susceptible than the aged, which are inconsistent with the findings of Taylor et al. [11]. This may be due to maternally derived PPR antibody that persists up to 4 months [23]. It is likely that antibody derived from sub-clinical infection in aged goats protected themselves as well as their young progenies. This observation was in accordance with those reported by Taylor et al. [24]. Some authors reported that more severe disease results from mixed infection of bacteria and viruses [17]. We did not take any attempt to isolate bacteria from these cases. In Bangladesh, when a goat is affected by PPR, veterinarians generally treat with antibiotic, antihistamine, dextrose saline and astringent mixtures. Treatment may help to reduce mortality from PPR due to (i) control of respiratory bacterial infections and (ii) counteracting shock by astringent mixture, dextrose saline and anti-histamine. Some goats that survived the acute stage of the disease died later, possibly due to immunosuppression induced by the PPRV. PPRV can cause severe lymphocytolysis in lymphoid tissues, such as tonsils, spleen, Peyer's patches, and mediastinal and mesenteric lymph nodes resulting in immunodeficiency [25-27]. Our observation also revealed lymphoid depletion in the lymphatic nodules and spleen.

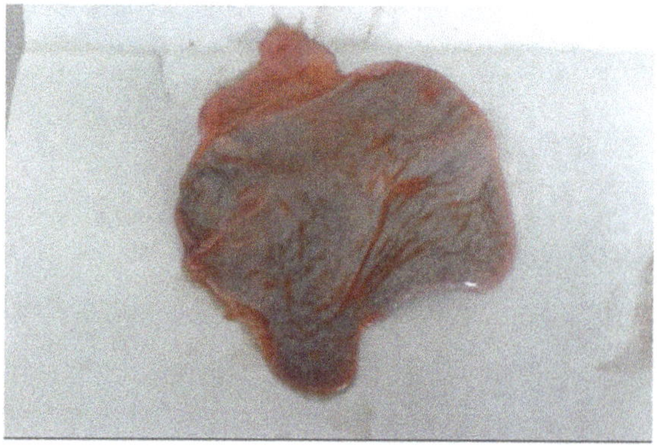

Figure 6 Spleen of a PPR virus infected goat. Severe spleen atrophy was present in a goat that died after 15 days of onset of clinical signs of PPR. The nasal swab was positive for PPR virus excretion.

In the present study in Black Bengal goats, characteristic erosive ulcerative lesions in the mouth and inflammatory lesions in the respiratory and gastrointestinal tract corroborate the findings of previous studies in sheep and other breeds of goats [6-8,12-17,27]. Cast of intra-luminal epithelial cells and macrophages in the lung tissue is a characteristic feature of morbillivirus infection. Immunohistochemically, PPRV were detected in the intra-luminal epithelial tissues and macrophages.

Histologically, proliferation of macrophages in different organs was seen, which indicates primarily non-purulent inflammation. Depletion of lymphocytes from lymph nodes and spleen may be due to affinity of the virus to lymphoid tissue and the involvement of lymphocytes in the pathogenesis of PPR [12]. The virus localizes in the lung parenchyma and causes diffuse interstitial pneumonia with eosinophilic intranuclear inclusion bodies in the pneumocytes [16]. Although we did not find intranuclear inclusion bodies with H&E, antigen was detected in pneumocytes and macrophages with immunohistochemistry. Brown et al. [28] used lung tissue for indirect immuno-histochemical methods and detected viral antigen in pneumocytes and alveolar macrophages. We were not able to detect PPRV antigen in tissues of other organs, the reason was not clear to us.

In this investigation, both blood and nasal swab samples were positive for virus in most cases. But 3 goats sampled at non-febrile stage 7 days after onset of clinical signs were positive only with nasal swabs. The febrile stage usually persists for 2 – 3 days and then the virus localizes in the respiratory and associated tissues and therefore excretes the virus through nasal secretion for longer period. Therefore the nasal swab can be a good choice for the PCR detection of PPR virus in infected animals both in febrile and non-febrile stages of the disease.

Conclusion

The striking histo-morphological diagnosis was acute pneumonia and severe gastro-enteritis. Since Bangladesh

Table 2 Histopathological findings in goats naturally infected with PPR virus

Carcass no	Lungs					Gastro intestinal changes		Lymphoid organs (depletion and necrosis)		Remarks
	Congestion	Proliferative changes in alveoli	Bronchitis/bronchiolitis	Presence of syncytia	Sero-fibrinous exudates	Desquamation and inflammation	Depletion in Payers patches	MLN	Spleen	
1	+	+	+	-	-	++	+	+	+	**
2	+++	-	++	-	+	-	-	-	-	*
3	+	+	+	-	-	+	+	+	+	***
4	++	-	+	-	-	-	-	+/–	+	*
5	+	+	+	-	-	+	+	-	-	**
6	+++	-	++	+	+	+	-	-	-	*
7	++	-	+	-	-	+	+	-	-	*
8	+	+	+	+	-	-	+	+	++	***
9	++	-	++	-	+	++	-	+	+	**
10	+	-	+	-	-	++	-	-	-	**
11	+	+	+	+	-	+	+	+	+	***
12	++		+	-	-	++	-	-	-	**
13	+	+	+	+	-	-	-	-	-	*
14	+	-	+	-	-	++	-	+	+	**
15	+	-	+	-	-	+	-	-	-	**

*Died within 24–48 hours, **= 3 – 5 days, ***Died after 7 days, MLN: Mesenteric lymph node, + = visible, ++ = prominent, +++ = severe.

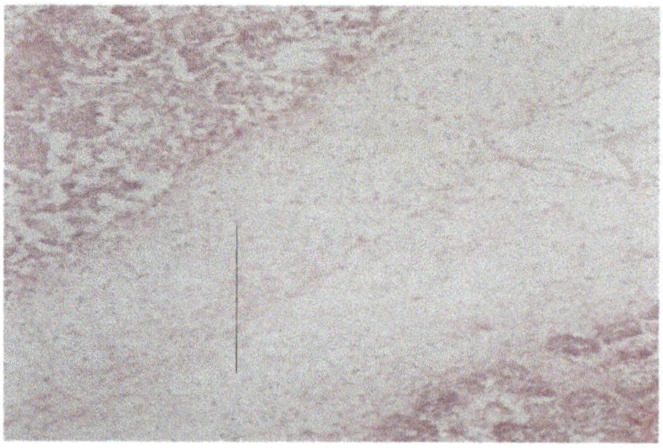

Figure 7 Histological section of a lung of a PPR infected goat. Accumulation of fibrin (line) and infiltration of inflammatory cells in the lung parenchyma, H&E X 82.5.

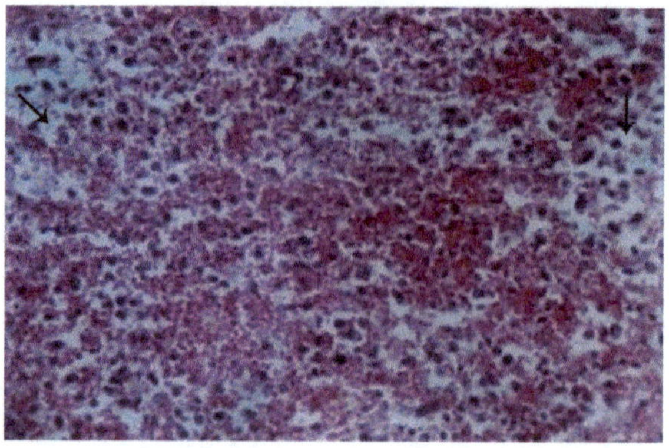

Figure 9 Histological section of spleen of a PPR infected goat. Spleen showed accumulation of extravagated Erythrocytes in the pulp and depletion of lymphocytes (arrow). H & E X 82.5.

is a PPR endemic country, stamping out is not practiced. Therefore, early supportive treatment based on the pathological findings, could reduce the mortality of PPR virus infected goats which is economic for the poor farmer. A detailed experimental pathological study of Black Bengal goats infected with different isolates is required.

Methods

Samples

A total of 28 PPR outbreaks from different parts of the country during December, 2008 – December, 2010 were included in this study (Table 1). The size of the affected flocks varied from 6 to 805 with a total of 1264 goats (Table 1). All the farms were in contact with veterinarians, who observed daily for morbidity, mortality and clinical signs and recorded body temperature of the affected goats. The veterinarians were in contact with the investigators and filled in the prescribed clinical examination form. From 15 outbreaks 21 dead goats were subjected to necropsy at the necropsy room of veterinary clinics or at the Department of Pathology, Bangladesh Agricultural University, Mymensingh. From the remaining 13 outbreaks, only nasal and blood smeared filter papers were received from the veterinarians with completed clinical examination form. The blood samples were collected from jugular vein by aseptic means. A few drops of blood were poured on the filter paper, from the base towards the tip, until it was completely soaked. Nasal swabs were collected with sterilized swab sticks, which were smeared on the filter paper. Smeared filter papers were air-dried avoiding direct sunlight and preserved in labelled sterilized Eppendorf tube. The papers and tissues were stored at −70°C at the laboratory until analysis.

Necropsy

Necropsies were performed on 21 goats of 15 outbreaks that were found dead at farms. None of them received any supportive treatment prior to death. These goats died 24 hours to 7 days after onset of clinical signs. Tissue samples from various organs were collected at necropsy and

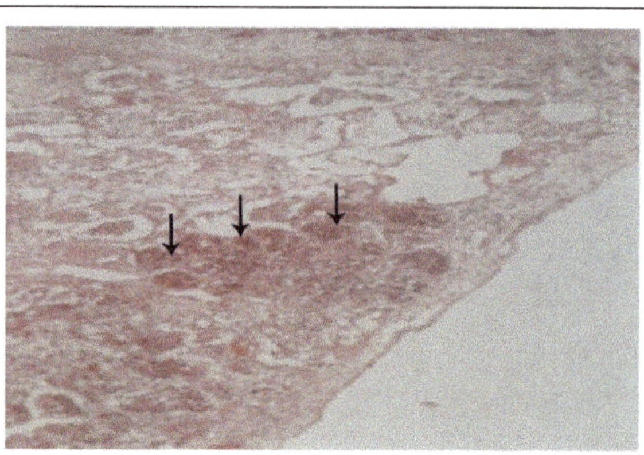

Figure 8 Histological section of a lung of a PPR infected goat. Lung alveoli filled with severe infiltration of inflammatory cells (arrow), H & E X 82.5.

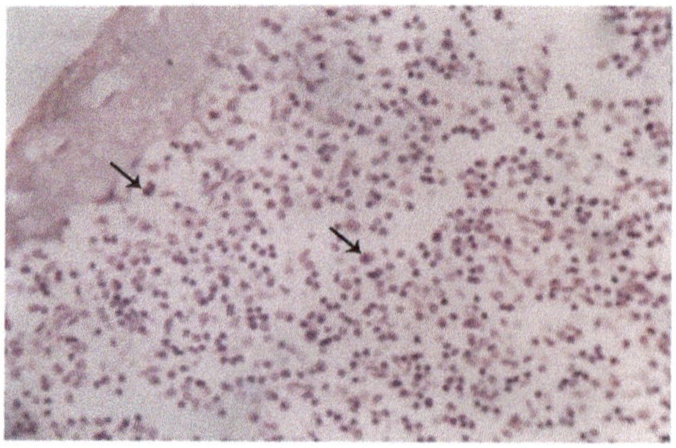

Figure 10 Histological section of Lymph node of a PPR infected goat. Lymph node revealed wide sinusoidal depletion of lymphocytes and proliferation of mononuclear cells (arrow). H & E X 330.

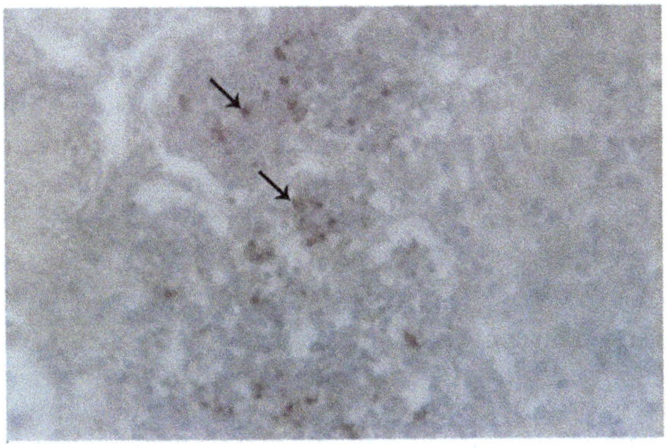

Figure 11 Immunochemical staining of lung tissues of a PPR infected goat. PPR virus antigen was detected in the macrophages accumulated in the lung alveoli (arrow) and epithelial cell of lung alveoli, counterstained with hematoxylin, x 82.5.

fixed in 10% neutral buffered formalin. Tissues from bronchial lymph node of dead animals were also collected aseptically for detection of viral RNA by RT-PCR.

Histopathology

Histopathology was performed on one goat from each of the 15 outbreaks, where necropsy was conducted. Formalin-fixed samples were processed and stained as described [29]. Briefly, the fixed tissues were trimmed and further fixed for 24 hrs. Tissues were kept in running tap water overnight to wash out formalin. The tissues were dehydrated in ascending grades of alcohol (50%, 70%, 80%, 95%) and three changes of absolute alcohol for one hour in each. Sections were cleared in chloroform by two changes, 1½ hours for each. The samples were embedded with molten paraffin wax at 56°C; two changes, 1½ hours for each, and then paraffin blocks were prepared using a template. The tissues were sectioned with a microtome at 5-μm thickness. The sections were allowed to spread on warm water bath (37°C) and taken on grease-free glass slides. A small amount of gelatin was added to the water bath for better adhesion of the section to the slide. The slides were air-dried and kept cool until staining.

The sectioned tissues were deparaffinized in three changes of xylene (three minutes in each) and rehydrated through descending grades of alcohol (three changes in

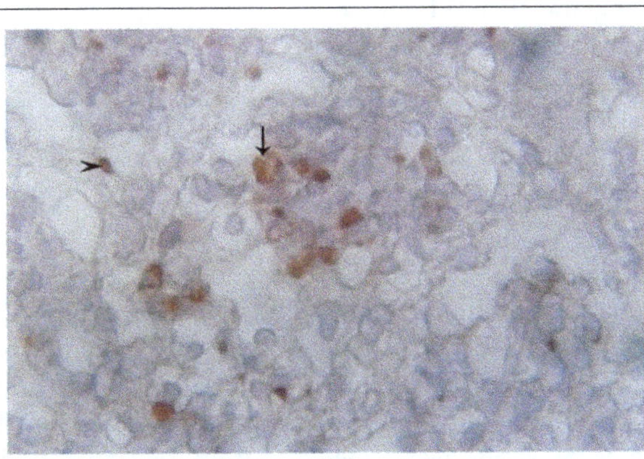

Figure 12 Immunochemical staining of lung tissues of a PPR infected goat. Higher magnification of Figure 11 that showed PPR virus antigen in the alveolar epithelial cells (arrow head) and macrophages in alveolar lumen (arrow), counterstained with hematoxylin, x 330.

Table 3 Samples tested from different outbreaks of PPR in Black Bengal goats

Outbreaks	Location	No. samples tested			No. of samples positive by RT-PCR		
		NSF	BSF	LH	NSF	BSF	LH
1	Chittagong	3	3	2	3	2	2
2	Narayangong	3	3	na	3	2	
3	Rajshahi	3	3	2	3	3	2
4	Dhaka	3	3	1	0	3	1
5	Narayangong	3	3	2	2	2	2
6	Chittagong	3	3	na	2	2	
7	Sylhet	3	3	1	3	3	1
8	Dhaka	3	3	na	3	2	
9	Dhaka	3	3	1	2	1	1
10	Sylhet	3	3	na	3	1	
11	Mymensingh	3	3	1	3	2	1
12	Dhaka	3	3	na	1	2	
13	Dhaka	3	3	na	2	2	
14	Sathkira	3	3	na	3	1	
15	Jessore	3	3	na	3	2	
16	Mymensingh	3	3	na	2	1	
17	Dhaka	3	3	2	2	2	2
18	Mymensingh	3	3	2	3	2	2
19	Dhaka	3	3	1	3	2	1
20	Dhaka	3	3	na	3	0	
21	Jessore	3	3	1	2	1	1
22	Dhaka	3	3	na	2	2	
23	Rajshahi	3	3	na	3	2	
24	Dhaka	3	3	1	2	3	1
25	Rajshahi	3	3	1	3	2	1
26	Mymensingh	3	3	2	3	2	2
27	Narayangong	3	3	1	2	2	1
28	Jessore	3	3	na	3	2	
Total	84	84	21	67 (79%)	59 (70%)	21 (100%)	

NSF: nasal swab smeared filter paper, BSF: Blood smeared filter paper, LH: Lymph node homogenates, na: not available, NSF and BSF samples originated from the same goats.

absolute alcohol, three minutes in each; 95% alcohol for two minutes; 80% alcohol for two minutes; 70% alcohol for two minutes) followed by distilled water for five minutes. The tissues were stained with Harris haematoxylin (MERCK, Germany) for fifteen minutes followed by washing in running tap water for 10–15 minutes. The tissues were differentiated in acid alcohol by 2 to 4 dips (1 part HCl and 99 parts 70% alcohol), washed in tap water for five minutes followed by 2–4 dips in ammonia water until sections were bright blue, followed by staining with eosin for one minute. Tissues were dehydrated in alcohol (95% alcohol: three changes, 2–4 dips each; absolute alcohol: three changes 2–3 minutes for each), and cleaned in xylene, three changes (five minutes each). Finally, the sections were mounted with cover slip using DPX (LOBA Chemie, India) and photographed using photo-micrographic camera (Olympus PM-C 35 Model).

Immunohistochemistry

The tissues were sectioned with a microtome at 5 μm thickness. Sections were allowed to spread on warm water bath (37°C) and taken on poly-L-lysine-coated slides (Thermoshandon). Afterwards the procedure was as follows:

(i) The sections were deparaffinized in fresh xylene (four changes, 5 minutes in each) and rehydrated through descending grades of alcohol (three changes in absolute alcohol, three minutes in each; 95% alcohol for 3 min; 80% alcohol for 3 min; 70% alcohol for 3 min and 50% for 3 min) followed by washing in running tap water for 20 minutes and in distilled water for 5 min. (ii) Sections were placed in a Coplin Jar containing 0.1% trypsin (Sigma-Aldrich) in Tris buffer, pH 7.8 (10 mM) and incubated for 10 minutes at 37°C in water bath, followed by washing in chilled PBS (0.01 M) in another Coplin jar (2 changes, 5 min in each). (iii) The trypsinized sections were fixed in air-free disposable cover plates and stacked in a immunostaining rack (Thermo Shandon). (iv) Endogenous tissue peroxidase was inactivated by applying 0.3% H_2O_2 to the sections at room temperature for 10 minutes followed by washing in PBS. (v) The sections were incubated with 100 μl blocking solution (non-immune goat serum) for 10 min, and washed again in PBS for 10 minute. (vi) The sections were incubated with primary antibody 1: 50 dilution of mAb (clone 38–4) against N protein overnight at 4°C in moist chamber (mAb was a kind gift from PPR Reference Laboratory, CIRAD France). (vii) After incubation with primary antibody, the sections were washed in PBS (three washes, each for 3 minutes). (viii) Remaining reaction was developed according to instruction of Histostain® plus Kits (LAB-SA Detection System, Invitrogen). (ix) The reaction was visualized by adding AEC (3-Amino-ethylcarbazole), 3 drops per section with incubation for 10 minutes. The sections were counter-stained with Meyer's haematoxylin for 5 minutes; excess haematoxylin was removed by washing in running tap water for 10 min and distilled water for 5 minutes. (x) Stained washed sections were mounted with glycerol gelatin (aqueous-based mounting medium, Aquaperm™, Thermo Shandon). Parallel negative (tissues from healthy goat) and positive (previously confirmed by RT PCR and histopathology) controls were run each time.

Reverse transcription - Polymerase chain Reaction

RNA was extracted from lymphnode tissue homogenates using RNeasy Kit (Qiagen, Germany) following the procedure described by the manufacturer. Reverse transcription-polymerase chain reaction (RT-PCR) was carried out with F and N gene-specific primer sets of PPRV as described by Forsyth and Barrett [22] and Qiagen one step RT-PCR kit. The pieces of smeared filter papers were directly used in PCR tubes as source of template RNA. The RT-PCR technique was used as described by Michaud et al. [30].

Sequencing and Analysis of nucleotide and deduced amino acid sequence data

One of the amplified RT-PCR products were sequenced directly using PCR primer specific for F and N genes as used before. The PCR products for both the genes were cleaned using the EZ-10 Spin column DNA Gel extraction kit (Bio Basic Inc., USA). The procedure was strictly followed as described by the manufacturer. Quantification of purified DNA, cycle amplification and sequencing of the products were done from 1st BASE Laboratories, Singapore. The nucleic acid sequences obtained from PCR products of F and N gene and their deduced amino acid sequences were aligned and studied for their divergence. The sequences of the isolate have been submitted to the GenBank. Homology and divergence among the Bangladeshi isolates have been studied. Sequenced data of Bangladeshi isolates were compared with other related sequences retrieved from the GenBank. Sequence editing, alignment, and homology study were carried out with the software package "Lasergene" (Modules - EditSeq and MegAlign; DNASTAR Inc., USA).

Ethical approval

The present study was not subject to ethical approval as Bangladesh laws don't require approval for studies not involving experimental inoculation. The samples originated from natural outbreaks and from dead animals. The nasal swabs were collected from sick animals by registered veterinarian. The post mortem was conducted by registered veterinarian as per country rule.

Competing interests

The authors declare that they have no competing interests.

Authors' contributions

All authors contributed to the design of the study. Necropsy was performed by ARB and MSAS. Histological examination was performed by EHC and ARB. Immunohistochemistry was done by ARB and EHC. RT-PCR was done ARB and MMR, phylogenetic analysis was done by MRI, EHC and ARB. All authors participated in drafting the manuscript and proofreading of the final manuscript. All authors read and approved the final manuscript.

Acknowledgements

SPGR, PIU, BARC, Dhaka Bangladesh and International Atomic Energy Agency, Vienna for providing funds and supporting research works.

Author details

[1]Department of Pathology, Faculty of Veterinary Science, Bangladesh Agricultural University, Mymensingh, Bangladesh. [2]Department of Livestock Services, Dhaka, Bangladesh.

References

1. Gibbs EPJ, Taylor WP, Lowman MJP, Bryant J: **Classification of peste des petits ruminants virus as the fourth member of the genus Morbillivirus.** *Intervirology* 1979, **1979**(11):268–274.
2. Barrett T, Romero CH, Baron MD, Yamanouchi K, Diallo A, Bostcok CJ, Black D: **The molecular biology of rinderpest and peste des petits ruminants.** *Ann Med Vet* 1999, **137**:77–85.
3. Banyard AC, Parida S, Batten C, Oura Kwiatek O, Libeau G: **Global distribution of peste des petits ruminants virus and prospects for improved diagnosis and control.** *J Gen Virol* 2010, **91**:2885–2897.
4. Dardiri AH, de Boer CI, Hamdy FM: **Response of American goats and cattle to PPR virus.** In *Proceedings of the 19th Annual Meeting of the American Association of Veterinary Laboratory Diagnosticians.* 1601 Mineral point Road, Madison, Wisconsin 55705: AAVLD; 1977:337.
5. Taylor WP: **The distribution and epidemiology of PPR.** *Prev Vet Med* 1984, **2**:157–166.
6. Bundza A, Afshar A, Dukes TW, Myers DJ, Dulac GC, Becker SA: **Experimental peste des petits ruminants (goat plague) in goats and sheep.** *Can J Vet Res* 1988, **52**:46–52.
7. Radostits OM, Gay CC, Blood DC, Hinchcliff KW: *Veterinary Medicine.* 9th edition. London: W.B. Saunders Company Limited; 2000:1059–1063.
8. Pawaiya RVS, Mishra N, Bhagwan PSK, Dubay SC: **Pathology and distribution of antigen in goats naturally infected with PPRV.** *Ind J Anim Sci* 2004, **74**:35–40.
9. Abu Elzein EME, Hassanien MM, Alfaleg AIA, Elhadi MAA, Housawi FMT: **Isolation of PPR virus from goats in Saudi Arabia.** *Vet Rec* 1990, **127**:309–310.
10. Lefevre PC, Diallo A: **Peste des petits ruminants virus.** *Rev Sci Tech Off Int Epiz* 1990, **9**:951–965.
11. Taylor WP, Abusaidy S, Barret T: **The epidemiology of PPR in the sultanate of Oman.** *Vet Micro* 1990, **22**:341–352.
12. Susan E, Aiello BS: *The Merck Veterinary Manual.* 8th edition. Whitehouse Station, N.J., U.S.A: Merck and Co., Inc; 1998:539–541.
13. Debasis J, Mousumi G: **Incidence of an explosive outbreak of Peste des petits ruminants (PPR) in Black Bengal goats in Bankura District of West Bengal.** *Ind Vet J* 2002, **79**:739–740.
14. Kumar GS, Rathore BS, Mehrotra ML: **Epidemiological observations on Peste-des petits ruminants in north India.** *Indian J Anim Sci* 1999, **69**:365–368.
15. Saliki JT: **Peste des petits ruminants.** In *Foreign Animal Diseases: the Gray Book. Part IV.* 6th edition. Richmond, VA: US Animal Health Association; 1998:344.
16. Aruni AW, Lalitha PS, Mohan AC, Chitravelu P, Anbumani SP: **Histopathological study of a natural outbreak of peste des petits ruminants in goats of Tamilnadu.** *Small Ruminant Res* 1998, **28**:233–240.
17. Osman NA, Ali AS, Rahman MEA, Fadol MA: **Pathological, serological and virological findings in goats experimentally infected with Sudanese peste des petits ruminants virus isolates.** *J Gen Molr Virol* 2009, **1**:1–6.
18. Islam MR, Shamsuddin M, Das PM, Dewan ML: **An outbreak of peste des petits ruminants in Black Bengal goats in Mymensingh, Bangladesh.** *The Bangladesh Vet J* 2001, **18**:14–19.
19. Islam MR, Sharma B, Dem P, Pattnaik B, Jha VC, Naeem K, Kothalawala KACHA: *Economic Impact of Transboundary Animal Diseases in SAARC Countries.* Dhaka: SAARC Agriculture Centre; 2013:96p.
20. Hammouchi M, Loutfi C, Sebbar G, Touil N, Chaffai N, Batten C, Harif B, Oura C, El Harrak M: **Experimental infection of alpine goats with a Moroccan strain of peste des petits ruminants virus (PPRV).** *Vet Microbiol* 2012, **160**:240–244.
21. Office International des Epizooties (OIE): **Chapter 2.77.11: Peste des petits ruminants.** In *Manual of Diagnostic Tests and Vaccines for Terrestrial Animals.* http://www.oie.int/international-standard-setting/terrestrial-manual/access-online/ (accessed on 6 November 2014).
22. Forsyth MA, Barrett T: **Evaluation of polymerase chain reaction for the detection and characterisation of rinderpest and peste des petits ruminants viruses for epidemiological studies.** *Virus Res* 1995, **39**:151–163.
23. Libeau G, Diallo A, Calvez D, Lefevre PC: **Competitive ELISA using anti- N monoclonal antibodies for specific detection of RP in cattle and ruminants.** *Vet Microbiol* 1992, **31**:147–160.
24. Taylor WP: **Serological studies with the virus of peste des petits ruminats in Nigeria.** *Res Vet Sci* 1979, **26**:236–242.
25. Rajak KK, Sreenivas P, Hosamani M, Singh RP, Singh SK, Bandyopadhyay SK: **Experimental studies on immunosuppressive effects of Pestte Des Petits Ruminants (PPR) virus in goats.** *Comp Immunol Microbiol J* 2005, **28**:287–296.
26. Emike BO, Ajisegiri WA: **The Response of Bronchial Associated lymphoid tissue to intratracheal administration of Peste Des Petits Ruminants virus and its co-infection with Mannheimia hemolytica in goats.** *Int J Morphol* 2011, **29**:1099–1103.
27. Madboli AA, Ali SM: **Histopathological and Immunohistochemical studies on the female genital system and some visceral organs in sheep and goat naturally infected by Peste des Petits Ruminants virus.** *Global Veterinaria* 2012, **9**:752–760.
28. Brown CC, Mariner JC, Olander HJ: **An immunohistochemical study of the pneumonia caused by peste des petits ruminant virus.** *Vet Pathol* 1991, **28**:166–170.
29. Luna LG: *Manual of Histologic Staining Methods for the Armed Forces Institutes of Pathology.* 3rd edition. New York: McGraw-Hill, Ink, Book Company; 1968.
30. Michaud V, Gil P, Kwiatek O, Prome S, Dixon L, Romero L, Potier M-FLE, Arias M, Couacy-Hymann E, Roger F, Libeau G, Albina E: **Long-term storage at tropical temperature of dried-blood filter papers for detection and genotyping of RNA and DNA viruses by direct PCR.** *J Virol Methods* 2007, **146**:257–265.

Emergence of porcine epidemic diarrhea virus in southern Germany

Julia Stadler[1*], Susanne Zoels[1], Robert Fux[2], Dennis Hanke[3], Anne Pohlmann[3], Sandra Blome[3], Herbert Weissenböck[4], Christiane Weissenbacher-Lang[4], Mathias Ritzmann[1] and Andrea Ladinig[5]

Abstract

Background: Over the last years, porcine epidemic diarrhea virus (PEDV) has caused devastating enteric diseases in the US and several countries in Asia, while outbreaks in Europe have only been reported sporadically since the 1980s. At present, only insufficient information is available on currently circulating PEDV strains in Europe and their impact on the European swine industry. In this case report, we present epidemic outbreaks of porcine epidemic diarrhea in three farms in South-Western Germany.

Case presentation: Epidemic outbreaks of diarrhea affecting pigs of all age groups were reported in three farms, one fattening farm and two piglet producing farms, in South-Western Germany between May and November 2014. In the fattening farm yellowish, watery diarrhea without evidence of mucus or blood was associated with a massive reduction of feed consumption. Severity of clinical signs and mortality in young suckling pigs varied significantly between the two affected sow farms. While mortality in suckling piglets reached almost 70 % in one sow herd, no increase in suckling piglet mortality was observed in the second sow farm. In all three cases, PEDV was confirmed in feces and small intestines by RT-qPCR. Phylogenetic analyses based on full-length PEDV genomes revealed high identity among strains from all three herds. Moreover, the German strains showed very high nucleotide identity (99.4 %) with a variant of PEDV (OH851) that was isolated in the United States in January 2014. This strain with insertions and deletions in the S-gene (so called INDEL strains) was reported to show lower virulence. Slightly lower identities were found with other strains from the US and Asia.

Conclusion: Phylogenetic information on the distribution of PEDV strains in Europe is severely lacking. In this case report we demonstrate that acute outbreaks of PEDV occurred in southern Germany in 2014. Current strains were clearly different from isolates found in the 1980s and were closely related to a PEDV variant found in the US in 2014. Moreover, the present case report indicates that variant strains of PEDV, containing insertions and deletions in the S gene, which were reported to be of lower virulence, might be able to cause high mortality in suckling piglets.

Keywords: Porcine epidemic diarrhea virus, Southern Germany, Phylogenetic analysis, S INDEL PEDV

Background

Porcine epidemic diarrhea virus (PEDV), an enveloped, single-stranded, positive-sense RNA virus, was identified as the causative agent of porcine epidemic diarrhea (PED) in 1978 [1]. It was subsequently placed into the order *Nidovirales,* the subfamily *Coronavirinae*, the family *Coronaviridae*, and the genus *Alphacoronavirus* [2]. PED was first described in the United Kingdom in 1971 [3]. While several outbreaks were reported across Europe in the 1970s, only sporadic outbreaks occurred in recent years [4, 5]. In contrast, PED has emerged as a devastating enteric disease causing severe economic losses in other major swine-producing countries, notably the United States and Asia, within the last years [6, 7]. Since the emergence of PEDV in the United States in April 2013, the disease has rapidly spread throughout the country, inducing explosive outbreaks of diarrhea with high mortality among infected suckling piglets [6, 8, 9]. Phylogenetic analysis of the original highly virulent US PEDV strain from April 2013 revealed high nucleotide identity to strains circulating in China in 2012 [6].

* Correspondence: j.stadler@med.vetmed.uni-muenchen.de
[1]Clinic for Swine at the Centre for Clinical Veterinary Medicine, Ludwig-Maximilians University, Oberschleissheim, Germany
Full list of author information is available at the end of the article

In January 2014, a new variant strain of PEDV (OH 851), containing insertions and deletions in the S gene (S INDEL), was identified in Ohio causing mild clinical signs and lower mortality rates in suckling piglets compared to other currently circulating PEDV strains in the US [10]. At present, both S INDEL and highly virulent non S INDEL strains are co-circulating in the US, though S INDEL strains are less frequently diagnosed [11] .

Fairly little information on the current situation on PED is available from European countries. Recently, several outbreaks of acute PED occurred in Germany. In this case report we describe acute outbreaks of PED in one fattening farm and two sow farms in South-Western Germany between May and November 2014.

Case presentation

Clinical presentation

Farm A (fattening farm)

In May 2014, an epidemic of diarrhea was reported in a 1200 head fattening farm located in an area with low pig density in Southern Germany. Two buildings separated by a distance of about 20 m are run in a continuous flow production, i.e. different age groups are housed in one barn. The pens are subdivided into an outdoor area with partially slatted floor and an indoor area equipped with concrete solid floor. On May 23, 2014, a new batch of 320 feeder pigs with an average weight of 30 kg was introduced into the fattening farm. The piglets had been purchased from a 14,000 head nursery facility in Northern Germany, which was single-sourced from a 5000 sow farrow to wean farm located in the Netherlands. On May 25, 2014 (two days after placement), the newly introduced pigs showed yellowish to greyish, watery diarrhea. According to the farmer, approximately 50 % of pigs from the youngest age group were affected. Feces contained undigested feed components but no mucus or blood. Vomitus was apparent in individual pigs. By the following day, all age groups within the same barn were affected. As of May 28, 2014, the disease had spread to the second barn. Within five to seven days after placement of the new group of feeder pigs, 95 % of all growing and finishing pigs developed diarrhea accompanied by anorexia and lethargy. The affected pigs showed varying degrees of weight loss and dehydration. Within the first ten days after the onset of clinical signs 20 pigs had died; 80 % of them originated from the youngest age group. Clinical signs subsided within three weeks in the older age groups, but recurrent diarrhea persisted in the youngest age group for up to 15 weeks. At the peak of clinical signs, five days after the onset of first clinical signs, feed consumption severely declined. Feed consumption returned to normal within six days in the older age groups but was compromised in the youngest age groups for several weeks. During the outbreak of PED an overall mortality rate of 4.5 %, an average daily gain (ADG) of 600 g and a prolonged fattening period of 30 days were documented. Prior to the outbreak, performance data accounted for 750 g ADG and 2 % mortality.

Farms B and C (sow farms)

The two sow farms are located in a pig dense area in South-Western Germany. In September 2014, farm B, which is producing piglets with 280 sows in a three week batch farrowing interval, was experiencing diarrhea in all age groups. First clinical signs were characterized by anorexia in lactating sows and diarrhea of the corresponding three week old piglets. Pasty diarrhea progressed to watery greyish feces with variable degrees of dehydration, affecting about 70 % of piglets from one farrowing batch. Two days after the first onset of diarrhea in suckling piglets, up to 100 % of the sows in the farrowing unit were affected by watery diarrhea. Within one week after the onset of first clinical signs, diarrhea had spread to all age groups of pigs present at the farm including boars and nursery pigs. During the outbreak, mortality ranged from 5.5 % in suckling piglets to 8.8 % in nursery pigs. Clinical signs were present for approximately four weeks and performance data returned to normal within six weeks after the outbreak of PED.

Clinical signs in farm C, a piglet producing farm with about 290 sows and a nursery unit for 700 piglets, started on October 30/November 1, 2014. The group of sows weaned on October 30 showed severely reduced feed intake for the first seven to eight days after weaning and had yellowish, watery diarrhea. More than 95 % of sows from that group were affected. Two to three days after the clinical signs had been observed in the breeding area, diarrhea and reduced to absent feed intake occurred in the farrowing unit in sows which were nursing piglets of about 2.5 weeks of age. Suckling piglets started with mild pasty, yellowish diarrhea but were not severely affected and only three piglets died before weaning. The next group of sows farrowed between November 7 and 9. Piglets from those sows were acutely affected and started to show yellowish, pasty to watery diarrhea about two days after birth. First piglet losses occurred on November 10. In total, 67.6 % of piglets from this farrowing group died or had to be euthanized before weaning. Diarrheic, gaunt and dehydrated piglets, covered with feces (Fig. 1), were found in 30 out of 35 (86 %) litters from this farrowing group. In addition to signs in piglets, sows had watery diarrhea and severely reduced feed intake. Pasty to watery diarrhea also occurred in the gestation unit where sows are housed in small groups of six to eight animals on slatted floor. Clinical signs in the nursery mainly consisted of severely reduced feed intake and diarrhea in individual pigs. Mortality in the nursery

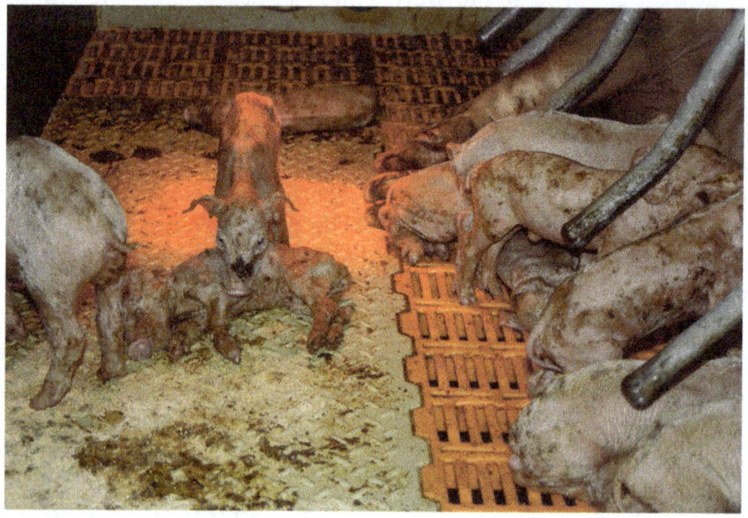

Fig. 1 Suckling piglets with severe diarrhea and dehydration. Seven-day-old piglets from a severly affected litter from farm C. Piglets, covered with feces, showing yellowish, pasty to watery diarrhea and varying degrees of dehydration

reached up to 7.1 % during the outbreak. Clinical signs subsided within four weeks after the onset of diarrhea. No diarrhea was observed in suckling piglets of the consecutive farrowing group born around November 26.

Laboratory findings

Severely affected animals from all three farms (Farm A: 3 feeder pigs, Farm B: 4 suckling piglets, Farm C: 25 suckling piglets) were submitted for pathological investigations. Gross lesions were limited to the intestines and characterized by distended, thin and transparent intestinal walls, mainly observed in the small intestines but partially also in the colon region (Fig. 2). The intestinal lumen contained yellow, watery and frothy fluid. In individual pigs intestinal contents were completely absent. Tissue samples from small intestines were fixed in 10 % neutral buffered formalin and embedded in paraffin wax. Tissue sections were stained with hematoxylin and eosin (H&E) for microscopic examination by standard methods. Histology was characterized by atrophic enteritis, which included shortening, blunting and fusion of the villi, occasionally with vacuolation and exfoliation of enterocytes (Fig. 3). There were individually differing grades of the lesions. In farm C a more detailed evaluation of histological lesions and an additional localization of viral nucleic acid within lesions was performed due to the availability of higher numbers of severely affected piglets. In four of the 25 investigated

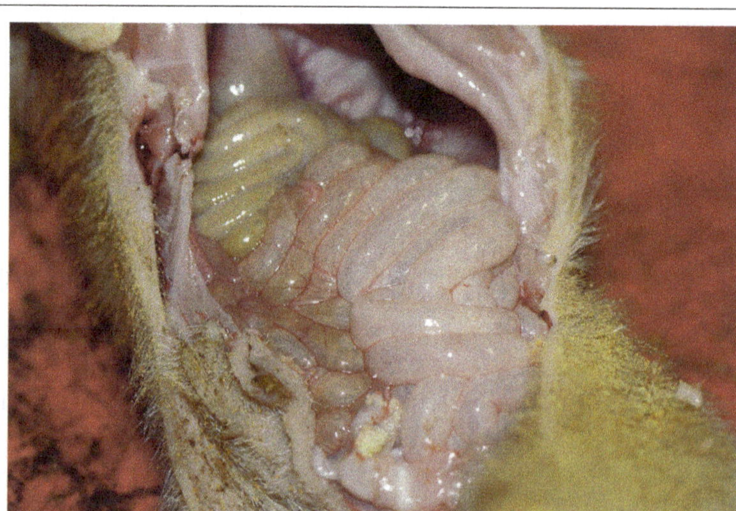

Fig. 2 Macroscopic changes in the small intestines from a suckling piglet of farm C. Gross lesions are characterized by thin and transparent intestinal walls and accumulation of large amounts of yellowish fluid in the intestinal lumen

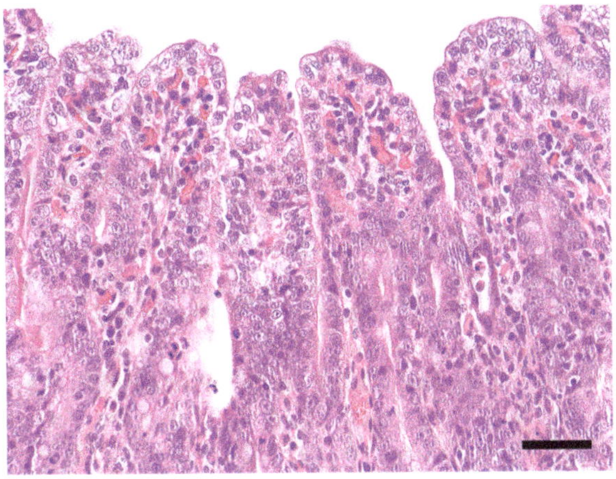

Fig. 3 Histological changes in the small intestines from a suckling piglet of farm C. There are shortened, blunted and partly fused villi. The cytoplasm of the villous enterocytes is markedly vacuolated. Haematoxylin and eosin staining, Bar = 80 µm

piglets lesions were categorized as severe, in nine piglets as moderate and in 12 piglets as mild (Table 1). A chromogenic *in situ* hybridization (ISH) procedure was developed for semi-quantitative analysis of viral nucleic acid present within enterocytes. An oligonucleotide probe with the potential to hybridize with all representatives of PEDV was designed. Probe design was based on extensive homology studies on available nucleocapsid gene sequences from GenBank using the software Sci Ed Central for Windows 95 (Scientific & Educational Software, Cary, NC, USA). The resulting probe sequence was: 5'-GCATCCTTGACAGCAGCCACCAGATCATC GCGTGAT-3'. The probe sequence was submitted to Basic Local Alignment Search Tool (BLAST) [12] to search against GenBank sequences and to exclude unintentional cross-reactivity with other organisms. The ISH procedure followed a previously published protocol [13]. The probe concentration was 35 ng/µl. As negative controls paraffin wax-embedded small intestinal tissue samples of a healthy piglet and of a piglet experimentally infected with transmissible gastroenteritis virus (TGEV), an unrelated alphacoronavirus, were used. The proportion of positive enterocytes was assessed semiquantitatively using the score +++ for abundant (between 75 % and 100 % of enterocytes positive), ++ for moderate (between 25 % to 75 % of enterocytes positive) and + for few (less than 25 % of enterocytes positive) signals. By ISH, viral signals were found exclusively in the cytoplasm of enterocytes (Fig. 4). The vast majority of infected cells was present in the villi but occasionally there were positive crypt epithelia too. In 9 piglets necropsied from farm C there were abundant ISH signals (+++) and in 8 cases each, moderate (++) or few (+) signals were

Table 1 Histological scores and in situ hybridization results of 25 piglets from farm C

Piglet No.	Histological score	ISH score
1	+	+++
2	+	+
3	++	++
4	+	++
5	++	+
6	+++	+++
7	++	+++
8	++	+++
9	++	+++
10	+	+
11	+	+
12	+	+
13	++	+
14	+	++
15	+	+
16	++	++
17	++	++
18	+++	+++
19	+++	++
20	+	+++
21	+	+++
22	+++	+++
23	+	++
24	+	+
25	++	+++

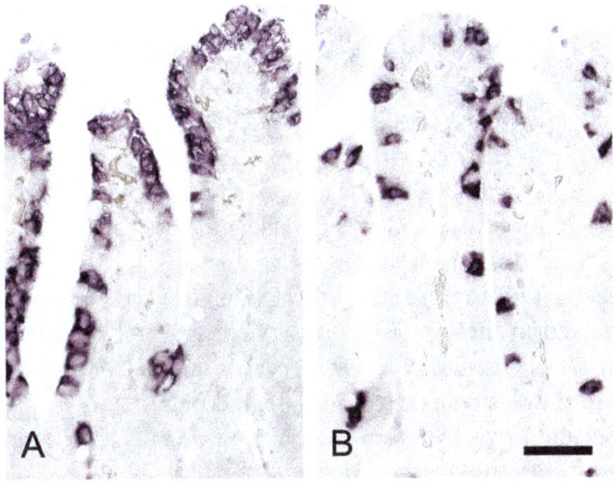

Fig. 4 Localization of viral nucleic acid in enterocytes by *in situ* hybridization. **a** The cytoplasm of the majority of villous enterocytes is positively labelled in a case with +++ score. **b** Only few, scattered enterocytes are positive in a case with + score. Bar = 80 µm

detected. The amount of positive cells did not exactly correspond with the histological scores (Table 1).

Electron microscopy was performed on fecal and tissue samples at the Institute for Infectious Diseases and Zoonosis, Ludwig-Maximilians University, Munich. Coronavirus-like particles were identified on the basis of their typical morphological characteristics.

For PEDV diagnosis pooled fecal samples (Farm A: n = 5 ; Farm B: n = 8; Farm C: n = 4) and small intestinal tissue samples (Farm A: n = 3; Farm B: n = 4; Farm C: n = 3) were investigated at the Institute for Infectious Diseases and Zoonosis, Ludwig-Maximilians University, Munich using two independent RT-qPCR systems targeting the PEDV N- and S-genes, respectively [14, 15]. The presence of PEDV-specific nucleotide sequences was confirmed in fecal and tissue samples of all three farms by RT-qPCR. All fecal samples were negative for TGEV, determined by RT-PCR [15]. For differential diagnosis fecal samples from all three farms were investigated for the presence of porcine Rotavirus, porcine Deltacoronavirus and porcine Norovirus by virus-specific RT-PCRs as described previously [16–18]. Additionally, fecal samples from both piglet producing farms were examined for porcine Sapovirus by RT-PCR [19]. All samples were negative for the aforementioned enteric viral pathogens. To further investigate concomitant infections, bacteriological investigations were performed on fecal samples from diarrheic pigs from all three farms. The following bacteria were isolated: *Salmonella derby* and *E. coli* (positive for F18 and Shigatoxin 2e) in farm A, ST-II and ST-IP producing *E. coli* in farm B, and *E. coli* without major virulence factors (including LT-1, ST-IP, ST-II, Shigatoxin 2e, F4, F5, F6, F18, F41 and Intimin) and *Clostridium perfringens* type A negative for the enterotoxin gene and the beta 2 toxin gene in farm C.

Subsequently, in farm A and farm B five pooled fecal samples, originating from different age groups, were tested for PEDV by RT-qPCR on a biweekly basis to monitor the on-farm infection dynamics. PEDV-specific nucleotide sequences could be detected in all fecal samples obtained from farm A up to 15 weeks after the onset of first clinical signs. Fecal samples from farm B collected four, six and eight weeks after the initial occurrence of diarrhea were negative for PEDV RNA. Nine weeks after the onset of clinical signs in farm B, diarrhea recurred in the group of pigs which was first affected by clinical signs. PEDV nucleic acid could be detected in fecal samples collected from affected pigs.

Selected positive fecal samples from all three farms were submitted to the Friedrich-Loeffler-Institute, Isle of Riems, Germany for full genome sequencing and virus isolation. PEDV was successfully isolated from one fecal sample of farm A following the protocol published by Oka *et al.* [20] with slight modifications. Supplemental investigations are ongoing. Full-length genomes were determined using next-generation sequencing as previously described [21]. Nucleotide sequence alignment analysis of the full-length genomes revealed up to 98.7 % nucleotide identities with currently circulating highly virulent US strains and strains from China. Highest similarity existed to the so-called S INDEL strains described in the US [10]. The German PEDV strains shared approx. 99.4 % identity with those strains (OH 851 as an INDEL prototype strain). Much lower overall similarity was found between the current German S INDEL strains and the European isolate CV777 from the late 1970s. Phylogenetic trees were constructed for complete genomes and Spike protein sequences using PhyML [22] in the Geneious software suite with a GTR substitution model and supported by 1000 bootstrapping replicates. Since the phylogenetic tree based on the Spike gene did not add more information than obtained from the full-length tree we decided not to include it in the manuscript. All German isolates clustered together and with OH 851 (Fig. 5). Based on the data obtained from all three farms no recombination events were observed.

Discussion

PEDV emerged and spread in the 1970s and 1980s in several European countries. The disease was characterized by watery diarrhea and affected all age classes of animals. However, the impact of PED on the European swine industry has remarkably decreased after the 1980s. Over the last ten years only sporadic outbreaks of PED combined with low mortality rates have been reported [4, 5, 23], thus requiring no active monitoring of PEDV in Europe. Moreover, serological data on the current prevalence of PEDV in Europe are scarce and further restricted by the limited sensitivity and specificity of the hitherto available diagnostic tests [24].

In contrast, PED has emerged as a devastating disease causing substantial economic losses in Asia and North America over the last years [8, 9]. Since the first introduction into the US in April 2013, PED has spread to 32 US states [25] and has also been introduced into Canada [26]. Soon after the emergence of PED in the US, sequence analyses revealed high nucleotide identity between North American and current Asian PEDV strains suggesting a common ancestor for PEDV in both continents [27, 28]. At the beginning of 2014, new variants of PEDV showing distinct genetic patterns in the S gene, i.e. deletions, an insertion and several mutations in the first 1170 nucleotides of the S1 region, were found in the US [10]. Those PEDV strains, also called S INDEL PEDV, were reported to be of lower virulence inducing mild to absent clinical signs and low mortality in suckling piglets [10]. PEDV strains described in this case report were most closely related to S INDEL PEDV.

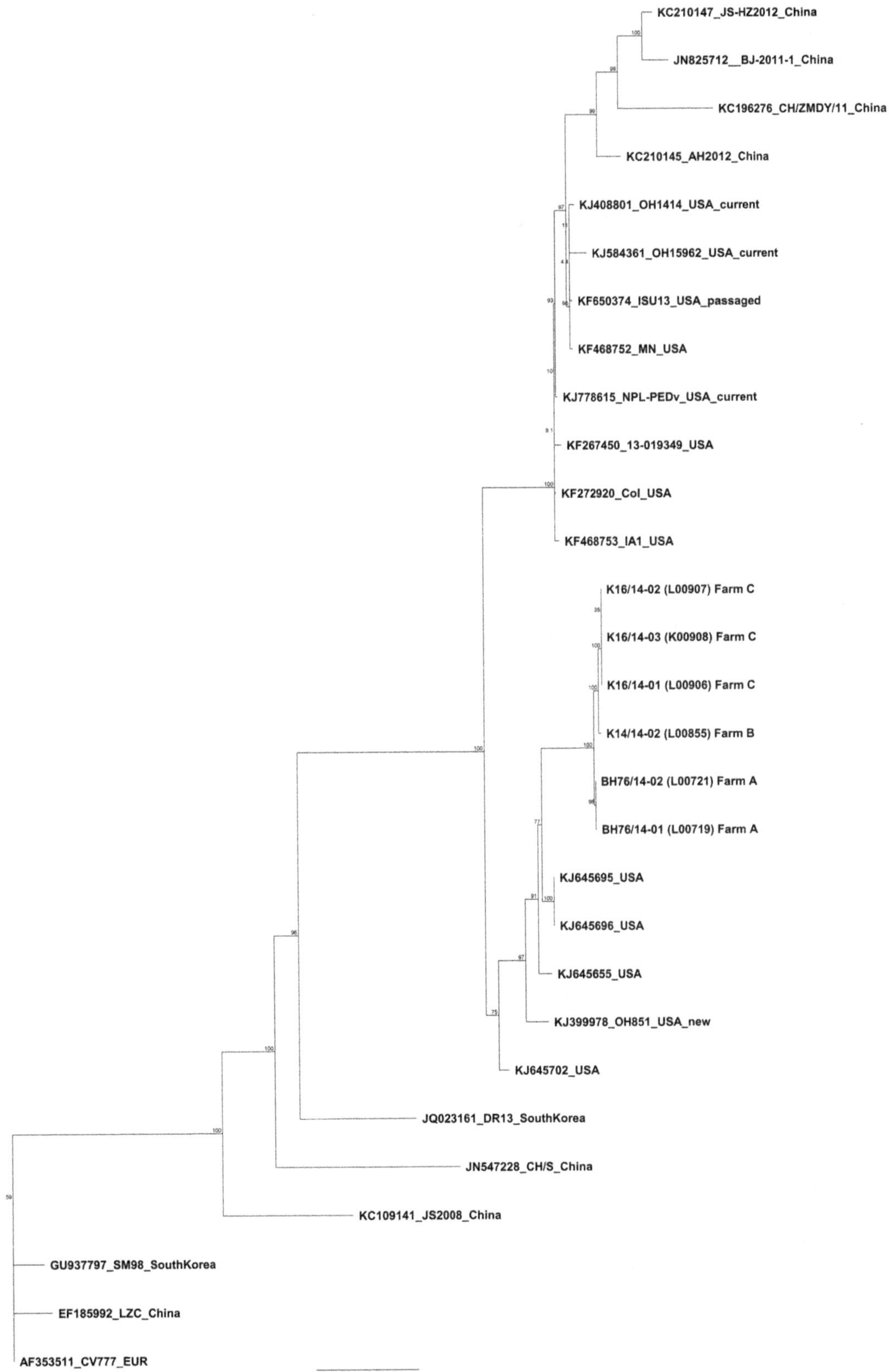

Fig. 5 (See legend on next page.)

(See figure on previous page.)

Fig. 5 Phylogenetic tree of current German PEDV strains compared with strains from the United States and China. Full genome sequences of German PEDV strains were aligned using MAFFT, and phylogenetic analyses were carried out using the maximum-likelihood method PhyML [22] with a GTR substitution model and tree reconstruction supported by 1000 bootstrapping replicates. All tools implemented in Geneious (vs. 8.0.5, Biomatters [30]). Strain derived from farm A are found as BH76/14, from farm B as K14/14, and farm C as K16/14

Similar strains were found in North-Western Germany, where outbreaks of PED characterized by high morbidity but no mortality occurred in three fattening farms in spring 2014 [29]. In contrast to the short duration of diarrhea observed in the North Western German fattening farms, diarrhea in the fattening farm described in this case report (Farm A) lasted up to 15 weeks after the initial outbreak and was associated with a massive decline in ADG and an increased mortality rate. This might be due to management and housing conditions in farm B, but could also be related to co-infections complicating the clinical disease.

Besides PED outbreaks in German fattening farms, the occurrence of PED in two sow farms in Southern Germany has unsettled German pig farmers. The severity of clinical signs observed in the two affected sow farms differed significantly, although sequence analyses revealed that strains found in both farms showed 99.9 % nucleotide identity based on full genome sequencing with 12 different nucleotides found in the genome, four of which were located in the spike protein coding sequence. The manifestation of the disease might vary between herds due to the level of immunity within the population, potential infectious co-agents as well as management and biosecurity reasons. Since no diarrhea occurred in suckling piglets in farm C prior to and after the acute outbreak of PED, we concluded that co-infections played a minor role in this farm, which is supported by the fact that no relevant enteric viral pathogens were found and bacteria isolated from diarrheic piglets were negative for known genes of major virulence factors.

Conclusion

In conclusion, the present case report reveals that PEDV strains similar to S INDEL PEDV are currently circulating in different farm types in Southern Germany. Severe clinical signs and high mortality rates in suckling piglets observed in one farm might indicate that the potential of virulence can vary between S INDEL PEDV strains. However, experimental studies to confirm the potential of high virulence of S INDEL PEDV are lacking to date.

Due to insufficient data on phylogenetic analysis of PEDV strains in Europe we cannot clarify if the reported strains were recently introduced from the US or have been circulating in Europe since the 1970s. Further molecular epidemiologic research is therefore needed to find temporal and geographic evidence for the exact origin and evolution of the recent PEDV strains in Germany.

Abbreviations

PEDV: Porcine epidemic diarrhea virus; PED: Porcine epidemic diarrhea; ADG: average daily gain; BLAST: Basic Local Alignment Search Tool; RT-qPCR: quantitative reverse transcriptase polymerase chain reaction; *E.coli*: *Escherichia coli*; LT-I: *Escherichia coli* heat-labile enterotoxin I; ST-IP: *Escherichia coli* heat-stable enterotoxin IP; ST-II: *Escherichia coli* heat-stable enterotoxin II; S INDEL: PEDV strains containing distinct insertions and deletions in the S gene.

Competing interests

The authors declare that they have no competing interests.

Authors` contributions

JS and AL wrote manuscript; JS, AL, SZ and MR were involved in farm visits including clinical examination and sample collection; RF was in charge of molecular diagnostics (RT-qPCR); SB, AP and DH provided virological expertise and performed phylogenetic analysis; CWL was responsible for development of the ISH assay; HW carried out pathological investigation. All authors read and approved the final manuscript.

Acknowledgements

The authors would like to recognize P. Zitzow, U. Kleinert and C. Dräger, Institute of Diagnostic Virology, Friedrich-Loeffler-Institut, for preparation of samples and technical assistance as well as Dr. D. Höper for sequence analyses. The excellent technical support of K. Fragner and K. Bittermann is gratefully acknowledged. We thank E. Liebler-Tenorio, Federal Research Institute for Animal Health Jena for the kind gift of TGEV control material. We are particularly grateful for assistance at farm visits provided by Dr. R. Hammer and Dr. A. Groschke, private veterinarians. The support of the farmers, who contributed to this study, is also greatly appreciated.

Author details

[1]Clinic for Swine at the Centre for Clinical Veterinary Medicine, Ludwig-Maximilians University, Oberschleissheim, Germany. [2]Institute for Infectious Diseases and Zoonosis at the Centre for Clinical Veterinary Medicine, Ludwig-Maximilians University, Munich, Germany. [3]Friedrich-Loeffler-Institut, Institute of Diagnostic Virology, Greifswald-Insel Riems, Germany. [4]Institute of Pathology and Forensic Veterinary Medicine, University of Veterinary Medicine Vienna, Vienna, Austria. [5]University Clinic for Swine, University of Veterinary Medicine Vienna, Vienna, Austria.

References

1. Pensaert MB, de Bouck P. A new coronavirus-like particle associated with diarrhea in swine. Archives of virology. 1978;58(3):243–7.
2. Carstens EB. Ratification vote on taxonomic proposals to the International Committee on Taxonomy of Viruses (2009). Archives of virology. 2010;155(1):133–46.
3. Oldham J: Letter to the editor. *Pig Farming* 1972:Oct suppl:72–73.
4. Martelli P, Lavazza A, Nigrelli AD, Merialdi G, Alborali LG, Pensaert MB. Epidemic of diarrhoea caused by porcine epidemic diarrhoea virus in Italy. The Veterinary record. 2008;162(10):307–10.
5. Rodak L, Valicek L, Smid B, Nevorankova Z. An ELISA optimized for porcine epidemic diarrhoea virus detection in faeces. Veterinary microbiology. 2005;105(1):9–17.
6. Stevenson GW, Hoang H, Schwartz KJ, Burrough ER, Sun D, Madson D, et al. Emergence of Porcine epidemic diarrhea virus in the United States: clinical signs, lesions, and viral genomic sequences. Journal of veterinary diagnostic

investigation : official publication of the American Association of Veterinary Laboratory Diagnosticians, Inc. 2013;25(5):649–54.
7. Gao Y, Kou Q, Ge X, Zhou L, Guo X, Yang H. Phylogenetic analysis of porcine epidemic diarrhea virus field strains prevailing recently in China. Archives of virology. 2013;158(3):711–5.
8. Cima G. Viral disease affects U.S. pigs: porcine epidemic diarrhea found in at least 11 states. Journal of the American Veterinary Medical Association. 2013;243(1):30–1.
9. Chen Q, Li G, Stasko J, Thomas JT, Stensland WR, Pillatzki AE, et al. Isolation and characterization of porcine epidemic diarrhea viruses associated with the 2013 disease outbreak among swine in the United States. Journal of clinical microbiology. 2014;52(1):234–43.
10. Wang L, Byrum B, Zhang Y. New variant of porcine epidemic diarrhea virus, United States, 2014. Emerging infectious diseases. 2014;20(5):917–9.
11. Vlasova AN, Marthaler D, Wang Q, Culhane MR, Rossow KD, Rovira A, et al. Distinct characteristics and complex evolution of PEDV strains, North America, May 2013-February 2014. Emerging infectious diseases. 2014;20(10):1620–8.
12. Altschul SF, Gish W, Miller W, Myers EW, Lipman DJ. Basic local alignment search tool. Journal of molecular biology. 1990;215(3):403–10.
13. Chvala S, Fragner K, Hackl R, Hess M, Weissenbock H. Cryptosporidium infection in domestic geese (Anser anser f. domestica) detected by in-situ hybridization. Journal of comparative pathology. 2006;134(2–3):211–8.
14. New rapid semi-quantitative RT-PCR assay developed to detect porcine epidemic diarrhea virus [http://www.cvm.umn.edu/sdec/prod/groups/cvm/@pub/@cvm/@sdec/documents/content/cvm_content_446628.pdf (2014)]
15. Kim SH, Kim IJ, Pyo HM, Tark DS, Song JY, Hyun BH. Multiplex real-time RT-PCR for the simultaneous detection and quantification of transmissible gastroenteritis virus and porcine epidemic diarrhea virus. Journal of virological methods. 2007;146(1–2):172–7.
16. Marthaler D, Raymond L, Jiang Y, Collins J, Rossow K, Rovira A. Rapid detection, complete genome sequencing, and phylogenetic analysis of porcine deltacoronavirus. Emerging infectious diseases. 2014;20(8):1347–50.
17. Pang XL, Cao M, Zhang M, Lee B. Increased sensitivity for various rotavirus genotypes in stool specimens by amending three mismatched nucleotides in the forward primer of a real-time RT-PCR assay. Journal of virological methods. 2011;172(1–2):85–7.
18. Vennema H, de Bruin E, Koopmans M. Rational optimization of generic primers used for Norwalk-like virus detection by reverse transcriptase polymerase chain reaction. Journal of clinical virology : the official publication of the Pan American Society for Clinical Virology. 2002;25(2):233–5.
19. Vinje J, Deijl H, van der Heide R, Lewis D, Hedlund KO, Svensson L, et al. Molecular detection and epidemiology of Sapporo-like viruses. Journal of clinical microbiology. 2000;38(2):530–6.
20. Oka T, Saif LJ, Marthaler D, Esseili MA, Meulia T, Lin CM, et al. Cell culture isolation and sequence analysis of genetically diverse US porcine epidemic diarrhea virus strains including a novel strain with a large deletion in the spike gene. Veterinary microbiology. 2014;173(3–4):258–69.
21. Juozapaitis M, Aguiar Moreira E, Mena I, Giese S, Riegger D, Pohlmann A, et al. An infectious bat-derived chimeric influenza virus harbouring the entry machinery of an influenza A virus. Nature communications. 2014;5:4448.
22. Guindon S, Dufayard JF, Lefort V, Anisimova M, Hordijk W, Gascuel O. New algorithms and methods to estimate maximum-likelihood phylogenies: assessing the performance of PhyML 3.0. Systematic biology. 2010;59(3):307–21.
23. Sozzi E, Luppi A, Lelli D, Martin AM, Canelli E, Brocchi E, et al. Comparison of enzyme-linked immunosorbent assay and RT-PCR for the detection of porcine epidemic diarrhoea virus. Research in veterinary science. 2010;88(1):166–8.
24. Gerber PF, Gong Q, Huang YW, Wang C, Holtkamp D, Opriessnig T. Detection of antibodies against porcine epidemic diarrhea virus in serum and colostrum by indirect ELISA. Veterinary journal (London, England : 1997). 2014;202(1):33–6.
25. Swine enteric coronavirus disease testing summary report [http://www.aphis.usda.gov/animal_health/animal_dis_spec/swine/downloads/swine_report_7_24_14.pdf (2014)]
26. Pasick J, Berhane Y, Ojkic D, Maxie G, Embury-Hyatt C, Swekla K, et al. Investigation into the role of potentially contaminated feed as a source of the first-detected outbreaks of porcine epidemic diarrhea in Canada. Transboundary and emerging diseases. 2014;61(5):397–410.
27. Marthaler D, Jiang Y, Otterson T, Goyal S, Rossow K, Collins J: Complete Genome Sequence of Porcine Epidemic Diarrhea Virus Strain USA/Colorado/2013 from the United States. *Genome announcements* 2013, 1(4):e00555-13.10.1128/genomeA.00555-13
28. Huang YW, Dickerman AW, Pineyro P, Li L, Fang L, Kiehne R, et al. Origin, evolution, and genotyping of emergent porcine epidemic diarrhea virus strains in the United States. mBio. 2013;4(5):e00737–00713.
29. Henniger T, Schwarz BA. Porcine Epidemic Diarrhoea-Neuausbrüche in deutschen Mastschweinebeständen. Tierärztliche Umschau. 2014;69:394–7.
30. Katoh K, Misawa K, Kuma K, Miyata T. MAFFT: a novel method for rapid multiple sequence alignment based on fast Fourier transform. Nucleic acids research. 2002;30(14):3059–66.

Inhibition of porcine reproductive and respiratory syndrome virus replication in vitro using DNA-based short antisense oligonucleotides

Longlong Zheng[1], Xiang Li[2], Lingyun Zhu[1], Wengui Li[1], Junlong Bi[3], Guishu Yang[1], Gefen Yin[1*] and Jianping Liu[4*]

Abstract

Background: Porcine reproductive and respiratory syndrome (PRRS) is caused by porcine reproductive and respiratory syndrome virus (PRRSV) and is an economically important disease in swine-producing areas. The objective of this study was to screen for effective antisense oligonucleotides (AS-ONs) which could inhibit PRRSV replication in MARC-145 cells and in pulmonary alveolar macrophages (PAM).

Results: Nine short AS-ON sequences against the well-conserved regions of PRRSV (5′-UTR, NSP9, ORF5 and ORF7) were selected. When MARC-145 cells or PAM were infected with PRRSV followed by transfection with AS-ONs, four AS-ON sequences targeting 5′-UTR, ORF5 or NSP9 were found to be the most effective oligonucleotides in decreasing the cytopathic effect (CPE) induced by PRRSV infection. Quantitative PCR and indirect immunofluorescence staining confirmed that ORF7 levels were significantly reduced both at RNA and protein levels. The PRRSV titration data furthermore indicated that transfection with AS-ON YN8 could reduce the PRRSV titer by 1000-fold compared with controls.

Conclusion: The results presented here indicate that DNA-based antisense oligonucleotides can effectively inhibit PRRSV replication in MARC-145 cells and in PAM. Furthermore, comparing with the reported hit rates (approximately 10-30 %), we achieved a higher success rate (44 %). The strategy we took to design the antisense sequences might be applied to select AS-ONs that more efficiently reduce the expression of target genes.

Keywords: Porcine reproductive and respiratory syndrome virus (PRRSV), Virus replication, Antisense oligonucleotides, Marc-145, Pulmonary alveolar macrophages (PAM)

Background

Porcine reproductive and respiratory syndrome (PRRS) is one of the most economically significant viral diseases in the swine industry, which is characterized by respiratory disorders in piglets and reproductive failure in sows [1]. This disease is due to the infection by porcine reproductive and respiratory syndrome virus (PRRSV), which belongs to the family *Arteriviridae*, genus *Arterivirus* [2]. PRRSV is an enveloped single-stranded positive-sense RNA virus. The genome of PRRSV is approximately 15 kb in length and consists of nine open reading frames (ORFs) [3]. ORF1a and ORF1b are located at the 5′ end of the genome and encode proteins with replicase and polymerase activities. NSP9 is a putative RNA-dependent RNA polymerase and plays important roles in viral replication [4]. ORFs 2–7 are located at the 3′-end of the genome and encode the structural proteins [2]. ORF5 encodes the GP5 protein, a receptor-binding protein [3, 5] which is a primary antigenic envelope glycoprotein. GP5 is targeted by the cellular immune response and is critical for viral neutralization functioning as. ORF7 encodes the nucleocapsid protein N which is important for the assembly and disassembly of the virion [6]. It is reasonable to speculate that antisense oligonucleotides targeting NSP9, ORF5 and ORF7, as well as 5′UTR, will result in degradation of the viral genome and inhibition of viral production.

* Correspondence: yingefen@ynau.edu.cn; Jianping.liu@ki.se
[1]Department of Veterinary Medicine, College of Animal Science and Technology, Yunnan Agricultural University, Kunming, China
[4]Present address: Karolinska Institute, Department of Biosciences and Nutrition, Novum, Huddinge, Sweden
Full list of author information is available at the end of the article

Antisense technology is one of the most promising technologies allowing the use of a short complementary oligonucleotide fragment to inhibit the expression of the target mRNA at transcriptional as well as at post-transcriptional levels. Antisense technology has the advantage that it shows high specificity and selectivity for the target gene sequence. Theoretically, antisense molecules could be used to treat any disease that is caused by the expression of a gene, e.g. viral infections, cancer growth, and inflammatory diseases [7–9].

Some highly pathogenic PRRSV strains of the North American type were found spread widely in more than 10 provinces in China and brought about four million fatal cases in 2006 [10]. Therefore, it is imperative to develop effective antiviral strategies to prevent and control this infection. In the interest of exploiting improved methods to control PRRS, we have applied the *in silico* oligo-walk method and *in vitro* biological approaches (cytopathic effect observation, quantitative PCR, virus titer assay and indirect immunofluorescence staining) to screen for protective antisense oligonucleotides that inhibit the replication of PRRSV in MARC-145 cells and in PAM.

Materials and methods

Ethics statement

Pigs used in this study did not undergo any manipulation prior to standard industrial slaughter according to the pertinent legislations. For this reason, no specific ethical approval was required. All animal experiments were performed with the approval of the Animal Care Committee of Yunnan Agricultural University, China.

Virus and cells

The PRRSV field strain YN-1 (GenBank accession number: KJ747052), a highly pathogenic PRRSV belonging to the North American genotype, was isolated in 2008 by our research group from the lungs of an infected pig in Yunnan province (China) during a severe PRRSV outbreak. It is known that the PRRSV can replicate in pulmonary alveolar macrophages (PAM) or in MARC-145 cells, thus both culture systems were applied in this study. The MARC-145 cell line was purchased from the Shanghai Cell Collection, Chinese Academy of Sciences (CAS), and cultured in Dulbecco's modified Eagle's medium (DMEM, Invitrogen) supplemented with 10 % heat-inactivated fetal bovine serum (FBS, GIBCO) (pH 7.4), 2 mM L-glutamine, 100 U/ml penicillin and 100 μg/ml streptomycin (Invitrogen). The cultures were maintained in a 5 % CO_2 humidified incubator at 37 °C. PAMs were obtained by *post mortem* lung lavage of 8-week-old PRRSV free pigs, and seeded into 96-well plates for 24 h incubation till further assays in RPMI-1640 supplemented with 10 % fetal calf serum (FBS), 2 mM L-glutamine, 0.1 mM non-essential amino acids, 1 mM sodium pyruvate and a mixture of antibiotics.

Selection of antisense oligonucleotide sequences

Bo et al. [11] developed a database named AOBase which stores 448 AS-ONs against the transcripts of 28 different target genes, and they found that the lengths of the AS-ON in the database range from 10 nt to 22 nt, with most of the AS-ONs 20 nt long. Therefore in this study we designed and synthesized all AS-ONs with a length of 20 nt.

Alignments of over 100 sequences (from NCBI database) of each gene region were carried out, respectively. Eight AS-ONs with 20 nt length (Table 1) directed against the well-conserved regions of PRRSV with 100 % sequence similarity (i.e., 5′-UTR, NSP9, ORF5 and ORF7) were selected using RNA Structure 5.6 [12, 13]. We selected the most frequently occurring secondary structure of the target RNA with minimal overall free energy as a potential AS-ON target site. Specificity of these sequences was verified by BLAST search. The positive AS-ON control (5UP2) studied by Patel et al. [14], which is not fully complementary to the corresponding 5′UTR region of the YN-1 strain used in this study, served as a negative control. This AS-ON control was also modified to 5′-**CGT**GGCATAGAGCCAACACC-3′ here to serve as a candidate sequence for the YN-1 strain(5UP2*, see Table 1). The AS-ONs were synthesized by Shengong (Shanghai, China).

The selection standards and procedures using RNAstructure were described in details by Mathews [12]. Briefly, for an oligonucleotide to tightly bind to its complementary sequence, the duplex free energy should be low and the magnitude of the cost of opening the target structure should also be minimized. The free energy of duplex formation and the oligonucleotide self-structure terms were previously shown to correlate with antisense oligonucleotide efficacy [15].

Virus infection and transfection

The cells were trypsinized and plated in 96-well plates (Corning) at 10^4 cells in 100 μl per well the day before PRRSV infection and AS-ON transfection. The cells were challenged with PRRSV YN1 strain (25 TCID50/well). After 90 min inoculation, the medium was removed and AS-ONs were transfected using 32 μM of AS-ONs in 100 μl of OPTI-MEM medium (Gibco) mixed with 1.5 μl/well of Lipofectamine 2000 (Invitrogen) according to the manufacturer's instructions. Four hours post-transfection, the transfection medium was replaced with fresh full DMEM medium till further analysis. Each treatment was performed in triplicates.

To measure the life time of AS-ONs in vitro, cy-3 labeled antisense oligonucleotide 5UP2 was used in the

Table 1 List of antisense oligonulceotides used in this study

Name of AS-ON	Sequence	Target gene	Position within the target gene	GC content (%)	Overall ΔG°37	Duplex ΔG°37	Break targ. ΔG°37	Oligo-self ΔG°37	Oligo-oligo ΔG°37	Tm (°c)
5UP2	5′-CAAGGCATAGAGCCAACACC-3′	2 nt mismatching	11–30 bp	55						
5UP2*	5′-CGTGGCATAGAGCCAACACC-3′	5′UTR	11–30 bp	60	−22.3	−24.9	0	−2.6	−6.8	68.9
YN1	5′-TGGGCTGTGCCAGTGGTCAC-3′	5′UTR	52–71 bp	65	−20.6	−41.1	−15.7	−4.8	−12.6	93.1
YN2	5′-GATTGAAGGCAGTCTGGATC-3′	ORF7	234–253 bp	50	−16.1	−22.6	−5.9	−0.3	−5.7	67.2
YN3	5′-TGCAACTCCGGAAGCAAGGT-3′	5′UTR	140–159 bp	55	−17.9	−25.4	−6.8	−0.5	−8	69.7
YN4	5′-CAGCTCACATAGCGTCAAAT-3′	ORF5	131–150 bp	45	−25.2	−36.1	−9.3	−1.5	−6.4	86.7
YN5	5′–CGTACGACGGTAGATGCTCT-3′	NSP9	1266–1285 bp	55	−23.5	−25	−0.4	−0.7	−7.8	69.6
YN6	5′-CGACGACAGACACAACTGCC-3′	ORF7	215–237 bp	60	−14.1	−24.5	−9.6	−0.6	−6.4	66.4
YN7	5′- CTGGATCGACAGACAGACACA-3′	ORF7	221–240 bp	55	−15.9	−38	−20.6	−1.4	−9.5	87.5
YN8	5′-TGCAGCATCCTCACAACCGT-3′	NSP9	704–723 bp	55	−23.1	−27.8	−4.7	0	−5.9	75.3

The thermodynamic parameters are free energy changes at 37 °C in kcal/mol. "Overall ΔG°37" is the total free energy change of binding for a structured target and structured oligonucleotide. "Duplex ΔG°37" is the free energy change of duplex formation between the oligonucleotide and target. "Break Targ. ΔG°37" is the free energy cost of opening target secondary structure. "Oligo Self ΔG°37" and "Oligo-Oligo ΔG°37" are the free energy costs of opening unimolecular and bimolecular self-structure in the oligonucleotide, respectively. The Tm is the melting temperature of duplex formation in °C, not accounting for self-structure in target or oligonucleotide

transfection. Cy-3 fluorescence signals were observed under the fluorescence microscopy (Olympus) at various time points (1, 2, 4 and 6 h post transfection) after removal of the old medium, PBS wash and addition of fresh medium.

Isolation of total RNA

Total RNA was isolated using the RNAiso Plus RNA isolation kit from Takara (Dalian, China), as per the manufacturer's instructions. The RNA was quantified using the absorbance at 260 nm and the purity assessed from the ratio of absorbance at 260 and 280 nm. The RNA used for all assays had a ratio of A260/A280 greater than 1.90.

Reverse transcription and qPCR analysis

Total RNA was isolated and subjected to reverse transcription and qPCR analysis. β-actin served as internal control. The primer pairs used in this study are: 5′-atcca ggctgtgctgtcc-3′ as forward primer and 5′-gaggatcttcatga ggtagtcg-3′ as reverse primer for β-actin; 5′-gaacgctccct ctgcttgc-3′ as forward primer and 5′-aaactcaacctgaaaacg ttaccttc-3′ as reverse primer for ORF7. The ΔΔCt method [16] for relative quantification of gene expression was used to determine viral RNA levels. For analyzing the inhibitory effect on RNA levels, SYBR Green real-time PCR was performed. Briefly, reverse transcription was carried out using Takara PrimerScript RT reagents kit in a volume of 10 μl at 37 °C for 15 min. One microliter of reverse transcription reaction mixture was used for qPCR by using gene-specific primers and master mix from SYBR Primer Ex Taq II kit (Takara). All reactions were performed in a 25 μl reaction volume. The reaction was carried out at 95 °C for 30 s, followed by 35 cycles at 95 °C for 30 s and 60 °C for 5 s. Relative amount of PRRSV RNA were normalized to β-actin mRNA. Amplification and detection of samples were performed with the CFX96 Touch Real-Time PCR Detection System (Bio-Rad).

Virus titration

Ten thousand Marc-145 cells were seeded into 96-well plates the day before infection and transfection. A Tenfold serial dilution of PRRSV YN-1 strain was made with medium. 100 μl/well of each dilution was added into six wells. Ninety minutes post infection, the transfection was performed as described above. CPE was monitored using the inverted microscope over a period of 4 days post transfection. Cell number was recorded and the 50 % tissue culture infected dose (TCID50) was determined by Reed–Muench method.

Indirect immunofluorescence staining

Sixty hours post PRRSV infection and transfection with AS-ONs, medium was removed and the MARC-145 cells were fixed with 100 μl/well of 4 % paraformaldehyde (PFA) at room temperature for 15 min followed by three washes with PBS (137 mM NaCl, 7 mM Na_2HPO_4, 1.5 mM KH_2PO_4, 2.7 mM KCl, pH 7.4), The fixed samples were permeabilized with PBS containing 0.3 % Triton X-100 for 15 min and blocked with PBS containing 1 % BSA for 2 h at 4 °C. The nuclei were stained with 5 μg/ml of Hoechst 33,342 (Life Technology) in PBS for 20 min at room temperature. Then the cells were incubated with 5 μg/ml of PRRSV antibody against N protein (encoded by ORF7) generated from mouse

(VMRD, Cat. no. 080728–004) at 4 °C overnight. Cells were washed three times with PBS and incubated with Alexa Fluor 488 conjugated goat anti-mouse IgG (H + L) antibody (Proteintech, Cat. no. 861163) at 5 µg/ml for 1 h at 37 °C. After three PBS washes the cells in the 96-well plates were protected from light until further analysis by fluorescence microscopy (Olympus).

Statistical analysis

Software SPSS 11.0 and Student's t-test were used to determine significant differences between treatments. A p-value <0.05 was considered statistically significant. n-values represent the number of independent experiments.

Results

Antisense oligonucleotide design

An effective AS-ON should be selected at the RNA regions which are accessible for hybridization [17, 18]. To select potent AS-ONs, the binding energy between the AS-ONs and RNA (ΔG°37) should be as low as possible (e.g., ≤ −8 kcal/mol), whereas the energy for binding between AS-ONs should be as high as possible (e.g., ΔG°37 ≥ −1.1 kcal/mol) [19]. After analyzing some data collected from > 1000 experiments, Matveeva et al. [15] found a positive correlation between AS-ON mediated RNA knockdown and the presence of CCAC, TCCC, ACTC, GCCA and CTCT motifs in the AS-ONs, while the presence of GGGG, ACTG, AAA and TAA motifs in AS-ONs showed negative correlations. Ho et al. [19] observed strong AS-ONs effects with a minimum of 11 G or C residues in 20 nt AS-ONs.

Nine AS-ONs were selected (Table 1) using the program OligoWalk from the package RNAstructure to calculate the binding energies of AS-ONs/AS-ONs and AS-ONs/RNA. We tried to keep the AS-ONs containing ≥ 11 G or C, or any of the positive motifs (e.g., GCCA in sequence 5UP2* and YN1) and to exclude the ones containing the negative motifs. Figure 1 illustrates the complementary sequences of the targeting gene regions for three AS-ONs showing prominent inhibitory effects on PRRSV replication and demonstrates that the local structures accessible to AS-ONs are those usually located at the terminal end, internal loops, joint sequences, hairpins and bulges of ≥10 consecutive nucleotides, as previously reported by Kretschmer-Kaxemi et al. [20].

Life time of antisense oligonucleotides in in vitro cell culture

To investigate how long AS-ONs are present in an in vitro cell culture system, the Cy-3 labelled antisense oligonucleotide 5UP2 was transfected into MARC-145 cells. At different time points (1, 2 , 4 and 6 h) post transfection, the medium was removed, the cells were washed with PBS, fresh medium was added into the wells, and cells were imaged. (Fig. 2). We found that the fluorescent signal from Cy-3 labelled antisense oligonucleotides was still detectable 6 h post transfection, although the signal decreased through the observation time period, demonstrating that the antisense oligonucleotide is not degraded prior to PRRSV mRNA transcription and thus can target to the viral mRNA for its degradation.

Inhibition of CPE by transfection with antisense oligonucleotides

To investigate whether AS-ONs can protect MARC-145 cells from the cytopathic effect (CPE) induced by PRRSV, cells were transfected with AS-ONs one and half hours post challenge with 25 TCID50 PRRSV per well. Treatments of no transfection, mock (Lipofectamin 2000 only, without any antisense sequence) and the 2 nt mismatching oligo 5UP2 served as negative controls. CPE was recorded daily. An image for each treatment was acquired 72 h post transfection and is shown in Fig. 3. Significant cytotoxic effects were observed neither in the mock well nor in the transfection well with 40 µM of 5UP2, but in the transfection well with 50 µM of 5UP2 (Fig. 3a), indicating that 40 µM of AS-ONs is a safe dose for the cells. Therefore the working concentration (32 µM) of AS-ONs in this study would not be toxic to the cells, ruling out the possibility of inhibitory effects due to the toxicity of different AS-ONs. In Fig. 3b, compared with the normal cells (neither PRRSV inoculation nor transfection was applied), the cells in the negative controls aggregated, rounded up and disintegrated. We found that cells transfected with 5UP2*, YN4, YN5 and YN8 manifested overtly less CPE. Other AS-ON-treated cells and the mock demonstrated the same typical PRRSV-induced CPE as cells infected only with virus (PRRSV only), which became pycnotic and detached from the monolayer, demonstrating that those antisense oligonucleotides do not show any obvious interference with viral replication.

Reduction of viral RNA levels by transfection with antisense oligonucleotides

To investigate whether AS-ONs inhibit PRRSV replication in MARC-145 cells and PAM, MARC-145 cells and PAM were transfected by the selected AS-ONs. Non-transfected MARC-145 cells and PAM challenged with PRRSV were used as neutral control. Mock and transfection with 5UP2 were applied as controls for nonspecific inhibition. When normalized to β-actin mRNA, similarly in both Marc-145 and PAM, the ORF7 RNA level in the cells transfected with AS-ONs YN8, 5UP2*, YN4 and YN5 were reduced by 85, 75, 70 and 70 %, respectively (Fig. 4). There was no significant inhibition in cells transfected with the other five AS-ONs and the 2 nt mismatching

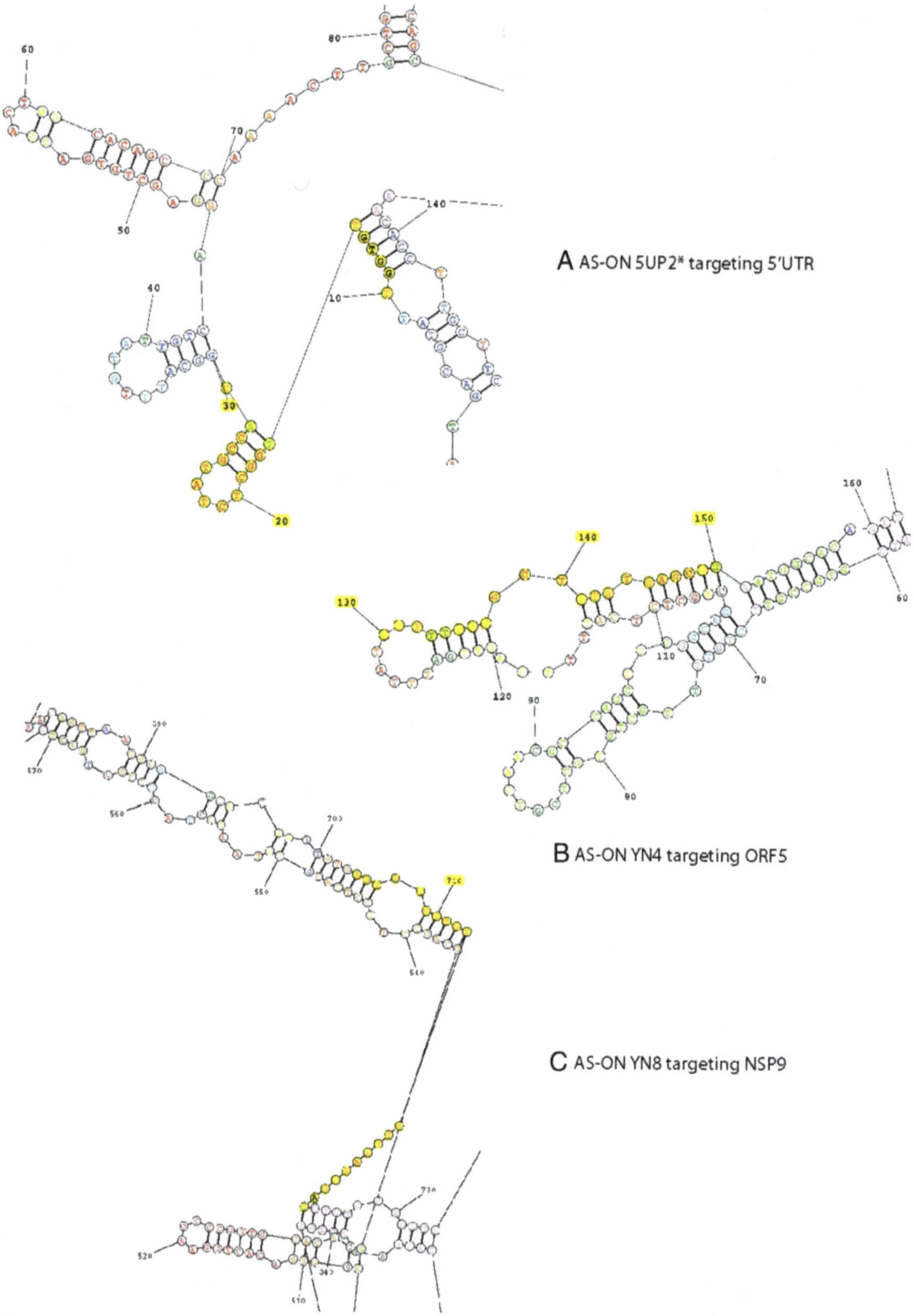

Fig. 1 (See legend on next page.)

(See figure on previous page.)

Fig. 1 Positions of the inhibitory AS-ON hits in the PRRSV gene regions. The lowest free energy secondary structures predicted for the PRRSV RNA regions were drawn by RNAstructure. The full RNA secondary structure of PRRSV 5'UTR is shown in A, while the partial RNA secondary structures of PRRSV ORF5 and NSP9 are shown in B and C, respectively. The complementary regions between the AS-On hits (5UP2*, YN4 and YN8) and their corresponding targets were highlighted in yellow: 5UP2* targeting 5'UTR, YN4 targeting ORF5 and YN8 targeting NSP9

oligo 5UP2, suggesting that the reductions in ORF7 RNA did not result from nonspecific inhibition or toxicity.

Reduction of viral titer by transfection with antisense oligonucleotides

In order to further determine the level of inhibition, CPE was monitored until 4 days post virus infection and transfection. Viral titers were measured by TCID50 assay. We found that compared to the mock and 2-nt mismatch 5UP2 control groups, transfection with antisense oligonucleotide sequence YN8 significantly protected Marc-145 cells from cytopathic effects (Fig. 5a) and reduced the viral titer by 1000-fold (Fig. 5b).

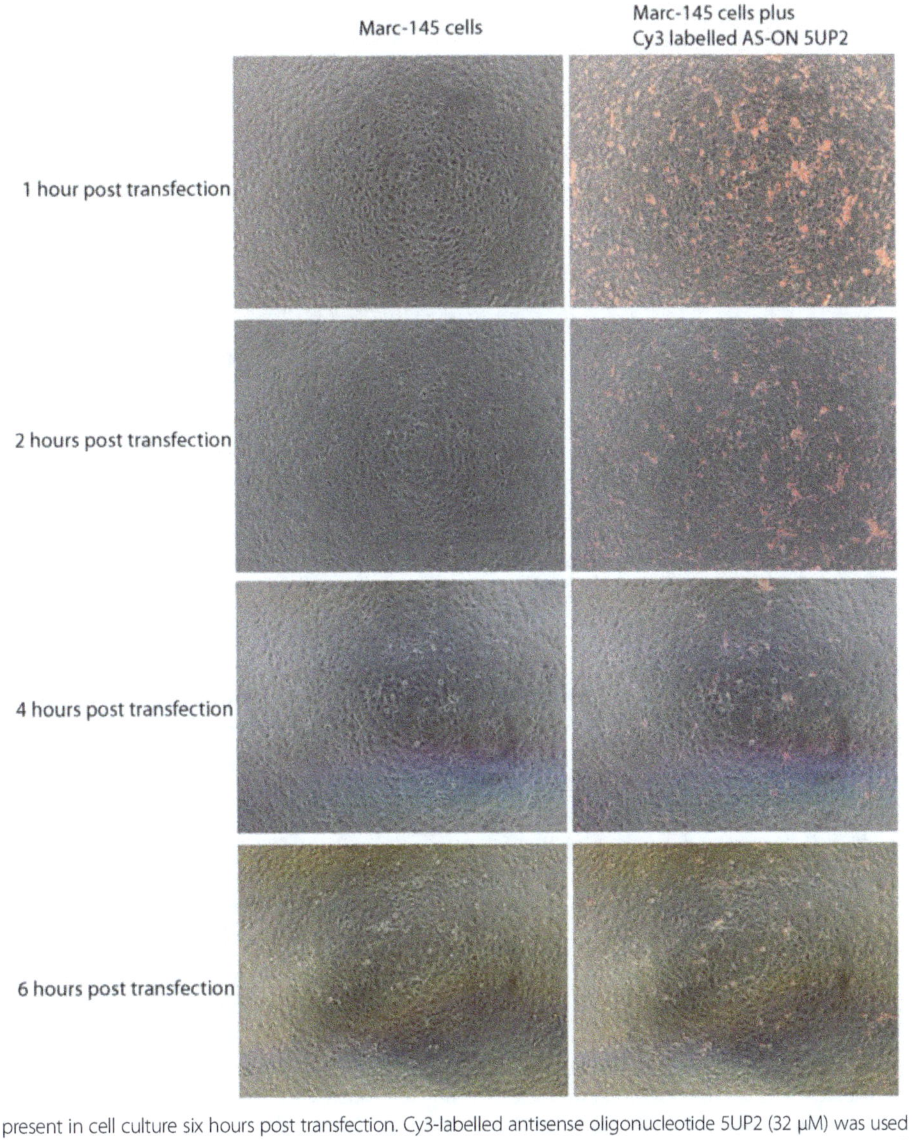

Fig. 2 AS-ON was present in cell culture six hours post transfection. Cy3-labelled antisense oligonucleotide 5UP2 (32 μM) was used in the transfection in Marc-145 cells. The fluorescent signals were recorded with fluorescence microscopy (Olympus) at various time points post transfection. Cells are shown to the left and the merged images (cells with fluorescent oligonucleotides) to the right. Although fluorescent signals decreased over the time, we could still clearly observe the signals even six hours post transfection, indicating that the antisense oligonucleotide persist in Marc-145 cells for sufficiently long time periods to induce the degradation of viral RNA and to inhibit PRRSV replication

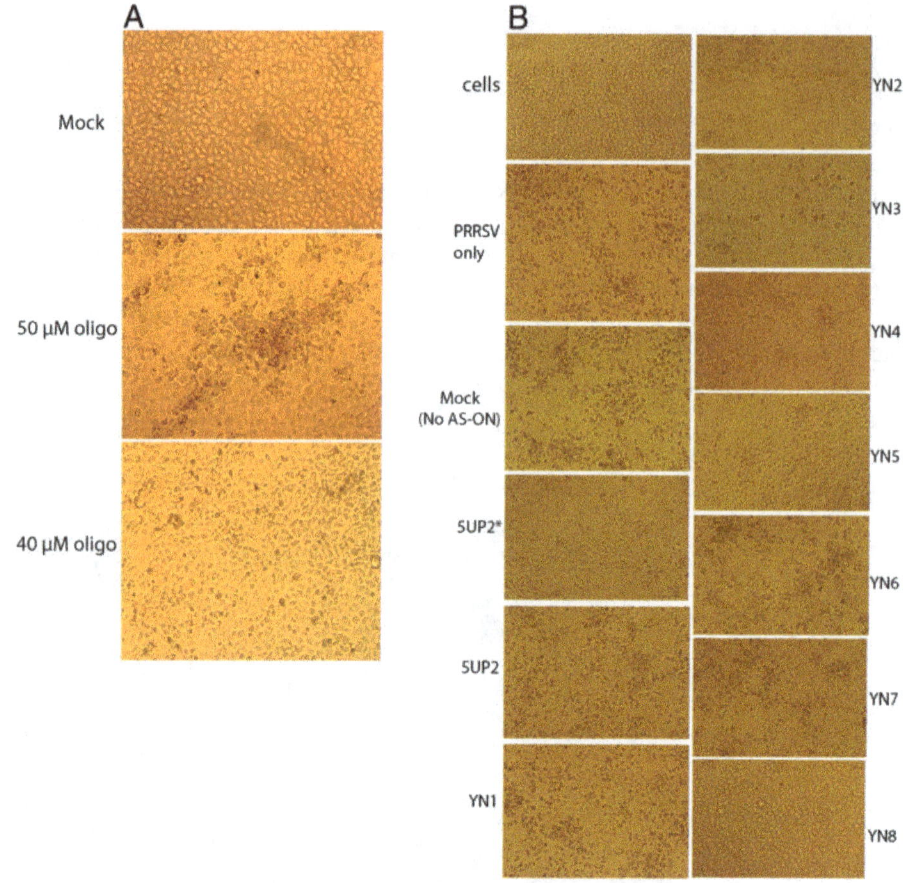

Fig. 3 Cytopathic effect (CPE) analysis of porcine reproductive and respiratory syndrome virus (PRRSV) in MARC-145 cells transfected with AS-ONs. **a**. Comparing with the mock treatment, transfection with 50 μM antisense oligonucleotide 5UP2 showed significant cytotoxicity, while transfection with 40 μM did not. **b**. Four out of nine selected antisense oligonucleotides demonstrated significant (5UP2* and YN8) or moderate (YN4 and YN5) protection from challenge with PRRSV YN-1 strain. Pictures were taken 72 h post infection with a Nikon E5400 camera mounted on an inverted microscope (Nikon TS100)

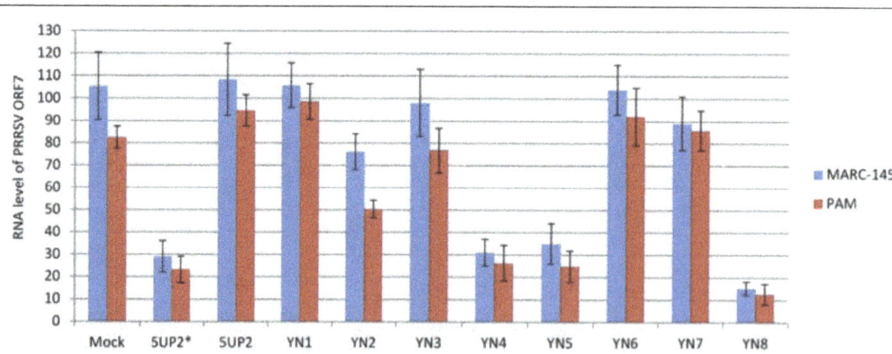

Fig. 4 Viral ORF7 RNA level was reduced by transfection with selected antisense oligonucleotides in both Marc-145 and PAM cells. Four of the nine selected antisense oligonucleotides (5UP2*, YN8, YN4 and YN5) significantly inhibited the RNA level of gene ORF7. After virus challenge and transfection with AS-ONs under the same conditions as in the CPE analysis experiment, total RNA was isolated and subjected to reverse transcription and qPCR analysis. The ΔΔCt method for relative quantification of gene expression was used to determine viral RNA levels. The Y-axis shows the relative RNA levels of the ORF7 gene for each treatment after normalization to the non-transfected reference sample using β-actin as internal control. The values shown are means of three independent experiments

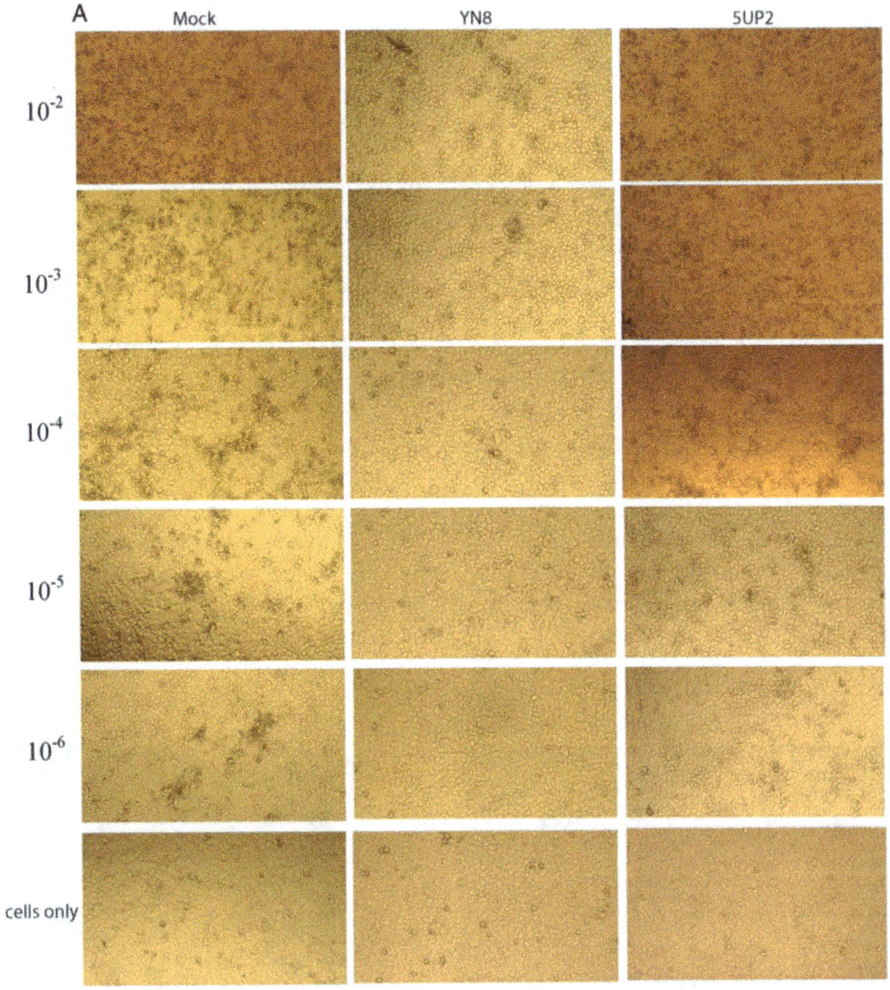

B

	$TCID_{50}$ determination
Mock	$10^{-5.6}$
YN8	$10^{-2.6}$
5UP2	$10^{-5.25}$

Fig. 5 The antisense oligonucleotide sequence YN8 protected PAM from cytopathic effects and reduced the viral titer by 1000 fold. Pulmonary alveolar macrophages (PAM) (10 000 cells per well) were seeded into 96-well plates the day before infection and transfection. Ten-fold serial dilution of PRRSV YN-1 strain was made with medium. 100 μl/well of each dilution was added into six wells. Ninety minutes post infection, the transfection was performed. CPE was monitored using the inverted microscope over a period of 4 days post transfection. The 50 % tissue culture infected dose (TCID50) was determined by Reed–Muench method. Comparing to the mock and 2-nt mismatch 5UP2control groups, transfection with antisense oligonucleotide sequence YN8 significantly protected the PAM from cytopathic effects (**a**) and reduced the viral titer by 1000-fold (**b**)

Abrogation of viral protein level by transfection with antisense oligonucleotides

To investigate the effect of AS-ONs on inhibiting the expression of viral protein, indirect immunofluorescence assays were performed with anti-N protein mAb (encoded by gene ORF7) 60 h post transfection. Indeed, fewer fluorescing cells were seen in the monolayers treated with YN8 and 5UP2* than in the other monolayers, while transfection with YN4 and YN5 mildly reduced the viral N protein level. In contrast, the infected cells in wells pre-transfected with YN1, YN2, YN3, YN6 and YN7 had equivalent or slightly less N protein-positive cells compared to that of controls (i.e., mock and transfection with the 2 nt mismatching oligo 5UP2, Fig. 6).

Discussion

PRRSV is recognized as one of the most important viruses for swine industry. It can persist in pigs for quite long time after initial infection, and infected animals with persistent infection can shed infectious virus for several months. Many scientists have been putting a lot of efforts into developing various shRNA or siRNA methods to suppress PRRSV replication in vitro and in vivo [21–27], and only few studies have used antisense technology [14, 28]. However, it is well known that antisense technology has outperformed siRNAs to some extent [29, 30], as it is easy and quick to design an antisense against a gene target, to produce the antisense sequence effectively in scale using standard equipment and procedures at lower cost and its modified derivatives that offer greater stability and efficacy, to deliver AS-ONs into cells.

Therefore, in this study we aimed to design AS-ONs targeting PRRSV regions of 5′UTR, ORF5, ORF7 and NSP9, and to test the inhibitory effects of these AS-ONs without any chemical modifications in cell culture. Under the conditions of this study, four out of the nine selected AS-ONs showed prominent inhibitory effectson PRRSV replication. The reasons for the ineffectiveness of the other AS-ONs are unclear, but could include the inaccessibility of the target sequence, or difficulties in secondary structure prediction of viral RNA. Alternatively, successful AS-ON/target RNA duplexing might not necessarily affect PRRSV replication. However, compared with the reported hit rates (approx. 10 % [31], 4/34 [32] or 4/12 [14]), we achieved higher 'success rate' (44 %). As shown in Table 1, the four effective AS-ONs have the lowest value of overall ΔG°37, indicating that the binding between the antisense oligonucleotide and its corresponding target sequence might be very stable. However, no obvious conclusions could be drawn regarding the efficacy and specific motifs or GC content in the AS-ON sequences. Larger sets of

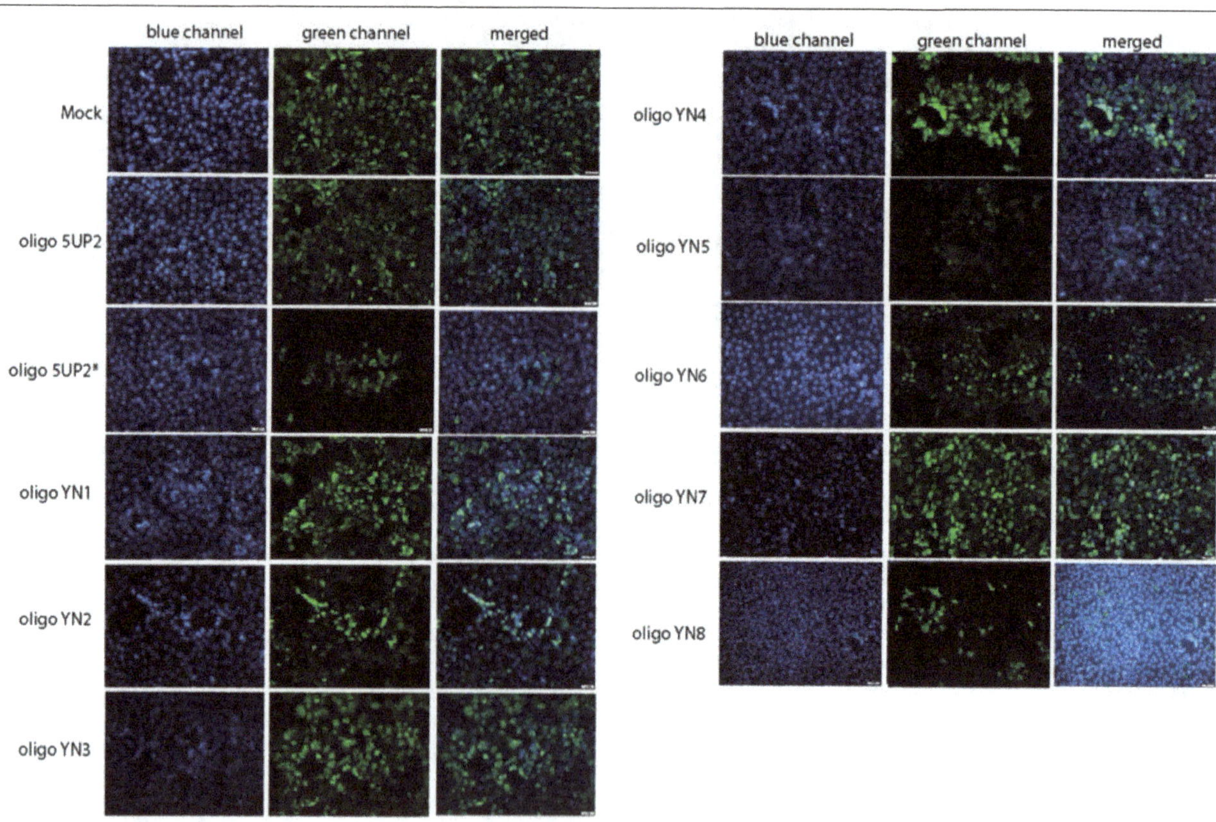

Fig. 6 Indirect immunofluorescence detection of PRRSV in MARC-145 cells transfected with or without AS-ONs. Transfection was performed 90 min post infection with PRRSV YN-1 strain (25 TCID50). Cells were fixed 60 h post transfection, reacted against anti-N monoclonal antibody (MAb) and then incubated with fluoresce in Alexa Fluo488 conjugated secondary antibody. Blue color stains nuclei to show the total number of cells. The green color indicates the expression of N protein in MARC-145 cells. The images of the same treatment from the two channels were merged. Treatment with YN8, 5UP2*, YN4 and YN5 resulted in reduction of virus replication, while 5UP2 and the other AS-ONs did not appear to have obvious effects under identical conditions

AS-ONs should be tested to obtain more statistically significant data.

Blasting the four inhibitory AS-ONs revealed that these sequences are highly conserved and hit more than 100 PRRSV strains of the Northern American type, with most of them reported from China. This suggests that that these AS-ONs should inhibit the replication of Northern American strains of PRRSV prevalent in China, not only limited to the YN-1 stain which was isolated from the southwest of China, and thus can be considered as potential drug candidates for use in PRRSV control.

Conclusion

In conclusion, this study demonstrates that DNA-based short antisense oligonucleotides can effectively inhibit PRRSV replication in MARC-145 cells and in PAMs. The experimental results which are based on the CPE experiments, measurement of the viral ORF7 RNA level and indirect fluorescence staining, demonstrated that MARC-145 cells transfected with AS-ON 5UP2* (targeting 5′-UTR) and YN8 (targeting NSP9) showed a significant decrease in virus replication when compared to the 2 nucleotide mismatching negative control (AS-ON 5UP2), indicating the specificity of the antisense oligonucleotides; while transfection with YN4 or YN5 also inhibited the PRRSV replication to some extents. It infers that 5′-UTR or NSP9 might be one of the optimal viral targets to design AS-ONs. However, the natural phosphodiester oligodeoxynucleotides (DNAs) used in this study could be relatively quickly degraded by nucleases. When it comes to the actual in vivo application of AS-ONs in therapeutic control of PRRSV, we plan to add some locked nucleic acid (LNA) modifications to the four promising AS-ON sequences for further studies both in vitro and in vivo, in order to increase the stability of AS-ONs and the cellular uptake, to enhance the hybridization affinity towards target mRNA and to reduce the toxicity, to investigate the techniques and efficiency of delivery, to study the temporary effects and to address the issue of emergence of escape mutants.

Abbreviations

PRRSV: Porcine reproductive and respiratory syndrome virus; PRRS: Porcine reproductive and respiratory syndrome; AS-ONs: Antisense oligonucleotides; UTR: Untranslated region; NSP: Non-structural protein; ORF: Open reading frame; CPE: Cytopathic effect; qPCR: Quantitative PCR; FBS: Fetal bovine serum; PAM: Pulmonary alveolar macrophages; TCID50: 50 % Tissue Culture Infective Dose; hr: Hour; hpi: Hours post infection; LNA: Locked nuclei acid.

Competing interests

The authors declare that they have no competing interests.

Authors' contributions

YGF and LJP conceived and designed the study. ZLL, ZLY, LX, LWG and YGS performed the experiments. BJL statistically analyzed the data. YGF and LJP wrote the paper with contributions from BJL. All authors read and approved manuscript.

Acknowledgments

The study was supported by grant from the National Natural Science Foundation of China (no. 31160509). The authors want to thank Dr. Bernhard Schmierer for proofreading this manuscript.

Author details

[1]Department of Veterinary Medicine, College of Animal Science and Technology, Yunnan Agricultural University, Kunming, China. [2]Present address: Wulan Institute for Animal Health, Lingyuan, Chaoyang City, Liaoning province, China. [3]Present address: Center for Animal Disease Control and Prevention of Chuxiong City, Chuxiong City, Yunnan province, China. [4]Present address: Karolinska Institute, Department of Biosciences and Nutrition, Novum, Huddinge, Sweden.

References

1. Pejsak Z, Markowska-Daniel I. Losses due to porcine reproductive and respiratory syndrome in a large swine farm. Comp Immunol Microbiol Infect Dis. 1997;20(4):345–52.
2. Meulenberg Janneke JM. PRRSV, the virus. Vet Res. 2000;31:11–21.
3. Dea S, Gagnon CA, Mardassi H, Pirzadeh B, Rogan D. Current knowledge on the structural proteins of porcine reproductive and respiratory syndrome (PRRS) virus: comparison of the North American and European isolates. Arch Virol. 2000;145(4):659–88.
4. Wang FX, Wen YJ, Yang BC, Liu Z, Shi XC, Leng X, et al. Role of non-structural protein 2 in the regulation of the replication of the porcine reproductive and respiratory syndrome virus in MARC-145 cells: effect of gene silencing and over expression. Vet Microbiol. 2012;161:58–65.
5. Verheije MH, Olsthoorn RC, Kroese MV, Rottier PJ, Meulenberg JJ. Kissing interaction between 3′ noncoding and coding sequences is essential for porcine arterivirus RNA replication. J Virol. 2002;76(3):1521–6.
6. Verheije MH, Kroese MV, Rottier PJ, Meulenberg JJ. Viable porcine arteriviruses with deletions proximal to the 3′ end of the genome. J Gen Virol. 2001;82(Pt 11):2607–14.
7. Kurreck J. Antisense technologies Improvement through novel chemical modification. Eur J Biochem. 2003;270:1628–44.
8. Crooke ST. Progress in antisense technology. Annu Rev Med. 2004;55:61–95.
9. Gleave ME, Monia BP. Antisense therapy for cancer. Nat Rev Cancer. 2005;5:468–79.
10. Tian K, Yu X, Zhao T, Feng Y, Cao Z, Wang C, et al. Emergence of fatal PRRSV variants: unparalleled outbreaks of atypical PRRS in China and molecular dissection of the unique hallmark. PLoS One. 2007;2(6):e526.
11. Bo X, Lou S, Sun D, Shu W, Yang J, Wang S. Selection of antisense oligonucleotides based on multiple predicted target mRNA structures. BMC Bioinformatics. 2006;7:122.
12. Mathews DH. RNA secondary structure analysis using RNAstructure. Curr Protoc Bioinformatics. 2006;Chapter 12:Unit 12.6.
13. Reuter JS, Mathews DH. RNAstructure: software for RNA secondary structure prediction and analysis. BMC Bioinformatics. 2010;11:129.
14. Patel D, Opriessnig T, Stein DA, Halbur PG, Meng XJ, Iversen PL, et al. Peptide-conjugated morpholino oligomers inhibit porcine reproductive and respiratory syndrome virus replication. Antiviral Res. 2008;77(2):95–107.
15. Matveeva OV, Tsodikov AD, Giddings M, Freier SM, Wyatt JR, Spiridonov AN, et al. Identification of sequence motifs in oligonucleotides whose presence is correlated with antisense activity. Nucleic Acids Res. 2000;28:2862–5.
16. Pfaffl MW. A new mathematical model for relative quantification in real time RT-PCR, Nucleic Acids Research, 29, 2002–2007, 2001ABI PRISM 7700 Sequence Detection System. 1999. User Bulletin # 2.
17. Ho SP, Bao Y, Lesher T, Malhotra R, Ma LY, Fluharty SJ, et al. Mapping of RNA accessible sites for antisense experiments with oligonucleotide libraries. Nat Biotechnol. 1998;16:59–63.
18. Ding Y, Lawrence CE. Statistical prediction of single-stranded regions in RNA secondary structure and application to predict effective antisense target sites and beyond. Nucleic Acids Res. 2001;29:1034–46.
19. Ho SP, Britton DH, Stone BA, Behrens DL, Leffet LM, Hobbs FW, et al. Potent antisense oligonucleotides to the human multidrug resistance-1mRNA are rationally selected by mapping RNA-accessible sites with oligonucleotide libraries. Nucleic Acids Res. 1996;24:1901–7.
20. Kretschmer-Kaxemi Far R, Nedbal W, Sczakiel G. Concepts to automate the theoretical design of effective antisense oligonucleotides. Bioinformatics. 2001;17:1058–61.

21. Huang J, Jiang P, Li Y, Xu J, Jiang W, Wang X. Inhibition of porcine reproductive and respiratory syndrome virus replication by short hairpin RNA in MARC-145 cells. Vet Microbiol. 2006;115(4):302–10.
22. He YX, Hua RH, Zhou YJ, Qiu HJ, Tong GZ. Interference of porcine reproductive and respiratory syndrome virus replication on MARC-145 cells using DNA-based short interfering RNAs. Antiviral Res. 2007;74(2):83–91.
23. Li G, Huang J, Jiang P, Li Y, Jiang W, Wang X. Suppression of porcine reproductive and respiratory syndrome virus replication in MARC-145 cells by shRNA targeting ORF1 region. Virus Genes. 2007;35(3):673–9.
24. Bao Y, Guo Y, Zhang L, Zhao Z, Li N. Inhibition of porcine reproductive and respiratory syndrome virus replication by RNA interference in MARC-145 cells. Mol Biol Rep. 2012;39(3):2515–22.
25. Yang M, Xiang Q, Zhang X, Li X, Sylla S, Ding Z. RNA interference targeting nucleocapsid protein inhibits porcine reproductive and respiratory syndrome virus replication in Marc-145 cells. J Microbiol. 2014;52(4):333–9.
26. Luo B, Ju S, Wang B, Rui R. A possible strategy to produce pigs resistant to porcine reproductive and respiratory syndrome virus. Antiviral Res. 2013;99(2):158–64.
27. Li L, Li Q, Bao Y, Li J, Chen Z, Yu X, et al. RNAi-based inhibition of porcine reproductive and respiratory syndrome virus replication in transgenic pigs. J Biotechnol. 2014;171:17–24.
28. Han X, Fan S, Patel D, Zhang YJ. Enhanced inhibition of porcine reproductive and respiratory syndrome virus replication by combination of morpholino oligomers. Antiviral Res. 2009;82(1):59–66.
29. Dove A. Antisense and sensibility. Nat Biotechnol. 2002;20:121–4.
30. Malik R, Roy I. Design and development of antisense drugs. Expert Opin Drug Discov. 2008;3(10):1189–207.
31. Gewirtz AM, Sokol DL, Ratajczak MZ. Nucleic acid therapeutics: state of the art and future prospects. Blood. 1998;92(3):712–36.
32. Myers KJ, Dean NM. Sensible use of antisense: how to use oligonucleotides as research tools. Trends Pharmacol Sci. 2000;21(1):19–23.

Permissions

All chapters in this book were first published in VR, by BioMed Central; hereby published with permission under the Creative Commons Attribution License or equivalent. Every chapter published in this book has been scrutinized by our experts. Their significance has been extensively debated. The topics covered herein carry significant findings which will fuel the growth of the discipline. They may even be implemented as practical applications or may be referred to as a beginning point for another development.

The contributors of this book come from diverse backgrounds, making this book a truly international effort. This book will bring forth new frontiers with its revolutionizing research information and detailed analysis of the nascent developments around the world.

We would like to thank all the contributing authors for lending their expertise to make the book truly unique. They have played a crucial role in the development of this book. Without their invaluable contributions this book wouldn't have been possible. They have made vital efforts to compile up to date information on the varied aspects of this subject to make this book a valuable addition to the collection of many professionals and students.

This book was conceptualized with the vision of imparting up-to-date information and advanced data in this field. To ensure the same, a matchless editorial board was set up. Every individual on the board went through rigorous rounds of assessment to prove their worth. After which they invested a large part of their time researching and compiling the most relevant data for our readers.

The editorial board has been involved in producing this book since its inception. They have spent rigorous hours researching and exploring the diverse topics which have resulted in the successful publishing of this book. They have passed on their knowledge of decades through this book. To expedite this challenging task, the publisher supported the team at every step. A small team of assistant editors was also appointed to further simplify the editing procedure and attain best results for the readers.

Apart from the editorial board, the designing team has also invested a significant amount of their time in understanding the subject and creating the most relevant covers. They scrutinized every image to scout for the most suitable representation of the subject and create an appropriate cover for the book.

The publishing team has been an ardent support to the editorial, designing and production team. Their endless efforts to recruit the best for this project, has resulted in the accomplishment of this book. They are a veteran in the field of academics and their pool of knowledge is as vast as their experience in printing. Their expertise and guidance has proved useful at every step. Their uncompromising quality standards have made this book an exceptional effort. Their encouragement from time to time has been an inspiration for everyone.

The publisher and the editorial board hope that this book will prove to be a valuable piece of knowledge for researchers, students, practitioners and scholars across the globe.

List of Contributors

Moses Tefula Dhikusooka and Chrisostom Ayebazibwe
National Animal Disease Diagnostics and Epidemiology Centre, Ministry of Agriculture Animal Industry and Fisheries, Entebbe, Uganda

Alice Namatovu
National Animal Disease Diagnostics and Epidemiology Centre, Ministry of Agriculture Animal Industry and Fisheries, Entebbe, Uganda
Department of Biotechnical and Diagnostic Sciences, College of Veterinary Medicine, Animal Resources and Biosecurity, Makerere University, Kampala, Uganda

Kirsten Tjørnehøj and Graham J. Belsham
National Veterinary Institute, Technical University of Denmark, Lindholm, Kalvehave DK 4771, Denmark

Hans Redlef Siegismund
Department of Biology, University of Copenhagen, Ole Maaløes Vej 5, DK 2200 Copenhagen N, Denmark

Sabenzia Nabalayo Wekesa
Foot-and-Mouth Disease Laboratory, Ministry of Livestock Development, Embakasi, Nairobi, Kenya
Department of, Environmental Management, College of Agricultural and Environmental Sciences, Makerere University, Kampala, Uganda

Vincent B. Muwanika and Sheila Nina Balinda
Department of, Environmental Management, College of Agricultural and Environmental Sciences, Makerere University, Kampala, Uganda

Jianye Wang, Jueyi Ling, Zhixian Wang, Yu Huang, Jianzhong Zhu and Guoqiang Zhu
College of Veterinary Medicine, Yangzhou University, 48 Wenhui East Road, 225009 Yangzhou, Jiangsu Province, People's Republic of China
Jiangsu Co-Innovation Center for Important Animal Infectious Diseases and Zoonoses, Yangzhou 225009, China

Zhanqin Zhao, Huisheng Liu, Ke Ding, Chunping Peng, Qiao Xue and Zuhua Yu
Lab of Veterinary Microbiology, College of Animal Science and Technology, Henan University of Science and Technology, Luoyang, China

Yun Xue
Lab of Medical Engineering, College of Medical Technology and Engineering, Henan University of Science and Technology, Luoyang, China

A. Javier Masot and Eloy Redondo
Unidad de Histología y Anatomía Patológica, Departamento de Medicina Animal, Facultad de Veterinaria, Universidad de Extremadura, Avda. Universidad s.n., Cáceres 10003, Spain

María Gil
Veterinary Teaching Hospital, University of Extremadura, Cáceres, Spain

David Risco
Innovación en Gestión y Conservación de Ungulados S.L., Cáceres, Spain

Olga M. Jiménez
Dirección General de Medio Ambiente, Consejería de Medio Ambiente y Rural, Junta de Extremadura, Spain

José I. Núñez
Institut de Recerca i Tecnologia Agroalimentàries (IRTA)-Centre de Recerca en Sanitat Animal (CReSA), UAB-IRTA, Campus de la Universitat Autònoma de Barcelona, Bellaterra, Cerdanyola del Vallès, Spain

Steven J. P. Tousignant, Laura Bruner and Jake Schwartz
Swine Vet Center, 1608 South Minnesota Avenue, St. Peter, MN 56082, USA

Fabio Vannucci, Stephanie Rossow and Douglas G. Marthaler
Department of Preventive Medicine, College of Veterinary Medicine, University of Minnesota, 1333 Gortner Avenue, St. Paul, MN 55106, USA

Nelson Henrique de Almeida Curi, Guilherme Ramos Demétrio and Marcelo Passamani
Postgraduate Programme in Applied Ecology, Department of Biology, Federal University of Lavras, Lavras, Brazil

Rodrigo Lima Massara and Ana Maria de Oliveira Paschoal
Postgraduate Programme in Ecology, Conservation and Management of Wildlife, Department of Biology, Institute of Biological Sciences, Federal University of Minas Gerais, Belo Horizonte, Brazil

Amanda Soriano-Araújo and Zélia Inês Portela Lobato
Laboratory of Viral Diseases, Department of Preventive Veterinary Medicine, School of Veterinary Medicine, Federal University of Minas Gerais, Belo Horizonte, Brazil

Adriano Garcia Chiarello
Department of Biology, University of São Paulo, Ribeirão Preto, Brazil

Xingyang Cui, Yunjia Shi, Chengwei Wei, Shanshan Wen and Shuang Xia
College of Veterinary Medicine, Northeast Agricultural University, Harbin 150030, China

Junwei Ge
College of Veterinary Medicine, Northeast Agricultural University, Harbin 150030, China
Northeastern Science Inspection Station, China Ministry of Agriculture Key Laboratory of Animal Pathogen Biology, Harbin 150030, China

Lili Zhao and Hongyan Chen
Laboratory Animal and Comparative Medicine Unit, Harbin Veterinary Research Institute, The Chinese Academy of Agricultural Sciences, No. 678 Haping Rd, Harbin 150069, China

Jelena Prpic, Tomislav Keros and Lorena Jemersi
Croatian Veterinary Institute, Savska cesta 143, 10 000 Zagreb, Croatia

Maja Lang Balija and Dubravko Forcic
Centre for Research and Knowledge Transfer in Biotechnology, University of Zagreb, Rockefellerova 10, 10 000 Zagreb, Croatia
Center of Excellence for Viral Immunology and Vaccines, CERVirVac, Zagreb, Croatia

Morten Tryland
Department of Arctic and Marine Biology, Arctic Infection Biology, UiT - The Arctic University of Norway, Stakkevollveien 23, 9010 Tromsø, Norway

Ingebjørg H. Nymo
Department of Arctic and Marine Biology, Arctic Infection Biology, UiT - The Arctic University of Norway, Stakkevollveien 23, 9010 Tromsø, Norway
Norwegian Veterinary Institute, Stakkevollveien 23, 9010 Tromsø, Norway

Javier Sánchez Romano
Department of Arctic and Marine Biology, Arctic Infection Biology, UiT - The Arctic University of Norway, Stakkevollveien 23, 9010 Tromsø, Norway
UiT - Arctic University of Norway, Arctic Infection Biology, Stakkevollveien 23, 9010 Tromsø, Norway

Torill Mørk
Norwegian Veterinary Institute, Stakkevollveien 23, 9010 Tromsø, Norway

Sauli Laaksonen
Department of Veterinary Biosciences, Faculty of Veterinary Medicine, University of Helsinki, Helsinki, Finland

Erik Ågren
Department of Pathology and Wildlife Diseases, Swedish National Veterinary Institute, 751 89 Uppsala, Sweden

Marianne Sunde
Norwegian Veterinary Institute, Ullevålsveien 68, 0454 Oslo, Norway

Akbar Dastjerdi
Animal and Plant Health Agency-Weybridge, New Haw, Addlestone, Surrey KT15 3NB, UK

Katharina Seilern-Moy and Falko Steinbach
Animal and Plant Health Agency-Weybridge, New Haw, Addlestone, Surrey KT15 3NB, UK
School of Veterinary Medicine, Faculty of Health and Medical Sciences, University of Surrey, Guildford GU2 7XH, UK

Karin Darpel
School of Veterinary Medicine, Faculty of Health and Medical Sciences, University of Surrey, Guildford GU2 7XH, UK

Fieke Molenaar
ZSL Whipsnade Zoo, Dunstable, Bedfordshire LU6 2LF, UK

Li-bin Wen, Shi-fu Wen and Kong-wang He
Institute of Veterinary Medicine, Jiangsu Academy of Agricultural Sciences, Nanjing 210014, China
Key Laboratory of Veterinary Biological Engineering and Technology, Ministry of Agriculture, Nanjing 210014, China
National Center for Engineering Research of Veterinary Bio-products, Nanjing 210014, China

Andrea Balboni, Francesca Bassi, Stefano De Arcangeli and Mara Battilani
Department of Veterinary Medical Sciences, Alma Mater Studiorum - University of Bologna, Via Tolara di Sopra 50, 40064 Ozzano dell'Emilia, BO, Italy

Rosanna Zobba, Carla Dedola and Alberto Alberti
Department of Veterinary Medicine, University of Sassari, Via Vienna, 2, Sassari 07100, Italy

Mohamed A. Shalaby and Ayman El-Deeb
Virology Department, Faculty of Veterinary Medicine, Cairo University, 12211 Giza, Egypt

Mohamed El-Tholoth
Virology Department, Faculty of Veterinary Medicine, Mansoura University, 35516 Mansoura, Egypt

Donata Hoffmann
Institute of Diagnostic Virology, Friedrich-Loeffler-Institute, 17493 Greifswald-Insel Riems, Germany

Ahmed Abd El Wahed and Claus-Peter Czerny
Division of Microbiology and Animal Hy giene, Department of Animal Sciences, Faculty of Agriculture Sciences, Georg-August-University, 37077 Goettingen, Germany

Frank T. Hufert
Institute of Microbiology & Virology, Brandenburg Medical School Fontane, 01968 Senftenberg, Germany

Manfred Weidmann
Institute of Aquaculture, University of Stirling, FK9 4LA Stirling, Scotland, UK

Estefania J. Valverde, Alejandro Labella, Juan J. Borrego and Dolores Castro
Departamento de Microbiología, Universidad de Málaga, 29071 Málaga, Spain

Irene Cano
CEFAS Weymouth Laboratory, Weymouth, Dorset DT4 8UB, UK

Huiqin Chen, Wei Li, Zhenzhan Kuang, Daxiang Chen, Xiaoqing Liao and Ming Li
Institute of Antibody Engineering, School of Laboratory Medicine and Biotechnology, Southern Medical University, Guangzhou 510515, People's Republic of China

Shuhong Luo
Institute of Antibody Engineering, School of Laboratory Medicine and Biotechnology, Southern Medical University, Guangzhou 510515, People's Republic of China
Department of Laboratory Medicine, School of Stomatology and Medicine, Foshan University, 5 Hebin Road, Foshan, Guangdong Province 528000, People's Republic of China

Wenbo Hao
Institute of Antibody Engineering, School of Laboratory Medicine and Biotechnology, Southern Medical University, Guangzhou 510515, People's Republic of China
Guangdong Provincial Key Laboratory of Tropical Disease Research, School of Public Health, Southern Medical University, Guangzhou 510515, People's Republic of China

Marlen Martinez-Gutierrez and Julian Ruiz-Saenz
Grupo de Investigación en Ciencias Animales GRICA, Universidad Cooperativa de Colombia, Calle 30A # 33-51, Bucaramanga, Colombia

Traimat Boonthai and Thomas P. Loch
Department of Pathobiology and Diagnostic Investigation, College of Veterinary Medicine, Michigan State University, 1129 Farm Lane, Room 174, East Lansing, MI 48824, USA

Matti Kiupel
Department of Pathobiology and Diagnostic Investigation, College of Veterinary Medicine, Michigan State University, 1129 Farm Lane, Room 174, East Lansing, MI 48824, USA
Comparative Medicine and Integrative Biology Program, College of Veterinary Medicine, Michigan State University, East Lansing, MI 48824, USA

Mohamed Faisal
Department of Pathobiology and Diagnostic Investigation, College of Veterinary Medicine, Michigan State University, 1129 Farm Lane, Room 174, East Lansing, MI 48824, USA
Comparative Medicine and Integrative Biology Program, College of Veterinary Medicine, Michigan State University, East Lansing, MI 48824, USA
Department of Fisheries and Wildlife, College of Agriculture and Natural Resources, Michigan State University, East Lansing, MI 48824, USA

Travis O. Brenden
Department of Fisheries and Wildlife, College of Agriculture and Natural Resources, Michigan State University, East Lansing, MI 48824, USA

Andrew D. Winters
Department of Microbiology, Immunology and Biochemistry, School of Medicine, Wayne State University, Detroit, MI 48201, USA

Coja J. Yamashita
Division of Fish Production Services, Pennsylvania Fish and Boat Commission, State College, PA 16801, USA

Geoffrey D. Smith
Division of Fisheries Management, Pennsylvania Fish and Boat Commission, Harrisburg, PA 17106, USA

Zhuo Ha
College of Veterinary Medicine, Northeast Agricultural University, Harbin 150030, China

Ning-yi Jin
College of Veterinary Medicine, Northeast Agricultural University, Harbin 150030, China
Institute of Military Veterinary medicine, Academy of Military Medical Sciences, Changchun 130122, China
Jiangsu Co-Innovation Center for the Prevention and Control of Important Animal Infectious Disease and Zoonoses, Yangzhou University, Yangzhou 225009, China

Shu-bo Wen and He Zhang
Institute of Military Veterinary medicine, Academy of Military Medical Sciences, Changchun 130122, China

Chang-zhan Xie
Institute of Military Veterinary medicine, Academy of Military Medical Sciences, Changchun 130122, China
College of Animal Science and Technology, Jilin Agricultural University, Changchun 130118, China

Wei Wang and Hui-jun Lu
Institute of Military Veterinary medicine, Academy of Military Medical Sciences, Changchun 130122, China
Jiangsu Co-Innovation Center for the Prevention and Control of Important Animal Infectious Disease and Zoonoses, Yangzhou University, Yangzhou 225009, China

Ying-cheng Guo
Jilin Fengman area Animal Prevention and Control Center, Jilin 132013, China

Jin-feng Li and Fu-long Nan
College of Veterinary Medicine, Jilin University, Changchun 130012, China

Ke-long Zhang
College of Animal Science and Technology, Guangxi University, Nanning 530004, China

Molin Chen and Xiuguo Hua
Shanghai Key Laboratory of Veterinary Biotechnology, School of Agriculture and Biology, Shanghai Jiao Tong University, Shanghai 200240, China

Wei Tang
Department of Library, Hunan University of Science and Engineering, Yongzhou 425199, People's Republic of China

Xian-Kai Wei, Yan Pan, Hai-Bo Tang, Xiao-Ning Li, Jing-Jing Liang and Ting Rong Luo
State Key Laboratory for Conservation and Utilization of Subtropical Agro-Bioresources, Guangxi University, Nanning 530004, Guangxi, China
Laboratory of Veterinary Microbiology and Animal Infectious Diseases, College of Animal Sciences and Veterinary Medicine, Guangxi University, Nanning 530004, Guangxi, China

Yi-Zhi Zhong and Cheng Liu Xiao-Xia He
Laboratory of Veterinary Microbiology and Animal Infectious Diseases, College of Animal Sciences and Veterinary Medicine, Guangxi University, Nanning 530004, Guangxi, China

Seung-Chai Kim, Salik Nazki, Sam Kwon, Jhung-Hyun Juhng, Kyeong-Hwan Mun, Do-Young Jeon, Chang-Gi Jeong, Amina Khatun and Won-Il Kim
College of Veterinary Medicine, Chonbuk National University, 79 Gobong-ro, Iksan 54596, Jeonbuk, Republic of Korea

Seog-Jin Kang
National Institute of Animal Science, Rural Development Administration, Cheonan 55365, South Korea

Jie Tong, Ying Yu, Linlin Zheng, Chong Zhang, Yabin Tu, Yonggang Liu, Jianan Wu, Hai Li, Shujie Wang, Chenggang Jiang, Gang Wang and Xuehui Cai
State Key Laboratory of Veterinary Biotechnology, Harbin Veterinary Research Institute of Chinese Academy of Agriculture Science, Harbin 150001, People's Republic of China

En-Min Zhou
Department of Preventive Veterinary Medicine, College of Veterinary Medicine, Northwest A&F University, Yangling, Shaanxi 712100, People's Republic of China

Index

www.ingramcontent.com/pod-product-compliance
Lightning Source LLC
LaVergne TN
LVHW080913210926
848485LV00004B/641